Chorionic Gonadotropin

Chorionic Gonadotropin

Edited by

Sheldon J. Segal

The Rockefeller Foundation
New York, New York

PLENUM PRESS · NEW YORK AND LONDON

Library of Congress Cataloging in Publication Data

Main entry under title:

Chorionic gonadotropin.

Proceedings of the Conference on Human Chorionic Gonadotropin, held at the Rockefeller Foundation Conference and Study Center, Bellagio, Italy, November 14–16, 1979.
Includes index.
1. Chorionic gonadotropin–Congresses. I. Segal, Sheldon Jerome, 1926-
II. Rockefeller Foundation. [DNLM: 1. Gonadotropin, Chorionic–Congresses. WK920 C551 1979]
QP572.C53C48   599.01'6   80-20274
ISBN-13: 978-1-4684-1064-8   e-ISBN-13: 978-1-4684-1062-4
DOI: 10.1007/978-1-4684-1062-4

Proceedings of the Conference on Human Chorionic Gonadotropin, held at the Rockefeller Foundation Conference and Study Center, Bellagio, Italy, November 14–16, 1979.

FOREWORD

This volume is devoted to the chemistry, immunology, molecular biology, and physiology of the human chorionic gonadotropin, hCG. For this glycoprotein molecule the course from discovery to chemical deciphering covered about fifty years. It was in 1928 that Ascheim and Zondek reported that urine from pregnant women contains something that stimulates the ovaries of mice or rats. This provided the basis for the famous A-Z test for pregnancy and for the "rabbit test" modification introduced by Friedman.

As researchers sought to find more sensitive responses to hCG, they used a wide variety of species including the South African aquatic toad, *Xenopus laevis*, the terrestrial toad of South America, *Bufo arinarus*, and the African weaver finch, *Euplectes afra*. The weaver finch feather reaction was particularly noteworthy, for it disclosed a non-gonadal response to hCG/LH. In retrospect, this may have been an important evolutionary clue to the realization that the designation of the hormone as a "gonadotropin" may have been only partially descriptive of the molecule's physiological function--a concept that is gaining attention, as the papers in this 1980 volume divulge.

With crude extracts to work with and only bioassays to measure activity, the early workers sought to understand the physiology and chemistry of the placental gonadotropin. Within the first ten years it was established that the human placental gonadotropin appears early in pregnancy, reaches its peak during the second month, and falls off rapidly thereafter. With the development of each more sensitive bioassay the date of hormone appearance in the urine moved closer and closer to the day of the first missed period. A similar hormone in the rhesus monkey was found only between the 18th and 25th day. In the blood of the pregnant mare a gonadotropic hormone was identified which also has a stimulating effect on the ovaries of test animals. Since this material was not found in the urine in significant amounts, it was concluded that it must be different chemically from the human hormone with similar action. By analyzing the difference in animal responses, researchers concluded that there must be dissimilarities between the gonadotropic hormone produced by the pituitary and the one produced by the placenta. Just 14 years after the Ascheim-Zondek discovery, the distinguished anatomist, George W.

Corner, could write a summary of the biology of hCG not very different from what can be said today. He also wrote, "The ovaries of the rat and the rabbit can distinguish [gonadotropins] better than the chemist. For the present we must content ourselves with being grateful for the pregnancy test and await the day when these troublesome substances yield themselves to chemical isolation."

As revealed by the papers in this volume, that day has now come. Modern chemistry has made it possible not only to isolate the hormone, but to describe fully the chemical structure of its molecule. Nevertheless, many questions about hCG remain as troublesome today as they were then. We can confirm that the human pituitary and placental gonadotropins are chemically different; and different still is the one produced by the pregnant mare. As yet, we cannot define the structural basis for similarities or differences in action. We can quantify with precision the time course of hCG production during pregnancy. By using highly sensitive radioligand assays the day of onset of production has been moved across the day-of-expected-menses milestone, delimited by the sensitivity of previous bioassays, to a point in the luteal phase of the fertile cycle when the hCG can rescue the failing corpus luteum. But, as in the past, the role played by the hormone later in pregnancy remains completely unsolved.

What was not evident before the emergence of the highly sensitive tests based on the antigenicity of hCG, is the surprising omnipresence of substances immunologically similar to hCG. In blood and urine samples of non-pregnant women, extracts of presumably normal tissue samples, or a number of non-trophoblastic tumors, scientists have found such substances. These observations, taken together with work establishing that some bacteria also can produce a factor with antigenic and biological properties similar to hCG, open a new phase in the course of hCG research. The scope of interest is now broadened beyond the endocrinology of pregnancy to include immunology, infectious disease, and oncology.

The rapid pace of these developments prompted the preparation of this comprehensive volume, the published proceedings of a conference held at the Rockefeller Foundation's Conference and Study Center, Bellagio, Italy, November 14-16, 1979. Many of the advances reported here depended for their achievement upon methodological improvements in the fields of protein chemistry, immunology, and radiochemistry. They would not, however, have been possible without the substantial knowledge base provided by those pioneering scientists who (using mice, rabbits, frogs, toads, and birds) learned so much about hCG.

Sheldon J. Segal
New York
May, 1980

CONTENTS

EARLY STUDIES OF CHORIONIC GONADOTROPIN AND ANTIHORMONES

Roy Hertz

Department of Pharmacology, The George
Washington University Medical Center
Washington, D.C. 20037, U.S.A.

INTRODUCTION

My aim in presenting this historical account is to share with
you something of my view of the initial development of our knowledge
of chorionic gonadotropin and of the antihormones. Accordingly,
this presentation will be purposefully retrospective and anecdotal,
so as to avoid encroachment upon subsequent papers which will deal
with more current and even future studies.

ORIGINAL OBSERVATIONS AND TECHNIQUES

The existence of a chorionic gonadotropin was first noted in
the human species. This original identification of a hormone in
man, prior to its recognition in animals, is a unique instance of
such initial discovery in endocrinological investigation. This may
have arisen from the relative difficulty of recovering the term
placenta from animals, as compared with the immediate availability
of massive amounts of human placenta at birth. For it was in working directly with fragments of human placenta that Hirose (1919;
1920) first demonstrated an effect of implanting such tissue on
the ovaries and uterus of the rabbit. These original studies were
largely repeated by Murata and Adachi (1927) who, in addition,
emphasized that luteinization of the rabbit ovary was optimally
produced when one used placental material from early pregnancy, which
we now know contains more hormone than is found at term.

From extended personal conversations with Dr. Bernhard Zondek
(Fig. 1), it is clear to me that the demonstration of a gondadotropic
substance in the urine of pregnant women by Ascheim and Zondek (1927)

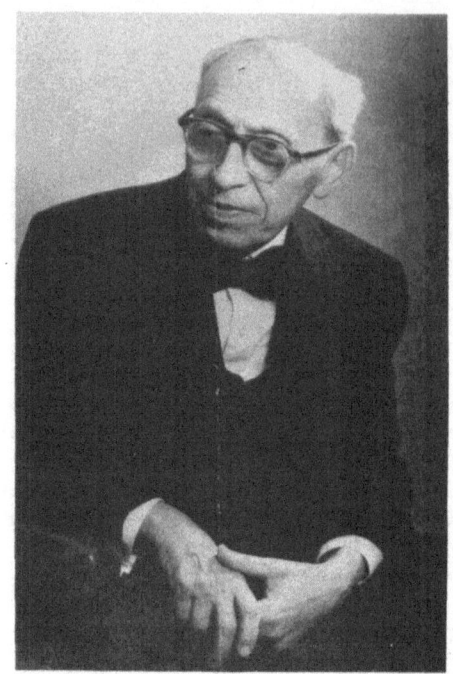

Dr. Bernhard Zondek (1891–1966)

Figure 1.

PROLAN IN HYPOPHYSECTOMIZED ANIMALS

PROTOCOL—*Concluded*

DATE	PROCEDURE	REMARKS
	Rat W-30, Female	
November 4, 1930	Total hypophysectomy —Mr. Pencharz	Age, $3\frac{3}{4}$ months; Weight, 171 grams
January 15, 1931	Operation to obtain control tissues	Left ovary, part of left uterine horn, one adrenal, and one thyroid removed. *Ovary*, infantile
January 19, 1931	Prolan injections begun	1 cc. daily, subcutaneously for 6 days. Prolan potency: 1/8 cc. = 1 R. U.
January 25, 1931	Prolan injections stopped	No change in vaginal lips or in vaginal smear during period of injection or subsequent to it
February 16, 1931	Prolan injections resumed	1 cc. daily, subcutaneously for 10 days
February 26, 1931	Injections stopped	No change in vaginal smear nor in lips of the vagina. Weight during injection period, 160 grams
May 11, 1931	Died	Weight, 148 grams. Ovary, infantile

Figure 2. Protocol on single hypophysectomized rat from Reichert et al., 1932, <u>Am. J. Physiol</u>. 100:157.

came about completely independently. He also recounted with good
humor how he chastised his technician for reporting a positive
pregnancy test with urine from a male patient, which was supposed
to serve as a control specimen. The matter was further complicated
in that this male's last name was the same as that of one of the
pregnant women in that group. When it finally was determined that
the male in question had a testicular tumor which was actually
producing chorionic gonadotropin, Zondek was obliged to make amends
and to never again doubt that technician's findings.

It is noteworthy that both Hirose's early report and Zondek's
initial investigations include the observation of the presence of
a gonadotropic substance in the urine not only of pregnant women,
but also of women with gestational trophoblastic disease -- actually,
hytadid mole and choriocarcinoma.

These early studies included rats, mice, and rabbits as test
animals. There then followed numerous reports concerning the responsiveness or lack of response in a variety of mammalian, avian,
and amphibian species. Many of these studies were oriented toward
the simplification of the original pregnancy test in rodents, which
had emerged from Ascheim's and Zondek's work. For soon the so-called
"A-Z test" became a household term -- even among the laity.

It is interesting that Zondek's perceptivity led him to consider the two major effects of pregnancy urine extracts on the rodent
ovary to consist of follicular development with occasional associated hemorrhage (the so-called "blutpunkte") and corpus luteum formation. These respective effects he attributed to two presumably
separate agents, which he called Prolan A and Prolan B. It should
be emphasized that this inference anteceded the first substantial
fractionation of anterior pituitary tissue into extracts, which
were predominantly follicle-stimulating and luteinizing (Fevold and
Hisaw, 1934). Indeed, the thesis that only one gonadotropic substance was produced by the pituitary was long quite firmly defended
by Smith and Engle (1927), who had initially shown the existence of
pituitary gonadotropin by the use of tissue implants.

Moreover, Zondek and Ascheim (1927) developed a feasible, but
laborious method for the concentration of hCG from urine. This consisted of precipitation of the filtered urine with eight volumes of
ethyl alcohol. This brought down a fairly floculent precipitate.
Most of the voluminous supernatant mixture of urine and alcohol was
then siphoned off and the remaining supernatant was removed by centrifugation. Zondek learned empirically that the toxicity of this
crude precipitate could be reduced by repeated washing with small
volumes of ether, which was then removed by centrifugation. The
washed precipitate was then injected in aqueous suspension or solution and the gonadotropic effect observed at autopsy. These extrac-

tion procedures taught us that hCG would probably prove to be a so-called "mucoprotein."

We are obliged to salute those workers who, during the very period when such laborious techniques were utilized, still managed to establish reasonably good quantitative curves of hCG excretion throughout pregnancy, and even of "total gonadotropin" throughout the normal menstrual cycle (Evans et al., 1937; McArthur et al., 1958).

DIFFERENTIATION BETWEEN CHORIONIC AND PITUITARY GONADOTROPIN

The true relationship between the urinary gonadotropin or gonadotropins found in the urine of pregnant women (PU) and that extracted from pituitary tissue, or from the urine of non-pregnant women or normal men, became a matter of heated debate and of extended experimentation. Zondek (1931) and others stressed the fact that most concentrates prepared from the urine of post-climacteric women contained only follicle-stimulating hormone. Also, the unresponsiveness of the avian gonad (Schockaert, 1933) and of the ovary of the immature rhesus monkey to PU (Engle, 1933), as contrasted with the response of these same species to pituitary gonadotropin, indicated a clear biological difference. The most crucial evidence came from the observation of Reichert et al. (1932) that the hypophysectomized rat was virtually unresponsive to PU, whereas pituitary extracts readily activated the atrophic ovary of such animals (Fig. 2).

Our statistical colleagues will be dismayed to note that this important observation of the Evans group rested on a single finding in one hypophysectomized rat. For at the time, hypophysectomy in the rat was done by directly traversing the naso-pharynx -- a frequently lethal step because of post-operative respiratory obstruction and a fatal pneumonia (Smith, 1927). Hypophysectomized rats were not readily produced in any number until Kenneth Thompson introduced the tracheotomy procedure, which obviates this complication and permits virtually 100% survival. This is a good example of how a minor technical improvement can advance a whole field.

In the foregoing, we have used the terms hCG and PU interchangeably. We must here define PU as the gonadotropin concentrate prepared from pooled pregnancy urine, whereas we now know that the term hCG relates to a specific chemical structure more recently elucidated (Canfield et al., 1971; Bahl et al., 1972). One wonders how justified such an assumption of equivalence of PU and hCG may be. May it not be that further exploration of the biological properties of these respective materials may yield as yet unidentified hormonal effects?

EARLY STUDIES ON AUGMENTATION

One of the major attempts to ascertain the suspected differences between chorionic and pituitary gonadotropin was the performance of so-called addition experiments. This was predicated on the assumption that 2 units of pituitary gonadotropin plus 2 units of chorionic gonadotropin should yield the same increment in ovarian weight as 4 units of either hormone alone. Evans et al. (1932) first noted the remarkable augmentation effect seen when PU preparations were added to pituitary extracts containing primarily follicle-stimulating hormone (FSH). They attributed this effect to a separate factor which they termed the "synergist" (Evans et al., 1933). Subsequent studies with more completely fractionated pituitary and urinary preparations attributed this phenomenon to the interaction between FSH and hCG (Fevold et al., 1933). This led to the use of the augmentation effect as an assay for the presence of small amounts of FSH in the presence of hCG (Bates and Schooley, 1942; Steelman and Pohley, 1953).

Having participated in these initial studies on the augmentation effect in Dr. Hisaw's laboratory, it was quite natural that some two decades later, when confronted with the massive ovarian enlargement seen in about one third of women with gestational trophoblastic disease, I inferred that this hyperstimulation effect consisting of theca-lutein cysts and corpora haemorrhagica may be due to the interaction of hCG from the tumor with endogenous FSH. Since earlier work had indicated that in normal gestation, pituitary FSH is suppressed (Philipp, 1930; Ehrhardt and Mayes, 1930), one could consider that an abnormal persistence of FSH production may play a role in the pathogenesis of gestational trophoblastic disease (Hertz, 1978). The more modern studies employing radioimmunoassay do confirm the remarkable suppression of FSH in early pregnancy. Presently available selective assays for β-subunit of hCG and FSH in normal pregnancy by specific radioimmunoassays should permit an adequate test of this hypothesis concerning the pathologic physiology in gestational trophoblastic disease.

A remarkable aspect of the augmentation phenomenon was concerned with the apparent lack of specificity of the effect, since it was noted very early that a wide variety of substances, notably heme, whole blood, and casein could enormously increase the gonadotropic effect of small doses of FSH (McShan and Meyer, 1937; Saunders and Cole, 1935; Casida, 1936). This created great consternation until it was noted that such augmentation occurred only if the augmentor and the hormone were mixed prior to injection. Further study of other means of augmentation, such as tannic acid precipitation, subsequently indicated that this type of non-specific augmentation was different, and that it was attributable to slowing of absorption from the injection site (Fevold and Hisaw, 1936). R. K. Meyer and I (unpublished data) confirmed this by comparing the effectiveness of a dose of FSH divided into hourly injections over a three day period with that of the same total dose given daily. The "augmentation" effect was enormous. The point of this digression is to emphasize that a physical artifact can be very misleading, when not properly interpreted. One wonders to what extent the current discrepancies in assay results between in vivo bioassays in mice and rats, in vitro bioassays in surviving cells in tissue culture, and radio-immunoassays in test tubes may hinge on such marked differences in the physical milieu in which hormones are expected to function in a totally equivalent manner.

The initial studies of augmentation with hCG required a detailed construction of a dose-response curve for hCG alone (Steelman and Pohley, 1953). It was soon appreciated that the ovarian weight response proved to be the most readily available test system. It was also soon appreciated that the ovarian weight response plateaued in a stubbornly fixed manner at a total dose of about 40 I.U. Even ten-fold increments in this dose yielded no further increase in ovarian weight, and for years it was considered that this ceiling could not be penetrated by hCG alone. However, Albert, after a lapse of some two decades, demonstrated that when this dose was increased fifty-fold, then further increments in ovarian weight could be obtained. The endogenous factors which may be involved in this extreme effect have not been elucidated.

Further analysis of both the augmentation phenomenon and of the unique character of the hCG dose response curve in terms of current concepts of receptor synthesis and regulation should aid in the elucidation of the mechanisms involved in these remarkable biological effects.

NON-HUMAN CHORIONIC GONADOTROPIN

It is historically interesting that the first non-human chorionic gonadotropin to be clearly identified was found in the horse, rather than in sub-human primate species (Cole and Saunders, 1935). I recall the excitement in our School of Agriculture at Wisconsin over the prospect of a reliable test for early pregnancy in common stock animals, especially those of fine pedigree. One by one, the dog, the cow, the sow, and the ewe proved disappointingly negative in this test. Paradoxically, even the horse proved usually negative in tests for gonadotropin in the urine. However, largely through the influence of Dr. Casida, there was set up a state-wide service for this new blood test for pregnancy in breeding mares. However, women were expected to surreptitiously seek out this service and the test was not infrequently obtained through persons prepared to provide an illegal abortion when desired.

The mare's enormous jugular vein could be readily entered with a sizeable trochar and several buckets of hormone rich blood could

be drawn without difficulty. Soon the pregnant mare became valued
as an adjunct to the pharmaceutical industry, and for several decades
physicians freely used so-called P.M.S. concentrates for gynecological
therapy and in cryptorchidism, without regard to its equine origin.
At that point, the FDA had not yet engaged its first immunologist.
Surprisingly, the general clinical tolerance to P.M.S. was remarkable,
although therapeutically quite dubious.

Nevertheless, P.M.S. proved to be a useful laboratory tool for
the production of primary follicular development in the immature rat
ovary, and this material became a standard reagent when followed by
hCG for later superovulation studies in this species.

There was a long period of controversy regarding the presence of
a chorionic gonadotropin in sub-human primates. Zondek (1930) had
described a positive test in the urine of several rhesus monkeys and
of an orangutan. There followed sporadic reports of both the presence
and absence of hormone in a variety of primate species. These
discrepancies arose from temporal differences in the urinary excretion, or plasma level of chorionic gonadotropin in the several species studied. However, chorionic gonadotropin is characteristic of
most primate species adequately tested. Much has been learned regarding the antigenic relationships between hormones of the respective primate species (Tullner, 1971). The remarkable parallelism
between the behavior of chimpanzee chorionic gonadotropin and hCG
stands in contrast to the discrepancies seen with that of other
species. However, the temporal pattern in relation to the course of
pregnancy in the chimpanzee fails to parallel that of women.

We have made attempts to correlate the temporal pattern in
chorionic gonadotropin secretion in the pregnant macacus rhesus with
observable histochemical changes in the trophoblast (Spicer and Hertz,
unpublished results). Employing such presumably carbohydrate specific stains as Schiff's reagent and Best's Carmine, no notable
change could be observed in the intensity or cellular distribution
of such stainable material, as pregnancy advanced past the usually
positive limit for urinary hormone excretion around the 35th day.
We inferred that the hormonal moiety of the histochemically demonstrable carbohydrate-containing material was too small to have an
effect in this system. This matter is raised here only to emphasize
that more exhaustive histochemical and ultramicroscopic study of the
trophoblast in various temporal patterns in a number of sub-human
primates may provide some clues to the cellular components involved
in chorionic gonadotropin synthesis.

THE ORIGIN OF THE ANTIHORMONES

The enormous impact of Berson and Yallow's (1958) genius in combining the exquisitely specific tools of immunology with the uniquely

sensitive mensuration of radio activity for radio-immunoassay empha-
sizes the importance of the antihormones. Moreover, there is emerging a vital area of research aimed at the exploitation of the antigenic potential of the hormones for fertility control, and one of
our sessions is to be devoted to this important development. It
would therefore seem instructive to review the genesis of our
knowledge of the anithormones, and of their probable relationship
to other antibodies.

It was a great privilege to have been in the laboratory of Dr.
Hisaw when he and his colleague, Dr. Harry Fevold, were embarking
on their initial studies of the chemistry of the gonadotropic hormones
of the anterior pituitary (Fevold et al., 1931). My assignment was
to extend to the immature rabbit the prior observations that had been
made in the rat, with the then emerging and newly named preparations
of FSH and LH. We selected the chinchilla rabbit, largely because
of its greater availability among the rabbit fanciers in our area.
With their cooperation, we ascertained that a four week old animal
was about as young a rabbit as could be transferred to the laboratory
and submitted to such procedures as daily injections and laporotomy
without undue loss. It was a great disappointment to find that these
month-old animals showed neither a gross nor histologically observable ovarian response to literally hundreds of rat units of either
unfractionated or fractionated sheep or pig pituitary extracts.
However, we noted that at this age the ovary was still made up
entirely of primordial follicles, which we inferred were unresponsive
to pituitary gonadotropin. Using progressively older rabbits, we
found that ovarian responsiveness to exogenous pituitary hormone
was not established until about 12 weeks of age. At that time,
numerous antrum-containing follicles were present, and extreme responses were readily elicited within five days of treatment. However,
we observed that despite sustained treatment with potent sheep pituitary extracts, the ovaries involuted and actually became atrophic.
This refractory state impressed us, but we were not circumspect
enough to attempt to try to find out why this occurred.

We were even more obtuse in our appreciation of the findings,
described in one of our reports as follows:

Desensitization to pituitary stimulation: We wished
to determine whether or not a refractory condition in the
ovary must be preceded by a maximal ovarian response. In
these experiments two litters of five animals and one
litter of four were employed. Twelve of these animals
were given follicle-stimulating extract as an equivalent
of 0.05 gram dried sheep pituitary twice daily for ten
days. Laporotomy on the 6th and 11th days after the
beginning of the injections revealed that this amount had
had no macroscopic effect upon the ovary, and in two

cases one ovary was removed for microscopic study. At this point all fourteen animals in this group were started on a dosage of follicle-stimulating extract ample to elicit an extreme ovarian response, namely 0.25 gram equivalent twice daily for 5 days. At autopsy the two animals which had not been previously treated with the sub-threshold dose showed the usual ovarian enlargement and follicular development already described. The remaining animals showed no appreciable gross or histological evidence of hypophyseal stimulation. The preliminary injection of the sub-threshold dose seemed to have rendered them insensitive to the hormone subsequently administered. (Hertz and Hisaw, 1934.)

While we were stupidly scratching our heads about this phenomenon, a bright person in Collip's laboratory, Dr. Evelyn Anderson, noted that the basal metabolic rate of rats treated with pituitary thyrotropin first rose, but then fell even to below normal levels after more prolonged treatment (Anderson and Collip, 1934). She promptly combined the serum of refractory rats with thyrotropin and showed that such sera completely neutralized the thyrotropic effect. Thus, the antihormones were born and it then became clear that both our refractory rabbits and our "desensitized" rabbits had formed antigonadotropic substances.

There ensued much controversy relating to two questions: (1) What was the relationship of the antihormones to such classical antibodies as the precipitins, agglutinins, or complement-fixing antibodies; and (2) What was the function of these inhibitory substances in normal physiology, if any?

Early in this period it was demonstrated that potent antihormonal sera could be precipitated with isologous non-hormonal antisera without reducing the hormonal inhibitory capacity of the remaining supernatant. Also, the temporal and quantitative relationship of the development of precipitins did not always parallel the development of the precipitin titre. Such discrepancies still plague our knowledge of the immunological identity of the antihormones, and hopefully our discussions here will deal with this complex problem.

It is of historical interest that Collip, who had already made the first potent extracts of parathormone and had also directed Banting and Best in their initial preparations of insulin, erroneously regarded the antihormones as having a distinct role in balancing the normal physiological functions of the body. He even postulated that the ebb and flow of the menstrual cycle could be under the control of a normal hormone-antihormonal balance. This view was in turn related to the "chalone" concept of intracellular inhibitors which had been postulated by Schaeffer (cf. Thompson, 1941). Thus, we must be aware that even a master experimentalist can trip badly on the hem of speculation. On the other hand, lack of imaginative exploitation of even as remarkable a phenomenon as we observed in our desensitization experiments, will leave the truly important discoveries for others to disclose.

Another instructive example of this loss of opportunity relates to the ingenious development of the immunoassay for hCG by Wide and Gemzell (1960). For we should realize that the essential ingredients of this assay, namely the agglutination reaction, the antigen, and the antisera were widely known to all of us for over two decades. However, the concept of a quantitative immunoassay for hCG had to wait upon the genius of these investigators for its expression.

HCG AS AN EVOLUTIONARY FOOTPRINT

The so-called rescue of the corpus luteum of early pregnancy was first suggested from the observations of Bradbury et al. (1950). They described the prolongation of the normal menstrual cycle following hCG administration in the luteal phase of the cycle. They utilized serial endometrial biopsies as well as the level of pregnandiol excretion as criteria of continued luteal function. It is interesting that they concluded that a daily dose of 5000 I.U. of hCG was required for this effect, and this is close to the dose of 3000 to 6000 I.U. hCG used for ovulation induction in women following FSH. treatment by Gemzell (1965) and others. However, it is interesting that in cases of induced ovulation by this method, the first dose is frequently followed by ovulation in 24 hours and only two additional days of hCG is sufficient to frequently lead to successful implantation and pregnancy. It may be inferred that by the time of implantation some five to seven days later, the exogenous hCG would have been expended and some endogenous mechanism for the persistence of the corpus luteum may have become initiated. This may be hCG already produced by the trophoblastic cells of the ovum prior to implantation. Croxatto et al. (1978) have offered data demonstrating the probable presence of hCG in the unimplanted human ovum by immunofluorescence studies. However, detectable plasma levels were first observed by Marshall et al. (1968) on day 9 following ovulation. An alternative explanation may be that some endogenous factor other than hCG comes into play between ovulation and implantation. Nevertheless, since human trophoblast cells in tissue culture can produce ample amounts of hCG without involvement of any maternal factor, it would seem more likely that the 99 trophoblast cells present in the 107 cell human blastocyst could already produce sufficient hCG to provide the necessary signal to the corpus luteum to endure.

Thus, hCG becomes the first clearly definable humoral agent identifiable in ontogenetic development. In keeping with the long held theory of biogenesis that ontogeny repeats phylogeny, this hormone must be regarded as primeval in its evolutionary origins. More recent observations demonstrating hCG in a wide variety of obviously embryonal and even unrelated neoplasms -- in normal testicular, gastro-intestinal and pituitary tissue, in spermatazoa, and even in bacteria -- attest to this early biological derivation of this important molecule.

For, particularly in relation to tumors, the ectopic production of hCG has been emphasized. Yet this phenomenon of ectopic hormonal production by tumors is now recorded for virtually every known peptide or protein hormone. In contrast, no instance of ectopic steroid production by tumors has been documented to date. This suggests that in evolutionary development the steroid hormones represent a more highly specialized element than the more primitive substances.

Accordingly, it is appropriate to ask in turn at what point in ontogeny do neoplasms first originate? It is indeed revealing that the trophoblast itself gives rise to a series of neoplasms with graded degrees of malignancy, namely hydatidiform mole, invasive mole, and choriocarcinoma. This spectrum of tumors has been given the name "gestational trophoblastic disease" and has been referred to by Hertig as "nature's first cancer" (Hertig, 1968; Hertz, 1978). HCG is the most distinctive and unfailing marker of these early tumors.

It is historically interesting that the concept of malignant tumors as representing a reversion to a primitive phase of early embryonal development was first expressed by Cohnheim in 1877, and independently by Hansemann in 1890. Perhaps in our newer knowledge of hCG, we have a biochemical verification of these earlier histo-pathological inferences.

I trust that all of this will bring home to us the conclusion that as investigators, we should not only look, but we should also look about and even occasionally look back.

REFERENCES

Anderson, E., and Collip, J. B., 1934, Preparation and properties of an antithyrotropic substance, Lancet 1:784.

Ascheim, S., and Zondek, B., 1928, Die schwangerschafts diagnose aus dem harn durch nachweis des hypophyenvorderslappen-hormone, Klin. Wchnschr. 7:1404.

Bahl, O. P., Carlson, R. B., Bellisaris, R., and Swaminathan, K., 1972, Human chorionic gonadotropin: Amino acid sequence of the alpha and beta subunits, 48:416.

Bates, R. W., and Schooley, J. P., 1942, Studies on the assay of pituitary gonadotropins using the augmentation reaction, Endocrinology 31:309.

Benson, S. A., and Yalow, R. S., 1958, Isotopic tracers in the study of diabetes, Adv. Biol. Med. Phys. 6:350.

Bradbury, J. T., Brown, W. E., and Guay, L. A., 1950, Maintenance of the corpus luteum and physiologic action of progesterone, Recent Prog. Horm. Res. 5:151.

Canfield, R. E., Morgan, J. F., Kammerman, S., Bell, J. J., and Agosto, G. M., 1971, Recent Prog. in Horm. Res. 27:121.

Casida, L. E., 1936, Relative gonadotropic augmentive action of plasma and formed elements from blood of cattle, Proc. Soc. Exp. Biol. Med. 33:570.

Cohnheim, J., 1877, Vorlesungen uber algemeine pathologie; ein handbuch fur aertzte und studierende, Verlag von August Hirschwald, Berlin.

Cole, H. H., and Saunders, F. J., 1935, Concentration of gonad-stimulating hormone in blood serum and of estrin in urine throughout pregnancy in the mare, Endocrinology 19:199.

Croxatto, H., 1978, Personal communication.

Ehrhardt, K., and Mayes, B. T., 1930, Beitrag zur hormongehalt des menschlichen und tierischen hypophysenvorderlappens, Zentrabl. J. Gynak. 54:2947.

Engle, E. T., 1933, Biological differences in response of the female macacus monkey to extracts of the anterior pituitary and of human pregnancy urine, Am. J. Physiol. 106:145.

Evans, H. M., Meyer, K., and Simpson, M. E., 1932, Relation of prolan to the anterior hypophyseal hormone, Am. J. Physiol. 100:141.

Evans, H. M., Simpson, M. E., and Austin, P. R., 1933, The hypophyseal substance giving increased gonadotropic effects when combined with prolan, J. Exp. Med. 57:897.

Evans, H. M., Kohls, C. L., and Wonder, D. H., 1937, Gonadotropic hormone in blood and urine of early pregnancy; normal occurance of transient extremely high levels, J. Am. Med. Assn. 108:287.

Fevold, H. L., and Hisaw, F. L., 1934, Interactions of gonad-stimulating hormones in ovarian development, Am. J. Physiol. 109:655.

Fevold, H. L., Hisaw, F. L., and Leonard, S. L., 1931, The gonad-stimulating and luteinizing hormones of the anterior lobe of the hypophysis, Am. J. Physiol. 97:291.

Fevold, H. L., Hisaw, F. L., Hellbaum, H., and Hertz, R., 1933, Anterior lobe or anterior lobe-like sex hormone combinations on growth of ovaries in immature rats, Proc. Soc. Exp. Bio. Med. 30:914.

Fevold, H. L., Hisaw, F. L., and Greep, R., 1936, Augmentation of the gonad-stimulating action of pituitary extracts by inorganic substances, particularly copper salts, Am. J. Physiol. 117:68.

Gemzell, C., 1965, Induction of ovulation with human gonadotropin, Recent Prog. Horm. Res. 21:179.

Hansemann, D., 1890, Uber asymmetrische zelltheilung in epithel-krebsen und deren biologische bedeutung, Virchows Arch. 119:299.

Hertig, A. T., 1968, *Human Trophoblast,* C. C. Thomas, Springfield, Illinois.

Hertz, R., 1978, *Choriocarcinoma and Related Trophoblastic Tumors in Women,* Raven Press, New York.

Hertz, R., and Hisaw, F. L., 1934, Effects of follicle stimulating and luteinizing pituitary extracts on the ovaries of infantile and juvenile rabbits, Am. J. Physiol. 108:1.

Hirose, T., 1919, Experimentalle histologische studie zur genese corpus luteum, Mitt. a.d. Med. Fakultd. t. Univ. Z. U. Tokyo 23:63.

Hirose, T., 1920, Exogenous stimulation of corpus luteum formation in the rabbit; influence of extracts of human placenta, decidua, fetus, hydatid mole and bovine corpus luteum on the rabbit gonad, J. Jpn. Gynecol. Soc. 16:1055.

Marshall, J. R., Hammond, C. B., Ross, G. T., Jacobson, A., Rayford, P., and Odell, W. D., 1968, Plasma and urinary gonadotropin during early human pregnancy, Obstet. and Gynecol. 37:760.

McArthur, J. W., Ingersoll, F. W., and Worcester, J., 1958, Urinary excretion of interstitial cell stimulating hormone by normal males and females of various ages, J. Clin. Endoc. 18:460.

McShan, W. H., and Meyer, R. K., 1937, Heme containing fractions of blood as related to the augmentation of pituitary gonadotropic extracts, Am. J. Physiol. 110:485.

Murata, M., and Adachi, K., 1927, Uber die kunstliche erzegung des corpus luteum durch injection der plazentasubstanz aus fruhen schwangerschaftsmonaten, A. tscher. f. Gentsch. U. Gynak. 92:45.

Philipp, E., 1930, Die bildungstatte des hypophysen vorderlappens-hormons in der graviditat, Zentrabl. f. Gynak. 54:1858.

Reichert, F. L., Pencharz, F. I., Simpson, M. E., Meyer, K., and Evans, H. M., 1932, Relative ineffectiveness of prolan in hypophysectomized animals, Am. J. Physiol. 100:157.

Saunders, F. J., and Cole, H. H., 1936, Means of augmenting the ovarian response to gonadotropic substances, Proc. Soc. Exp. Biol. Med. 33:505.

Schochaert, J. A., 1933, Difference between anterior pituitary sex stimulating hormones and pregnancy urine substances in the male mammal and bird, Am. J. Physiol. 105:497.

Smith, P. E., 1927, The disabilities caused by hypophysectomy and their repair, J. Am. Med. Assoc. 88:158

Smith, P. E., and Engle, E. T., 1927, Experimental evidence regarding the role of the anterior pituitary in the development and regulation of the genital system, Am. J. Anat. 40:159.

Steelman, S. L., and Pohlman, J. M., 1953, Assay of the follicle stimulating hormone based on the augmentation with human chorionic gonadotropin, Endocrinology 53:604.

Thompson, K. W., 1941, Antihormones, Physiol. Rev. 21:588.

Tullner, W. W., 1971, Chorionic gonadotropin in non-human primates, Symposium on the Use of Non-Human Primates for Research, Sukumi, U.S.S.R., Dec.

Wide, L., and Gemzell, C., 1960, An immunological pregnancy test, Acta Endoc. 35:261.

Zondek, B., 1930, Hormonale schwangerschafts raction aus dem harn bei mensch und tier, Klin. Wchuschr. 9:2285.

Zondek, B., 1931, Die Hormone des Ovariums und des Hypophysenvorderlappens, Springer, Berlin.

Zondek, B., and Ascheim, S., 1927, Das hormon des hypophysenvorderlappens. Darstellung, chemische eigenschaften, biologische wirkung, Klin. Wchuschr. 7:831.

PRIMARY AND SECONDARY BIOLOGIC ACTIVITIES

INTRINSIC TO THE HUMAN CHORIONIC GONADOTROPIN MOLECULE

Bruce C. Nisula, George S. Taliadouros,
and Pierre Carayon

Developmental Endocrinology Branch, National
Institute of Child Health and Human Development,
National Institutes of Health, Bethesda, MD, U.S.A.

INTRODUCTION

The hypothesis that follicle-stimulating activity (FSA) and thyroid-stimulating activity (TSA) are intrinsic to the human chorionic gonadotropin (hCG) molecule is one aspect of a broad controversy nearly as old as the discovery, more than 50 years ago, that the urine of pregnant women contains gonadotropic activity. At the heart of this controversy is the observation that urine rich in hCG stimulates follicular growth, as well as interstitial repair in the ovaries of hypophysectomized rats (Evans et al., 1953; Lyons et al., 1953). The unsettled issue is whether one accounts for the FSA in pregnancy urine on the basis of follicle-stimulating hormone (hFSH) of pituitary origin, on the basis of a putative separate factor with FSA secreted by the placenta, or potentially even on the basis of the hCG molecule having intrinsic FSA. There is reason to suspect that all three may contribute, making the FSA in pregnancy urine heterogeneous in nature. Kulin et al. (1979) have recently found low, but measurable levels of pituitary hFSH-like material in pregnancy urine by radioimmunoassay. Ashitaka et al. (1970) have separated two glycoprotein fractions from pregnancy urine, one of which is richer in FSA than the other. Albert (1969) has shown that FSA is not lost when hCG is purified seven-fold, suggesting that FSA represents an intrinsic property of the hCG molecule. A controversy, similar in nature, has gone on concerning what substances account for the TSA in pregnancy urine (Lyon et al., 1953). Possible candidates include thyroid-stimulating hormone (hTSH) of pituitary origin (Burger, 1967), a putative separate factor with TSA secreted by the placenta (Akasu et al., 1955; Hennen, 1965;

Hershman and Starnes, 1969; Kitagaki, 1977; Tojo et al., 1978), or
the hCG molecule on the basis of its hypothetical intrinsic TSA.
Again, some combination of these may actually account for the TSA
in extracts of pregnancy urine.

A key aspect of these controversies is the question whether
FSA and TSA are intrinsic to the hCG molecule, and hence, whether
the hCG molecule contributes to the FSA and TSA apparent in the
urine of pregnant women. In this chapter, we review recent investigations aimed at examination of this question; the evidence adduced
indicates that FSA and TSA are intrinsic to the hCG molecule.

BIOLOGIC ACTIVITIES OF THE HCG MOLECULE

Bioassay of Purified hCG Preparations

In addition to interstitial cell-stimulating activity (ICSA),
purified hCG preparations exhibit FSA (Simpson, 1961; Albert, 1969;
Louvet et al., 1976) and TSA (Nisula et al., 1974; Nisula and Ketelslegers, 1974; Uchimura et al., 1975). Not only hCG preparations
derived from the urine of pregnant women, but also hCG preparations
extracted from hydatidiform mole exhibit FSA (Ashitaka et al., 1972)
and TSA (Kenimer et al., 1975). In general, the various in vivo
assays used to assess the biologic activities of purified hCG preparations are based on the following responses: 1) For ICSA, increase
in weight of the ventral prostate in hypophysectomized immature rats,
2) For FSA, increase in weight of the ovaries in hypophysectomized
immature rats, and 3) For TSA, increase in blood radioactivity in
mice which have been given radioiodine to label the thyroid. The
starting preparations, purification procedures, and physicochemical
properties of the purified hCG preparations from Dr. Robert Canfield's laboratory, with which much of the work has been accomplished,
are outlined elsewhere (Canfield et al., 1971; Morgan et al., 1974;
Canfield and Ross, 1976). In so far as the detection and relative
proportions of ICSA, FSA, and TSA are concerned, the purified hCG
preparations (CR115, CR117, and CR119) are quite similar. While the
bioassay data summarized in this chapter reflect experience with
these three preparations, the data with respect to the radioligand-
receptor assays is for the CR119 batch of hCG. The Center for Population Research of the National Institute of Child Health and Human
Development provided many of the preparations used in these studies.

Contamination with Pituitary Hormones

At the outset, it is essential to exclude contamination of the
purified hCG preparation with small amounts of the pituitary hormones,
hFSH and hTSH. That such contaminants could be the source of the
biological activities, FSA and TSA, apparent in purified hCG has

TABLE I: Examination of the purified hCG (CR119) preparation in
biological assays for FSA and TSA, and in radioimmunoassays for
hFSH and hTSH, to show that the secondary biologic activities in
the purified hCG are not due to contamination with pituitary
glycoprotein hormones.

Activity	Bioassay Potency	Immunoassay Potency	Biologic/Immunologic Potency Ratio
hFSH-like (IU/mg)^a	19.5	0.02	975
hTSH-like (mIU/mg)^b	4.0	<0.006	>667

^{a}Potency is expressed in terms of Second IRP-hMG.

^{b}Potency is expressed in terms of First IRP-hTSH.

troubled investigators for many decades (Simpson, 1961). Although
hCG has a substantially larger molecular size than hFSH or hTSH,
which would make copurification unlikely, the levels of contamination could be quite low and still account for the FSA or TSA. A
simple approach to showing that the pituitary hormones do not account
for either the FSA or the TSA in purified hCG preparations is to
measure their levels by radioimmunoassay. The details of our
radioimmunoassay procedures are given elsewhere for hFSH (Siris et
al., 1978) and for hTSH (Nisula and Louvet, 1978). Indeed, examination of the purified hCG (CR119) preparation in biological assays
for FSA and TSA and in radioimmunoassays for pituitary hFSH and
hTSH, shows that the FSA and TSA are not due to contamination with
the pituitary hormones (Table I). In Fact, there is 975 times more
FSA in the purified hCG preparation than can be accounted for by
contamination with the pituitary hormone hFSH, and more than 667
times greater TSA than can be accounted for by contamination with
the pituitary hormone hTSH. Another way of excluding contamination
with pituitary hFSH is to assess neutralization of the apparent FSH-
like activity in the purified hCG preparations with antiserum to
hFSH. In agreement with the results obtained by direct radioimmunoassay, such antiserum fails to neutralize the FSH-like activity in
the purified hCG preparation (Siris et al., 1978).

Contamination with Putative Placental Hormones

The possibility that the purified hCG preparation is contaminated with putative placental hormones, which account for its FSA and TSA, is a more difficult problem with which to contend. This is because there is no general agreement concerning the existence, not to mention the chemical and immunological properties, of these putative placental hormones. For instance, one laboratory has recently reported failure to reproduce its earlier work on the isolation from placenta of the putative so-called chorionic thyrotropin (Harada and Hershman, 1978). Regardless, the original characterization of preparations of chorionic thyrotropin extracted from placenta showed that their factor with TSA elutes from Sephadex G-100 columns in a position corresponding to a molecular size much smaller than that of hCG (Hershman and Starnes, 1969). In contrast, the TSA apparent in purified hCG preparations co-elutes with the hCG molecule on Sephadex G-100 chromatography (Taliadouros et al., 1978). In addition, the fact that the ratio of ICSA to TSA in pooled fractions from the ascending limb of the hCG protein peak was the same as that from the descending limb, gives further indication that the ICSA and TSA are properties of either the same molecule , or of molecules of similar apparent size on gel chromatography.

The finding that hCG preparations fail to cross-react in radioimmunoassays for the putative chorionic thyrotropin is additional evidence against contamination of the purified hCG with this substance (Ketelslegers et al., 1975).

Recombination of Purified Subunits

To date, the most critical test of the hypothesis that FSA and TSA are intrinsic to the hCG molecule, rather than to contaminants in the purified hCG preparations, has been to assess whether there is exclusion of these activities during purification of the hCG subunits. The initial possibity for consideration is whether the FSA and TSA are detectable in the purified subunits themselves. However, the purified subunit preparations are devoid of activity in bioassays for FSA, TSA, and ICSA (Figure 1), and thus it is clear that the purified subunit preparations are not contaminated with the putative intact placental hormones. Therefore, when one recombines the subunit preparations to make the recombinant hCGα+β preparation, the activities which are regained are not due to contaminants carried along with the subunits during the purification procedures. Should the recombinant hCGα+β preparation be lacking in either the FSA or the TSA which was apparent in the starting purified hCG preparation, one would conclude that the activity was not a property of the hCG molecule. Based on this rationale, the TSA (Nisula et al., 1974) and the FSA (Louvet et al., 1976) of purified hCG preparations have

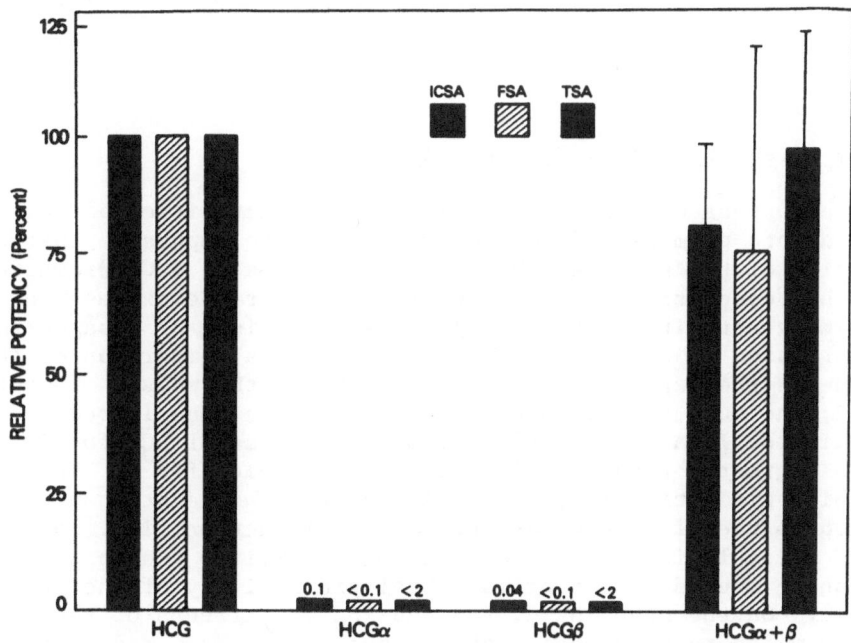

Figure 1. Relative potencies of the purified hCG, the hCGα subunit, the hCGβ subunit, and the recombined subunits in biological assays for ICSA, FSA, and TSA. The hCGα and hCGβ subunit preparations were derived from the dissociation of the purified hCG (CR119) preparation and further purified prior to assessing their individual activities and those resulting from their recombination. The error brackets indicate the 95% confidence limits for the relative potency estimate.

been put to the test. For these experiements, the purified hCG is dissociated, and the hCGα and hCGβ subunits are purified on DEAE Sephadex and on Sephadex G-100 (Morgan et al., 1974). The critical finding is that in the recombinant hCGα+β preparation, all three biological activities are regained to a degree comparable to that of the purified hCG preparation from which the subunits were derived (Figure 1). This finding that the ICSA, the FSA, and the TSA have indistinguishable β-subunit as well as α-subunit structures strongly indicates that they are activities intrinsic to the same native molecule. Conversely, with these results the possibility that the FSA and TSA apparent in hCG preparations is due to contamination with putative placental hormones becomes extremely remote, if not untenable. Since either of the putative placental hormones, the one with the FSA or the one with the TSA, could have been excluded by purification of the subunits, the recovery of both activities further reinforces the conclusion that the FSA and the TSA are intrinsic properties of the hCG molecule.

Primary versus Secondary Biologic Activities

The purpose of classifying the biologic activities of the hCG molecule into primary and secondary types is to emphasize that for expression of the secondary biologic activities of hCG, dramatically higher hCG concentrations are required than for the expression of its primary activity. Table II gives a comparison of dosages for the expression of ICSA and FSA in the rat and a comparison of the dosages for the expression of ICSA and TSA in the mouse. To obtain the FSA, one must give a 1000-fold greater dose than is required to obtain the ICSA. Similarly, in mice the dose of hCG for TSA is 5000-fold greater than that for its gonadotropic effect. Thus, of hCG's biologic activities, the ICSA requires the least dosage, and compared to the pituitary hormones with this action (i.e., hLH), the hCG molecule is quite potent in this activity. On this basis, ICSA can be viewed as the primary biologic activity of the hCG molecule. On the other hand, FSA and TSA are effects of the hCG molecule which require much higher dosages, and compared to the pituitary hormones with these activities (i.e., hFSH and hTSH), the hCG molecule is considerably less potent. Thus, in this classification scheme, the FSA and TSA of the hCG molecule are viewed as secondary biological activities because they are relatively weak activities.

TABLE II: Comparison of the minimum dose of purified hCG at which it manifests its primary biologic activity (ICSA) with the minimum dose at which it manifests its secondary biologic activities (FSA, TSA).

| Test Animal | Minimum Dose for | | | Secondary/Primary Ratio |
	Primary ICSA	Secondary FSA	TSA	
Mouse	0.1^a	–	500	5,000
Rat	0.4	400	–	1,000

[a]Numbers given in table are approximate values in terms of IU of hCG (CR119); its potency is 13500 IU/mg relative to Second IS-hCG.

MECHANISM OF THE SECONDARY BIOLOGIC ACTIVITIES OF HCG

Interaction with Glycoprotein Hormone Receptors

The current picture of the mechanism of action of the glyco-protein hormones on their primary target cells depicts the hormone interacting with a receptor in the plasma membrane. Presumably, the selectivity of this interaction between hormone and target cell is reflected by structural compatability between the receptor and the hormone. Thus, the hCG molecule is structurally most compatible with the glycoprotein receptors of interstitial cells, the LH/CG receptors, and through this interaction, hCG expresses its primary biologic activity -- ICSA. The expression of the secondary biologic activities of hCG, not surprisingly, seems to operate through the same type of mechanism. The available data is consistent with the notion that the hCG molecule binds to the FSH receptor and TSH receptor with an affinity appropriately diminished in accordance with the relatively weak nature of its secondary biologic activities. Further, as with the more potent ligands, hFSH and hTSH, the quarternary structure of the hCG molecule is key for the interaction in FSH and TSH radioligand-receptor assays. Effectively, the subunits of the high affinity glycoprotein ligands and the subunits of hCG are bereft of binding activity. Hence, the quarternary structure of the glycoprotein hormone is required for relevant interaction with the receptor, whether the interaction is occurring with the primary receptor or the secondary receptor.

The interactions of purified hCG, its purified subunits, and recombined hCG have been systematically studied with rat testis membranes (Siris et al., 1978). This is a logical system in which to study the receptor mechanism because FSA is evident in bioassays with the rat species. The results in the bioassay for FSA show good agreement with the results obtained in FSH-like activity in the FSH radioligand-receptor assay just as it does in the bioassay for FSA; and, in both assays, activity is quite weak relative to pitui-tary hFSH preparations (Siris et al., 1978). Further, the purified hCG preparation and the recombinant $hCG\alpha-hCG\beta$ preparation exhibit comparable effects on FSH binding, while the subunits themselves are essentailly devoid of activity (Figure 2).

While the TSA of hCG preparations has been worked out in the mouse thyroid bioassay, the TSH receptor interactions have not been studied in this species. The data concerning the interaction of purified hCG and its subunits with the TSH receptor have been gener-ated with bovine thyroid membranes (Amir et al., 1977; Azukizawa et al., 1977; Pekonen and Weintraub, 1979) and with porcine thyroid membranes (Davies et al., 1979). Interpretation of the results with bovine membranes has been hampered because the results seem to vary from laboratory to laboratory; this probably reflects

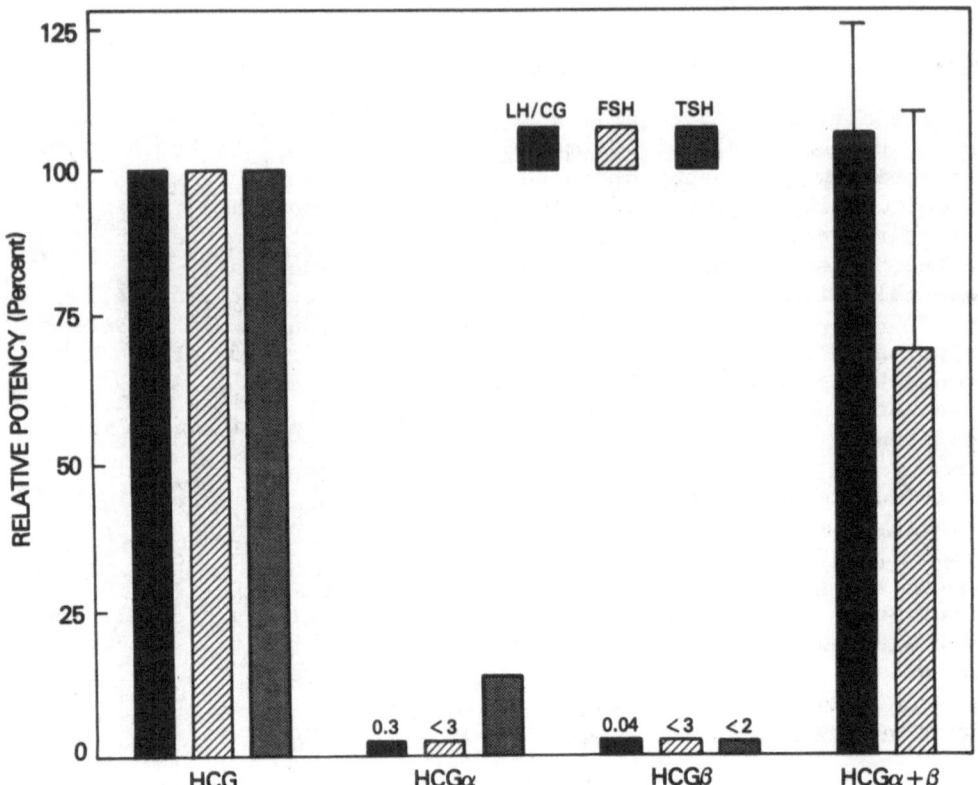

Figure 2. Relative potencies of the purified hCG, the hCGα subunit, the hCGβ subunit, and the recombined subunits in radioligand-receptor assays for LH/CG, FSH, and TSH. The hCGα and hCGβ subunit preparations were derived from the dissociation of the purified hCG (CR119) preparation and further purified prior to assessing their individual activities and those resulting from their recombination. The error brackets indicate the 95% confidence limits for the relative potency estimate.

differences in assay conditions (Pekonen and Weintraub, 1979). The data obtained with porcine thyroid membranes does not show the sort of variability shown by bovine membranes under assay conditions differing in temperature and osmolarity (Davies et al., 1979). It is notable that the more recent studies show agreement between bovine and porcine systems, providing the assays are performed at physiologic pH and temperature (Pekonen and Weintraub, 1979; Davies et al., 1979). Accordingly, the data shown in Figure 2 reflects the findings obtained under the more physiologic conditions. The notable finding is that the purified hCG (CR119) preparation inhibits TSH binding to porcine thyroid membranes much more potently than do its subunits (Figure 2). The small amount of TSH binding inhibition activity observed in the hCGα preparation may be non-specific in nature, considering the quantity of protein added to the assay system. Since the native hCG gives much more TSH binding inhibition than either subunit, quarternary structure is evidently the predominant factor in the interaction. From these data, it can be reasoned that the lack of biologic activity in the subunit preparations in vivo is not simply due to increased metabolic clearance rates of the subunits, but is also attributable to a deficiency of receptor interaction.

Structural Basis of the Secondary Biologic Activities

The structural features of the hCG molecule that determine its secondary biologic activities are unknown. However, the glycoprotein hormones, hCG, hLH, hFSH, and hTSH, comprise a group of structural congeners; not only are their α-subunits nearly identical in structure, but their β-subunits have many areas of homology of primary structure. Detailed comparisons of primary structure can be found elsewhere (Pierce, 1976). Based on the results of the glycoprotein hormone receptor studies outlined earlier in this chapter, it seems reasonable to postulate that hCG behaves as an FSH and TSH agonist because it is a structural congener of these hormones. Further development of this line of thought yields the prediction that the LH molecule, which is structurally and functionally quite similar to hCG, should exhibit intrinsic FSH-like and TSH-like actions. To adequately test this prediction, an LH preparation virtually uncontaminated with FSH or TSH is required. By recombining highly purified hCGα with highly purified ovine LHβ, one creates an LHβ-containing hybrid molecule preparation which has potent luteinizing activity, but which lacks detectable contamination with pituitary FSH or TSH. As predicted, this LHβ-containing molecule interacts with the FSH receptor (Siris et al., 1978) and exhibits TSA in the mouse thyroid bioassay (Taliadouros et al., 1978). That this LHβ-containing hybrid molecule, a structural congener of hCG, posses intrinsic FSH-like and TSH-like activities further extends and supports the conclusion that FSA and TSA are intrinsic to the hCG molecule. Since the major structural difference between hLH and hCG is the presence of the extra 30 amino acids at the carboxy-terminus of hCGβ, the results with the LH are not attributable to the unique carboxy-terminal region.

Copurification of the Activities in Crude hCG

The notion that FSA and TSA are intrinsic to the hCG molecule prompts one to consider the extent to which the hCG content of crude

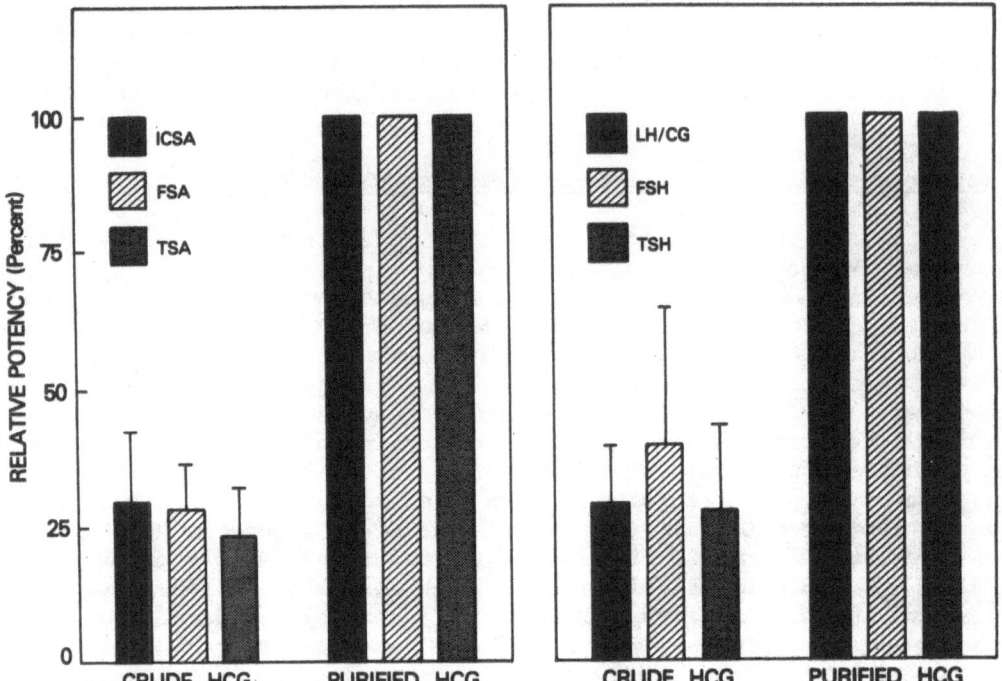

Figure 3. Relative potencies of crude commercial hCG (Organon) and the derived purified hCG preparation in biological assays for ICSA, FSA, and TSA (left panel) and in radioligand-receptor assays for LH/CG, FSH, and TSH (right panel). In the TSH radioligand-receptor assay, a different batch of crude hCG with a similar LH/CG potency was employed. The error brackets indicate the 95% confidence limits for the relative potency estimate.

hCG. To examine this issue, one can compare the ratio of the FSA to the ICSA in crude hCG with that in purified hCG, expecting to find a much higher ratio of FSA to ICSA in the crude hCG, if there are substantial amounts of substances with FSA other than hCG in the crude preparation. A similar argument can be applied to the ratio of TSA to ICSA in crude hCG versus that in purified hCG preparations. A comparison of the relative levels of these activities in crude and purified hCG is presented in Figure 3. It is evident that the relative levels of FSA, TSA, and ICSA in crude hCG are not significantly different from the relative levels in the purified hCG preparation. Data obtained with radioligand-receptor assays are in complete agreement with these bioassay findings (Figure 3). Thus, the starting crude commercial hCG preparation (Organon) from which purified hCG is derived, gives no evidence for molecules separate from hCG to account for its content of FSA and TSA. In addition, that these three biologic activities co-purify with one another is yet more evidence to support the conclusion that FSA and TSA are properties of the hCG molecule. Several other activities in crude hCG preparations have been studied, but these do not appear to co-purify with the hCG molecule. These include immunosuppressive activity (Morse et al., 1976), porphyrin synthesis inhibitory activity (Rifkind et al., 1976). and NAD-glycohydrolase activity (Moss et al., 1978).

It should be emphasized that these observations are not inconsistent with the concept that there are placental hormones with FSA and TSA in extracts of trophoblastic tissues or in the urine of pregnant women. The purification procedures used to derive the crude hCG employed in these studies may exclude or alter these other putative molecules. It is obvious, then, that while hCG can account for the FSA and TSA in the crude hCG used in our studies, other hCG preparations or the tissue and biologic fluids of pregnancy could contain substances, in addition to hCG, with intrinsic TSA and FSA.

THYROID-STIMULATING ACTIVITY INTRINSIC TO HCG

Unique Nature of the Thyroid-stimulating Activity

The thyroid-stimulating activity intrinsic to the hCG molecule is qualitatively quite different from that of the hTSH molecule and that of the long acting thyroid stimulator. In suitably prepared mice (Nisula et al., 1973), the level of blood radioactivity is measured at 2, 9, and 22 hours after injection of the test preparation. The mouse thyroid bioassay performed in this manner reveals the unique nature of the time course of the response obtained with each of these thyrotropic factors (Nisula and Ketelslegers, 1974). The maximum response to hCG is observed at 9 hours, while that to hTSH is observed at 2 hours, and that to the long acting thyroid

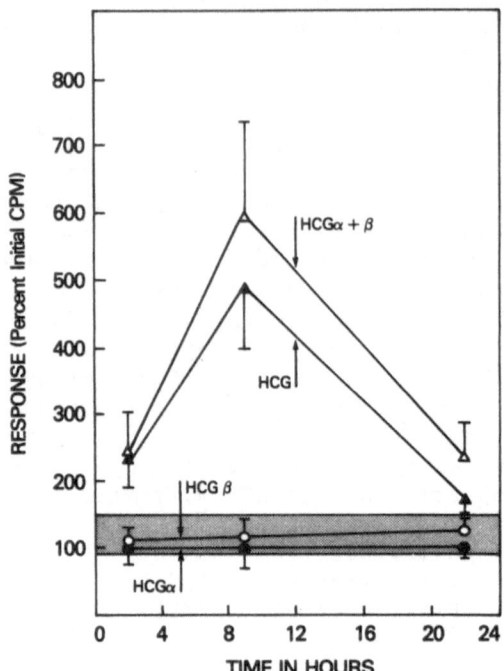

Figure 4. Time course of the biological response obtained with purified hCG (125 µg), hCGα (1000 µg), hCGβ (1000 µg), and recombinant hCG (125 µg) in the mouse thyroid bioassay. The shaded area indicates the control response obtained with the injection of the physiological saline vehicle. The brackets indicate the SE of the mean response of 5 mice.

stimulator is observed at 22 hours. This unique intermediate response is obtained not only with purified hCG, but also with the recombinant hCG molecule (Figure 4). Thus, the qualitative nature of the TSA in purified hCG is recovered in the recombinant preparation. Also, the purified subunits are devoid of biological activity at each time point (Figure 4), indicating that dissociation results in a loss of activity, rather than a shift in the time course of the response. This intermediate response pattern is seen with biologic specimens which contain sufficient levels of hCG, whether obtained from normal pregnant women, men with hCG-secreting neoplasms, or women with gestational trophoblastic diseases, such as hydatidiform mole or choriocarcinoma (Nisula and Ketelslegers, 1974).

Another feature of the behavior of hCG in the mouse thyroid bioassay worth noting is the magnitude of the response evoked.

The maximum response obtained with purified hCG preparations occurs at 9 hours after injection and is about 2000%, while the maximum response obtained with hTSH 2 hours after injection is about 1000%. Thus, although the response to hCG peaks at a later time, it is actually much greater in magnitude than the response to hTSH. The dose-response relationships with respect to the time of the peak response and the maximum response obtained at this time provides a biologic basis on which to judge whether a given unknown sample from a patient has the unique characteristics of hTSH or those of hCG. Further, given that the responses of hTSH and hCG are so different from each other, one needs to consider whether it is logical to express the TSA of hCG preparations in terms of TSH reference standards. From the theoretical standpoint, it seems logical to assess the time course of the response and then express the potency obtained in terms of an hTSH standard, or in terms of an hCG standard, depending on whether the response was hTSH-like or hCG-like, respectively.

Effects on Human Thyroid in Vitro

It is obvious that the finding that the hCG molecule exhibits TSA in the mouse does not prove that it is a thyrotropic factor in the human. To appreciate the problem, one need only consider the heterologous nature of the assay system for TSA -- a human gonadotropin acting on the mouse thyroid. It is heterologous with respect to the animal species and with respect to the responding organ. For comparison, prolactin is a peptide hormone whose biologic activity varies, depending on the animal species to which it is administered. Also, interspecies variability in structure-function relationships have been well-established for the gonadotropins in nonmammalian vertebrate species (Licht et al., 1977). Thus, while the hCG molecule may have secondary biological actions in the mouse and the rat, independent data concerning these actions must be sought regarding the human. The activities of adenylate cyclase in the thyroid membrane is considered to be a consequence of appropriate interaction with the TSH receptor. Indeed, crude commerical hCG preparations have been shown to stimulate cyclase activity in slices of human thyroid tissue (Silverberg et al., 1978), but whether the hCG or some other factor in the crude hCG accounts for the apparent TSA in this system has not been determined. To assess this problem, some fractionation procedures should be employed, such as G-100 chromatography on which hCG can be separated from potential pituitary and/or putative placental contaminants. Using purified human thyroid membranes prepared as described elsewhere (Carayon et al., 1979), we find that the TSA in crude hCG cochromatographs with the hCG molecule (Figure 5). Further, to show the comparability of the action of hCG on the mouse thyroid with that on the human thyroid, crude hCG was chromatographed on Sephadex G-100 and the eluted fractions assayed for their ability to stimulate adenylate cyclase activity

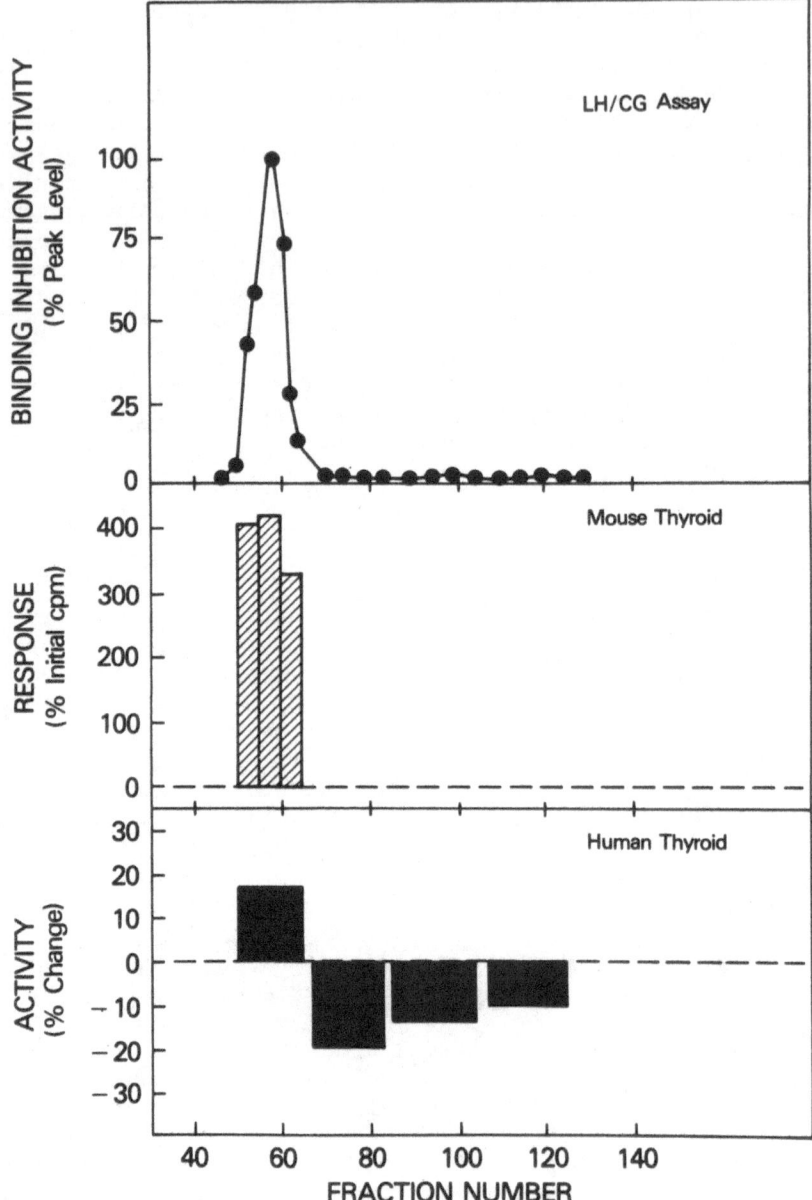

Figure 5.   Gel filtration of crude hCG on G-100 Sephadex.   The
position in which the thyrotropic activity eluted corresponds with
the postion of the hCG.   The upper panel indicates the activity in
the LH/CG radioligand-receptor assay; the middle panel indicates
the fractions with activity in the mouse thyroid bioassay; and the
bottom panel indicates the effect of the pooled fractions from
various positions, on adenylate cyclase activity in purified human
thyroid membranes.

in human purified thyroid membranes and for their ability to
stimulate the mouse thyroid. In Figure 5, it can be seen that the
activity in the human thyroid adenylate cyclase assay and that the
TSA in the preparation co-elutes with the hCG molecule as measured
by radioligand-receptor assay. Importantly, there is no thyroid
stimulating factor present, either for the mouse or the human, other
than that which co-eluted with the hCG. Rather, there is inhibition
of adenylate cyclase activity obtained with the substances eluted
after the hCG molecule (Figure 5). These observations are consistent
with hCG being a thyrotropic factor for the human as well as the
mouse. These data also confirm that there are no detectable human
thyrotropic factors of a molecular size similar to pituitary hTSH or
chorionic thyrotropin in the crude hCG preparation (Organon) which
was employed in these studies.

Clinical Relevance

To assess the clinical relevance of the TSA intrinsic to hCG,
one must look to the experiments of nature. This is because the
TSA of the hCG molecule is relativley weak and to obtain blood levels
sufficiently high to expect an effect on human thyroid function, one
would have to administer more purified hCG than is currently available. A systematic study of the correlation of human thyroid function
and blood hCG level would be a useful alternative, although it must
be remembered that putative factors other than hCG with TSA may also
be secreted by the pituitary or the tissue which secretes the hCG.
It has been well established that pregnant women are not thyrotoxic;
clearly, levels of hCG up to 100 IU/ml, which can be seen in normal
pregnancy, are not sufficient to cause hyperthyroidism. Patients
with levels of hCG exceeding those of pregnancy would be the logical
ones to scrutinize. Figure 6 shows peripheral thyroid hormone
levels in patients with gestational trophoblastic disease in whom
the serum hCG level may be quite high. In the occasional patient,
the serum hCG level can be many-fold greater than in normal pregnancy;
and in such patients (Figure 6), accelerated thyroid function and
symptomatic thyrotoxicosis are seen. As predicted, serum thyroid
hormone levels show a correlation with the serum hCG level in those
patients with hCG levels higher than that of normal pregnancy (i.e.,
>100 IU/ml). These results are consistent with the hypothesis that
the TSA intrinsic to the hCG molecule mediates the increased thyroid
function seen in patients with gestational trophoblastic disease.
That extremely high levels of hCG are required seems to indicate
that what the hCG molecule lacks in potency as a thyrotropic factor,
it can more than compensate for by the high blood concentration it
can achieve.

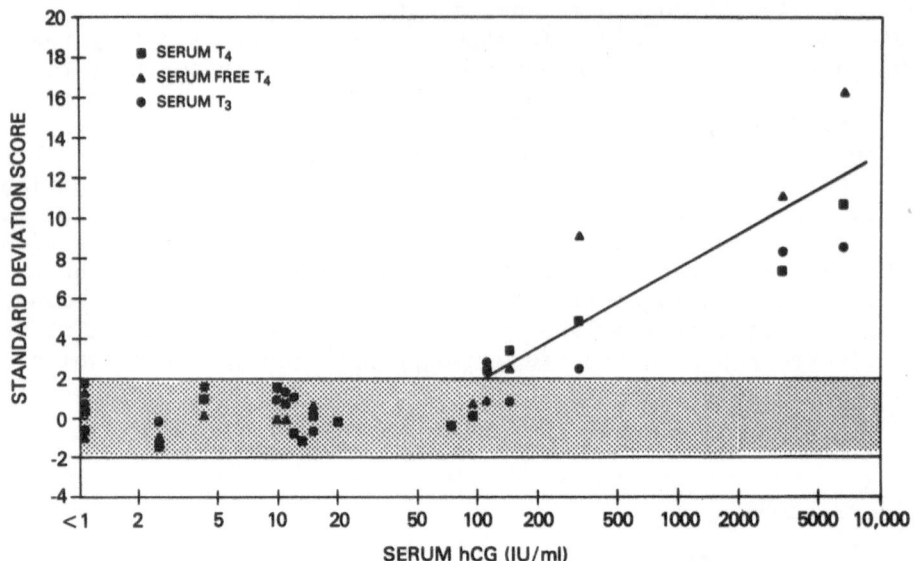

Figure 6. Correlation of the serum hCG level and the serum thyroid level in patients with gestational trophoblastic disease. For comparison, the levels of hCG in normal pregnant women do not exceed 100 IU/ml. Serum hCG was measured by radioimmunoassay using an antiserum to the carboxy-terminal peptide of hCGβ. The standard deviation score was calculated by subtracting the patient value from the normal mean value and dividing the result by the standard deviation of the normal range.

CONCLUSIONS

The hypothesis that FSA and TSA are intrinsic to the hCG molecule has been explored. Purified hCG preparations exhibit FSA and TSA, which are not due to contamination with pituitary hormones. The TSA cochromatographs with the ICSA in purified hCG. The ICSA, FSA, and TSA of our crude hCG preparations copurify with one another. Purified hCG subunits, devoid of these activities, regain ICSA, FSA, and TSA when recombined. Investigation of the mechanism of the secondary activities of the hCG molecule shows that purified hCG inhibits FSH and TSH binding in radioligand-receptor assays with activity appropriately diminished in accordance with hCG's weak activity in the bioassays for FSA and TSA. The molecular basis of the interactions with the secondary receptors may be found in the rather high degree of structural homology evident among the glycoprotein hormones. The finding that the target organ specificity of human hormones in rodent bioassays is relative, not complete, raises question of the relevance to human thyroid physiology. Results of

studies with human thyroid tissue in vitro correlate with the results
of the mouse thyroid bioassay, indicating that the TSA in the hCG
molecule acts on both the mouse and the human thyroid. Observations
of patients with gestational trophoblastic disease are consistent
with the hypothesis that the hCG molecule is the thyrotropic factor
which mediates the thyrotoxicosis associated with gestational trophoblastic disease.

REFERENCES

Akasu, F., Kawaraha, S., Ohki, H., Harano, M., and Tejima, Y., 1955,
    Thyroid stimulating hormone extracted from human placenta,
    Endocrinol. Jap. 2:297.
Albert, A., 1969, Follicle stimulating activity of human chorionic
    gonadotropin, J. Clin. Endocrinol. Metab. 29:1504.
Amir, S. M., Uchimura, H., and Ingbar, S. H., 1977, Interactions of
    bovine thyrotropin and preparations of human chorionic gonado-
    tropin with bovine thyroid membranes, Endocrinology 45:280.
Ashitaka, Y., Tokura, Y., Tane, M., Mochizuki, M., and Tojo, S.,
    1970, Studies on the biochemical properties of highly purified
    hCG, Endocrinology 87:233.
Ashitaka, Y., Mochizuki, Y. M., and Tojo, S., 1972, Purification and
    properties of human chorionic gonadotropin from the tropho-
    blastic tissue of hydatidiform mole, Endocrinology 99:609.
Azukizawa, M., Kurtzman, G., Pekary, E., and Hershman, J., 1977,
    Comparison of the binding characteristics of bovine thyrotropin
    and human chorionic gonadotropin to thyroid plasma membranes,
    Endocrinology 101:1880.
Burger, A., 1967, Further studies on a thyroid stimulating factor in
    crude chorionic gonadotropin preparations and in urine, Acta
    Endocrinol. 55:600.
Canfield, R. E., Morgan, F. J., Kammerman, S., Bell, J. J., and
    Agosto, G. M., 1971, Studies on human chorionic gonadotropin,
    Recent Progr. Horm. Res. 27:121.
Canfield, R. E., and Ross, G. T., 1976, A new reference preparation
    of human chorionic gonadotropin and its subunits, Bull. WHO
    54:463.
Carayon, P., Guibot, M., and Lissitzky, S., 1979, The interaction of
    radioiodinated TSH with human plasma membranes from normal and
    diseased thyroid glands, Ann. Endocrinol. (Paris) 40:211.
Davies, T. F., Taliadouros, G., Catt, K., and Nisula, B. C., 1979,
    Assessment of urinary TSH-competing activity in choriocarcinoma
    and thyroid disease: Further evidence for hCG interacting at
    the thyroid cell membrane, J. Clin. Endocrinol Metab. 49:353.
Evans, H. M., Simpson, M., Austin, P., and Ferguson, R., 1933,
    Peculiarities of the prolan-like substance in urine in a case
    of embryonal carcinoma of the testis, Proc. Soc. Exp. Biol. Med.
    31:21.

Harada, A., and Hershman, J. M., 1978, Extraction of human chorionic thyrotropin (hCT) from term placentas: Failure to recover thyrotropic activity, J. Clin. Endocrinol. Metab. 47:681.

Hennen, G., 1965, Detection and study of a human chorionic thyroid-stimulating factor, Arch. Int. Phys. Bio. 73:689.

Hershman, J. M., and Starnes, W. R., 1969, Extraction and characterization of a thyrotropic material from the human placenta, J. Clin. Invest. 48:923.

Kenimer, J. G., Hershman, J. M., and Higgins, H. P., 1975, Thyrotropin in hydatidiform moles is human chorionic gonadotropin, J. Clin. Endocrinol. Metab. 40:482.

Ketelslegers, J. M., Nisula, B. C., and Kohler, P., 1975, Investigation of choriocarcinoma clonal cell lines in vitro and choriocarcinoma transplants in the hamster for the secretion of a thyroid-stimulating factor, Endocrinology 96:808.

Kitagaki, S., 1977, Studies on the purification and biochemical properties of human chorionic thyrotropin, Acta Obstet. Gynaec. Jpn. 29:601.

Kulin, H., Santner, S., and Mann, W., 1979, Urinary follicle-stimulating hormone during pregnancy: Relationship to sex of fetus, J. Clin. Endocrinol. Metab. 48:736.

Licht, P., Papkoff, H., Farmer, S., Muller, C., Tsui, H., and Crews, D., 1977, Evolution of gonadotropin structure and function, Rec. Progr. Horm Res. 33:169.

Louvet, J. P., Harman, S. M., Nisula, B. C., Ross, G. T., Birken, S., and Canfield, R. E., 1976, Follicle stimulating activity of human chorionic gonadotropin: effect of dissociation and recombination of subunits, Endocrinology 99:1126.

Lyon, R. A., Simpson, M. E., and Evans, H. M., 1953, Qualitative changes in urinary gonadotropins in human pregnancy during the period of rapid increase in hormone titer, Endocrinology 53:674.

Morgan, F. J., Canfield, R. E., Vaitukaitis, J. L., and Ross, G. T., 1974, Properties of the subunits of human chorionic gonadotropin, Endocrinology 94:1601.

Moss, J., Ross, P. S., Agosto, G., Birken, S., Canfield, R. E., and Vaughn, 1978, Mechanism of action of choleragen and the glycopeptide hormones: Is the nicotinamide adenine dinucleotide glycohydrolase activity observed in purified hormone preparations intrinsic to the hormone?, Endocrinology 102:415.

Morse, J. H., Stears, G., Arden, J., Agosto, G. M., and Canfield, R. E., 1976, The effects of crude and purified human gonadotropin on in vitro stimulated human lymphocyte cultures, Cell Immunol. 35:178.

Nisula, B. C., Kohler, P. O., Vaitukaitis, J. L., Hershman, J. M., and Ross, G. T., 1973, Neutralization of human thyrotropin by antisera to subunits of glycoprotein hormones, J. Clin. Endocrinol. Metab. 37:664.

Nisula, B. C., and Ketelslegers, J. M., 1974, Thyroid stimulating activity and chorionic gonadotropin, J. Clin. Invest. 54:494.

Nisula, B. C., Morgan, F. J., and Canfield, R. C., 1974, Evidence that chorionic gonadotropin has intrinsic thyrotropic activity, Biochem. Biophys. Res. Commun. 59:86.

Nisula, B. C., and Louvet, J. P., 1978, Radioimmunoassay of thyrotropin concentrated from serum, J. Clin. Endocrinol. Metab. 46:729.

Pierce, J. G., 1976, Amino acid sequences of proteins: Hormones of the anterior pituitary and placenta. CRC Handbook of Biochemistry and Molecular Biology, G. D. Fashman, ed., 3rd edition, Proteins Vol. III, pp. 385-398.

Pekonen, F., and Weintraub, B. D., 1979, Thyrotropin receptors on bovine thyroid membranes: Two types with different affinities and specificities, Endocrinology 105:352.

Rifkind, A. B., Canfield, R. E., and Kappas, A., 1976, Inhibition chemical induction of porphyrin synthesis in chick embryo liver cells by partially purified human chorionic gonadotropin, Biochem. Biophys. Res. Commun. 68:503.

Silverberg, J., O'Donnell, J., Sugenoya, A., Row, V., and Volpe, R., 1978, Effect of chorionic gonadotropin on human thyroid tissue in vitro, J. Clin. Endocrinol. Metab. 46:420.

Simpson, M. E., 1961, Comparison of follicle-stimulating and interstitial cell-stimulating properties of gonadotropins from pituitary and non-pituitary sources, in Human Pituitary Gonadotropins, Albert, A., ed., C. Thomas, Illinois p. 123.

Siris, E. S., Nisula, B. C., Catt, K. J., Horner, K., Birken, S., Canfield, R. E., and Ross, G. T., 1978, New evidence for intrinsic follicle stimulating hormone-like activity in human chorionic gonadotropin and luteinizing hormone, Endocrinology 102:1356.

Taliadouros, G. S., Canfield, R. E., and Nisula, B. C., 1978, Thyroid stimulating activity of chorionic gonadotropin and luteinizing hormone, J. Clin. Endocrinol. Metab. 47:855.

Tojo, S., Mochizuki, M., Ashitaka, Y., and Kanazawa, S., 1978, Biological aspects of placental protein hormones, in Proceedings of the 6th Asia and Oceania Congress of Endocrinology, Lim Pin, ed., pp. 206-216.

Uchimara, H., Nagataki, S., Tabuchi, T., Mizuno, M., and Ito, K., 1975, The thyroid stimulating activity of highly purified preparations of human chorionic gonadotropin, Seventh International Conference, Boston, Exerpta Medica ICS, p. 37.

CHORIONIC GONADOTROPIN IN RODENTS

Leif Wide, Bruce Hobson, and Mariann Wide

Department of Clinical Chemistry, University Hospital
Institute of Zoology and Department of Anatomy
University of Uppsala, Uppsala, Sweden
Department of Obstetrics and Gynaecology, Royal Infirmary
Edinburgh, Scotland

INTRODUCTION

The nature of the luteotropic factor in rodent placentae has been a matter of controversy. Most textbooks in reproductive endocrinology claim that chorionic gonadotropin (CG) is found only in the human (hCG) and in some ape and monkey placentae, and that the luteotropic hormone in the rodent placenta is different, having both luteotropic and mammotropic activity. The results of our studies indicate that rodent placentae contain a gonadotropin very similar in structure to hCG.

It would appear that the first evidence for the presence of a placental gonadotropin in rodents was presented exactly 50 years ago, in November 1929, by Ljuba Mirskaia in Edinburgh. This author concluded that "The difference between the mouse placenta, on the one hand, and the human placenta on the other, appears not to be so fundamental as might have been expected. The mouse placenta and human placenta and certain pituitary extracts, have one effect in common: the incitement of the second phase of ovarian secretion, that is, the production of beta hormone. Whether the factor which is responsible for this action is identical with Rho 2 of the anterior lobe remains to be seen." (The beta hormone was later named 'progesterone' and the Rho 2 'luteinizing hormone.')

Nine years later, Astwood and Greep (1938) demonstrated the presence of a corpus luteum-stimulating substance in the rat placenta. They employed the deciduoma reaction as a test for corpus luteum function and used animals hypophysectomized on the fourth day of pseudopregnancy. For many years it was thought that the luteotropin in the rat placenta also had a lactogenic and mammotropic activity (Matthies, 1967; Shintani et al., 1966). However, studies on rat chorionic mammotropin by Kelly et al. (1975) suggested that the lactogenic and the luteotropic activities derive from two different entities.

Linkie and Niswender (1973) confirmed earlier reports which indirectly identified luteotropic activity in serum and placentae of the pregnant rat, and extended the latter observations by quantitating progesterone levels in the serum of hypophysectomized animals injected with placental extracts. They found that the biological component(s) was characterized as a heat-labile protein of approximately 25,000-50,000 molecular weight. The biologically active placental extracts had no activity in a radioimmunoassay (RIA) for rat pituitary LH or FSH. Further evidence for a difference between the pituitary LH and the placental gonadotropin in the rat was obtained by Haour et al. (1976) who found that placental extracts had significant activity in a radioreceptor assay (RRA) utilizing ^{125}I-labeled hCG and no detectable activity in an RIA for rat pituitary LH.

Our studies on rodent placentae indicate that they contain a chorionic gonadotropin and that this hormone in the rat, mouse, and hamster is structurally similar to human CG with its alpha and beta subunits (Wide and Hobson, 1977; Wide and Hobson, 1978; Wide and Wide, 1979). Our most recent studies, on the guinea pig, indicate that extracts made from the placenta of this rodent contain a CG which is similar to hCG (Humphreys, Wide and Hobson, unpublished). The present communication reviews our previous work on rodent placental CG, including some unpublished results.

BIOLOGICAL POTENCY OF RODENT PLACENTAE

The biological gonadotropic activity of rat (day 18 of pregnancy), hamster (day 16 of pregnancy), and guinea pig placentae (varying from day 15 to day 60 of pregnancy) was assayed by injecting placental extracts into immature mice and using the increase in uterine weight as the index of response. The extracts were made by precipitating the gonadotropins with acetone and ether and then dissolving the dried precipitate in saline (Hobson, 1972). The completeness of the extraction method for the removal of steroid material was checked in ovariectomized estrone-primed mice. All placental extracts had significant activity in the bioassay. There was no significant difference between parallelism of the dose-response lines of the 2nd International Standard for hCG and the placental material. The gonadotropic activity was equivalent to 5.77 IU/per placenta or 13.2 IU/g of placental tissue for the rat. The corresponding figures for the hamster were 0.82 IU or 2.72 IU, respectively. The activities of the guinea pig placentae varied from 0.15 to 33.9 IU/g, depending on the day of pregnancy. Thus, the concentration of gonadotropins in the rat, hamster, or guinea pig placentae was similar to that for human placentae at term (range 2.9–42.4 IU/g), using the same bioassay method (Hobson and Wide, 1974).

IMMUNOASSAY OF RODENT PLACENTAE FOR HCG-LIKE ACTIVITY

When these extracts, together with a number of extracts of mouse placentae from different days of pregnancy, were assayed in the solid-phase RIA systems (Wide, 1969) for hCG, hCG α-subunit, and hCG β-subunit, they were found to have significant activity in all three systems. However, such an activity could be a non-specific inhibition of the immunological reaction. To obtain more information about the nature of these activities, the extracts were tested after chromatography on Sephadex G-200 and the elution patterns were compared with those from similar chromatographic studies of human placental extracts and of purified preparations of hCG and its subunits. Some rodent placental extracts were also examined in a similar way after zone electrophoresis.

The chromatographies were made on a 26 x 930 mm Sephadex G-200 column, equilibrated with 0.1 M Tris-HCl buffer of pH 7.5 with 0.2 M NaCl, and the flow was against gravity with a rate of 9 ml per hour with 3 ml fractions collected. The degree of retardation of immunoreactive material on the columns was expressed in K_{av} values (Laurent and Killander, 1964). The eluted material was treated for immunoreactivity in three RIA systems. The hCGα- and hCGβ-subunits and their antisera (SA-6 and SB-6) used in the RIA were supplied by NIAMDD, National Institutes of Health, Bethesda. The sensitivity of the assay was adjusted by varying the amount of test sample analyzed and the time of incubation before the labeled antigen was added.

The elution patterns obtained after chromatography of purified preparations of hCG and of its two subunits are shown in Figure 1. The immunological activities are plotted in relation to elution volume, K_{av} values. These values for hCG, hCGα, and hCGβ preparations were 0.40, 0.48, and 0.63, respectively. The activities and elution profiles, obtained after chromatographic separation of different rodent placental extracts, were plotted in a manner similar to that of the purified preparations. Two of these elution profiles, from the rat and the hamster, are shown in Figures 2 and 3. A considerable variation in the relative CG, CGα-subunit, and CGβ-subunit activity between placentae from the different animal species was found. Because of this the position and profile of these activities are deliberately accentuated by the use of different scales in the figures. The elution patterns of the extracts of different rodent placentae were very similar in position to that of purified hCG,

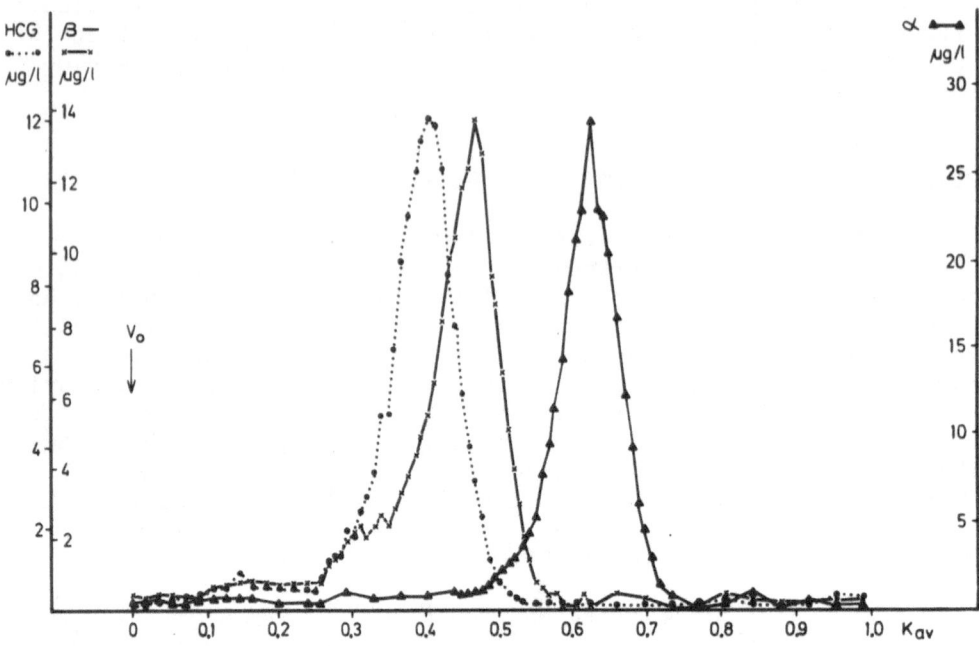

Figure 1. Elution patterns for purified hCG, hCGα, and hCGβ preparations mixed and chromatographed on Sephadex G-200. Each fraction was assayed in hCG, hCGα, and hCGβ RIAs.

hCGα, and hCGβ preparations, or of extracts of human placentae (Figure 4). CG activities were eluted around K_{av} 0.40 and CGα activities, around 0.60-0.65. The K_{av} values of the CGβ activities showed a larger variation. This was probably due to a cross-reactivity between CG and CGβ-subunits in the CGβ assay and to the existence of more than one molecular form with CGβ activity. In addition to the presence of CGβ activity in the same position as that of purified hCGβ-subunits, a second more retarded form was observed in extracts of the rat, hamster, mouse, and human placentae. Such a retarded form was very prominent in extracts of implantation sites taken on days 6 and 7 of pregnancy in the mouse (Figure 5). A molecular form of hCGβ more retarded than the hCGα has also been reported in extracts of pregnancy urine and placentae after chromatography on Sephadex G-100 (Good et al., 1977).

These chromatographic studies thus showed that the immunological activities of extracts of rat, hamster, mouse, and guinea pig placentae, as measured in the three RIA systems, were eluted in positions

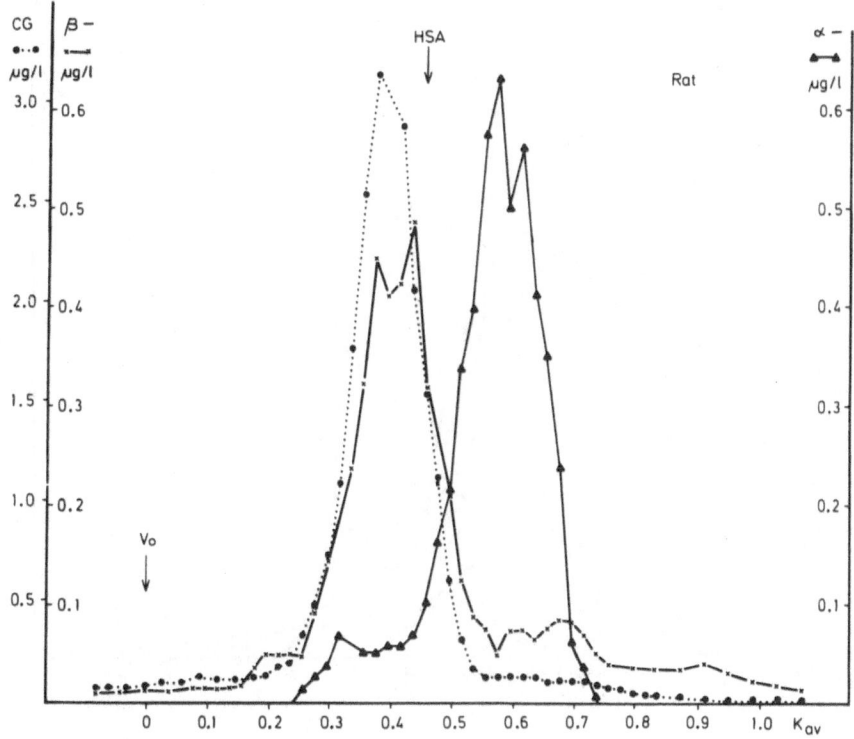

Figure 2. Elution profile of an extract of 350 mg of rat placental tissue, equivalent to 0.8 of a placenta, chromatographed on Sephadex G-200. Each fraction was assayed in hCG, hCGα, and hCGβ RIAs. The position for human serum albumin (HSA) is indicated. (From Wide and Hobson, 1978.)

similar to that of human placentae. The results indicate structural similarities between CG, CGα-subunits and CGβ-subunits in these rodents and humans.

ELECTROPHORETIC MOBILITY OF RAT PLACENTAL CG

The electrophoretic mobility of CG in a rat placental extract was compared with that of purified hCG preparations and hCG in placental extracts, serum, and urine. Zone electrophoresis in a column (0.9 cm x 65 cm) with 0.17% agarose suspension was performed in 0.075 M sodium Veronal$^{T.M.}$ buffer (pH 8.6) according to the technique described by Hjertén (1963). Before being added to the column, the

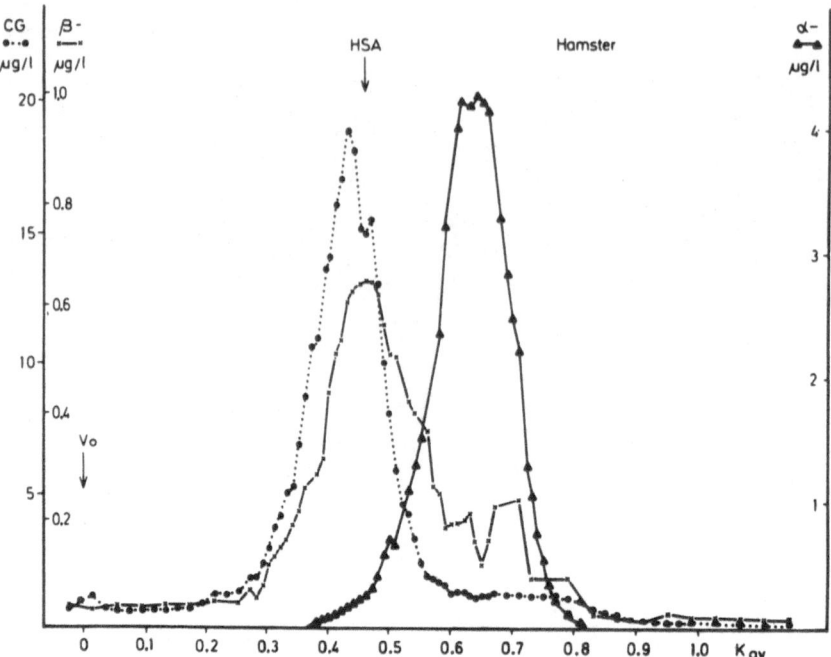

Figure 3.   Elution profile of an extract of 456 mg of hamster placental tissue, equivalent to 1.5 placentae, chromatographed on Sephadex G-200.   Each fraction was assayed in hCG, hCGα, and hCGβ RIA.   The position for human serum albumin (HSA) is indicated. (From Wide and Hobson, 1978.)

material to be tested was mixed with ^{125}I-labeled hCG and serum from a child (without detectable hCG activity).   After electrophoresis, 1 cm fractions were collected, the agarose removed by centrifugation, and the CG activity in the supernatants was measured.   The mobility of purified hCG (CR-119) and of hCG in pregnancy urine (first trimester) were very similar to ^{125}I-labeled hCG (Figure 6).   HCG in placental extract and in serum (taken early in pregnancy), had a similar but different mobility from that of purified hCG and hCG in urine specimen (Figure 7).   CG in rat placental extract had a mobility similar to that of hCG in human placental extract (Figure 8). This finding indicates further the similarity between rat and human placental CG.   The difference in mobility between purified (urinary) hCG and hCG in urine, on the one hand, and the hCG found in serum and in placental extract, on the other, suggests structural differences between hCG from the various sources.   The hCG in urine may be

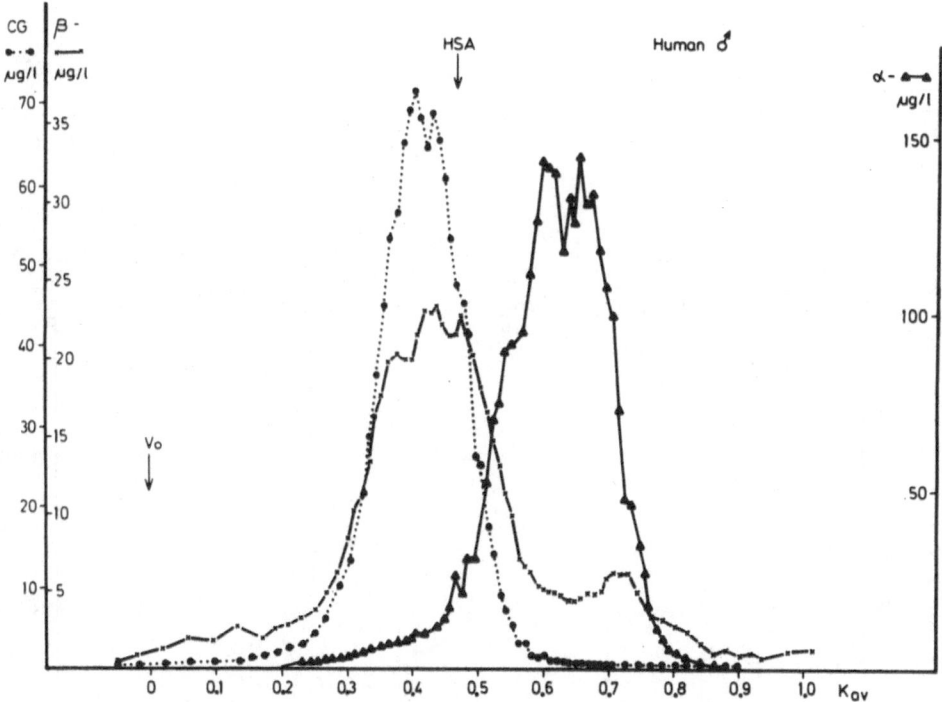

Figure 4. Elution profile of an extract of 420 mg of human placental tissue, equivalent to 0.001 of a placenta, chromatographed on Sephadex G-200. Each fraction was assayed in hCG, hCGα, and hCGβ RIAs. The position for human serum albumin (HSA) is indicated.

regarded as a waste product with a majority of molecules not identical to those circulating in the body or present in the placenta.

Extracts of rat placentae were treated with 8 and 10 M urea for 2 hr at 37°C and after that chromatographed on a Sephadex G-25 column. After urea treatment, there were significant increases in both CGα and CGβ activities, and a decrease in the CG activity. This further supports the concept that rat CG, like the human CG, consists of an α- and a β-subunit bound by noncovalent forces.

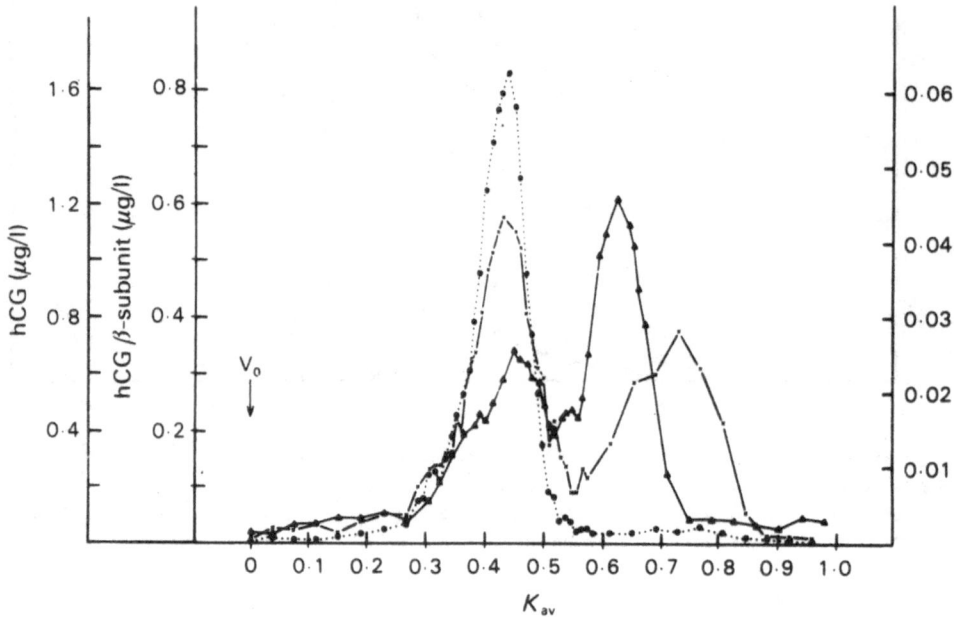

Figure 5. Elution profile of an extract of a pool of 35 Day-6 and 23 Day-7 implantation sites, chromatographed on Sephadex G-200. Each fraction was assayed in hCG (●), hCGα (▲), and hCGβ (x) RIAs. (From Wide and Wide, 1979.)

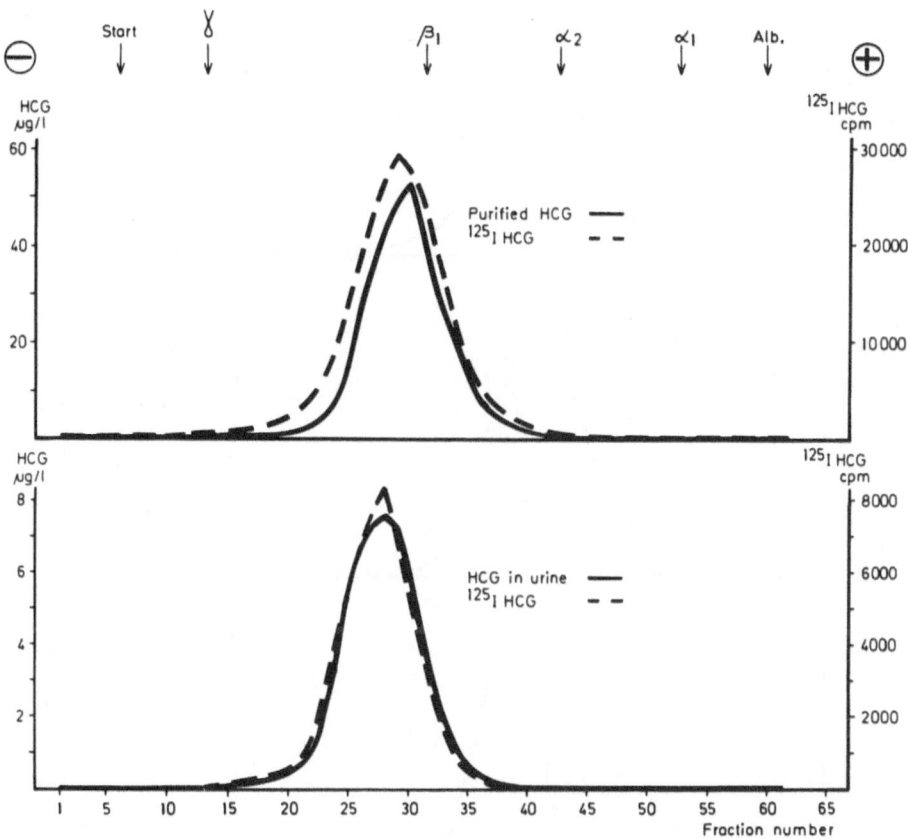

Figure 6. Electrophoresis in 0.17% agarose suspension. Upper part: purified hCG, unlabeled and labeled with ^{125}I. Lower part: hCG in urine and ^{125}I-labeled purified hCG.

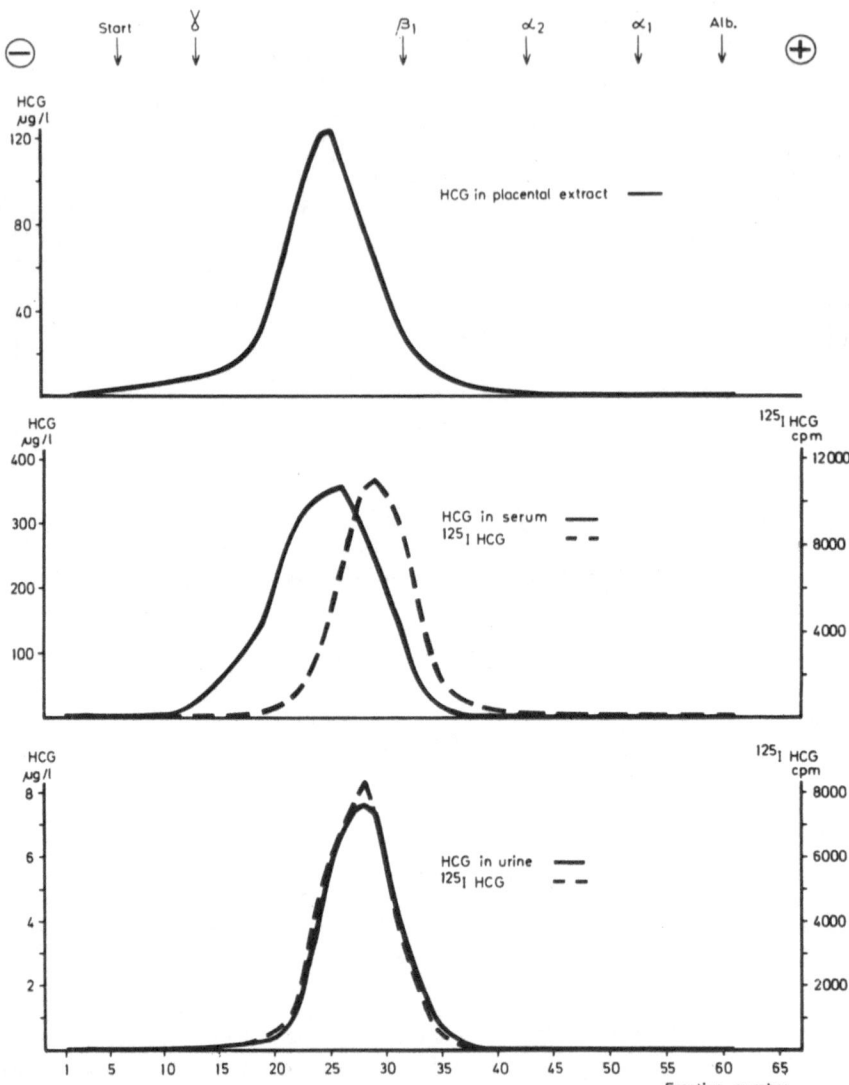

Figure 7. Electrophoresis in 0.17% agarose suspension. Upper part: hCG in placental extract. Middle part: hCG in serum and ^{125}I-labeled purified hCG. Lower part: hCG in urine and ^{125}I-labeled purified hCG.

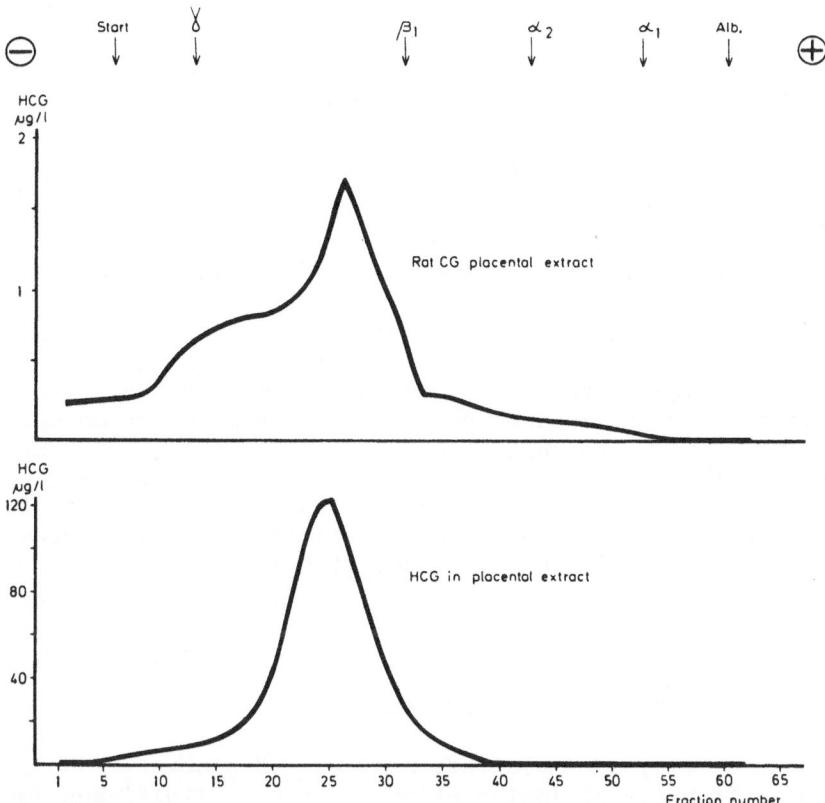

Figure 8. Electrophoresis in 0.17% agarose suspension. Upper part: CG in rat placental extract. Lower part: CG in human placental extract.

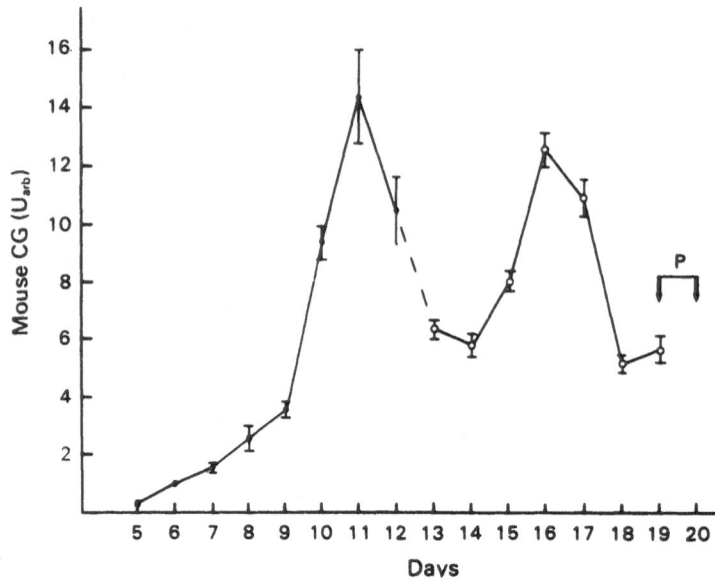

Figure 9.   Average content of mouse CG per implantation site (●)
or per placenta (O) from early pregnancy to term in the mouse.
Estimates were made with an RIA on extracts of pooled implantation
sites (Days 5-12) and of placentae (Day 13-19).   The average content
of a Day-6 implantation site was designated 1 U_{arb}.   The 95% fiducial
limits, as estimated from intra-assay variation, are indicated.
P = parturition.   (From Wide and Wide, 1979.)

TEMPORAL ASPECTS OF RAT CG PRODUCTION

    The CG activity in implantation sites and placentae was studied
in the mouse from day of implantation to term.   Significant amounts
of CG were detected in extracts of implantation sites or placentae
throughout the period of gestation investigated.   The pattern for
CG content per implantation site or per placenta from days 5 to 19
is illustrated in Figure 9.   CG content rose from day 5 until a
maximum level was reached on day 11, after which a rapid fall in
gonadotropin concentration occurred.   This was followed by a second
but lower peak on day le, and a further decline in CG concentration
was found in placentae obtained during the last two days of pregnancy.
Using a bioassay, Linkie and Niswender (1973) found detectable levels
of a 'luteotropic factor' in the rat placenta on days 11, 12, and 13,
with a maximum on day 12.   Haour et al. (1976) measured the gonadotropic activity in rat placentae by the use of a radioreceptor assay
(RRA) and found the highest concentration on day 13 of pregnancy.

Our results indicate that the peak values for the placental gonadotropin in the mouse occur at a stage of pregnancy similar to that
in the rat.

No CG activity was detected in an extract of 98 mouse blastocysts flushed from the uteri on day 5 of pregnancy (Wide and Wide,
1979). Wiley (1974) reported the presence of a gonadotropin on the
surface of mouse embryos in the 8-cell and morula stages. However,
he was not able to detect any gonadotropic activity on the surface
of uncultured mouse blastocysts or in mouse placental tissue. A
gonadotropic factor was detected in pre-implantation rabbit blastocysts by Haour and Saxena (1974) and by Fujimoto et al. (1975), but
Sundaram et al. (1975) and Holt et al. (1976) were unable to confirm
these results. Recently, Ellinwood et al. (1979) presented results
indicating that the factor present in rabbit blastocysts and active
in RRAs using labeled hCG as a reagent, has a molecular size much
larger than that known for gonadotropins and that this factor was
also present in uterine fluid of pseudo-pregnant rabbits. The
question whether the pre-implantation mouse or rabbit blastocysts
synthesize a gonadotropin has still to be determined.

CONCLUSION

A structural similarity between human CG and CG in extracts
from placentae of apes, monkeys, and a lemur was shown by Hobson
and Wide (1980). These observations, together with those showing
the presence of CG in rodent placentae, lead us to expect gonadotropin similar in structure and function to be found in the placentae
of other mammalian species.

REFERENCES

Astwood, E. B., and Greep, R. O., 1938, A corpus luteum-stimulating
    substance in the rat placenta, Proc. Soc. Exp. Biol. Med. 38:716.
Ellinwood, W. E., Seidel, D. E., and Niswender, G. D., 1979, Secretion
    of gonadotropic factors by the preimplantation rabbit blastocyst,
    Proc. Soc. Exp. Biol. Med. 161:136.
Fujimoto, S., Euker, J. S., Riegle, G. D., and Dukelow, W. R., 1975,
    On a substance cross-reacting with luteinizing hormone in the
    preimplantation blastocyst fluid of the rabbit, Proc. Jap. Acad.,
    51:123.
Good, A., Ramos-Uribe, M., Ryan, R. J., and Kempers, R. D., 1978,
    Molecular forms of human chorionic gonadotropin in serum, urine,
    and placental extracts, Fertil. Steril. 28:846.
Haour, F., and Saxena, B. B., 1974, Detection of a gonadotropin in
    rabbit blastocyst before implantation, Science, 185:444.
Haour, F., Tell, M. G., and Sanchez, P., 1976, Mise en évidence et

dosage d'une gonadotropin chorionique chez le rat (rCG), C. R. Acad. Sci. Paris, 282:1183.

Hjertén, S., 1963, Zone electrophoresis in columns of agarose suspensions, J. Chromatog. 12:510.

Hobson, B. M., 1972, Gonadotrophin concentrations in the placentae of man, the rhesus monkey and the marmoset, Folia primat. 18:35.

Hobson, B. M., and Wide, L., 1974, Chorionic gonadotrophin in the human placenta in relation to the sex of the foetus at term, J. Endocrin. 60:75.

Hobson, B. M., and Wide, L., 1980, The similarity of chorionic gonadotrophin and its subunits in term placentae from man, apes, old and new world monkeys and a prosimian, Folia primat., In press.

Holt, J. A., Heise, W. F., Wilson, S. M., and Keyes, P. L., 1976, Lack of gonadotropic activity in the rabbit blastocyst prior to implantation, Endocrinology 98:904.

Kelly, P. A., Shiu, R. P. C., Robertson, M. C., and Friesen, H. G., 1975, Characterization of rat chorionic mammotropin, Endocrinology 96:1187.

Laurent, T. C., and Killander, J., 1964, A theory of gel filtration and its experimental verification, J. Chromatog. 14:317.

Linkie, D. M., and Niswender, G. D., 1973, Characterization of rat placental luteotropin. Physiological and physiochemical properties, Biol. Reprod. 8:48.

Matthies, D. L., 1967, Studies on the luteotropic and mammotropic factor found in trophoblast and maternal peripheral blood of the rat at mid-pregnancy, Anat. Rec. 159:55.

Mirskaia, L., 1929, On the presence of a myogenic substance in the mouse placenta, Proc. Roy. Soc. (Edinburgh) 50:104.

Shintani, S., Glass, L. E., and Page, E. W., 1966, Studies of induced malignant tumors of placental and uterine origin in the rat, Am. J. Obstet. Gynecol. 95:559.

Sundaram, K., Connell, K. G., and Passantino, T., 1975, Implication of absence of hCG-like gonadotropin in the blastocyst for control of corpus luteum function in pregnant rat, Nature (Lond.) 256:739.

Wide, L., 1969, Radioimmunoassays employing immunosorbents, Acta Endocr., Copenh., Suppl. 142:207.

Wide, L., and Hobson, B. M., 1977, Presence of chorionic gonadotropin and free alpha- and beta-subunits in placental extracts of the rat, mouse, and hamster, Acta Endocr. Suppl. 212:31.

Wide, L., and Hobson, B., 1978, Chromatographic studies on a chorionic gonadotropic activity in the placenta of the rat, mouse, and hamster, Uppsala J. Med. Sci. 83:1.

Wide, L., and Wide, M., 1979, Chorionic gonadotropin in the mouse from implantation to term, J. Reprod. Fert. 57:5.

Wiley, L. D., 1974, Presence of a gonadotropin on the surface of preimplanted mouse embryos, Nature (Lond.) 252:716.

ACKNOWLEDGEMENTS

This research was supported by the Swedish Medical Research Council. We thank Mrs. J. Flockhart and Mr. Christer Bengtsson for technical assistance; and N.I.A.M.D.D., National Institutes of Health, Bethesda, for supply of subunit preparations and antisera to these compounds.

PATTERNS OF SECRETION AND ANTIGENIC SIMILARITIES AMONG PRIMATE

CHORIONIC GONADOTROPINS: SIGNIFICANCE IN FERTILITY RESEARCH

Gary D. Hodgen

Pregnancy Research Branch, National Institute of
Child Health and Human Development, National
Institutes of Health, Bethesda, Maryland, U.S.A.

INTRODUCTION

In women and several species of nonhuman primates, prolonged
steroid hormone secretion from the corpus luteum, especially
progesterone, is essential for establishment and maintenance of
pregnancy in the peri- and post-implantation interval. Later,
steroids provided by the conceptus are sufficient to sustain normal
gestation autonomous from luteal secretions in these primates,
although the time of this luteo-placental shift may differ among
species.

Existing evidence indicates that the primary biological role
of chorionic gonadotropin, thought to be secreted by the syncytiotrophoblast at implantation (Wislocki and Streeter, 1938), is to
extend the functional life-span of the corpus luteum in the fertile
menstrual cycle. That is, to sustain the steroid hormone secretory
capacity of the corpus luteum until the conceptus is able to function
independent of ovarian steroid secretions. Although some evidence
suggests that chorionic gonadotropin may influence intrauterine
immune privilege, fetal gonadal development, or placental metabolism,
these additional effects of chorionic gonadotropin remain tentative.

Clearly, manipulation of the functional status of the corpus
luteum in the peri-implantation interval of the menstrual cycle may
be useful either for enhancement of fertility in individuals with
infertility due to luteal phase defects or, alternatively, to
suppress normal fertility where avoidance of pregnancy is desired.
Since the biological actions of chorionic gonadotropin upon the
corpus luteum are imperative for early maternal recognition of
pregnancy, the reproductive event called the "rescue" of the corpus

luteum (Neill et al., 1969) is the subject of extensive investigations in women and laboratory primates. These and related subjects
involving chorionic gonadotropins of women and nonhuman primates
will be considered here. Some previous reviews cover portions of
this topic (Knobil, 1973; Ross, 1978; Hodgen, 1979). Here, emphasis
is placed on more recent developments concerning primate chorionic
gonadotropins and the relevant application of these primate models
in the study of problems in human reproduction.

PATTERNS OF SECRETION OF CHORIONIC GONADOTROPIN AMONG PRIMATES

That chorionic gonadotropin secretion is a uniform characteristic of pregnancy among primates seems assured. To varying degrees,
the patterns of chorionic gonadotropin secretion have been described
in women (Taymor, 1967); chimpanzees (Nixon et al., 1972; Clegg and
Weaver, 1972; Hodgen et al., 1976; Reyes et al., 1975); gorillas
(Tullner, 1974); orangutans (Hodgen et al., 1977b); baboons (Hodgen
et al., 1975); macaques, including rhesus and cynomolgus monkeys
(Hodgen et al., 1972; Hodgen et al., 1974; Hodgen et al., 1975;
Atkinson et al., 1975; Hobson, 1975; Hodgen et al., 1977a); squirrel
monkeys (Hodgen et al., 1978); marmosets (Hodgen et al., 1976);
tamarins (Kleinmann et al., 1978); and owl monkey (Hall and Hodgen,
1979). Although the patterns of chorionic gonadotropin secretion
among these primates are as different as their natural geographic
distributions, existing reports describe the presence of chorionic
gonadotropin during some portion of gestation in every primate yet
studied (Table I). To some extent, the sensitivity and specificity
of the varied assays applied for measurement of chorionic gonadotropins have influenced our perception of secretory patterns.
Whereas the bioassays, both in vivo and in vitro, and radio-receptor
assays are useful for quantitation of seemingly all primate chorionic
gonadotropins, without specificity, radioimmunoassays (Hodgen et al.,
1974; Niswender et al., 1970) are highly specific depending on the
antigen, the antigenic response to it, and the tracer hormone
utilized.

Generalizing, these observations suggest that three basic
patterns of chorionic gonadotropin secretion are known. In humans
and apes, chorionic gonadotropin in blood or urine is detectable
virtually coincident with implantation, is present at maximal levels
in the first trimester, and continuously throughout gestation, including a few days postpartum (Taymor, 1967; Midgely and Jaffe, 1968;
Nixon et al., 1972; Hodgen et al., 1976; Hodgen et al., 1977b).

Among baboons and macaques (rhesus and cynomolgus), they too
manifest chorionic gonadotropin secretion almost simultaneous with
implantation (Neill et al., 1969; Hodgen et al., 1972; Hodgen et
al., 1974), but unlike women and apes, the levels of chorionic

TABLE I: Comparative patterns of chorionic gonadotropin secretion among primates.

Primate	Span of Detectable Chorionic Gonadotropin Levels in Pregnancy	Remarks
Woman	~ day 10 to parturition	Highest levels during the 1st trimester

Apes
  Gorilla
  Chimpanzee
  Orangutan
	~ day 10 to parturition	Highest levels during the 1st trimester

Baboon	~ day 10 up to ~ day 50	Peak levels about day 26; levels near or below limits of detection in mid and late gestation

Macaques
  Rhesus
  Cynomolgus
	~ day 10 up to ~ day 40	Peak levels about day 21; levels near or below limits of detection in mid and late gestation

South American Monkeys Marmoset	From ~ day 25 to ~ day 100	Peak levels near mid-pregnancy; levels near or below limits of detection during final weeks of gestation
Tamarin	From ~ day 25 to ~ day 90	Peak levels near mid-pregnancy; levels near or below limits of detection during final weeks of gestation
Squirrel monkey	From ~ day 25 to ~ day 80	Peak levels near mid-pregnancy; levels near or below limits of detection during final weeks of gestation
Owl monkey	From ~ day 15 to parturition	Peak levels near mid-pregnancy; detectable levels until the final week of gestation

gonadotropin in circulation during mid and late gestation decline to near or below the limits of detection in existing assay systems.

Still different are the patterns of chorionic gonadotropin secretion among squirrel monkeys, marmosets, owl monkeys, and tamarins, all native to South America. Although existing descriptions on these primates are less thorough and considerably more tentative, they seem to manifest a later appearance of detectable chorionic gonadotropin in blood and urine, relative to the estimated time of fertilization. Further, the peak interval of chorionic gonadotropin secretion occurs in mid-pregnancy, with a rapid decline before parturition (Hodgen et al., 1976; Hodgen et al., 1978; Hall and Hodgen, 1979). We can expect that new information will rapidly change this initial appraisal regarding patterns of chorionic gonadotropin secretion in South American monkeys.

Quantitatively, peak concentrations of chorionic gonadotropin in blood or urine are highest in women, perhaps 10 times lower in apes, and 100 to 1000 times less among baboon, macaques, and South American monkeys.

RESCUE OF THE CORPUS LUTEUM BY CHORIONIC GONADOTROPIN IN THE FERTILE MENSTRUAL CYCLE

The course of events during the peri-implantation interval (Table II), when the functional life-span of the corpus luteum is extended in the presence of chorionic gonadotropin, has been evaluated at some length only in women (Ross, 1979) and rhesus monkeys (Neill et al., 1969; Hodgen et al., 1974; Hodgen et al., 1975; Goodman and Hodgen, 1979). In both instances, it seems clear that coincident with the initiation of implantation and detection of chorionic gonadotropin in blood or urine, the levels of progesterone in circulation are sustained at a time when the spontaneous demise of the corpus luteum already has begun. Evidence that progesterone is the essential hormone to secure implantation and avoid loss of the endometrium and the early conceptus is compelling (Goodman and Hodgen, 1979). Indeed, among women using a copper IUD, hCG-like activity has been detected transiently in the late luteal phase at a frequency indicative of normal conception rates (Hodgen et al., 1978; Landesman et al., 1976; Beling et al., 1976), even though the sera from these women do not show a concurrent increase in progesterone or chorionic gonadotropin (Klein and Mishell, 1977). Whether or not hCG is detectable in these IUD users remains controversial (Sharpe et al., 1977).

TABLE II: The time-course of reproductive events in the fertile menstrual cycle of the rhesus monkey.

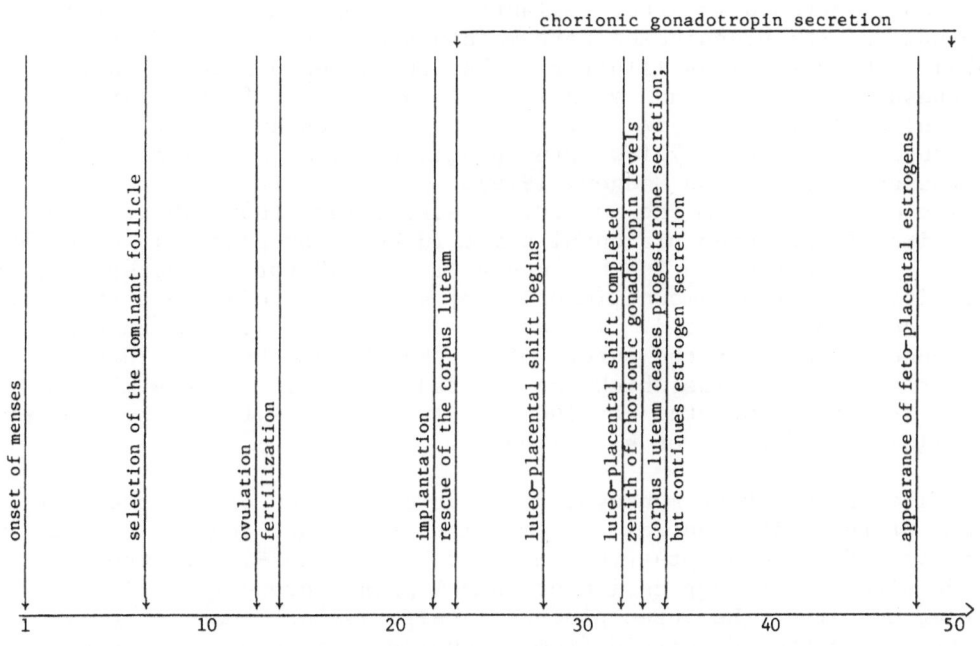

DAYS OF THE FERTILE MENSTRUAL CYCLE

TIME OF THE LUTEO-PLACENTAL SHIFT

The time of the luteo-placental shift has been investigated
at length only in women and rhesus monkeys (Csapo et al., 1973;
Goodman and Hodgen, 1979). Although some evidence points to species
differences in the transition from dependence on ovarian steroids
to those of the conceptus, this issue is unresolved. Whereas an
earlier report described a more lengthy dependence on progesterone
of luteal origin in women (Csapo et al., 1973), the data are very
clear that neither the ovaries nor the corpus luteum of pregnancy
are necessary beyond the 3rd week after fertilization to sustain
normal gestation in rhesus or cynomolgus monkeys (Hodgen and Tullner,
1975; Williams and Hodgen, 1978). In fact, recent evidence shows
that despite luteectomy or bilateral ovariectomy of rhesus monkeys
as soon as seven days after implantation (pregnancy day 16), fully
one-half of the pregnancies were maintained (Goodman and Hodgen,
1979). These findings illustrate that the luteo-placental shift
in rhesus monkeys begins as early as 14 days after fertilization
and uniformly is completed before day 21 of pregnancy. It is of
interest that even very low serum progesterone may not compromise
pregnancy (Goodman and Hodgen, 1979). On this point, the woman
may be different from the monkey. Clearly, more thorough study of
the time of the luteo-placental shift in human pregnancy is necessary.
With regard to application of "menses inducers" for contraception,
this issue is of paramount importance, since the induced menstruation
must occur when expected. Indeed, there is sufficient circumstantial
evidence to question the surety of our knowledge, because in women
secretions of steroids which can be credited to the corpus luteum
apart from the conceptus decline rapidly about the fourth week after
fertilization (Strott et al., 1969).

The use of these monkey models for evaluation of interceptive
means of fertility control in women must take into account the early
autonomy of the conceptus (Goodman and Hodgen, 1979). Further,
since significant suppression of luteal progesterone secretion
during and after the luteo-placental shift may not lead to early
abortion, we should refrain from assessing anti-luteal agents on
the basis of circulating progesterone levels during the menstrual
cycle as an independent indicator of their contraceptive potency.
For example, investigations of anti-chorionic gonadotropic sera,
prostaglandins, or estrogens, all aimed at induction of luteolysis,
must take into account both the timing of these events and possible
direct effects on the conceptus.

ANTIGENIC SIMILARITIES AMONG PRIMATE CHORIONIC GONADOTROPINS

The significance of similarities in the molecular structures
of primate chorionic gonadotropins (Table III), and their pituitary
gonadotropins as well (especially LH), is important mainly in two

TABLE III: Cross reactivity of primate chorionic gonadotropins in radioimmunoassay systems with ^{125}I-CG.

Antiserum	Antigen	hCG*	ChCG	GCG	OrCG	PaCG	MCG	MaCG
H26	oLHβ	+†	+	+	+	+	+	+
H80	hCG	+	+	+	+	±	±	-
Sb6	hCGβ	+	+	+	+	-	-	-
H93	CTP–hCGβ	+	+	+	-	-	-	-

*hCG, human chorionic gonadotropin; ChCG, chimpanzee chorionic gonadotropin; GCG, gorilla chorionic gonadotropin; OrCG, orangutan chorionic goandotropin; PaCG, baboon (Papio) chorionic gonadotropin; MCG, rhesus (Macaca) chorionic gonadotropin; MaCG, marmoset chorionic gonadotropin; oLHβ, ovine luteinizing hormone, β subunit; hCGβ, human chorionic gonadotropin, β subunit; CTP–hCGβ, carboxyl terminal peptide, human chorionic gonadotropin, β subunit.

†+, complete; ±, incomplete; -, undetectable.

(Chen HC, Hodgen GD: J Clin Endocrinol Metab 43: 1414–1417, 1976)

areas: 1) the development and application of radioimmunoassay systems, and 2) the use of surrogate primates for evaluations of the antigenicity of reagents and efficacy of anti-chorionic gonado-tropin sera. Clearly, there are patterns of antigenic similarities, such as the very high degree of crossreactivities between chorionic gonadotropins of apes and antisera to hCG, α or β subunits of hCG, or even the carboxyl-terminal peptide of $hCG\beta$. The chorionic gonado-tropins of lower primates often crossreact with such antisera only poorly, or not at all (Chen and Hodgen, 1976). That this generali-zation is not uniformly applicable, points out the risks in predict-ing antigenic responses and binding affinities of the antisera generated. For example, a certain antiserum made against $oLH\beta$ (Hodgen et al., 1974; Hodgen, 1979) displays near uniform cross-reactivity with the chorionic gonadotropins of at least 12 species of primates, including man, although there is markedly less crossreactivity with hLH. In contrast, an antiserum to oLH (Niswander et al., 1970) binds pituitary LH of many species very efficiently, crossreacts well with the chorionic gonadotropin of rhesus monkeys, but has low affinity for hLH and hCG. Further, the majority of anti-hCG sera bind the chorionic gonadotropins of lower primates with markedly less affinity than hCG itself. Accordingly, how can antigenicity and contraceptive action be assessed for any antigen or antiserum aimed at human application? What nonhuman primate model is best suited? What antigen should be used? What dose and regimen should be applied? How should the titer, affinity, and specificity be assessed? How should side effects be evaluated? These very difficult questions remain.

SUMMARY

Despite known differences between the patterns of secretion and antigenicities of primate chorionic gonadotropins, perhaps even the time of the luteo-placental shift, there are extensive similarities among these paradigms of man. Clearly, surrogate laboratory primates are a key component in developing and utilizing our knowledge of chorionic gonadotropin secretion and its biological role in the human reproductive process. Future research must be directed toward broader experiences with more laboratory primates, placing emphasis on those models which provide maximal insight and predictive value for either enhancement or suppression of human fertility.

REFERENCES

Atkinson, L. E., Hotchkiss, J., Fritz, G. R., Surve, A. H., and Knobil, E., 1971, Circulating levels of luteinzing (LH), chorionic gonadotropin (CG), estrogens (E), and progesterone (P) during pregnancy in the rhesus monkey, Biol. Reprod. 5:95-101.

Beling, C. G., Cederqvist, L. L., and Fuchs, F., 1976, Demonstration of gonadotropin during the second half of the cycle in women using intrauterine contraception, Am. J. Obstet. Gynecol. 126:855.

Chen, H. C., and Hodgen, G. D., 1976, Primate chorionic gonadotropins: Antigenic similarities to the unique carboxyl-terminal peptide of hCGβ subunit, J. Clin. Endocrinol. Metab. 43:1414.

Clegg, M. T., and Weaver, M., 1972, Chorionic gonadotropin secretion during pregnancy in the chimpanzee, Proc. Soc. Exp. Biol. Med. 139:1170.

Csapo, A. I., Pulkkinen, M. O., and Wiest, W. G., 1973, Effects of luteectomy and progesterone replacement therapy in early pregnant patients, Am. J. Obstet. Gynecol. 115:759.

Goodman, A. L., and Hodgen, G. D., 1979, Corpus luteum-conceptus-follicle relationships during the fertile cycle in rhesus monkeys: Pregnancy maintenance despite early luteal removal, J. Clin. Endocrin. Metab. 49:469.

Hall, R. D., and Hodgen, G. D., 1979, Pregnancy diagnosis in owl monkeys (Aotus trivivgatus): Evaluation of the hemagglutination inhibition test for urinary chorionic gonadotropin, Lab. Anim. Sci. 29:345.

Hobson, W., Faiman, C., Dougherty, W. J., Reyes, F. I., and Winters, J. S. D., 1975, Radioimmunoassay of rhesus monkey chorionic gonadotropin, Fertil. Steril. 26:93.

Hodgen, G. D., 1979, Primate models for pregnancy hormone secretion in man: Fetal, maternal, and placental factors, in Animal Models for Research on Contraception and Fertility, N. Alexander, ed., pp. 425-436, Harper and Row, Washington, D. C.

Hodgen, G. D., and Neimann, W. H., 1975, Application of the subhuman primate pregnancy test kit to pregnancy diagnosis in baboons, Lab. Anim. Sci. 25:757.

Hodgen, G. D., and Tullner, W. W., 1975, Plasma estrogens, progesterone and chorionic gonadotropin in pregnant rhesus monkeys (Macaca mulatta) after ovariectomy, Steroids 25:275.

Hodgen, G. D., Chen, H. C., Dufau, M. L., Klein, T. A., and Mishell, D. R., 1978, Transistory hCG-like activity in the urine of some IUD users, J. Clin. Endocrinol. Metab. 46:698.

Hodgen, G. D., Stouffer, R. L., Barber, D. L., and Nixon, W. E., 1977a, Serum estradiol and progesterone during pregnancy and the status of the corpus luteum at delivery in cynomolgus monkeys (Macaca fascicularis), Steroids 30:295.

Hodgen, G. D., Turner, C. K., Smith, E. E., and Bush, R. M., 1977b, Pregnancy diagnosis in the orangutan (Pongo pygmaeus) using the subhuman primate pregnancy test kit, Lab. Anim. Sci. 27(1):99.

Hodgen, G. D., Neimann, W. H., Turner, C. K., and Chen, H. C., 1976, Diagnosis of pregnancy in chimpanzees using the nonhuman primate pregnancy test kit, J. Med. Primatol. 5:247.

Hodgen, G. D., Wolfe, L. G., Ogden, J. D., Adams, M. R., Descalzi, C. C., and Hildebrand, D. F., 1976, Diagnosis of pregnancy in

marmosets: Hemagglutination inhibition test and radioimmuno-
assay for urinary chorionic gonadotropin, Lab. Anim. Sci. 26:224.
Hodgen, G. D., Neimann, W. H., and Tullner, W. W., 1975, Duration of
chorionic gonadotropin production by the placenta of the rhesus
monkey, Endocrinology 96:789.
Hodgen, G. D., Tullner, W. W., Vaitukaitis, J. L., Ward, D. N., and
Ross, G. T., 1974, Specific radioimmunoassay of chorionic
gonadotropin during implantation in rhesus monkeys, J. Clin.
Endocrinol. Metab. 39:457.
Hodgen, G. D., Dufau, M. L., Catt, K. J., and Tullner, W. W., 1972,
Estrogens, progesterone and chorionic gonadotropin in pregnant
rhesus monkeys, Endocrinology 91(4):896.
Klein, T. A., and Mishell, D. R., Jr., 1977, Absence of circulating
chorionic gonadotropin in wearers of intrauterine contraceptive
devices, Am. J. Obstet. Gynecol. 129:626.
Knobil, E., 1973, On the regulation of the primate corpus luteum,
Biol. Reprod. 8:246.
Landesman, R., Coutinho, E. M., and Saxena, B. B., 1976, Detection
of human chorionic gonadotropin in blood of regularly bleeding
women using copper intrauterine contraceptive devices, Fertil.
Steril. 27:1062.
Midgley, A. R., and Jaffe, R. B., 1968, Regulation of human gonadotropins: II disappearance of human gonadotropin following
delivery, J. Clin. Endocr. Metab. 28:1712.
Neill, J. D., Johansson, E. D. B., and Knobil, E., 1969, Patterns
of circulating progesterone concentration during the fertile
menstrual cycle and the remainder of gestation in the rhesus
monkey, Endocrinology 84:45.
Niswender, G. D., Monroe, S. E., Peckham, W. D., Midgley, A. R., Jr.,
Knobil, E., and Reichert, L. E., Jr., 1971, Radioimmunoassay
for rhesus monkey luteinizing hormone (LH) with anti-ovine LH
serum and ovine LH-^{131}I, Endocrinology 88:1327.
Nixon, W. E., Hodgen, G. D., Neimann, W. H., et al., 1972, Urinary
chorionic gonadotropin in middle and late pregnancy in the
chimpanzee, Endocrinology 90:1105.
Reyes, F. I., Winter, J. S. D., Faiman, C., and Hobson, W. C., 1975,
Serial serum levels of gonadotropins, prolactin and sex steroids
in the nonpregnant and pregnant chimpanzee, Endocrinology 96:1447.
Ross, G. T., 1979, Human chorionic gonadotropin and maternal recog-
nition of pregnancy, in Maternal Recognition of Pregnancy,
J. Whalen, ed., pp. 191-201, Excerpta Medica, London.
Sharpe, R. W., Wrixon, W., Hobson, B. M., Corker, C. S., McLean,
H. A., and Short, R. V., 1977, Absence of hCG-like activity in
the blood of women fitted with intrauterine contraceptive
devices, J. Clin. Endocrinol. Metab. 45:496.
Strott, C. A., Yoshimi, T., and Ross, G. T., 1969, Ovarian physiology:
Relationship between plasma and steroidogenesis by the follicle
and corpus luteum effect of hCG, J. Clin. Endocr. Metab., 29:1157,

Taymor, M. L., 1967, Bioassay and immunoassay of human chorionic gonadotropin, Clin. Obstet. Gynec. 10:303.

Tullner, W. W., 1974, Comparative aspects of primate chorionic gonadotropins, Contr. Primatol. 3:235, Karger, Basel.

Williams, R. F., Johnson, D. K., and Hodgen, G. D., 1978, Ovarian estradiol secretion during early pregnancy in monkeys: Luteal versus extra-luteal secretion and effect of chorionic gonadotropin, Steroids 32:539.

Wislocki, G. B., and Streeter, G. L., 1938, On the placentation of the macaque (Macaca mulatta) from the time of implantation until the formation of the definitive placenta, Carnegie Contrib. Embryol. 27:1-66.

CHEMISTRY AND IMMUNOCHEMISTRY OF HUMAN CHORIONIC GONADOTROPIN

Steven Birken and Robert E. Canfield

Department of Medicine, Columbia University
College of Physicians and Surgeons
New York, New York, U.S.A.

INTRODUCTION

This symposium marks the end of a decade of fruitful research related to the chemistry of the glycoprotein hormones. Ten years ago their similarities in subunit structures had just begun to be appreciated; six years ago their primary structures were delineated. The question that confronts investigators now looking toward the next decade in this field is how to extend this new knowledge of the chemistry of these molecules along avenues of either basic science or of clinical application.

Work in our own laboratory has focused on human chorionic gonadotropin (hCG). Early studies of hCG purification were aided by the establishment of a NICHHD program to provide standardized preparations of the purified hormone and its subunits to other investigators (Morgan et al., 1974) and this also provided a sufficient supply of hormone to allow a determination of its primary structure. Two proposals for the structure of hCG have been put forth: one from this laboratory (Morgan et al., 1973; 1975), and the other from Dr. O. P. Bahl and his colleagues (Bellisario et al., 1973; Carlsen et al., 1973). A re-examination of the structure of the COOH-terminal region of the β-subunit (Birken and Canfield, 1977; Keutmann and Williams, 1977) has produced results leading to general agreement concerning the entire structure of this molecule. In the first portion of this paper we review some of these features of the chemistry of the hormone, as well as evidence relating to the presence of biosynthetic precursor forms of the subunits.

As a consequence of the structural studies of hCG, a number of investigators embarked upon efforts to produce a state of infertility

65

either in women or other primates, by immunization with the β-subunit or fragments thereof (Stevens, 1975; Talwar, 1976; Stevens, 1976). In a sense, these studies were ahead of their time, since the conceptual basis for this kind of experimentation probably requires much more knowledge of the immuno-chemical behavior of this molecule than is presently available. We believe the acquisition of such knowledge should be a principal focus for research in the future.

The major applications of knowledge of the chemistry of hCG to date have been related to measurement of the hormone and the development of antisera that are specific for hCG. Dr. J. Vaitukaitis and her colleagues initiated this phase of research with the demonstration that the β-subunit of hCG could be used as an immunogen to provide discrimination between human luteinizing hormone (hLH) and hCG (Vaitukaitis et al., 1972). The demonstration that hCG is synthesized in many neoplastic states followed soon thereafter (Braunstein et al., 1973; see chapter by Dr. Braunstein), and recent evidence suggests that minute quantities of hCG are synthesized by normal, nonpregnant individuals (Chen et al., 1976; Yoshimoto et al., 1979). Thus, a great deal of diagnostic as well as therapeutic information can be obtained from highly specific and sensitive hCG assays. In the quest for better antisera to accomplish this task, the emphasis turned away from immunization with the whole β-subunit to employment of the unique 30 amino acid fragment at the COOH-terminus of the β-subunit (Louvet et al., 1974; Chen et al., 1976; see chapter by Dr. Chen). Hence, studies of the immunologic characteristics of this portion of the molecule are of considerable interest, and we discuss some of our more recent findings related to this in the second part of this paper.

CHEMISTRY

Purification of hCG from Pregnancy Urine

The preparations of human choriogonadotropin purified by this laboratory under a contract from the National Institute of Child Health and Human Development (Morgan et al., 1974) employed as starting material, commercial preparations of urinary hCG (2-3,000 IU/mg) purchased from Organon (OSS, Netherlands). The purification of the hormone was carried out by a series of gel filtration and ion-exchange procedures which have been described in detail elsewhere (Canfield and Morgan, 1973a). The resultant purified hormone was homogenous in protein content by amino acid analysis, structural analysis (except for the heterogeneity of the NH_2-terminus of hCG), and electrophoretic techniques, and exhibited a biological activity of the order of 12,000 IU/mg. The heterogeneity that is consistently noted on electrophoresis and isoelectric focusing was presumably due to carbohydrate differences--chiefly, varying quantities of sialic acid--since most of the heterogeneity disappeared upon desialylation (Gershey and Kaplan, 1974). The issue of sialic acid content is of particular importance because it is known that partial or complete removal of sialic acid drastically reduces the biological half-life of hCG, due to uptake of the asialo hormone via liver receptors which recognize the exposed underlying galactose residues (Van Hell et al., 1966; Kawasaki and Ashwell, 1976). Therefore, purified preparations of hCG with a higher content of sialic acid may have significantly increased biopotency estimates.

The hCG subunits are held together by noncovalent forces (electrostatic and hydrophobic) and are not easily disassociated in urea at neutral pH, as indicated by studies with the fluorescent probe anilino-naphthalene-sulfonate (Aloj et al., 1973). They are separated in acidified urea and purified by step-wise ion-exchange (Canfield and Morgan, 1973). The isolated subunits are not biologically active, but can be reassociated in ammonium bicarbonate to regenerate nearly 100% of the hormone's original biological activity (Aloj et al., 1973; Morgan et al., 1974).

Hormone Structure and Chemical Properties

The primary structure of hCG was proposed by our laboratory (Morgan et al., 1973b) and that of Dr. O. P. Bahl (Bellisario et al., 1973; Carlsen et al., 1973). The two proposals were nearly identical, except for the amino acid alignment and sites of carbohydrate attachment in the COOH-terminal region of hCGβ. This is a difficult region to sequence because of the high proline, serine, and carbohydrate content (Morgan et al., 1975). Reinvestigation of the structure of this region has yielded the same results (Birken and Canfield, 1977), with confirmation provided by Keutmann and Williams (1977) and Kessler et al. (1979).

The amino acid sequence of the α-subunit appears in Figure 1. The sequence of the β-subunit of hCG, compared with the β-subunit of hLH is shown in Figure 2. The identity of the α-subunits and the great similarity of the hCGβ and hLHβ subunits is of importance for immunological measurement of hCG in the presence of hLH. The only major primary structure difference between the two subunits is the presence of a peptide of 30 amino acids at the hCGβ COOH-terminus, which is absent in hLH.

The structures of the subunits of the four homologous glycoprotein hormones have been carefully examined by Stewart and Stewart (1977), who searched for constant and variable regions. They found three variable regions which, when identified by the enumeration of hCGβ, are residue numbers 1-15, 39-55, and 101-to end of molecule. The two constant regions reside at 16-38 and 56-100. Presumably, the constant regions provide the structure for subunit-subunit

ALPHA SUBUNIT

```
 1                                                           10
ALA - PRO - ASP - VAL - GLN - ASP - CYS - PRO - GLU - CYS - THR - LEU -

                                                    20
GLN - GLU - ASP - PRO - PHE - PHE - SER - GLN - PRO - GLY - ALA - PRO -

                                  30
ILE - LEU - GLX - CYS - MET - GLY - CYS - CYS - PHE - SER - ARG - ALA -

                      40
TYR - PRO - THR - PRO - LEU - ARG - SER - LYS - LYS - THR - MET - LEU -

           50              CHO                                      60
VAL - GLN - LYS - ASN - VAL - THR - SER - GLU - SER - THR - CYS - CYS -

                                              70
VAL - ALA - LYS - SER - TYR - ASN - ARG - VAL - THR - VAL - MET - GLY -

                            CHO         80
GLY - PHE - LYS - VAL - GLU - ASN - HIS - THR - ALA - CYS - HIS - CYS -

                            90
SER - THR - CYS - TYR - TYR - HIS - LYS - SER
```

Figure 1 (above). The amino acid sequence of the alpha subunit of human choriogonadotropin. The NH_2-terminus is heterogeneous and begins at one of the three amino acids which are underlined. Carbohydrate groups are indicated by "CHO."

Figure 2 (opposite). The amino acid sequences of the beta subunit of human choriogonadotropin (upper straight letters) and human luteinizing hormone (lower slanted letters) are shown as aligned by the position of 1/2 cystine residues. The regions of identity appear in the boxes. Carbohydrate groups are indicated by "CHO."

association, while the variable regions probably specify the structure necessary for different target cell receptor recognition. These assumptions are supported by experimental studies that have been performed by Drs. Cheng and Pierce (1972, 1973) and Ward (1979) and their associates.

HCG is composed of approximately 30% carbohydrate. Two large branched-chain carbohydrate groups are attached to the subunit by N-asparagine linkage at residue numbers 52 and 78 (Figure 1). The β-subunit contains six carbohydrate groups. Two branched-chain moieties are attached to asparagines 13 and 30, and six small linear sugar groups are attached via O-serine linkages to serines within the unique hCG COOH-terminal peptide at residues 121, 127, 132, and 138 (Figure 2). The structure of the carbohydrate groups shown in Figure 3 has been proposed by Kessler et al., (1979a, b) and is basically the same as that of Dr. Endo and colleagues, as described within this volume.

A summary of some properties of hCG appears in Table I. The hormone is approximately 1/3 carbohydrate, which leads to a large Stokes' radius in aqueous solution, causing the hormone to elute with an apparent molecular weight of 65-70,000 on gel filtration instead of its true weight of 37,000. It is important to employ the molar extinction coefficient for accurate determination of the concentration of a solution of hCG, not only because absorbed water and salts make a weight determination inaccurate, but also because variations in carbohydrate content would lead to errors.

The question as to whether urinary hCG accurately reflects serum hCG has not yet been answered, due to the inability to accumulate sufficient serum or placental hCG for structural analysis. However, since the urinary preparation of hCG is highly active biologically and appears to be nearly identical in structure to pituitary hLH, it is likely that the differences observed in serum hCG (by electrophoresis or isoelectric focusing) result chiefly from small carbohydrate differences.

BIOSYNTHESIS OF HCG

We have been engaged in a collaboration with the laboratory of Dr. I. Boime and associates (see chapter in this volume) to determine the structure of hPL (Birken et al., 1977) and the subunits of hCG (Birken et al., 1978) translated from placental mRNA in vitro. The results indicated that α- and β-subunits are translated from separate messengers and that both are synthesized as precursors (Daniels-McQueen, 1978). The pre-hCGα NH$_2$-terminal signal peptide has been sequenced nearly completely, and has recently been confirmed and completed, based on the structure of complementary DNA made to the hCGα message (Fiddes et al., 1979). The latter sequence agrees

CARBOHYDRATE MOIETY ATTACHED TO ASPARAGINES (2 in hCGα; 2 in hCGβ)

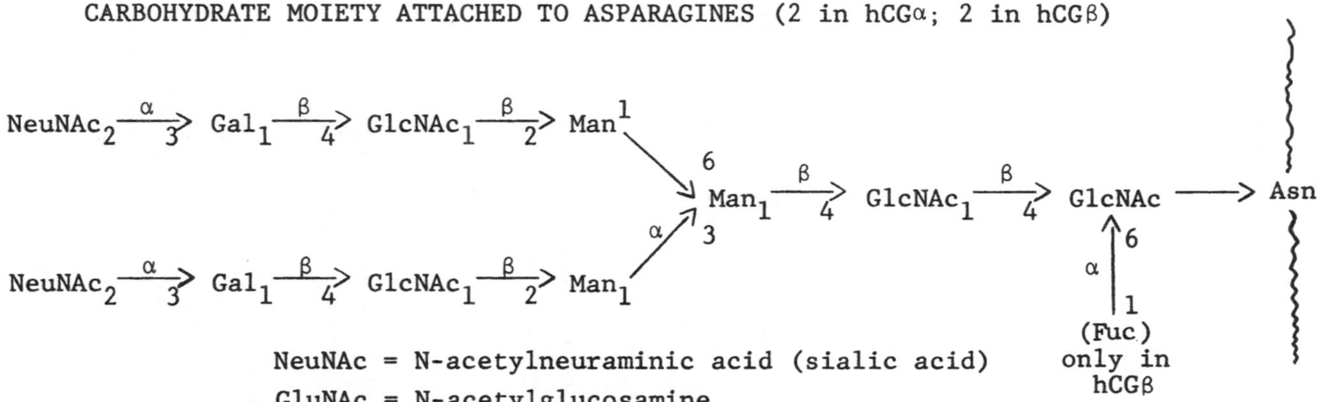

$$NeuNAc_2 \xrightarrow[3]{\alpha} Gal_1 \xrightarrow[4]{\beta} GlcNAc_1 \xrightarrow[2]{\beta} Man_1$$

$$NeuNAc_2 \xrightarrow[3]{\alpha} Gal_1 \xrightarrow[4]{\beta} GlcNAc_1 \xrightarrow[2]{\beta} Man_1$$

$$\xrightarrow{6} Man_1 \xrightarrow[4]{\beta} GlcNAc_1 \xrightarrow[4]{\beta} GlcNAc \longrightarrow Asn$$

$$\xrightarrow[3]{\alpha}$$

$$\xleftarrow[\alpha]{6}{1} (Fuc) \text{ only in } hCG\beta$$

NeuNAc = N-acetylneuraminic acid (sialic acid)

GluNAc = N-acetylglucosamine

Fuc = Fucose

CARBOHYDRATE MOIETY ATTACHED TO SERINES (4 in hCGβ COOH-TERMINUS)

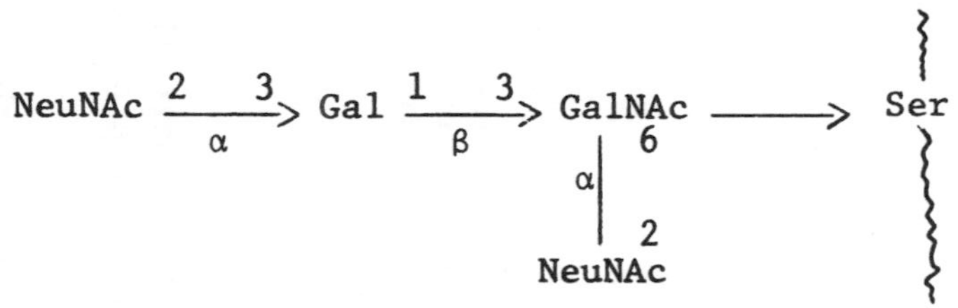

$$NeuNAc \xrightarrow[\alpha]{2 \quad 3} Gal \xrightarrow[\beta]{1 \quad 3} GalNAc \longrightarrow Ser$$

$$\xleftarrow[\alpha]{6}{2} NeuNAc$$

GalNAc = N-acetylgalactosamine

Figure 3. The structure of the large-branched-chain carbohydrate groups attached by N-asparagine linkage to hCGα and β appears in the upper part of this figure (Kessler et al., 1979a,b). The small carbohydrate groups attached to the hCGβ-terminal region by 0-serine linkage is shown in the lower part of the figure (Kessler et al., 1979b).

TABLE I: Properties of hCG and its subunits.

	Native hCG	hCGα	hCGβ
Molecular weight of protein portion	25,690	10,185	15,505
Average total molecular weight	36,700	14,500	22,200
% carbohydrate	29–31%	26–32%	28–36%
Molecular extinction ($M^{-1}cm^{-1}$)	1.41×10^{4a}	0.64×10^4	0.56×10^4
Concentration of protein in water solution based on O.D. of 1.0 measured at 280 nm <u>moles</u>	70.9 nmol/ml^a	156 nmol/ml	178 nmol/ml
<u>mass</u>	2.77 mg/ml	2.32 mg/ml	4.76 mg/ml

^{a}The molar extinction coefficient should always be employed to measure the concentration of hCG or its subunits in solution, since it is most accurate. Use of dry protein weight will lead to errors of 10% or more in concentration and is not reproducible or reliable.

completely with the partial structure we had proposed earlier, based on translation of mRNA and microsequence techniques (Birken et al., 1978).

The structure of the subunit of hCG shown in Figure 1 indicates that its NH_2-terminus is heterogeneous. The origin of such hetero-geneity was unclear, especially since the β-subunit was homogeneous and was purified from the same source material. We examined several preparations of hCGα and found consistent NH_2-terminal heterogeneity as detailed in Table II. The major polypeptide chain commenced with alanine, while minor chains apparently resulted from removal of two or three amino acids from the NH_2-terminus of the subunit.

The in vitro mRNA translation system presented an opportunity to test for one possible origin of this NH_2-terminal heterogeneity:

TABLE II: Heterogeneity of the α-subunit as determined by amino acid sequencing of several preparations of hCGα.

Lot number of hCGα	Mole percent of amino acids recovered at step 1^a		
	alanine	valine	aspartic acid
CR 117	73%	16%	11%
CR 119	73%	20%	7%
CR 123	83%	12%	7%

^{a}The mole % figures shown are based on hydrolysis of the PTH-amino acids resulting from one cycle of Edman degradation in a Beckman sequencer followed by amino acid analysis. Several subsequent steps agreed with the relative chain percentages indicated at cycle 1.

In summary the polypeptide sequences present in hCG are:

```
              1    2    3    4    5    6    7    8    9
   73-83%:   Ala- Pro- Asp- Val- Gln- Asp- Cys- Pro- Glu
                        3    4    5    6    7    8    9
    7-11%:             Asp- Val- Gln- Asp- Cys- Pro- Glu
                             4    5    6    7    8    9
   12-20%:                  Val- Gln- Asp- Cys- Pro- Glu
```

i.e., heterogeneous cleavage of the signal peptide leader sequence by the signal peptidase. We had already shown that hCGα was translated in vitro with an NH_2-terminal precursor piece of 24 amino acids. The question we sought to answer was whether the heterogeneity observed in urinary hCGα had resulted from cleavage of the precursor piece at three different positions instead of one. The results of translation of the α message with and without the membranes containing the peptidase appear in Figure 4. The study was conducted by in vitro translation of first-trimester mRNA in the presence of ^3H-proline, followed by immuno-precipitation of the product by an anti-RCM (reduced and carboxy-methylated)α antiserum and microsequencing. It is clear that the peptidase cleaves at only one position (before alanine) at the NH_2-terminus of the major polypeptide chain of hCGα and is therefore not responsible for the observed heterogeneity. Hence, it seems likely that this represents

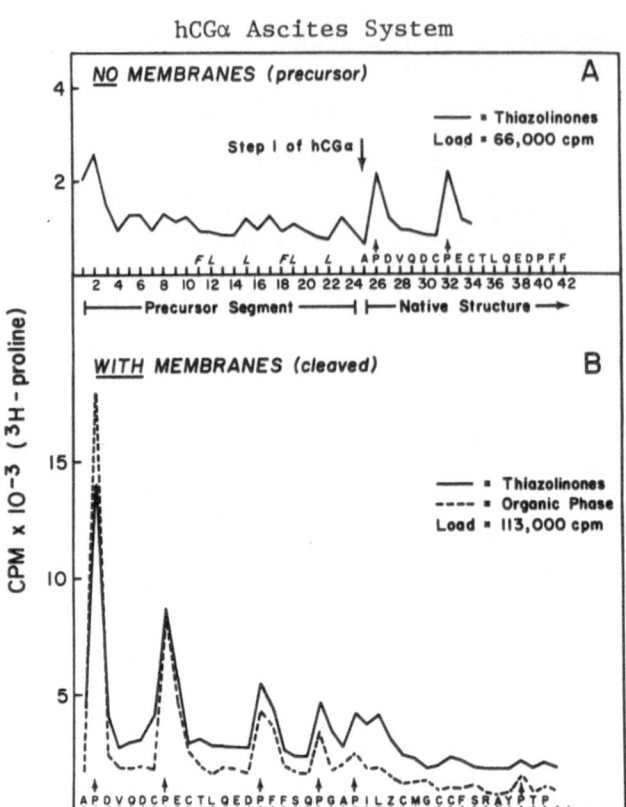

Figure 4.   Determination of the structure of the in vitro translation product of first-trimester mRNA encoding for the α-subunit of
hCG. The upper figure (A) indicates that translation of mRNA with
^{3}H-proline in the absence of membranes results in synthesis of a
24-amino acid NH_2-terminal signal peptide leader piece which does
not contain proline. The proline peaks at sequence cycles 26 and
32 correspond to 2 and 8 in native hCGα. When translation of the
message is performed in the presence of membranes containing the
signal peptidase (panel B) only the native sequence beginning at
alanine (prolines at 2, 8, 16, 21, 24, 38) was observed. (Birken
et al., 1978, Biochem. Biophys. Res. Comm. 85:1247.)

degradation of the placental hormone in plasma or urine and represents one minor difference in the structure of the hormone as it
is synthesized versus the form in which it is recovered from urinary
concentrates.

IMMUNOCHEMISTRY

Two immunogens have been successfully employed in an effort to generate antisera specific to hCG. One is purified hCGβ which was used for the generation of SB6-type antisera (Vaitukaitis et al., 1972) and the second was the unique hCGβ COOH-terminal peptide (Louvet et al., 1974; Chen et al., 1976). There have also been reports that partially reduced and alkylated hCGβ may sometimes elicit antisera with good specificity for hCG (Pandian and Bahl, 1977). Problems exist with antisera generated to all of these immunogens. For example, antisera made to hCGβ only rarely exhibit good specificity and sensitivity for hCG (Vaitukaitis et al., 1972). They generally cross-react to a signigicant extent with the very similar hLHβ structure (see Figure 2). In addition, these antisera frequently react much better with β-subunit than with hCG, resulting in lower sensitivity to hCG (Swaminathan and Braunstein, 1978). Lerario et al. (1978) have used a novel approach to this problem by combining hCGβ with a pituitary α-subunit from a non-cross-reacting animal species.

Antisera made in response to the carrier-conjugated hCGβ COOH-terminal peptide are always specific to hCG (i.e., with no hLH cross-reactivity) if the peptide used for immunization is free of contaminants from the rest of the hCG molecule. However, these antibodies usually have lower affinity and consequently a lower sensitivity (1-2%) to hCG than antisera raised against the whole subunit. The use of reduced and alkylated β as immunogen appears only rarely to generate antisera which bind well to hCG (as shown below).

Anti-hCGβ Sera

We have begun to examine a variety of hCG immunogens in a systematic manner. The first series of antisera were obtained by immunization of five rabbits with purified hCGβ. Titrations of three of these sera, as well as SB-6, using iodinated tracers, indicated all of the antibodies for hCG were conformationally directed. Also, the presence or absence of sialic acid made little difference to ligand binding and all of the antisera-bound hLH tracer. A summary of the results of these titrations appears in Table III. The inferences derived from the titration data were confirmed by competition assays performed using two β antisera with ^{125}I-hCG as tracer and five competitors, as shown in Figure 5. It is clear that desialylation of the β-subunit makes little difference to the binding sites recognized by antisera to hCG, since native β and asialo-β react equally well. Reduction and alkylation (i.e., RCM-β and As.-RCMβ) destroys the determinants recognized by the major antibody populations in these antisera, since the unfolded subunit did not compete at all in the dose range employed in these assays.

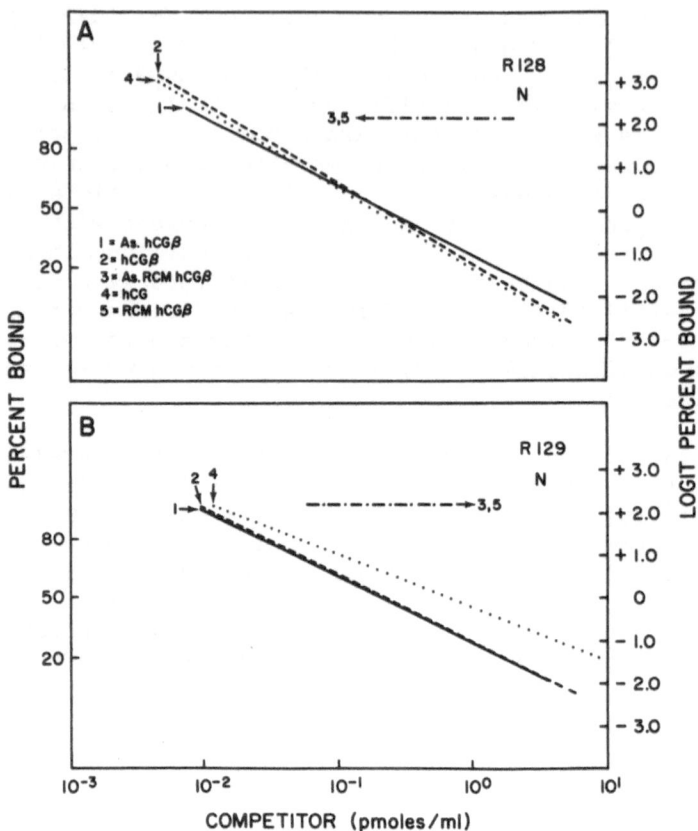

Figure 5.   Competition studies using two typical anti-hCGβ
sera (R128 and R129), ^{125}I-hCGβ tracer, and five competitors
are shown.   Competitor 1 (As.hCGβ), 2 (hCGβ), and 4 (hCG) all
retain conformational determinants and compete equally well,
while competitors 3 (As.RCMβ) and 5 (RCMβ) are both reduced
and alkylated (RCM), and do not compete at the doses shown in
this figure.   Desialylation of competitor (As.) makes no
difference in competing ability of any of the ligands assayed
with these antisera.

TABLE III: Summary of the results of titration of four hCGβ antisera with five tracer proteins.

Antiserum	Binding of tracers relative to 50% binding of ^{125}I-hCGβ[a]			
	hCGβ	As.hCGβ	hLH	RCMβ+As.RCMβ
SB-6	100	120	20	< 5
R126	100	120	36	< 5
R128	100	114	38	< 5
R129	100	110	34	< 5
Mean±2S.D.	100 Ref.	116±8.4	32±14.2	

[a]The above titrations indicate that:
1. The antisera require native structure, i.e., conformationally directed.
2. The presence or absence of sialic acid makes little difference.
3. Significant cross-reactivity with hLH universally occurs.

Unique Conformational Determinants in hCGβ

Since immunization with whole hCGβ elicited antisera to conformational determinants which are unrelated to the unique COOH-terminal peptide, the question of the presence of two distinct hCGβ-specific antigenic sites was raised. Swaminathan and Braunstein (1978) showed that synthetic COOH-terminal peptides did not compete with ^{125}I-hCG for the SB-6 binding site. However, their studies did not exclude the possibility that the peptide, when attached to β may be folded in a conformational determinant within hCGβ, and thus form an hCG unique determinant. Therefore, the question of the presence of two distinct hCG-specific determinants (i.e., one conformational in nature and the other specific to the COOH-terminal peptide) was not completely answered by the Swaminathan and Braunstein study.

In order to prove the presence of two such determinants, we separated the COOH-terminal portion from the conformational site and performed competition studies using SB-6 with an hCGβ fragment

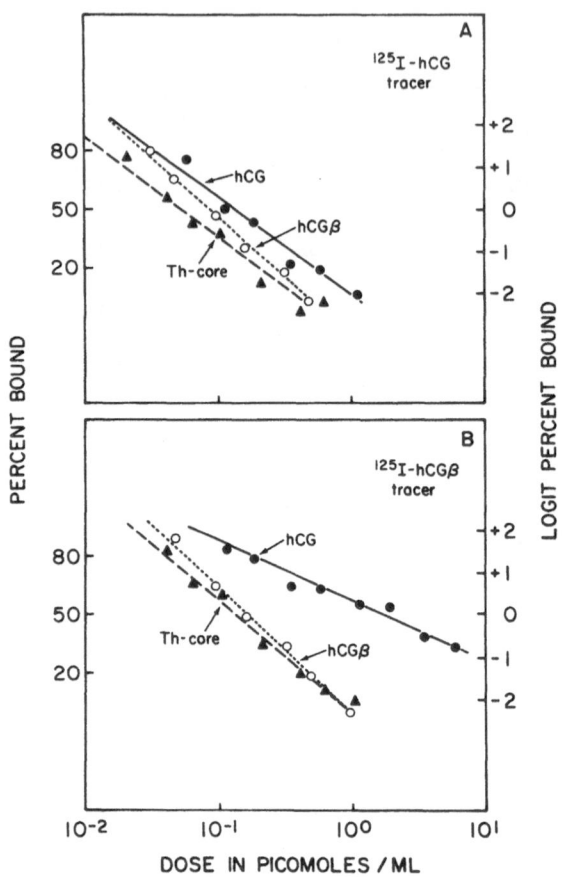

Figure 6.   Competition studies as shown using the SB-6 antiserum (1:120,000) and (A) ^{125}I-hCG or (B) ^{125}I-hCGβ as tracers are shown above. The immunopotency of the thermolytic core (Th-core) which lacks the COOH-terminal 30 amino acids of hCGβ is compared to hCGβ and hCG. The dose on the X-axis represents picomoles/ml in the standard solutions of which 20% is the quantity added to each assay tube (Figure from Birken et al., 1980 with permission of Endocrinology.)

TABLE IV: Immunoreactivity of hCGβ core with SB-6.

Tracer: ^{125}I-hCG

Competitor	Slope	ED_{50}(pmoles/ml)^a
hCG	-1.01	0.05 < 0.13 < 0.32
hCGβ	-1.2	0.05 < 0.09 < 0.15
Th-core	-1.2	0.03 < 0.05 < 0.10

Tracer: ^{125}I-hCG β

Competitor	Slope	ED_{50}(pmoles/ml)^a
hCG	-0.6	0.70 < 1.71 < 4.23
hCGβ	-1.3	0.12 < 0.17 < 0.24
Th-core	-1.1	0.08 < 0.14 < 0.24

^{a}The ED_{50} is bracketed by its 95% confidence interval calculated from the data entered in the assay. All curves for each tracer were performed within a single assay (Table from Birken et al., 1980, with permission of Endocrinology.)

devoid of its tail peptide. The results of this experiment appear in Figure 6 and Table IV, which show the data of several competition assays using SB-6 and ^{125}I-hCG or ^{125}I-hCGβ as tracer and hCG, hCGβ, and the des-COOH-terminalβ core (Th-core) as competitor. It is clear that the core fragment of the β-subunit competes as well as, or better than, the entire subunit and this conclusively shows that the COOH-terminal portion plays no role in determinants recognized by the SB-6 type of antiserum. This confirms the hypothesis that there are at least two distinctly separate regions of the hCGβ subunit that could be exploited to produce antisera which are specific to hCG.

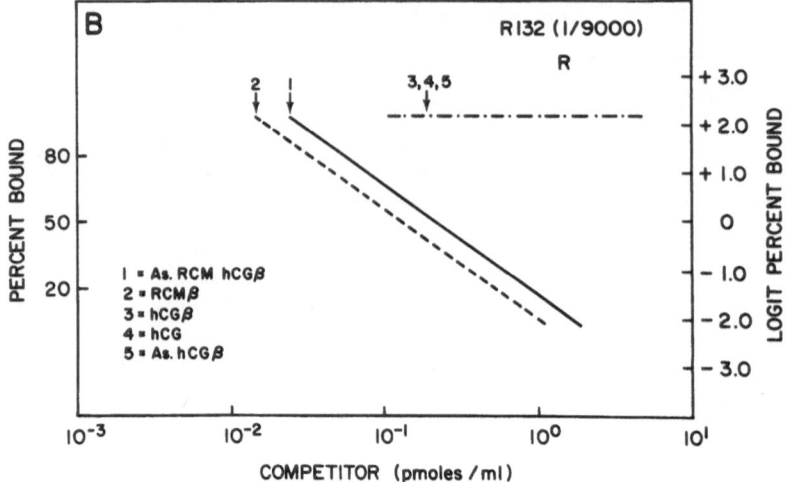

Figure 7.   Competition studies of a typical antiserum to asialo, reduced and alkylated hCGβ (R132) is shown above. When ^{125}I-As.RCMβ is used as tracer, only reduced and carboxy-methylated (RCM) competitors will compete at these dose ranges, while disulfide-linked β or hCG do not compete (Competitors 3-5). Desialylation (As.) of ligands makes no difference in their ability to compete with the tracer.

Antisera to Asialo, RCMβ

Two groups of antisera were raised against the reduced and alkylated beta subunit (RCMβ); one group of rabbits received this molecule alone as the immunogen and another group of rabbits was immunized with RCMβ conjugated to ovalbumin. Our objective was to study a group of antisera that reacted mostly with primary structure determinants. When these antisera were studied for binding to hCG, as shown by a representative dose-response curve in Figure 7, it was apparent that there was essentially no cross-reactivity with the native molecule. In this instance, the presence or absence of sialic acid did not appear to make a difference in reactivity in contrast to studies noted below with antisera elicited to the asialo COOH-terminal portion of this immunogen. Despite almost total lack of recognition of the native hormone, these antisera have proven to be of great value in studies of hCG precursors made by in vitro translation of mRNA in biosynthetic systems. The fact that these antisera efficiently immuno-precipitate the product adds evidence to the concept that native subunit conformation is probably not achieved until the precursor piece is cleaved.

TABLE V: Summary of titrations performed with antisera to Asialo β COOH-terminal peptide (residues 123-145).

Antiserum	Binding of tracers relative to 50% binding of ^{125}I-As.RCMβ^a			
	As.RCMβ	As.hCGβ	hCGβ	hLH
R141	100	90	< 10	0
R142	100	96	< 10	0
JPL-8	100	85	50	0
H-93	100	89	68	0
Mean ± 2 S.D.		90±7.8		

^{a}Inferences derived from above data:
1. Presence of sialic acid in native hCGβ impairs reactivity with this group of antisera.
2. No significant contaminating hCG "core" materials were present in the immunogen (there is no binding of hLH).

Antisera to an Asialoβ COOH-Terminal Peptide: Importance of Sialic Acid

Study of the characteristics of several antisera elicited to an asialoβ COOH-terminal peptide (residues 123-145) yielded data with different results from those described above. First, these antisera, as well as several antisera elicited from synthetic peptides, all appeared to have similar determinants and affinity to hCG (Matsuura et al., 1978, 1979) (see chapter by Dr. Chen). Second, when we examined four of these antisera (two generated in New York, R-141 and R-142, and two donated by Drs. Louvet (JPL-8) and Hodgen (H-93) made against the same asialo tryptic peptide, we found a significant effect of sialic acid upon ligand binding to these antisera. Table V, taken from a series of titrations, first suggested this significant impairment of binding of sialic acid-containing tracers by R-141 and R-142, while reduction and akylation had little effect on binding. This was further explored in a quantitative fashion, as shown in Figure 8, in a series of dose-response curves using asialo-hCG as tracer and the tryptic

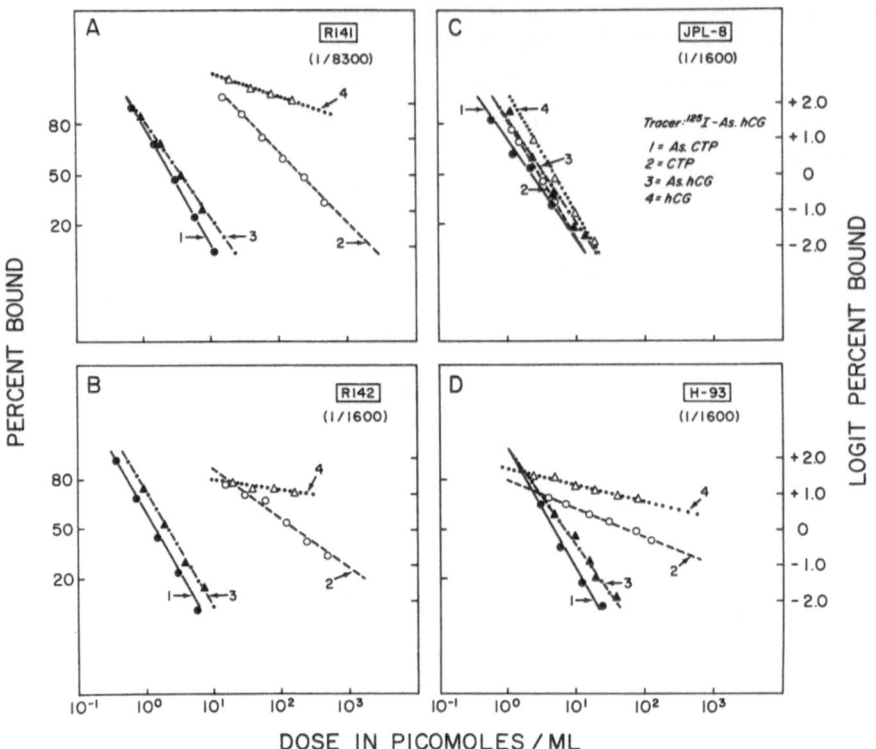

Figure 8.   Competition studies of four anti-asialo β COOH-terminal antisera employing ^{125}I-asialo hCG as tracer. Final dilutions of each antiserum appears on the figure. Competitors used are: (1) asialoβ peptide 123-145; (2) β peptide 123-145 with native content of sialic acid; (3) asialo hCG; (4) hCG. Dose refers to concentration of standard solutions of which 20% is added to each assay tube. (Reproduced from Birken et al., 1980, with permission of Endocrinology.)

peptide 123-145 or whole hormone as competitors with or without sialic acid. For the antisera shown in panels A, B, and D, it is clearly seen that sialic acid-containing competitors bind poorly to that population of antibodies which recognize asialo hCG. Desialylation of hCG exposes all the determinants available in the asialo tryptic peptide immunogen. Hence, use of a desialylated peptide prepared from hCG had elicited antibodies to sites available on the asialo peptide and on asialo hCG, but masked by sialic acid in the native hormone. Presumably, a synthetic peptide would produce a comparable result. Antiserum JPL-8 did not contain such sialic

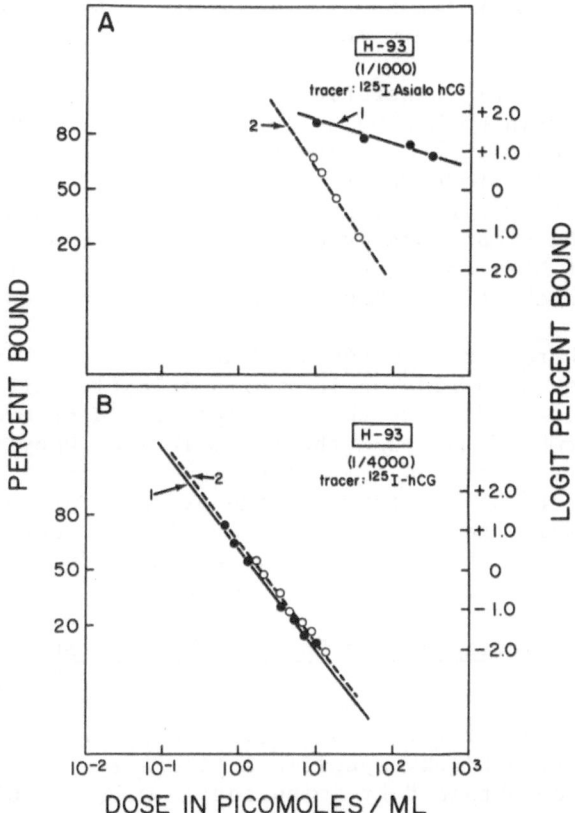

Figure 9. Competition studies of antiserum H-93, an anti-asialoβ COOH-terminal serum, using (A) ^{125}I-asialo hCG tracer and (B) ^{125}I-hCG tracer. Final antiserum dilution appears on the figure. Competitor (1) is hCG and (2) is asilalo hCG. Dose refers to concentration of standard solutions of which 20% is added to each assay tube.

acid-sensitive antibodies. Antiserum H-93 contained a major population of antibodies which, like JPL-8, bound native hCG. When an RIA was performed using native hCG tracer, H-93 failed to distinguish native from asialo hCG (Figure 9B). However, H-93 also contained a population of antibodies resembling the R-141 type which preferred asialo hCG to native hCG. This is illustrated in Figure 9, which shows immunoassays using: (A) the sialic acid-sensitive antibodies (asialo hCG tracer) at 1:1000 antibody dilution, and (B) the "native" antibodies at 1:4000 dilution using hCG tracer. On the other hand, R-141 and R-142 bound asialo hCG at high titers and bound native hCG only at very low dilutions (1:300).

These studies imply generation of two distinct antibodies, one to a site that is masked by sialic acid in the COOH-terminal region of the β-subunit, and a second to a determinant available in both the asialo peptide and the native hormone. It was conceivable that this latter site may be more immunogenic than the hCG specific site, which Matsuura et al. (1978) have mapped to the last 15 amino acids of hCG, and this may be one reason for the low response rate of rabbits to this immunogen when titered with hCG.

Recently, there has been renewed interest that hCG is synthesized and secreted by a wide variety of neoplastic cells, and the suggestion has been made that these ectopic forms of hCG, unlike the placental hormone, may lack their complete carbohydrate structure. Since the antisera described above are highly specific for hCG, and since they appear to be sensitive to the presence or absence of sialic acid which is the terminal residue of these carbohydrate chains, they may have their greatest value in studying this issue.

Antisera to a COOH-Terminal Beta Subunit Peptide with Sialic Acid Intact

As a consequence of the studies cited earlier, we reasoned that the best quality highly specific antisera for detection of native hCG might be obtained by immunization with the COOH-terminal region of the beta subunit with its complement of sialic acid intact. Such sialic acid-containing peptides were produced by tryptic digestion of the hCGβ subunit and separated from the larger molecular weight residual subunit by gel filtration. In order to eliminate any immunogenic potential from small residual quantities of disulfide-linked core contaminants that might contaminate fractions containing the COOH-terminal peptides, the product was reduced and carboxymethylated, and subjected again to gel filtration to further purify the COOH-terminal fragment.

One of the products, a sialic acid-containing peptide composed of residues 115-145, was conjugated by carbodiimide to thyroglobulin. Examination of the conjugated product by gel filtration and RIA, using a COOH-terminal antiserum, indicated that only about 10% of the peptide existed as dimers or polymeric material with the major component eluting as free, but probably modified peptide. This low coupling yield was unexpected and deserves further study in relation to such efforts to generate antisera. It is conceivable that the high content of sialic acid in this region (as much as 8 residues) of the molecule may hinder conjugation. Injection of free, unconjugated peptide failed to generate hCG antibodies in eight rabbits, while the conjugation mixture described above induced hCG antibodies

TABLE VI: Comparison of immunoreactivity and sensitivity of hCGβ COOH-terminal antisera.

Antiserum (Final Dilution)		Competitor			
		hCG		Asialo hCG	
		Slope	ED_{50}	Slope	ED_{50}
Tracer: $^{125}I\text{-}hCG$					
JPL-8	(1/3,800)	-1.3	2.4^1	-1.3	2.3 } $Asialo^2$
H-93	(1/2,600)	-1.0	2.7	-1.1	2.8
R-524	(1/1,500)	-1.5	1.0	-1.0	2.9
R-525	(1/10,000)	-1.5	0.8	-1.0	1.2 } $Native^3$
R-528	(1/2,000)	-1.2	0.8	-0.8	1.4
R-529	(1/2,500)	-1.3	0.4	-1.0	0.6
Tracer: $^{125}I\text{-}As.hCG$					
JPL-8	(1/1,000)	-1.3	4.7	-1.3	3.6
H-93	(1/1,000)	-0.3	>1000.0	-1.3	4.7 } $Asialo$
R-141	(1/12,000)	-0.4	>1000.0	-1.2	3.7
R-142	(1/2,500)	-0.4	>1000.0	-1.6	3.7
R-524	(1/2,000)	-0.6	0.9	-0.8	0.8
R-525	(1/2,000)	-1.1	0.6	-0.8	0.6 } $Native$
R-528	(1/1,500)	-0.7	0.6	-0.7	1.0
R-529	(1/2,500)	-1.1	0.6	-0.8	0.6

[1] pmoles/ml of standard solution at the 50% point of the curve; each assay tube contains 20% of this quantity

[2] asialo refers to use of a desialylated hCGβ COOH-terminal peptide for generation of these antisera

[3] native refers to use of hCGβ COOH-terminal peptide with its native content of sialic acid

in six out of eight rabbits. Four of the best antisera were examined for sensitivity to hCG and to asialo hCG, using both forms of the molecule as tracers; the data appear in Table VI. It was observed that all of these new antisera (R524-R529) were three to six times more sensitive to hCG at the 50% point than the best of the larger number of antisera that had been generated to an asialo COOH-terminal peptide. In addition, none of the antisera displayed the population of sialic acid-sensitive antibodies that three out of four of the earlier antisera (R-141, R-142, H-93) had displayed. Therefore, we infer that the use of the sialic acid-containing β COOH-terminal peptides are preferred as immunogens to produce high sensitivity antisera that are also specific for hCG.

REFERENCES

Aloj, S. M., Edelboch, H., Ingham, K. C., Morgan, F. J., Canfield, R. E., and Ross, G. T., 1973, The rates of dissociation and reassociation of the subunits of human chorionic gonadotropin, Arch. Biochem. Biophys. 159:497.

Bellisario, R., Carlsen, R. B., Bahl, O. P., 1973, Human chorionic gonadotropin: Linear amino acid sequence of the subunit, J. Biol. Chem. 248:6797.

Birken, S., and Canfield, R. E., 1977, Isolation and amino acid sequence of COOH-terminal fragments from the beta subunit of human choriogonadotropin, J. Biol. Chem. 252:5386.

Birken, S., Fetherston, J., Desmond, J., Canfield, R. E., and Boime, I., 1978, Partial amino acid sequence of the preprotein form of the alpha subunit of human choriogonadotropin and identification of the site of subsequent proteolytic cleavage, Biochem. Biophys. Res. Comm. 85:1247.

Birken, S., Smith, D. L., Canfield, R. E., and Boime, I., 1977, Partial amino acid sequence of human placental lactogen precursor and its mature hormone form produced by membrane-associated enzyme activity, Biochem. Biophys. Res. Comm. 74:106.

Braunstein, G. D., Vaitukaitis, J. L., Carbone, P. P., and Ross, G. T., 1973, Ectopic production of human chorionic gonadotropin by neoplasms, Ann. Intern. Med. 78:39.

Canfield, R. E., and Morgan, F. J., 1973a, Human chorionic gonadotropin (hCG): 1. Purification and biochemical characterization, in Methods in Investigative and Diagnostic Endocrinology, S. A. Berson and R. S. Yalow, eds., pp. 727-733, North Holland Publishing Co., Amsterdam.

Chen, H. C., Hodgen, G. D., Matsuura, S., Lin, L. J., Gross, E., Reichert, L. E., Birken, S., Canfield, R. E., and Ross, G. T., 1976, Evidence for a gonadotropin from nonpregnant subjects that has physical, immunological, and biological similarities to human chorionic gonadotropin, Proc. Natl. Acad. Sci. U.S.A. 73:2885.

Cheng, K. W., and Pierce, J. G., 1972, The reaction of tetranitro-methane with pituitary, luteinizing and thyroid-stimulating hormones, J. Biol. Chem. 247:7163.

Cheng, K. W., Glazer, A. N., and Pierce, J. G., 1973, The effects of modification of the COOH-terminal regions of bovine thyro-tropin and its subunits, J. Biol. Chem. 248:7930.

Daniels-McQueen, S., McWilliams, D., Birken, S., Canfield, R. E., Landefeld, T., and Boime, I., 1978, Identification of mRNAs encoding alpha and beta subunits of human chorionic gonadotropin, J. Biol. Chem. 253:7109.

Fiddes, J. C., and Goodman, H. M., 1979, Isolation, cloning and sequence analysis of the cDNA for the α-subunit of human chorionic gonadotropin, Nature 281:351.

Gershey, E. L., and Kaplan, I., 1974, A method for the preparation of desialylated human chorionic gonadotropin and its subunits, Biochem. et Biophys. Acta 342:322.

Kawasaki, T. and Ashwell, G., 1976, Chemical and physical properties of an hepatic membrane protein that specifically binds asialo-glycoproteins, J. Biol. Chem. 251:1296.

Kessler, M. J., Reddy, M. S., Shah, R. H., and Bahl, O. P., 1979a, Structures of N-glycosidic carbohydrate units of human chorionic gonadotropin, J. Biol. Chem. 254:7901.

Kessler, M. J., Mise, T., Ghai, R. D., and Bahl, O. P., 1979b, Structure and location of the O-glycosidic carbohydrate units of human chorionic gonadotropin, J. Biol. Chem. 254:7809.

Keutmann, H., and Williams, R., 1977, Human chorionic gonadotropin amino acid sequence of the hormone-specific COOH-terminal region, J. Biol. Chem. 252:5393.

Lerario, A. C., Pierce, J. C., and Vaitukaitis, J. L., 1978, Effect of conformation on hCG on generation of hCG-specific antibody, Endocr. Res. Comm. 5:43.

Louvet, J. P., Ross, G. T., Birken, S., and Canfield, R. E., 1974, Absence of neutralizing effect of antisera to the unique structural region of human chorionic gonadotropin, J. Clin. Endocrin. Metab. 39:1155.

Matsuura, S. H., Chen, C., and Hodgen, G. D., 1978, Antibodies to the carboxyl-terminal fragment of human chorionic gonadotropin β-subunit: synthetic peptide analogues, Biochemistry 17:575.

Matsuura, S. H., Ohashi, M., Chen, H. C., and Hodgen, G. D., 1979, A human chorionic gonadotropin-specific antiserum against synthetic peptide analogs to the carboxyl-terminal peptide of its β-subunit, Endocrinology 104.

Morgan, F. J., Canfield, R. E., Vaitukaitis, J. L., and Ross, G. T., 1973a, Preparation and characterization of the subunits of hCG, in Methods of Investigative and Diagnostic Endocrinology, Part III, Non-Pituitary Hormones, S. A. Berson and R. S. Yalow, eds., pp. 733,

Morgan, F. J., Birken, S., and Canfield, R. E., 1973b, Human chori-onic gonadotropin: A proposal for the amino acid sequence, Mol. Cell. Biochem. 2:97.

Morgan, F. J., Canfield, R. E., Vaitukaitis, J. L., and Ross. G. T., 1974, Properties of the subunits of human chorionic gonadotropin, Endocrinology 94:1601.

Morgan, F. J., Birken, S., and Canfield, R. E., 1975, The amino acid sequence of human chorionic gonadotropin: The α-subunit and β-subunit, J. Biol. Chem. 250:5247.

Pandian, M. R., and Bahl, O. P., 1977, Immunological properites of the subunit of hCH: Preparation of specific antibodies and their properites, Abstr. Endocr. Soc. Mtg. (59th), Abstr. No. 12.

Stevens, V. C., 1975, Female contraception by immunization with hCC-Prospects and status, in Immunization with Hormones in Reproductive Research, E. Nieshlag, ed., pp. 217-231, North Holland Publishing Co., Amsterdam.

Stevens, V. C., 1976, Antifertility effects from immunisations with intact subunits and fragments of hCG, in Physiological Effects of Immunity Against Reproductive Hormones, R. G. Edwards and M. H. Johnson, eds., pp. 249-274, Cambridge University Press, Cambridge.

Stewart, M., and Stewart, F., 1977, Constant and variable regions in glycoprotein hormone beta subunit sequences: Implications for receptor binding specificity, J. Mol. Biol. 116:175.

Swaminathan, N., and Braunstein, G. D., 1978, Location of major antigenic sites of the subunit of human chorionic gonadotropin, Biochemistry, 17:5832.

Talwar, G. P., Sharma, N. C., Dubey, S. K., Salahuddin, M., Ramakrishnan, S., Kuman, S., Das, C., and Hingorani, V., 1976, Isoimmunization against human chorionic gonadotropin with conjugates of processed β-subunit of the hormone and tetanus toxoid, Proc. Natl. Acad. Sci. U.S.A. 73:218.

Vaitukaitis, J. L., Braunstein, G. D., and Ross, G. T., 1972, A radioimmunoassay which specifically measures human chorionic gonadotropin in the presence of human luteinizing hormone, Am. J. Obstet. Gynec. 113:751.

Van Hell, H. Goverde, B. C., Schuurs, A. H. W. M., DeJager, E., Matthijsen, R., and Homan, J. D. H., 1966, Purification, characterization, and immunochemical properties of human chorionic gonadotropin, Nature 221:261.

Ward, D. N., 1979, Chemical approaches to the structure-function relationships of luteinizing hormone (Lutropin), in Structure and Function of the Gonadotropin, pp. 31-45, Plenum Press, New York.

Yoshimoto, Y., Wolfsen, A. R., Hirose, F., and Odell, W. D., 1979, Human chorionic gonadotropin-like material: Presence in normal human tissues, Am. J. Obstet. Gynecol. 134:729.

ACKNOWLEDGEMENT

This work was supported in part by National Institutes of Health grants AM09579 and HD13496.

CHORIONIC GONADOTROPINS: COMPARATIVE STUDIES AND

COMMENTS ON RELATIONSHIPS TO OTHER GLYCOPROTEIN HORMONES

William T. Moore, Jr., Bruce D. Burleigh, and
Darrell N. Ward

Department of Biochemistry, The University of Texas
System Cancer Center, M. D. Anderson Hospital and
Tumor Institute, Houston, Texas, U.S.A.

INTRODUCTION

Chorionic gonadotropins have been detected during pregnancy in
the human (Ascheim and Zondek, 1927; Braunstein et al., 1976), non-
human primates (Hamlett, 1937; Van Wagenen and Simpson, 1955; Delfs,
1941; Chen and Hodgen, 1976; Hobson and Wide, 1972), the equidae
(Cole and Hart, 1930; Rowlands, 1949; Wide and Wide, 1963; Allen,
1969), recently in rodents (Wide and Hobson, 1978; Wide and Wide,
1979; Haour et al., 1976), possibly in sheep (Rowson and Moor, 1967;
Martal et al., 1979; Lacroix and Martal, 1979), and rabbits (Haour
and Saxena, 1974; Channing et al., 1978; and Elinwood et al., 1979),
suggesting a fundamental luteotropic and/or other role for these
hormones in the placental animals. To date, only human chorionic
gonadotropin (hCG) has been extensively examined and defined at the
chemical level. A full understanding of the primary amino acid
sequence of both the alpha and beta subunits is available (Bellisario
et al., 1973; Carlsen et al., 1973; Morgan et al., 1973, 1975; Birken
and Canfield, 1977; Keutman and Williams, 1977; and Kessler et al.,
1979b), as well as a nearly complete understanding of the chemical
structure of the N and O glycosidic-linked carbohydrate moieties
(Endo et al., 1979; Kessler et al., 1979a, 1979b). In this chapter
we will summarize the current status of our structural studies on
the polypeptide moieties of the α- and β-subunits of pregnant mare
serum gonadotropin (PMSG) and compare the sequence information that
we have obtained with that proposed for the other well characterized
chorionic and pituitary gonadotropins. Stewart et al. (1977) and
Farmer and Papkoff (1979) have suggested that PSMG be better termed
as equine chorionic gonadotropin, or more specifically, as mare
chorionic gonadotropin, on the basis of its trophoblastic origin

(Allen and Moor, 1972; Allen et al., 1973). Our chemical data presented herein should further solidify the designation of PSMG as an equine chorionic gonadotropin (eCG). Furthermore, we will present our biological characterization of the FSH–LH duality of PMSG that is clearly demonstrable in rodents and offer a hypothetical molecular basis for the expression of both the LH and FSH activities intrinsic to PMSG.

PURIFICATION AND COMPOSITIONAL ANALYSIS

Intact PMSG

Since the PMSG content of high titer serum usually does not exceed 6 mg/liter (Legault–Demare and Clauser, 1961; Gospodarowicz and Papkoff, 1967), the purification of PMSG from serum or plasma requires the elimination of the bulk of inactive proteins comprising 99.9% of the blood proteins. Therefore, the preparation of highly purified PMSG requires combination of fractionation techniques:

(1) Protein precipitation with either salts or organic solvents.
(2) Ion exchange chromatography and/or adsorption chromatography.
(3) Gel filtration.

Several purification schemes have been described in the literature; however, only those methods that have yielded pure products as assessed by extensive biological and chemical analysis will be discussed.

To date, the purification scheme that has been most widely used has been that developed by Gospodarowicz and Papkoff (1967). This three-phase procedure has also been employed to purify the gonadotropin from endometrial cups (Papkoff et al., 1979). The initial stage of the procedure incorporates the metaphosphoric acid precipitate step of Rimington and Rowlands (1941) and an ethanol fractionation similar to that described by Cartland and Nelson (1937). The two subsequent steps incorporate gel filtration and ion exchange chromatography on SE-Sephadex, the order of the last two steps being interchangeable. The last two steps may be employed for the purification of PMSG from partially purified commercially available PMSG preparations (Gospodarowicz, 1972) also.

Recently, Christakos and Bahl (1979) have described an efficient purification method involving three column procedures utilizing Sephadex G-200, DEAE-Sephadex and hydroxylapatite for the purification of the hormone from a partially purified commercial preparation of PMSG. In their scheme the most efficient purification step was ion exchange chromatography on DEAE Sephadex, the second step of the procedure. Hydroxylapatite was used as a final step to remove the remaining minor contaminants.

Hydroxylapatite chromatography has also been utilized to purify PMSG (Moore, 1978; Moore and Ward, 1980a). This study, however, differs significantly from that of Christakos and Bahl (1979) in that hydroxylapatite chromatography was exploited as the most efficient purification step. In fact, when purifying hormone from materials having starting potencies of approximately 2000 IU/mg, this step may be utilized exclusively if care is taken to optimally load the column.

The chromatographic pattern obtained for an optimal hydroxyla-patite run is shown in Figure 1. Approximately 23% of the PMSG activity in the form of highly purified hormone emerged from the column unadsorbed in the starting buffer (0.5 mM sodium phosphate, pH 6.8). An additional 15% of the total activity representing a slightly desialylated form eluted as a flattened unimpressive peak with a protracted development with the second buffer (1 mM sodium phosphate, pH 6.8). The use of slightly increased ionic strength to sharpen the resolution of buffer II eluted material is not recommended, since weakly adsorbed contaminants are released from the hydroxylapatite with 2 mM phosphate buffer. The remainder of

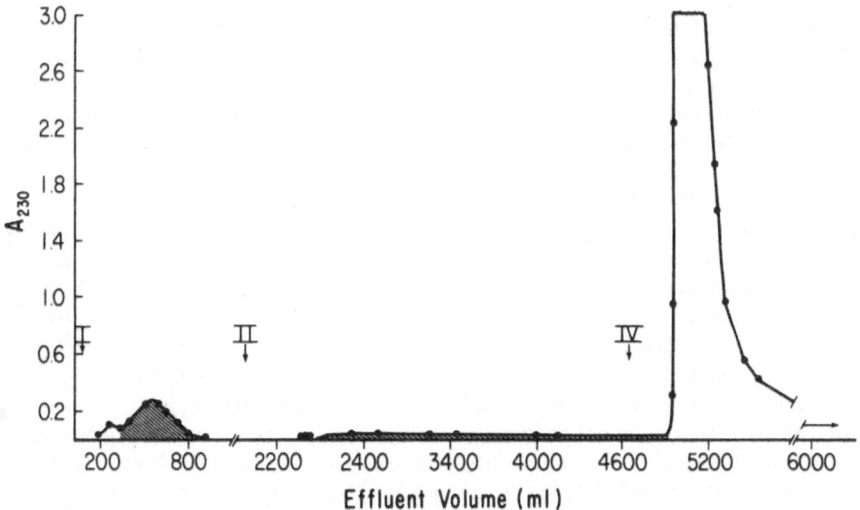

Figure 1. Chromatography of a 2000 IU/mg Ayerst preparation on a column of hydroxylapatite (Biogel HTP) at 4°C. Stepwise elution with sodium phosphate buffers, pH 6.8. Buffer I: 0.5 mM; II: 1.0 mM; IV: 100 mM. Active fractions denoted by cross-hatching.

the activity was tightly bound to the column and was eluted with
100 mM phosphate buffer, along with the bulk of inactive contaminants.
Highly purified forms of PMSG having in vivo potencies on the order
of 12,000 IU/mg (95% confidence limits 10,400-14,300; λ = 0.11) and
possessing only two NH_2-termini can be obtained. The only differences
detected between the nonabsorbing fraction (Buffer I, Figure 1) and
the Buffer II eluted material were in sialic content and in vitro
potency, as assessed by a PMSG radioligand assay. The nonadsorbed
PMSG designated in Figure 1 had a sialic acid content of 108.4 ± 0.3
μg/mg (mean ± S.D. of four determinations), whereas the sialic acid
content of the 1 mM sodium phosphate eluted PMSG was 101.8 ± 0.4
μg/mg (mean ± S.D. of four determinations). This difference in
content represents only one or two sialic acid residues per molecule
of PMSG. Thus, the PMSG eluted by the 1 mM sodium phosphate is a
slightly higher in vitro potency (13,000 IU/mg) in a PMSG radioligand
assay than that of the nonadsorbing fraction (12,200 IU/mg). That
the sialic acid content of the β-subunit of PMSG dictates the
behavior of the intact hormone on hydroxylapatite was suggested by
the observations that α-subunit and enzymatically desialylated PMSG
adsorbed tightly to hydroxylapatite, and that free β-subunit does
not absorb to hydroxylapatite. This behavior is consistent with the
behavior of other highly sialylated glycoproteins (i.e., submaxillary
mucins 30% sialic acid by weight) on hydroxylapatite (Tettamonti and
Pigman, 1968).

Subunit Isolation

Several methods can be used to effect adequate separation of
PMSG subunits based on the fact that isolated α-subunit behaves
differently from the β-subunit and intact hormone in every chromatographic system tested. α-subunit adsorbs to hydroxylapatite and can
be eluted with 100 mM sodium phosphate buffer, whereas, the β-subunit
does not adsorb. In addition, when a solution of PMSG which has been
dissociated with 8 M urea is applied to Sephadex-QAE in 0.01 M
ammonium acetate buffer, pH 5.5, α-subunit fails to bind and passes
through with the urea in the void volume of the column. The β-subunit
is eluted at the same ionic strength as the intact hormone (0.25 M
ammonium acetate pH 5.5). However, Sephadex G-75 (Figure 2) or
Sephacryl S-200 chromatography of 6 M guanidine-HCl-treated PMSG
has become the method of choice since subunits are well resolved
from each other and denatured in a single chromatographic step
(Moore and Ward, 1980a). Although anion exchange chromatography
methods were directly used for the purification of PMSG subunits,
in the recent studies of Papkoff et al. (1978) and Christakos and
Bahl (1979), these workers also recognized the potential facility of
employing only gel filtration.

The chromatographic behavior (Figure 2) and lyophilization of
recovered subunits indicate that the subunits are dissimilar in size.

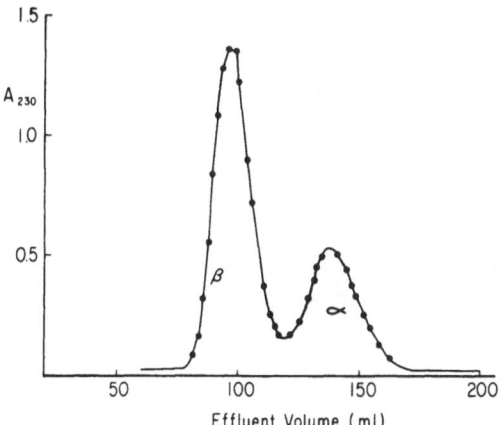

Figure 2. Separation of PMSG subunits on a column of Sephadex G-75. Elution buffer: 0.126 M ammonium bicarbonate, pH 8.0. Prior to column chromatography, purified PMSG was incubated at room temperature for 24 hr in a 6 M guanidine-HCl solution.

The weight of the β-subunit fraction was approximately three times that of the α-subunit. Analysis by SDS-polyacrylamide gel electrophoresis of PMSG subunits attests to the high degree of subunit purity achieved with the Sephadex G-75 chromatography (Moore and Ward, 1980a). The PMSG radioligand assay indicated that the β-subunit is 1% contaminated with PMSG. Since intact hormone and purified β-subunit behave similarly in several chromatographic systems (hydroxylapatite, Sephadex G-75, and Sephadex-QAE), to avoid obtaining a β-subunit fraction contaminated with intact hormone, dissociation conditions must be designed to insure disruption of the intact hormone. On the basis of Ferguson plot data, Christakos and Bahl (1979) estimated the molecular weights of intact PMSG, α-subunit and β-subunits to be 64,000, 17,000, and 44,000, respectively. On the basis of analytical data and spectrophotometric data (Moore and Ward, 1980a), we have estimated the mol. wt. to be 50,000 to 60,000 for intact hormone and 16,500 and 38,200 for α- and β-subunits, respectively.

Compositional Analysis of PMSG and Subunits

A single broadly diffuse band (a pattern characteristic of most, if not all, purified glycoproteins) was obtained after subjecting highly purified PMSG (12,000 IU/mg) to analytical polyacrylamide gel electrophoresis, indicating the existence of a single component.

TABLE I: Amino acid composition of PMSG and subunits.^{a} (Part 1)

Amino Acid	INTACT PMSG			PMSG α		
	Moore & Ward (1980a)	Papkoff et al. (1978)	Christakos & Bahl (1979)	Moore & Ward (1980a)	Papkoff et al. (1978)	Christakos & Bahl (1979)
Aspartic	12.9	13.2	12.5	6.2	6.2	6.4
Threonine	20.0	20.5	23.4	9.1	9.5	7.0
Serine	16.9	19.2	20.7	5.0	4.8	6.5
Glutamic	17.8	20.2	16.9	8.4	8.3	9.2
Proline	31.0	30.0	32.0	5.8	6.1	7.0
Glycine	12.2	12.2	12.5	4.4	4.3	4.7
Alanine	17.0	18.0	18.8	4.7	4.2	4.7
Cysteine	18.0	18.0	20.0	8.1	9.7	6.7
Valine	12.1	11.0	12.5	5.2	4.8	6.0
Methionine	5.7	4.1	3.4	2.4	2.0	1.9
Isoleucine	11.4	11.5	12.0	4.9	4.4	4.9
Leucine	14.0	15.1	14.4	5.1	4.1	4.6
Tyrosine	7.0	5.8	6.0	4.8	4.9	4.6
Phenylalanine	8.4	9.6	9.6	5.5	5.8	6.5
Histidine	3.4	6.0	3.6	4.0	3.0	2.8
Lysine	9.5	13.2	10.1	8.8	9.0	8.2
Arginine	12.8	14.5	11.3	5.4	6.1	4.6
% Protein	41	35	58.3	Total 97.8	97.2	96.8

TABLE I (continued): Amino acid composition of PMSG and subunits.[a] (Part 2)

Amino Acid	PMSG β		
	Moore & Ward (1980a)	Papkoff et al. (1978)	Christakos & Bahl (1979)
Aspartic	6.4	7.0	5.4
Threonine	12.1	11.0	8.4
Serine	13.6	14.5	15.5
Glutamic	10.1	10.4	8.8
Proline	22.3	23.0	23.6
Glycine	8.0	8.7	7.4
Alanine	12.4	13.2	13.1
Cysteine	8.6	10.0	15.7
Valine	7.4	6.8	7.8
Methionine	3.3	3.7	1.3
Isoleucine	7.4	6.8	7.1
Leucine	10.8	10.6	9.9
Tyrosine	2.2	2.3	1.9
Phenylalanine	3.4	4.3	4.1
Histidine	3.9	2.3	1.9
Lysine	5.2	4.5	4.1
Arginine	8.7	9.3	8.8
Total	145.8	148.4	144.8

[a] Data reported as number of residues per mole (54,700).

TABLE II: Carbohydrate composition of PMSG and subunits.[a]

PMSG	Moore & Ward (1980a)	Papkoff et al. (1978)	Christakos & Bahl (1979)
Fucose	0.2	0.6	0.8
Mannose	2.1	2.8	2.3
Galactose	14.1	9.6	11.6
Glucosamine	13.6	14.0	9.2
Galactosamine	4.1	3.6	3.3
Sialic Acid	11.0	10.8	14.5
Total	45.1	41.4	41.7
PMSG α			
Fucose	0.1	0.8	0.5
Mannose	3.4	3.9	2.5
Galactose	3.9	8.7	8.5
Glucosamine	7.8	3.7	5.1
Galactosamine	1.7	2.0	0
Sialic Acid	6.3	4.5	5.0
Total	23.2	18.6	21.6
PMSG β			
Fucose	trace	0.6	0.3
Mannose	2.3	2.7	1.6
Galactose	14.7	12.5	13.5
Glucosamine	14.3	14.6	9.9
Galactosamine	9.6	3.6	2.8
Sialic Acid	12.9	21.3	18.0
Total	48.8	55.3	46.1

a = data expressed as g/100g, not corrected for moisture or ash.

Amino terminal analysis of intact PMSG yielded the residues phenyl-alanine and serine, while NH_2-terminal analysis of isolated α and β yielded phenylalanine and serine, respectively. Our NH_2-terminal determinations are in complete agreement with Papkoff et al. (1978).

The best estimates of the amino acid compositions of hydroxy-apatite purified PMSG and its subunits are presented in Table I. As can be seen, values for the number of individual amino acids obtained by amino acid analysis or protein sequencing (α-subunit: Moore et al., 1980; β-subunit: Burleigh et al., 1980) and by amino acid analysis in the studies of Papkoff et al. (1978) and Christakos and Bahl (1979) are comparable.

The carbohydrate composition of intact PMSG and its subunits is summarized in Table II. The total carbohydrate composition of the intact hormone was approximately 45% on a weight basis (uncorrected for moisture content). Similar carbohydrate compositional analyses have been reported by Papkoff et al. (1978) and Christakos and Bahl (1979) and are included in Table II for comparative purposes. The bulk of the carbohydrate appears to be associated with the β-subunit. Noteworthy are the particularly high contents of galactose, glucosamine, and sialic acid.

DEMONSTRATION OF THE LH-FSH DUALITY

In Vivo

Crude PMSG induces a complete gonadotropic stimulation of the reproductive tract of the immature female rat (Hamburger, 1957). Follicular and uterine growth are induced, interstitial tissue is stimulated, and discernable luteinization occurs. A complete gonado-tropic response is also obtained in the immature male rat. PMSG induces an increase in testicular weight and enlargement of seminal vesicles and prostate (Cole et al., 1932; Raacke et al., 1957). Cole and his colleagues (Cole et al., 1940; Goss and Cole, 1940; Pencharz et al., 1940) were the first to suggest that the dual gonadotropic activity of PMSG was dependent on a single substance, since they were unable to separate the FSH and LH activities in PMSG by fractional precipitations.

In contrast, however, PMSG appears to act primarily as a luteo-tropin of pregnancy in the mare. The first evidence that PMSG had a profound LH effect in the mare was provided by Cole et al. (1931), who observed that the formation of several secondary corpora lutea were coincident with the period of gestation when PMSG activity was detectable in serum. Recently, Squires and Ginther (1975) confirmed the observations of Cole et al. (1931) by critically evaluating ovarian events in pregnant mares. In addition, Squires and Ginther

(1975) observed that PMSG maintains the primary corpus luteum of
pregnancy as well as stimulates the formation of secondary corpora
lutea. The most significant observation was that PMSG did not appear
to influence follicular growth during pregnancy. No difference in
follicular development was noted between pregnant and day-3, post-
coital, hysterectomized mares. These findings suggest that PMSG is
monofunctional in the mare and that its role is analogous to that of
hCG in the human--that is, primarily a luteotropin of pregnancy. The
marked difference in the ovarian FSH responses in rodents and mares
raises the interesting question of whether a difference in perception
exists between equine and rodent FSH receptors.

In Vitro

The LH-FSH duality of PMSG has also been substantiated by assaying impure preparations of PMSG in in vitro bioassay systems specific
for either LH activity (Dufau et al., 1976: RICT steroidogenesis assay;
Stewart et al., 1976: LH radioligand assay) or FSH activity (Means and
Vaitukaitis, 1972: inhibition of H-hFSH binding to rat testis mince;
Stewart et al., 1976: FSH radioligand assay; Strickland and Beers,
1976: plasminogen-activator production by rat ovarian granulosa cells).
In addition, highly purified preparations of PMSG have been shown to
possess FSH and LH activities in similar in vitro bioassays for specific LH activity (Gospodarowicz, 1973: inhibition of ^{125}I-oLH binding
to bovine corpora lutea membranes; Christakos and Bahl, 1979: inhibition of ^{125}I-hCG binding to rat testicular homogenate; Farmer et al.,
1977: rat interstitial cell testosterone production; Combarnous et
al., 1978: inhibition of ^{125}I-pLH binding to porcine testis membranes;
Moyle et al., 1978: rat Leydig cell testosterone and cAMP production)
and FSH activity (Reichert and Bhalla, 1974: inhibition of ^{125}I-hFSH
binding to rat testis tubule homogenates; Farmer and Papkoff, 1978:
cAMP production of rat testis tubules; Combarnous et al., 1978:
inhibition of ^{125}I-pFSH binding to porcine testis membranes; Moyle
et al., 1978: cAMP production by granulosa cells of DES fed rats),
thereby further substantiating the hypothesis that the dual activities
associated with PMSG arise from a single substance.

We (Moore and Ward, 1980b) have also examined the LH-FSH duality
of our preparations of PMSG in in vitro LH and FSH specific-response
systems and will review our findings here since they will pertain to
the discussion of our chemical findings.

The intrinsic LH activity of PMSG was assessed by two in vitro
bioassay systems: (1) the inhibition of ^{125}I-oLH binding to rat
testis homogenates, and (2) stimulation of testosterone production
by collagenase dispersed Leydig cells. The results of the binding
assay are presented in Figure 3. The oLH radioligand assay has been
described previously by Liu et al. (1974) and is essentially that of
Leidenberger and Reichert (1972). Comparison of the 50% inhibition

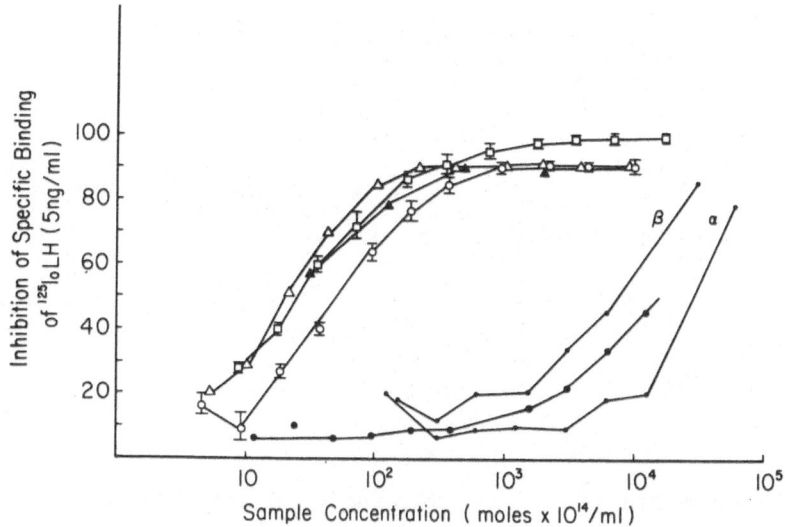

Figure 3. Demonstration of LH activity in PMSG. Inhibition of ^{125}I-oLH binding in the radioligand receptor assay (RRA) by increasing quantities of PMSG (O——O); oLH (□——□); hCG (△——△); 70% desialylated PMSG (▲——▲); oFSH (●——●); PMSG α-subunit (α); and PMSG β-subunit (β).

dosages on a molar basis indicate that our highly purified PMSG possessed 50% of the LH activity of a highly purified oLH preparation (2.32 x NIH-LH-S18), whereas partially (70%) desialylated PMSG was as active as the oLH. The inability of intact oFSH (AFP-1176-C; 35 x NIH-FSH-S1) and PMSG subunits to significantly inhibit the binding of ^{125}I-oLH attests to the specificity of the LH radioligand assay system. The high level of LH activity intrinsic to our PMSG was also demonstrated by the ability of the hormone to stimulate testosterone production in collagenase dispersed rat Leydig cells according to the method described by Moyle and Ramachandran (1973) incorporating the modification of Ascoli et al. (1975). Again, as shown in Figure 4, PMSG was less active than oLH, having a relative potency of 0.345 (0.294-0.401; 95% confidence limits) with respect to oLH and partially (70%) desialylated PMSG was nearly as active as oLH.

We assessed the intrinsic FSH activity of our PMSG by examining the ability of PMSG to (1) inhibit the specific binding of ^{125}I-oFSH and ^{125}I-hFSH to rat testis and (2) to stimulate plasminogen-activator production by rat granulosa cells. The results presented in Panel A of Figure 5 demonstrate that on a molar basis PMSG is 0.5 times as active as a highly purified preparation of oFSH (AFP 1176-C; 35 x

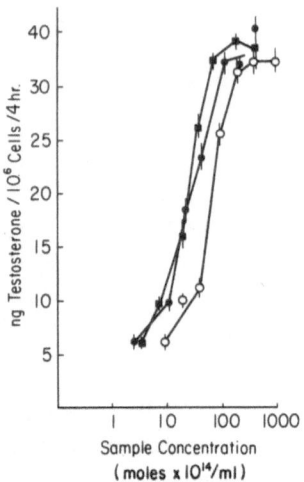

Sample Concentration
(moles x 10^{14}/ml)

Figure 4.   Demonstration of the intrinsic LH activity of PMSG by
the stimulation of testosterone production in collagenase dispersed
rat Leydig cells.   Intact PMSG (0——0); 70% desialylated PMSG (●——●);
oLH (■——■).   Each point is the mean of duplicate determinations.
The bars represent the spread between the two values for each point.

NIH-FSH-S1) and that partially (70%) desialylated PMSG is nearly as
potent as the oFSH preparation utilized.   In Panel B, Figure 5, where
the ability of PMSG to inhibit the binding of ^{125}I-hFSH is presented,
it is shown that the FSH activity of PMSG is approximately 0.50 times
as potent as the highly purified hFSH utilized (AFP-574-C; 68 x NIH-
FSH-S1) and 250 times more potent than the minor intrinsic FSH
activity present in hCG (CR-117; 11.8 x NIH-LH-S1).   The failure of
PMSG subunits, hCG, and oLH to significantly inhibit either labeled
oFSH or hFSH binding attests to the specificity of the FSH radioligand
assays.

The FSH activity intrinsic to highly purified PMSG was also
demonstrated by monitoring the ability of PMSG to stimulate plasminogen activator production in rat granulosa cells, a response that
has recently been shown to be FSH-specific (Strickland and Beers,
1976; Beers and Strickland, 1978).   The in vitro plasminogen activator assay was performed by Dr. Sidney Strickland of the Rockefeller
University, New York.   Briefly, for the assay of hormone activity,
rat granulosa cells were allowed to attach to ^{125}I-fibrin coated
culture cells.   Increasing amounts of sample dissolved in culture
media made with plasminogen depleted serum were then allowed to
incubate with the cell cultures for 10 hr.   Following the incubation
period, the cells were washed and exposed to medium containing

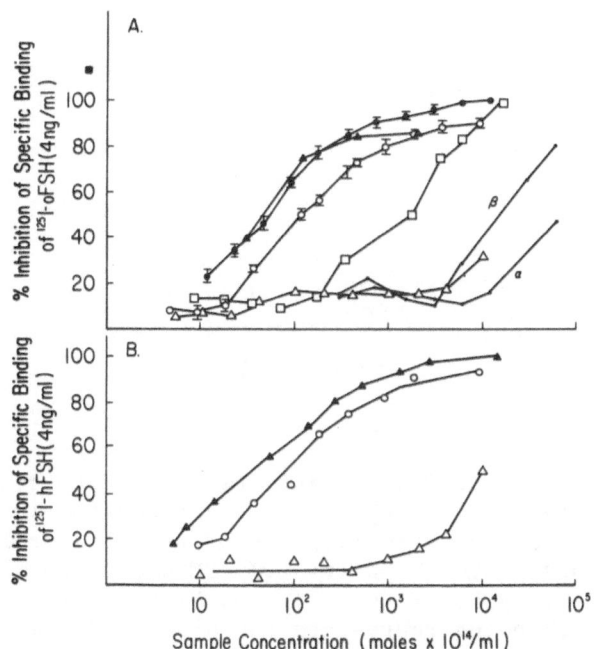

Figure 5. Demonstration of FSH activity in PMSG. Panel A: Inhibition of ^{125}I-oFSH binding in the radioligand assay by increasing quantities of PMSG (O——O); oFSH (●——●); oLH (□——□); hCG (△——△); 70% desialylated PMSG (▲——▲); PMSG α-subunit, and PMSG β-subunit. Panel B: Inhibition of ^{125}I-hFSH binding in the radioligand receptor assay by increasing quantities of PMSG (O——O); hFSH (▲——▲); and hCG (△——△).

plasminogen. After an additional 15 hr incubation period, aliquots of the supernatant were taken for counting. Hormonally stimulated granulosa cells secrete plasminogen activator which catalytically converts plasminogen to plasmin. This conversion causes lysis of the ^{125}I-fibrin coat and subsequent release of ^{125}I-fibrin peptides into the supernatant. The percentage solubilization of the ^{125}I-fibrin layer is therefore a quantitative measure of the hormonally induced production of plasminogen activator.

The results presented in Figure 6 indicate that on a weight basis, intact and partially desialylated (70%) PMSG were approximately 7 and 29 times as active as NIH-FSH-S1, respectively. The 70% desialylated PMSG, therefore, would be comparable to an oFSH having 83% of the activity of the highly purified oFSH (35 x NIH-FSH-S1) used

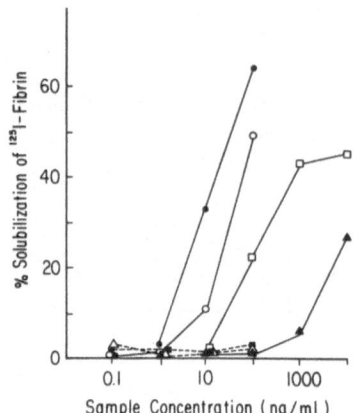

Figure 6.   Demonstration of the intrinsic FSH activity of PMSG by
the stimulation of plasminogen activator production in rat granulosa
cells in vitro.   The in vitro response of granulosa cells to PMSG
(O——O), 70% desialylated PMSG (●——●), PMSG α-subunit (Δ——Δ),
PMSG β (■——■), NIH-FSH-S11 (□——□), and NIH-LH-S19 (▲——▲) is
illustrated.   Each point represents the mean of duplicate samples.
Assays were kindly performed by Dr. Sidney Strickland of Rockefeller
University, New York.

in the binding assays.   PMSG subunits were inactive at the levels
examined.

Characterization of the FSH-like Binding Activity of PMSG in Rat Testis Versus Equine Testis

Since the in vivo studies in pregnant mares (Squires and Ginther,
1975) suggested that PMSG may not be a potent FSH in the pregnant
mare, we chose to determine whether the equine FSH receptor would
recognize PMSG as a potent FSH by examining the ability of PMSG to
inhibit ^{125}I-eFSH binding to equine testis homogenate.   The inability
of PMSG to significantly inhibit the specific binding of ^{125}I-eFSH
to equine testis is shown in Figure 7.   Panel A depicts the percent
inhibition of ^{125}I-eFSH to rat testis homogenate by increasing
amounts of eFSH (80-90 x NIH-FSH-S1, a gift from Dr. Thomas Landefeld,
University of Michigan), PMSG, and 70% desialylated PMSG.   Panel B
illustrates the percent inhibition of ^{125}I-eFSH binding to partially
purified equine testis homogenate [a 100,000 x g pellet of testis
homogenate prepared according to method described by Cheng (1975) for

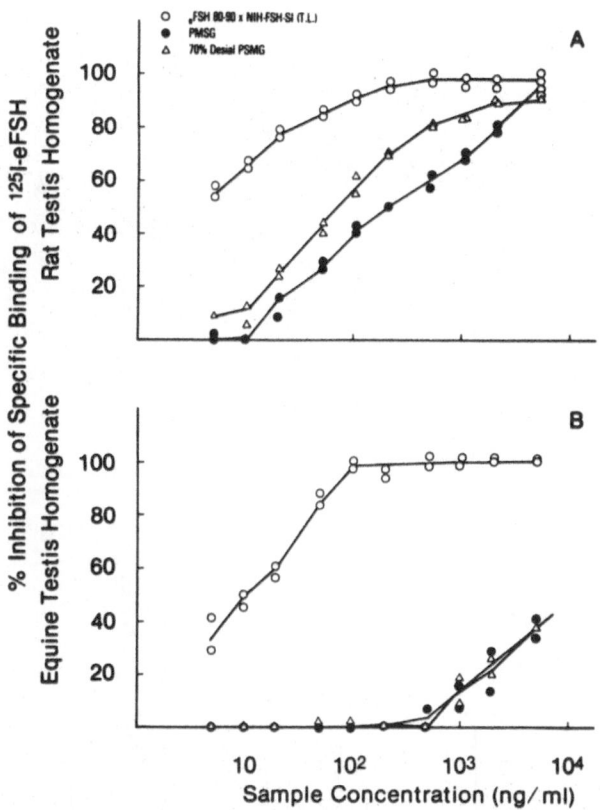

Figure 7. FSH-like binding activities of intact PMSG and 70% desialylated PMSG as characterized in rat and equine testis homogenates. Panel A: Inhibition of ^{125}I-eFSH binding to rat testis homogenate by increasing quantities of eFSH (O——O), PMSG (●——●), and 70% desialylated PMSG (△——△). Panel B: Inhibition of ^{125}I-eFSH binding to equine testis homogenate by the identical hormone preparation.

preparation of crude bovine testis membrane fractions] by identical hormone solutions. Comparison of the relative degree of displacements of inhibition curves of PMSG and 70% desialylated PMSG with

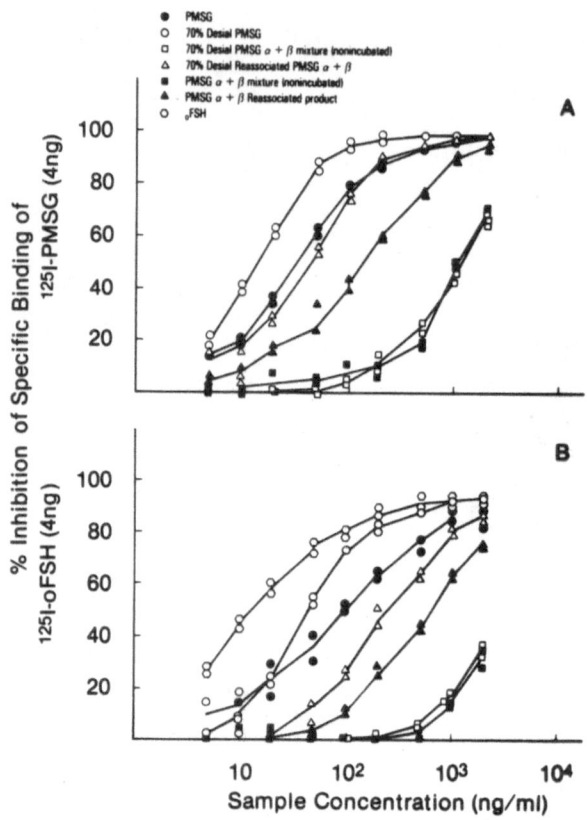

Figure 8.   Regeneration of the LH and FSH-like activities of PMSG
upon reassociation of PMSG α- and β-subunits. Panel A: Inhibition
of ^{125}I-PMSG binding rat testis homogenate by increasing quantities
of native PMSG (●——●), Native PMSG subunit reassociation product
(▲——▲), a mixture of dissociated native PMSG subunits (■——■). 70%
desialylated intact PMSG (O——O), 70% desialylated PMSG subunit
reassociation product (△——△), and a mixture of dissociated 70%
desialylated PMSG subunits (□——□).   Panel B: Inhibition of
^{125}I-oFSH binding rat testis homogenate by identical hormone
preparations. The binding assays for both LH-like activity (Panel
A) and FSH-like activity (Panel B) were performed simultaneously,
using identical conditions and materials, except for the radioligands.

respect to that of eFSH in rat testis homogenate versus equine testis homogenates, indicates that intact PMSG and 70% desialylated PMSG are 15 and 68 times, respectively, more potent FSH-like substances in the rat testis homogenate assay system than in the equine testis homogenate assay system. This result indicates that the affinity of PMSG for the equine FSH receptor is dramatically less than the affinity of PMSG for the rat FSH receptor. This result suggests that PMSG is not effectively perceived by the equine FSH receptor as an FSH-like molecule and that PMSG probably does not have an FSH role in the pregnant mare, as the study of Squires and Ginther (1975) appears to indicate. Thus, the role of PMSG in the mare is most likely restricted to its luteotropic action.

Selective Liability of FSH Activity in PMSG

The converse situation in which iodinated PMSG was used as a tracer was enigmatic in that only cold LH showed competition-binding. FSH was as ineffective as PMSG subunits (Moore and Ward, 1980b). We interpret this as indicating that iodination specifically attacks a sensitive site in the FSH-receptor-binding region of the PMSG molecule. This possibility will be studied further. However, it should be noted that while the FSH activity of PMSG appears to be selectively destroyed by iodination, such treatment does not prevent the detection of FSH-specific binding in eFSH, oFSH, and hFSH molecules. Therefore, this selective loss of FSH activity in radioiodinated PMSG appears to be a property unique to PMSG.

Another indication of the "selective" liability of the FSH activity of PMSG was observed in our subunit reassociation studies. Two reassociation experiments were performed, one employing subunits derived from native PMSG, and the other utilizing subunits obtained from 70% desialylated PMSG. For the reassociation of the subunits obtained from intact PMSG, 2 mg of beta were incubated with 4 mg of alpha in 1 ml of 0.5 M sodium acetate buffer, pH 6.0, for 24 hr at 37°C. At the end of the incubation period, the mixture was subjected to Sephacryl S-200 (1 x 87 cm) chromatography in order to separate excess α-subunit from the reassociated product.

For the desialylated PMSG α- and β-subunit reassociation experiment, subunits obtained from the dissociation of 4 mg of 70% desialylated PMSG were pooled after separation on Sephacryl S-200, lyophilized, and then dissolved in 1.0 ml sodium acetate buffer, pH 6.0, and incubated for 24 hr at 47°C. Nearly complete reassociation of these subunits was verified by the observance of a single major peak having the elution volume of intact PMSG. The partial restoration of the LH and FSH-like activities of reassociated subunits are presented in Figure 8. In both cases, partial restoration of both FSH and LH activities was obtained. However, the level of activities were markedly less than that for the intact hormones from which the

subunits were derived. The native PMSG subunit reassociation product possessed only 25.2% (20.3-31.3%; 95% confidence limit) of the
original LH-like activity (Panel A, Figure 14) and possessed only
17.1% (14.0-20.6%; 95% confidence limit) of the original FSH-like
activity (Panel B, Figure 14). The 70% desialylated PMSG subunit
reassociation product possesed 34.1% (32.2-36.2%; 95% confidence
limit) of the original LH-like activity and 18.6% (15.8-21.6%; 95%
confidence limit) of the original FSH-like activity. Note in both
cases the restoration of the FSH-like activity was significantly
less than the restoration of the LH-like activity. Although we
have interpreted the greater loss of FSH activity upon recombination
in PMSG to be indicative of a selective lability of FSH activity in
PMSG, it should be noted that Christakos and Bahl (1979) have measured the FSH and LH activities of reassociated PMSG and have found
that FSH activity was restored to a greater degree (62.4%) than LH
activity (27.5%). The reason for this discrepancy is unclear and
warrants further investigation.

AMINO ACID SEQUENCES OF THE PMSG ALPHA AND BETA SUBUNITS

Alpha Subunit Primary Structure

    The complete details of the methodology and peptide characteri-
zations will not be presented here, since they will be described in
a separate publication (Moore et al., 1980).

    The primary structure of the PMSG α-subunit was deduced from
several lines of evidence, primarily by the sequence analysis of
overlapping peptides obtained from tryptic and chymotryptic digests
and automatic sequence analysis of reduced and alkylated PMSG α. A
two dimensional paper mapping technique previously described by
Burleigh et al. (1976) was used to isolate the tryptic and chymotryptic peptides. Figure 9 summarizes the sequence information we have
obtained for the α-subunit. Comparison of the PMSG α primary
structure with gonadotropin α-subunits derived from other species
indicate that PMSG α shares a 70-80% chemical identity with the other
α-subunits (Figure 10). The degree of chemical similarity is higher
(78-89%) if conservative substitutions are taken into consideration.
Although there is a high degree of similarity between PMSG α and α-
subunits from other species, there is a unique structural feature
which is specific to the equine species. This feature, which we
refer to as the COOH-terminal region "tyrosine-histidine" transposi-
tion, is indicated by the asterisks in Figure 10, positions 87 and
93. Sequence studies published to date which do not involve the
equine species have placed a histidinyl residue at position 87 and
a tyrosinyl residue at position 93. PMSG α and eFSH α (Rathnam et
al., 1978) have a tyrosyl residue at position 87 and a histidinyl
residue at position 93.

Phe-Pro-Asp-Gly-Glu-Phe-Thr-Thr-Glu-Asx-Cys-Pro-Glu-Cys-Lys-Leu-Arg-Glu-Asn-Lys-Tyr-Phe-Phe-Lys-Leu-Gly-Val-Pro-Ile-Tyr-
                                        10   20   30

Gln-Cys-Lys-Gly-Cys-Cys-Phe-Ser-Arg-Ala-Tyr-Pro-Thr-Pro-Ala-Arg-Ser-Arg-Lys-Thr-Met-Leu-Val-Pro-Lys-Asn-Ile-Thr-Ser-Glx-
                                        40   50   *60

Ser-Thr-Cys-Cys-Val-Ala-Lys-Ala-Phe-Ile-Arg-Val-Thr-Val-Met-Gly-Asn-Ile-Lys-Leu-Glx-Asn-His-Thr-Glx-Cys-Tyr-Cys-Ser-Thr-
                                        70   *80   90

Cys-Tyr-His-His-Lys-Ile.
96

Figure 9.   The primary structure of PMSG alpha.

```
                              10              20              30           40
hCG
h FSH
h LH  (4)  - - - - A P D V    T Q D P F   S Q P   L E  M              L  K
p LH  (3)  - - - - - -   M G  K Q D       S       E  M                   K
o,b LH (2)              M G   K D         S P D A   M                     K
PMSG  (1)  F P D G E F T T E B C P E C K L R E N K Y F F K L G V P I Y Q C K G C C F S R A Y P T P A R S R


              50          60          70          80           90      96
(4)                     Q  V         S Y N       G F V(E)     A H    Y  S.
(3)                        A         T K A       (N)A R V(E) S (E) H  Y  S.
(2)                        A         T K A       (N)V R V(E)         H  Y  S.
(1)  K T M L V P K N I T S E S T C C V A K A F I R V T V M G B I K L Z N H T Z C Y C S T C Y H H K I.
                                                              *         *
```

Figure 10. The amino acid sequence of the α-subunits of several mammalian gonadotropins. The sequences are identical with PMSGα unless a different amino acid is indicated along the line designated. Numbers refer to the PMSG sequence presented. The single letter code for the amino acid designation has been employed. The sequences which have been compared to PMSGα were taken from the following sources: oLHα and bLHα, Liu et al. (1972); Ward and Liu (1971); pLHα, Maghuin-Rogister et al. (1973); hCGα, Morgan et al (1973); hLHα, Sairam et al. (1972b); hFSHα, Rathnam et al. (1975). The symbol ▼ indicates a carbohydrate attachment site.

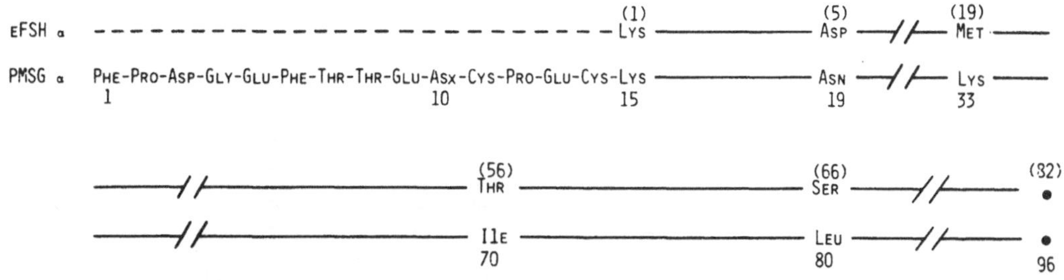

*RATHNAM EI AL. JBC 253: 5355 (1978)

Figure 11. Comparison of PMSG α sequence with eFSH α.* Solid lines denote areas of common identity. Only differences have been indicated.

The recent study by Rathnam et al. (1978) has allowed the intraspecies comparison between PMSG α and eFSH α. Figure 11 summarizes the differences between their sequence proposal and ours. The high degree of identity denoted by the solid lines was expected. However, the differences indicated, especially the 14 residues at the NH_2-terminal region, and at positions 19, 33, 70, and 80 of these PMSG molecules were unexpected since other intraspecies comparisons have indicated identical sequence information for the α-subunit (Liu and Ward, 1975; Pierce, 1971) supporting a single gene hypothesis for the origin of this peptide moiety. It is important to note that the NH_2-terminal region, where no sequence information was found in the equine FSH α, includes two half-cystine placements in PMSG and other α-subunits. It is known that all half-cystine residues in the α-subunits of gonadotropins are involved in disulfide bond formation. If Rathnam et al. (1978) did indeed isolate a form of active eFSH having an α-subunit deficient in the first 14 residues, two significant implications follow. The first is that the NH_2-terminal region not observed is not necessary for the expression of biological activity in FSH, and second, that a disulfide bond would exist between cysteinyl residues 11 and 14. The second implication seems unlikely in the light of several independent α-subunit disulfide studies (Chung et al., 1973; Combarnous and Hennen, 1974; Cornell and Pierce, 1974). Although there is disagreement on the disulfide placement, none of the results obtained from these studies suggests that a disulfide exists between half-cystine 11 and 14. Furthermore, Giudice and Pierce (1979) have recently demonstrated that the first disulfide to be reduced in bLH α occurs between half-cystine 11 and 35, and that a second disulfide is probably located between positions 14 and 36. Our sequence data for PMSG α, the various disulfide placement studies, and the discrepancy between the results for NH_2-terminal analysis on intact eFSH [i.e., Nuti et al., 1972, reported that phenylalanine and either

hCG - β Ser Lys Glu Pro Leu Arg Pro Arg Cys Arg Pro Ile Asn Ala Thr Leu Ala Val Glu Lys Glu Gly Cys Pro Val Cys Ile Thr Val Asn Thr Thr Ile Cys Ala

eCG - β Ser Arg Gly Pro Leu Arg Pro Leu Cys Arg Pro Ile Asn Ala Thr Leu Ala Ala Glu Lys Gln Ala Cys (Ser Lys) Cys (X X X) Thr Ile Cys Ala

hCG - β Gly Tyr Cys Pro Thr Met Thr Arg Val Leu Gln Gly Val Leu Pro Ala Leu Pro Gln Val Val Cys Asn Tyr Arg Asp Val Arg Phe Glu Ser Ile Arg Leu Pro

eCG - β Gly Tyr Cys Pro Ser Met Val Arg Val Thr Pro Ala Ala Leu Pro Ala Ile Pro Gln Pro Val Cys Thr Tyr Arg Glu Leu Arg Phe Ala Ser Ile Arg Leu Pro

hCG - β Gly Cys Pro Arg Gly Val Asn Pro Val Val Ser Tyr Ala Val Ala Leu Ser Cys Gln Cys Ala Leu Cys Arg Arg Ser Thr Thr Asp Cys Gly Gly Pro Lys Asp His Pro Leu

eCG - β Gly Cys Pro Gly Val Asx Pro (Arg) Val Ser Phe Gly Val Ala Leu Ser Cys Asx Cys Gly Pro Cys Glx Ile Lys Thr Thr Asp Cys Gly Val Phe Arg Asn Glu Pro Leu

hCG - β Thr Cys Asp Asp Pro Arg Phe Gln Asp Ser Ser Ser Lys Ala Pro Pro Pro Ser Leu Pro Ser Pro Ser Arg Leu Pro Gly Pro Ser Asp Thr Pro Ile Leu Pro Gln

eCG - β Ala Cys Asp Pro Pro Ser Glx Leu Thr Ser (Thr, Ser, Arg) Ala Pro Pro Pro Glx Thr Ser Pro Pro Lys (Gly, Pro, Pro, Ser, Arg) (Asx, Ser, Ala, Leu, Pro, Gln)

Figure 12.   Comparative summary of currently available
structural information on PMSGβ as compared
to hCGβ. The hCG sequence is taken from
Morgan et al., 1973. Our current data for
PMSGβ allow 82% of the sequence to be placed
by direct sequencing, 15% placed by peptide
composition and homology with hCGβ, and 3%
for which no data are available (positions
27-30). The latter gap results from failure
to isolate the missing glycopeptide in
sufficient quantity and purity to define
composition.

aspartic acid or asparagine were NH_2-termini, whereas Rathnam et al.
(1978) reported that lysine and either aspartic acid or asparagine
were NH_2-termini] suggest that the sequence proposed for eFSHα does
not represent the sequence of <u>native</u> eFSHα-subunit. Therefore, we
believe that our proposal for the PMSGα represents the first complete
amino acid sequence of a native equine α-subunit. The remaining four
differences, which correspond to PMSG positions 19, 33, 70, and 80,
suggest that separate genes may exist for eFSHα and PMSGα, or perhaps
that the sequence in these positions requires further study.

Beta Subunit Primary Structure

     The details of the sequence analysis will not be presented
since they will be described elsewhere (Burleigh et al., 1980).
Approximately 80% of the primary structure of PMSGβ has been rigidly
established by sequencing intact PMSGβ tryptic peptides isolated
from performic acid oxidized, aminoethylated, HF-deglycosylated-
aminoethylated PMSGβ derivatives, and chymotryptic peptides isolated
from carboxymethylated PMSGβ. Figure 12 presents our proposal for
the PMSGβ-subunit compared to that for hCGβ. Figure 12 shows the
remarkable homology of PMSGβ to hCGβ. Besides sharing the overall
LH-like information that hCG shares with the other LH's for which
sequence data are available, PMSGβ shares several similarities that
have previously been thought to be unique to hCGβ. The most striking
hCGβ-like feature of PMSGβ is the 35 amino acid residue extension
at the COOH-terminus. In the tail-piece region where we have definite
sequence data, PMSGβ shares a 39% identity with hCGβ. Although we
have placed several basic residues in this region (Arg-122, Lys-134,
and Arg-139) we have not obtained the putative tryptic peptides in
any detectable yield, presumably because this region is protected
from proteolysis by the carbohydrate moieties attached in this region.
This conclusion is supported by the fact that an intact COOH-terminal
fragment having an NH_2-terminal sequence of Ala-Pro-Pro compromising
residues 123-145 can be isolated as the largest molecular weight
fraction by gel filtration from a tryptic digest of aminoethylated
PMSGβ. Additional sequence information in this area was not obtained
until tryptic peptides from an HF deglycosylated PMSGβ were isolated
and characterized. Besides the COOH-terminal extension PMSGβ shares
a few unique residue substitutions that have until now only been
observed in hCGβ. At position number 10, hCGβ and PMSGβ share an
arginine substitution, whereas all other gonadotropin β-subunits
sequenced to date, including hLH, contain either glu or gln. At
position number 51, hCGβ and PMSGβ share an alanine substitution,
whereas all the other gonadotropins sequenced to date contain proline.
At position number 83, hCGβ and PMSGβ share the similar hydrophobic
residues alanine and glycine, respectively, whereas the others--
including hLH--share proline. Finally, at position 89, hCGβ and
PMSGβ share a possible amide placement, whereas all the others share
either histidine or--in the case of hLH--arginine. The significance

of these unique chorionic β-subunit substitutions and COOH-terminal extensions is not yet clear. The positions in parentheses represent areas where we have only peptide composition, but no direct sequence data. The gap at position 26-30 represents a glycopeptide which has not been purified adequately to define composition.

Figure 13 shows the amino acid sequence similarities and dissimilarities that the LH-like and FSH-like β-subunits share with the primary structure of PMSGβ. Half-cystine placements were used as positional points of reference. As expected from the close similarity of PMSGβ to hCGβ, a superficial examination of Figure 13 indicates that PMSGβ more closely resembles the β-subunits of the LH-like hormones. The average percentage of chemical similarity of PMSG to the other LHβ-subunits is 85%, if conservative substitutions are taken into consideration. PMSGβ therefore, on the basis of its overall structure, appears to be a luteotropin.

MOLECULAR BASIS FOR FSH ACTIVITY IN PMSG--THE DETERMINANT LOOP HYPOTHESIS

Since it has been demonstrated that the biological and binding activities of glycoprotein hormones are only optimally mainfested when α- and β-subunits form an intact complex, Ward (1978) has postulated that the receptor binding region of a gonadotropin is comprised of a collection of functional groups belonging to both subunits. Furthermore, since various subunit recombination studies (Pierce, 1977; Liu and Ward, 1975) have indicated that the β-subunit is responsible for conferring hormonal specificity, it must follow that the subset of functional groups comprising the receptor binding region that arise from the unique structural features offered by each β-subunit constitute a hormone specificity determinant.

It is not yet clearly understood what role the carbohydrate moiety has in the storage of hormone specificity information. Our laboratory is prepared only to address the function of the polypeptide moiety at this time, and therefore the discussion that will follow will be limited to addressing the possible role of the protein moiety. If hormone specificity determinants do indeed lie in the polypeptide moiety, comparison of the PMSGβ primary structure with that of the LH-like and FSH-like hormones should permit the recognition of candidate areas which could be considered as molecular determinants for FSH and LH activity. As discussed above, the PMSGβ primary structure is overwhelmingly LH-like in character. No significant direct FSH homology (sequence information) has been observed. This finding suggests that the FSH information that is recognized at best by rat receptors, if it is located in the polypeptide, must be very subtly expressed. However, if this subtle FSH information recognized by rat FSH receptors can be identified, an important

```
pLH-β (1)                    R/Z                 D       P V   I T F T   S                   R     L           P V                     I       S
oLH-β (2)                    Q                           P V   I T F T   S                   K     L   V I     P M     R         H             V
hCG-β (3)    K Q         R                   V       G   P V   I T V"N"                  T   T     L Q G V       L     V     N     D V     E
                             10                  20                  30                  40                  50                  60                  70
eCG-β (4)  S R G P L R P L C R P I"N"A T L A A E K E A C(S K)C X X X X T T(I C)A G Y C P S M V R V T P A A L P A I P Q P V C T Y R E L R F A S I R L P
hFSH-β (5) - - - - - - N S   E L T   I   I   I       E   R F   L T I"N"    W           Y T R D L   Y K N P A R P K I   K T   F T K     V Y E T V   V
                                         V       L                                    G
pFSH-β (6) - - - - - - - -   Z L T   I   I T V Q K───C T F   I S I"N"    W           T T R B L   Y K B P A R P B I   K T             V Y E T V K V
eFSH-β (7) - - - - - - N S   Z L T   I   I A V E K   G   R F   I T I"N"    W           Y T R D L   Y K D P A R P K I Q K T   F K     V Y E T V K V

(1)                    D   T       P           H         R L S S S       P G   A Q           R   P L P G L L.
(2)                        M       P           H         R L S S         P G   T Q           H   P L P D T L.
(3)              R         V     Y A           Q   A L   R R S           G P K D H     T     D   R F E D S   S K         "S"L P S P "S"R L P G P S D T P I L P Q.
                             80                  90                  100                 110                 120         130           140
(4)        G C P P G V B P(R)V S F G V A L S C B C G P C Z I K T T D C G V F R N E P L A C D P P S Z T L T S(T, S)R A P P P Z T S P(S, T, P)K(G P P S R)(B, S, A, L, P, Q).
(5)            A H H A   S L Y T Y P     T Q   H     K   D S D S       T   R G L G   S Y   S F G E M K Q Y P   A L S Y.
(6)            A H H A   S L Y T Y P     T Z   H     K   B S B S       T   R G L G   S Y   S F G E.
            G
(7)        P C A H H A   S L Y T Y P     T Z   H     K   B S D S   B   T   R G L G   S Y   S F G D M K Z Y P V A L S Y.
```

Figure 13. The amino acid sequences of the beta subunits of several mammalian gonadotropins. The sequences are identical with PMSGβ unless a different amino acid is indicated along the line designated. Numbers refer to the PMSGβ sequence presented. The single letter code for amino acid residue designation has been employed. (-) represents a missing residue. An X represents an unknown residue. Quotation marks indicate a carbohydrate attachment site. The underscored regions of the PMSGβ sequence correspond to those positions in hLH that have been proposed by Stewart and Stewart (1977) to be responsible for the determination of receptor interaction specificity in LH. The sequences which have been compared to PMSGβ were taken from the following sources: hCG, Morgan et al.,1973; oLH, Liu et al., 1927b; pLH, Maghuin-Rogister and Hennen, 1973; hFSH, Saxena and Rathnam, 1976; pFSH, Closset et al., 1978; eFSH, Fujiki et al., 1978.

implication would be that the region under question may constitute a hormone specificity determinant region of primary importance in the glycoprotein hormone family.

A careful comparative examination of the primary structures of PMSGβ, the LH and FSH/TSH-like β-subunits, reveals a limited area comprising residues 92-102 where conspicuous hormone-specific (radical vs. conservative) substitutions exist. Figure 14 compares the sequence of PMSGβ with that of the other glycoprotein β-subunit in this specific area under discussion. The LH-like β-subunits (o, b, p, h, LH) have proline, a neutral hydrophobic, at position 92, Arg, a positively charged residue, at position 94 (hLH and hCG have arginine at position 95 as well), and serine, a polar neutral, at position 96. In contrast, the FSH/TSH-like β-subunits have lysine, a positively charged residue, at position 92, and acidic, negatively charged residues, at positions 94 and 96. The sequence of PMSGβ in this region is neither obviously LH-like nor FSH-like. The PMSGβ primary structure reveals a compromise, LH-like β-subunit substitutions, a possible FSH-like β-subunit substitution, and a substitution that is unique to PMSGβ. No obvious overall homology between PMSGβ and either the LH-like β-subunits or the FSH/TSH-like β-subunits is observed in this limited region (Figure 14). The location of a potential acidic residue glutamic acid (Glx = Glu or Gln) at position 94 and Val at position 102 suggest an FSH/TSH-like β similarity. However, an LH-like β similarity is suggested by Pro at position 92 and the Ile at position 95. The presence of a basic residue Lys at position 96 is totally unique to PMSGβ.

An additional property which makes this area of particular interest is the presence of a disulfide bond between the half-cystines at positions 93 and 100. This disulfide placement has been established for LHβ in the laboratories using three different techniques (Chung et al., 1975; Reeve et al., 1975; Tsunasawa et al., 1977). One study has also established this disulfide placement in bTSHβ (Reeve et al., 1975). This disulfide bond also has the unique property of being the one most accessible to reducing agents. In studies involving LH and TSHβ-subunits, Reeve et al. (1975) demonstrated that only this disulfide of the six present in the molecule (β-subunit) is reduced with dithioerythyritol (DTE) (2.4-fold excess of DTE to total protein disulfide, at pH 7) in the absence of denaturant. The fact that this disulfide bond is so readily accessible to reducing agents suggests that the octapeptide loop is probably located at the surface of the β-subunit.

Indirect evidence which further attests to the potential importance of the octapeptide loop region has been provided by the recent studies of Mori et al. (1977). They have shown that a 10-fold molar excess of DTT (in the absence of denaturant) results in the reduction of two disulfide bonds in the α-subunit of intact hCG. An S-carboxy-

Figure 14. Comparison of residues 84–105 of PMSGβ with the corresponding regions of the LH–like and FSH/TSH-like beta subunits. These regions contain the suggested determinant loops (residues 93–100) for the respective hormones. The sequences are identical with PMSGβ unless a different amino acid is indicated in the column designated. The boxed residues are indicated to emphasize the putative FSH-like and LH-like substitutions in PMSGβ. The symbol ** indicates a PMSGβ specific substitution. The symbol * indicates the TSHβ specific substitution in the octapeptide loop.

methyl (SCm) derivative of the partially reduced hCG retained full biological activity in an in vivo bioassay. Using a 40-fold molar excess of DTT, a third disulfide bond confined to the β-subunit of intact hCG was reduced. The SCm derivative of this partially reduced hCG resulted in an 80% loss of the biological activity. Although these authors did not locate the exact position of the β-subunit disulfide, the data of Reeve et al. (1975) suggest that the crucial disulfide is probably the one formed between half-cystines 93 and 100. Therefore, it appears that the integrity of the octapeptide loop is of crucial importance to the biological activity of the glycoprotein hormones (LH, FSH, TSH, hCG, and PMSG).

The net charge on the octapeptide loop, a consequence of the hormone specific residue substitutions, is postulated to be the chemical basis for the expression of hormone specificity. It may be suggested that expression of LH-like character requires a positive charge (Arg) at position 94 (as in o, b, and pLH) or at 94 and 95 (as in hLH and hCG), an octapeptide loop net charge of 0 or +1, and that FSH-like character (that at least detected by rat FSH receptors) requires a negative charge (Asp) at positions 94 and 96 or an octapeptide loop net charge of -3. According to this scheme, TSH (an Asp at 94 and 96, and an octapeptide loop net charge of -3) should have an FSH-like character. However, as indicated in Figure 21, TSH has a unique substitution at position 97, tyrosine. We suggest that this substitution may prevent the TSH loop from mimicking the action of the FSH loop. If a Glu is present at position 94 (Glx) in the PMSG β octapeptide loop the net charge would be -1, intermediate to that of the human LH-like hormones (hLH and hCG) and the FSH/TSH-like hormones. It is postulated that PMSG has significant FSH activity in rats on account of this intermediate octapeptide loop net charge. The chemical uniqueness of each loop probably is not the only distinguishable feature the hormone has to offer the receptor; however, present knowledge of the PMSG β structure with its overall LH-like similarity suggests that it may be a principal determinant or receptor binding contact site, since PMSG is readily detected by rat FSH receptors.

That some octapeptide loop net charges may be more readily adopted by the LH and FSH receptor octapeptide loop binding domains is suggested by the differences in the relative potencies and binding characteristics of oLH and the human LH-like molecules (hLH and hCG). It has been shown in this study and also by others (Farmer et al., 1977; Moyle et al., 1978) that hCG is more potent than oLH in in vitro LH bioassays. The determinant loop hypothesis would attribute the greater potency of hLH and hCG in the in vitro LH bioassays to the presence of the additional Arg at position 95 in the human series.

Additional support for the determinant loop hypothesis has been recently provided by Stewart and Stewart (1977). These workers have used computer methods to critically examine the relationship between the primary structures of the β-subunits of human LH, FSH, CG, and TSH. From their variable versus constant region computer analysis, they have identified regions in the hLHβ-subunit which they tentatively believe are responsible for the expression of LH specificity. The analogous region in PMSGβ that corresponds to the regions they putatively designate as LH hormone specificity determinants are underscored in Figure 13. It is of interest to note that the corresponding regions in PMSGβ are for the most part homologous to LH, except for one position out of the 28 positions indicated. The one excepted position is number 94, a "determinant loop" position, Glx.

It is important to determine whether Glu or Gln exists at position 94 in PMSGβ. It is also important to determine whether the possibility exists that highly purified PMSG, although a single gene product, is actually a heterogeneous mixture of position 94 deamidated and intact molecules. Our evidence suggests that a glutamine residue probably exists at position 94; however, it must be noted that glutamine residues can undergo a post-synthetic modification to glutamic acid residues through hydrolytic deamidation (Robinson et al., 1970; Robinson and Rudd, 1974). If some deamidation has occurred involving glutamine 94 in PMSGβ, it is possible that highly purified PMSGβ derived from serum, although a single gene product, is actually a heterogeneous mixture of deamidated and intact molecules. Therefore, the possibility exists employing the "determinant loop" net charge argument, that intact PMSG molecules (Gln at position 94) express only LH activity (net charge similar to o, b, p, LH) while deamidated PMSG molecules (Glu at position 94) express either FSH alone or both FSH and LH activity in rats. Substantiation of this proposal requires a demonstration of this possible heterogeneity and a demonstration that this heterogeneity is connected with the separate FSH and LH activities.

CONCLUSION

Our studies on the in vitro biological and chemical characterization of PMSG have been summarized and indicate that: 1) The intrinsic FSH and LH activities of PMSG can be clearly demonstrated in rat bioassay systems; 2) The intrinsic FSH activity of PMSG is undetectable in an equine assay system suggesting that the equine FSH receptor does not perceive PMSG as an FSH, unlike the rat FSH receptor; 3) The intrinsic FSH activity of PMSG as defined in rat assay systems is more unstable than the intrinsic LH activity. The selective loss of FSH activity upon iodination and the failure to generate the FSH activity to the same degree as LH activity of PMSG upon subunit reassociation supports this contention; 4) The PMSGα-subunit primary structure is highly similar to that observed for α-subunits of other species. However, significant differences exist between our PMSGα primary structure proposal and the eFSHα proposal of Rathnam et al. (1978). It is important to substantiate these differences, since

these observations suggest that separate genes may exist for
chorionic and pituitary derived α-subunits; 5) The overall primary
structure of PMSGβ closely resembles that of the LH-like gonadotropins. Furthermore, PMSGβ shares chemical features that were
previously thought to be unique to hCG (an hCG-like COOH-terminal
tail piece and "chorionic gonadotropin specific" substitutions at
positions 10, 23, 51, and 89). These findings offer a chemical
basis to the designation of PMSG as eCG, as originally suggested
by Stewart et al. (1977) and Farmer and Papkoff (1979), on account
of its trophoblastic origin.

A "determinant loop hypothesis" has been presented to explain
the molecular basis of FSH activity of PMSG clearly demonstrable in
rats. If this structural feature is indeed responsible for the
expression of FSH activity of PMSG in rats, this area should be
considered as a hormone specificity determinant of capital importance
in all the glycoprotein hormones. The dramatic hormone specific
differences that exist in this area within the glycoprotein hormone
family support this argument.

To conclude, we believe that our studies indicate that PMSG is
an equine choriogonadotropin, probably having a physiological role
in the mare analogous to that of hCG in the human--i.e., primarily
a luteotropin of pregnancy. Our studies suggest that the designation
of PMSG as an FSH-like substnace is an "historical artifact" arising
from defining FSH activity in rat bioassays. However, this "historical artifact" has provided the biochemical endocrinologist with an
intriguing natural analogue that should prove useful in the endeavor
to define glycoprotein hormone specificity determinants.

REFERENCES

Aggarwall, B. B., Farmer, S. W., Papkoff, H., and Allen, W. R., 1979,
    Isolation of a gonadotropin secreted by horse trophoblast cells
    in culture: Comparison with PMSG. Proceedings of the Endocrine
    Society, 61st Annual Meeting. Abstract No. 936.
Allen, W. R., 1969, The immunological measurement of pregnant mare
    serum gonadotropin, J. Endocrinol. 43:593.
Allen, W. R., Hamilton, D. W., and Moor, R. M., 1973, The origin of
    equine endometrial cups. II. Invasion of the endometrium by
    trophoblast, Anat. Record 177:485.
Allen, W. R., and Moor, R. M., 1972, The origin of equine endometrial
    cups. I. Production of PMSG by foetal trophoblast cells, J.
    Reprod. Fertil. 29:313.
Ascheim, S., and Zondek, B. 1927, Hypophysenvorderlappen-hormone und
    ovarial hormonė in horn von Schwangeren, Klin. Wochschr. 6:1322.
Ascoli, M., Liddle, R. A., and Puett, D., 1975, The metabolism of
    luteinizing hormone plasma clearance, urinary excretion, and
    tissue uptake, Molec. Cell. Endocrinol. 3:21.

Beers, W. H., and Strickland, S., 1978, A cell culture assay for follicle-stimulating hormone, J. Biol. Chem. 253:3877.

Bellisario, R., Carlsen, R. B., and Bahl, O. P., 1973, Human chorionic gonadotropin: Linear amino acid sequence of the alpha subunit, J. Biol. Chem. 248:6797.

Birken, S., and Canfield, R. E., 1977, Isolation and amino acid sequence of COOH-terminal fragments from the beta subunit of human choriogonadotropin, J. Biol. Chem. 252:5386.

Braunstein, G. D., Rasor, J., and Adler, D., 1976, Serum human chorionic gonadotropin levels throughout normal pregnancy, Am. J. Obstet. Gynecol. 126:677.

Burleigh, B. D., Liu, W. K., and Ward, D. N., 1976, Reaction of tetranitromethane with luteotropin, oxytocin, and vasopressin, J. Biol. Chem. 251:308.

Burleigh, B. D., Moore, W. T., and Ward, D. N., 1980, The amino acid sequence of the beta subunit of pregnant mare serum gonadotropin, submitted to J. Biol. Chem.

Carlsen, R. B., Bahl, O. P. and Swaminathan, N., 1973, Human chorionic gonadotropin: Linear amino acid sequence of the beta subunit, J. Biol. Chem. 248:6810.

Cartland, G. F., and Nelson, J. W., 1937, The preparation and purification of extracts containing the gonad stimulating hormone of pregnant mare serum, J. Biol. Chem. 119:59.

Channing, C. P. Stone, S. L., Sakai, C. W., Haour, F., and Saxena, B. B., 1978, A stimulatory effect of the fluid from preimplantation rabbit blastocysts upon luteinization of monkey granulosa cell cultures, J. Reprod. Fert. 54:215.

Chen, H. C., and Hodgen, G. D., 1976, Primate chorionic gonadotropins: antigenic similarities to the unique carboxyl-terminal peptide of hCG beta subunit, J. Clin. Endocrinol. Metab. 43:1414.

Cheng, K. W., 1975, Properties of follicle-stimulating hormone receptor in cell membranes of bovine testis, Biochem. J. 149:123.

Christakos, S., and Bahl, O. P., 1979, Pregnant mare serum gonadotropin purification and physicochemical, biological and immunological characterization, J. Biol. Chem. 254:4253.

Chung, D. Sairam, M. R., Li, C. H., 1973, The primary structure of ovine interstitial cell-stimulating hormone. III. Disulfide bridges of the alpha subunit, Arch. Biochem. Biophys. 159:678.

Chung, D., Sairam, M. R., and Li, C. H., 1975, The primary structure of ovine interstitial cell stimulating hormone. IV. Disulfide bridges of the beta subunit, Intl. J. Peptide Prot. Res. 7:487.

Closset, J., Maghuin-Rogister, G., Hennen, G., Strosberg, A. D., 1978, Porcine follitropin. The amino acid sequence of the beta subunit, Eur. J. Biochem. 86:115.

Cole, H. H., Guilbert, H. R., and Goss, H., 1932, Further considerations of the properties of the gonad-stimulating principle of mare serum, Am. J. Physiol. 102:227.

Cole, H. H., and Hart, G. H., 1930, The potency of blood serum of mares in progressive stages of pregnancy effecting the sexual maturity of the immature rat, Am. J. Physiol. 93:57.

Cole, H. H., Howell, C. E., and Hart, G. H., 1931, The changes occurring in the ovary of the mare during pregnancy, Anat. Rec. 49:199.

Cole, H. H., Pencharz, R. L., and Goss, H., 1940, On the biological properties of highly purified gonadotropin from pregnant mare serum, Endocrinology 27:548.

Combarnous, Y., and Hennen, G., 1974, The disulfide bridges of porcine luteinizing hormone alpha subunit, Biochem. Soc. Trans. 2:915.

Combarnous, Y. Hennen, G., and Ketelsleger, J. M., 1978, Pregnant mare serum gonadotropin exhibits higher affinity for luteotropin than follitropin receptors of porcine testis, FEBS Letters 90:65.

Cornell, J. S., and Pierce, J. G., 1974, Studies on the disulfide bonds of glycoprotein hormones. Locations in the alpha chain based on partial reductions and formation of ^{14}C-labeled S carboxymethyl derivatives, J. Biol. Chem. 249:4166.

Delfs, E., 1941, Serum chorionic gonadotropin in the rhesus monkey, Abstr. #123, Anat. Rec. (suppl. 2) 79:17.

Dufau, M. L., Pock, R., Neubauer, A., and Catt, K. J., 1976, In vitro bioassay of LH in human serum: The rat interstitial cell testosterone (RICT) assay, J. Clin. Endocrinol. Metab. 42:958.

Ellinwood, W. E., Seidel, G. E., Niswender, G. D., 1979, Secretion of gonadotropic factors by the preimplantation rabbit blastocyst, Proc. Soc. Exp. Biol. Metab. 161:136.

Endo, Y., Yamashita, K., Tachibana, Y., Tojo, S., and Kobata, A., 1979, Structures of the asparagine-linked sugar chains of human chorionic gonadotropin, J. Biochem. (Tokyo) 85:669.

Farmer, S. W., and Papkoff, H., 1978, Pregnant mare serum gonadotrophin and follicle stimulating hormone. Stimulation of cyclic AMP production in rat seminiferous tubule cells, Endocrinology 76:391.

Farmer, S. W., and Papkoff, H., 1979, Immunochemical studies with mare serum gonadotropin, Biol. Reprod. 21:425.

Farmer, S. W., Suyama, A., and Papkoff, H., 1977, Effects of diverse mammalian and nonmammalian gonadotropins on isolated rat Leydig cells, Gen. Comp. Endocrinol. 32:488.

Fujiki, Y., Rathnam, P., Saxena, B. B., 1978, Amino acid sequence of the beta subunit of the follicle-stimulating hormone from equine pituitary glands, J. Biol. Chem. 253:5363.

Gospodarowicz, D., 1972, Purification and physicochemical properties of the pregnant mare serum gonadotropin (PMSG), Endocrinology 91:101.

Gospodarowicz, D., 1973, Properties of the luteinizing hormone receptor of isolated bovine corpus luteum plasma membranes, J. Biol. Chem. 248:5042.

Gospodarowicz, D., and Papkoff, H., 1967, A simple method for the isolation of pregnant mare serum gonadotropin, Endocrinology 80:699.

Goss, H., and Cole, H. H., 1940, Further studies on the purification of mare gonadotropin hormone, Endocrinology 26:244.

Gray, W. R., 1972, Sequence analysis with dansyl chloride, in *Methods in Enzymology XXV*, S. P. Colowick and N. O. Kaplan, eds., pp. 333-344, Academic Press, New York.

Guidice, L. C., and Pierce, J. G., 1979, Studies on the disulfide bonds of glycoprotein hormones formation and properties of 11,35-Bis(Salkyl) derivatives of the alpha subunit, J. Biol. Chem. 254:1164.

Hamburger, C., 1957, The assay of gonadotropin hormones. A survey, Acta Endocrinol. (Suppl.) 31:59.

Hamlett, G. W. D., 1937, Positive Friedman tests in the pregnant rhesus monkey, *Macaca mulatta*, Amer. J. Physiol. 118:664.

Haour, F., and Saxena, B. B., 1974, Detection of a gonadotropin in rabbit blastocyst before implantation, Science 185:444.

Haour, F., Tell, G., and Sanchez, P., 1976, Presence and assay of rat chorionic gonadotropin (rCG), C. R. Acad. Sci., Paris, Series D, 282:1183.

Hartley, B. S., 1970, Strategy and tactics in protein chemistry, Biochem. J. 119:805.

Hobson, B. M., and Wide, L., 1972, A comparison between chorionic gonadotropins extracted from human, rhesus monkey and marmoset placentae, J. Endocrinol. 55:363.

Isler, G. V., 1974, Purification de la gonadotrofina endometrial de yegua prenda, Acta Physiol. latinoam. 24:235.

Kessler, M. J., Mise, T., Ghai, R. D., and Bahl, O. P., 1979b, Structure and location of the O-glycosidic carbohydrate units of human chorionic gonadotropin, J. Biol. Chem. 254:7909.

Kessler, M. J., Reddy, M. S., Shah, R. H., Bahl, O. P., 1979a, Structures of N-glycosidic carbohydrate units of human chorionic gonadotropin, J. Biol. Chem. 254:7901.

Keutman, H., and Williams, R., 1977, Human chorionic gonadotropin amino acid sequence of the hormone-specific COOH-terminal region, J. Biol. Chem. 252:5393.

Lacroix, M. C., and Martal, J., 1979, Evidence and evolution of chorionic gonadotropin in ewes, C. R. Acad. Sci., Ser. D. 288:771.

Legault-Demare, J., and Clauser, H., 1961, Gonadotropine serique de jument gravide (PMSG), in *Etudes d'endocrinologie*, R. Courrier and M. Jutisz, eds., pp. 69-91, Hermann, Paris.

Leidenberger, F. L., and Reichert, L. E., 1972b, Evaluation of a rat testis homogenate radioligand receptor assay for human pituitary LH, Endocrinology 91:901.

Liu, W. K., Nahm, H. S., Sweeney, C. M., Lamkin, W. M., Baker, H. N., and Ward, D. N., 1972a, The primary structure of ovine luteinizing hormone. I. The amino acid sequence of the reduced and S-carboxymethylated S-subunit (LH-alpha), J. Biol. Chem. 247:4351.

Liu, W. K., Nahm, H. S., Sweeney, C. M., Holcomb, G. N., and Ward, D. N., 1972b, The primary structure of ovine luteinizing hormone. II. The amino acid sequence of the reduced, S-carboxymethylated A-subunit (LH-beta), J. Biol. Chem. 247-4365.

Liu, W. K., and Ward, D. N., 1975, The purification and chemistry of pituitary glycoprotein hormones, Pharmac. Therap. B. B., Vol. 1, 3:545.

Liu, W. K., Yang, K. P., Nakagawa, Y., and Ward, D. N., 1974, The role of the amino acid group in subunit association and receptor site interaction for ovine luteinizing hormone as studied by acylation, J. Biol. Chem. 249:5544.

Maghuin-Rogister, G., Combarnous Y., and Hennen, G., 1973, The primary structure of the porcine luteinizing hormone alpha-subunit, Eur. J. Biochem. 39:255.

Maghuin-Rogister, G. and Hennen, G., 1973, Luteinizing hormone: The primary structures of the beta-subunit from bovine and porcine species, Eur. J. Biochem. 39:235.

Martal, J., Lacroix, M. C., Loudes, C., Saunier, M., and Wintenberger-Torres, S., 1979, Trophoblastin an antiluteolytic protein present in early pregnancy in sheep, J. Reprod. Fert. 56:63.

Means, A. R., and Vaitukaitis, J., 1972, Peptide hormone "receptors": Specific binding of ^{3}H-FSH to testis, Endocrinology 90:39.

Moore, W. T., 1978, Biological and chemical characterization of pregnant mare serum gonadotropin-consideration of the origin of its two activities, Ph.D. dissertation, University of Texas Health Science Center at Houston Graduate School of Biomedical Sciences.

Moore, W. T., and Ward, D. N., 1980a, Pregnant mare serum gonadotropin: Rapid chromatographic procedures for the purification of intact hormone and isolation of subunits, submitted to J. Biol. Chem.

Moore, W. T., and Ward, D. N., 1980b, Pregnant mare serum gonadotropin: An in vitro biological characterization of the lutropin-follitropin dual activity, submitted to J. Biol. Chem.

Moore, W. T., Ward, D. N., and Burleigh, B. D., 1980, The amino acid sequence of the alpha subunit of pregnant mare serum gonadotropin, submitted to J. Biol. Chem.

Morgan, F. J., Birken, S., and Canfield, R. E., 1973, Human chorionic gonadotropin: A proposal for the amino acid sequence, Mol. Cell. Biochem. 2:97.

Morgan, F. J., Birken, S., and Canfield, R. E., 1975, The amino acid sequence of human chorionic gonadotropin: The alpha subunit and beta subunit, J. Biol. Chem. 250:5247.

Mori, K. F., Hum, V. G., Botting, H. G., 1977, Partial reduction with dithiothreitol of disulfide bonds in human chorionic gonadotropin, Molec. Cell. Endocrinol. 6:181.

Moyle, W. R., Erickson, G., Bahl, O. P., Christakos, S., and Gutowski, J., 1978, Action of PMSG and asialo-PMSG on rat Leydig and granulosa cells, Am. J. Physiol. 235:E218.

Moyle, W. R., and Ramachandran, J., 1973, Effect of LH on steroidogenesis and cyclic AMP accumulation in rat Leydig cell preparations and mouse tumor Leydig cells, Endocrinology 93:127.

Nuti, L. C., Grimek, H. J., Braselton, W. E., and McShan, W. H., 1972, Chemical properties of equine pituitary follicle-stimulating hormone, Endocrinology 91:1418.

Papkoff, H., Bewley, T. A., and Ramachandran, J., 1978, Physicochemical and biological characterization of pregnant mare serum gonadotropin and its subunits, Biochim. Biophys. Acta 532:185.

Papkoff, H., Farmer, S. W., and Cole, H. H., 1978, Isolation of a gonadotropin (PMEG) from pregnant mare endometrial cups: Comparison with PMSG, Proc. Soc. Exptl. Biol. Med. 158:373.

Pencharz, R. L., Cole, H. H., and Goss, H., 1940, Response of hypophysectomized rats to highly purified extracts of pregnant mare serum, Proc. Soc. Exptl. Biol. Med. 43:932.

Pierce, J. G., 1971, Eli Lilly Lecture. The subunits of pituitary thyrotropin--their relationship to other glycoprotein hormones, Endocrinology 89:1331.

Pierce, J. G., 1977, Structural homologies of glycoprotein hormones, Excerpta Med. Int. Congr. Ser., No. 403, Proceedings of the V. International Congress of Endocrinology, V. H. Janus, ed., Vol. 2, pp. 93-103, Excerpta Medica, Amsterdam.

Raacke, I. D., Lostroh, A. J., Boda, J. M., Li, C. H., 1957, Some aspects of the characterization of pregnant mare serum gonadotropin, Acta Endocrinol. 26:377.

Rathnam, P., Fujiki, Y., Landefeld, T. D., and Saxena, B. B., 1978, Isolation and amino acid sequence of the alpha subunit of follicle stimulating hormone from equine pituitary glands, J. Biol. Chem. 253:5355.

Rathnam, P., and Saxena, B. B., 1975, Primary amino acid sequence of follicle-stimulating hormone from human pituitary glands. I. Alpha subunit, J. Biol. Chem. 250:6735.

Reeve, J. R., Cheng, K. W., and Pierce, J. G., 1975, Partial reduction of disulfide bonds in the hormone-specific subunits of TSH and LH, Biochem. Biophys. Res. Commun. 67:149.

Reichert, L. E., and Bhalla, V. K., 1974, Development of a radioligand tissue receptor assay for human follicle-stimulating hormone, Endocrinology 94:483.

Rimington, C., and Rowlands, I. W., 1941, Serum gonadotropin. I. Preparation of a stable concentrate from pregnant mare's serum, Biochem. J. 35:736.

Robinson, A. B., McKerrow, J. H., and Cory, P., 1970, Controlled deamidation of peptides and proteins: An experimental hazard and a possible biological timer, Proceed. Natl. Acad. Sci. 66:753.

Robinson, A. B., and Rudd, C. J., 1974, Deamidation of glutaminyl and asparaginyl residues in peptides and proteins, in Current Topics in Cellular Regulation, B. L. Horecker and E. R. Stadtman, eds., Vol. 8, pp. 247-295.

Rowlands, I. W., 1949, Serum gonadotrophin and ovarian activity in the pregnant mare, J. Endocrinol. 6:184.

Rowson, L. E. A., and Moor, R. M., 1967, The influence of embryonic tissue homogenate infused into the uterus on life-span of the corpus luteum in the sheep, J. Reprod. Fert. 13:511.

Sairam, M. R., Papkoff, H., and Li, C. H., 1972, Human pituitary interstitial cell stimulating hormone: Primary structure of the subunit, Biochem. Biophys. Res. Commun. 48:530.

Saxena, B. B., and Rathnam, P., 1976, Amino acid sequence of the beta subunit of follicle stimulating hormone from human pituitary glands, J. Biol. Chem. 251:993.

Squires, E. L., and Ginther, O. J., 1975, Follicular and luteal development in pregnant mares. J. Reprod. Fert., Suppl. 23:429.

Stewart, F., Allen, W. R., and Moor, R. M., 1976, Pregnant mare serum gonadotrophin: Ratio of follicle-stimulating hormone and luteinizing hormone activities measured by radioreceptor assay, J. Endocrinol. 71:371.

Stewart, F., Allen, W. R., and Moor, R. M., 1977, Influence of foetal genotype on the follicle stimulating hormone: luteinizing hormne ratio of pregnant mare serum gonadotrophin, J. Endocrinol. 73: 419.

Stewart, M., and Stewart, F., 1977, Constant and variable regions in glycoprotein hormone beta subunit sequences: Implications for receptor binding specificity, J. Molec. Biol. 116:175.

Strickland, S., and Beers, W. H., 1976, Studies in the role of plasminogen activation in ovulation, J. Biol. Chem. 251:5694.

Tettamanti, G., and Pigman, W., 1968, Purification and characterization of bovine and ovine submaxillary mucins, Arch. Biochem. Biophys. 124:41.

Tsunasawa, S., Lou, W. K., Burleigh, B. D., and Ward, D. N., 1977, Studies of disulfide bond location in ovine lutropin beta subunit, Biochim. Biophys. Acta 492:340.

Van Wagenen, G., and Simpson, M. E., 1955, Gonadotrophic hormone excretion of the pregnant monkey (Macaca mulatta), Proc. Soc. Exptl. Biol. Med. 90:346.

Ward, D. N., 1978, Chemical approaches to the structure-function relationships of luteinizing hormone (lutropin), in Structure and Function of the Gonadotropins, K. W. McKerns, ed., pp. 31-4o, Plenum Press, New York.

Ward, D. N., and Liu, W. K., 1971, The chemistry of ovine and bovine luteinizing hormone, in Protein and Polypeptide Hormones, M. Margolies and F. C. Greenwood, eds., Part I, Ser. 241, pp. 80-90,

Wide, L. and Hobson, B., 1978, Chromatographic studies on a chorionic gonadotropic activity in the placenta of the rat, mouse, and hamster, Upsala J. Med. Sci. 83:1.

Wide, L., and Wide, M., 1979, Chorionic gonadotropin in the mouse from implantation to term, J. Reprod. Fert. 57:5.

Wide, M., and Wide, L., 1963, Diagnosis of pregnancy in mares by an immunological method, Nature, Lond. 198:1017.

STRUCTURES OF THE ASPARAGINE-LINKED SUGAR CHAINS OF

HUMAN CHORIONIC GONADOTROPIN

Yoshinori Endo, Yoshihiko Ashitaka, Akira Kobata,
and Shimpei Tojo

Department of Obstetrics and Gynecology and
Department of Biochemistry, Kobe University
School of Medicine, Ikuta-ku, Kobe, Japan

INTRODUCTION

From the viewpoint of the physiological function of the carbohydrate moieties of glycoproteins, glycohormones and glycoenzymes
are of current interest. These molecules have sugar components
widely found in all glycoproteins.

The structure of human chorionic gonadotropin (hCG) has
been thoroughly studied by many workers (Bell et al., 1969; Bahl,
1969a; Bahl, 1969b; Swaminathan and Bahl, 1970; Merz et al., 1974).
It is composed of α-subunit (MW=14,000) and β-subunit (MW=24,000).
Both subunits contain more than 30% of carbohydrate. The linear
amino acid sequences of α- and β-subunits were determined by two
research groups (Bellisario et al., 1973; Carlsen et al., 1973;
Morgan et al., 1975). Both subunits contain two asparagine-linked
sugar chains. In addition, β-subunit also contains four serine-
linked sugar chains. The structures of two different asparagine-
linked sugar chains of hCG was proposed by Bahl (1969b). However,
the structures were attained only by sequential exoglycosidase
digestion, and no methylation analysis was performed. Since there
are several evidences (Moyle et al., 1975) indicating the important
roles of asparagine-linked sugar chains for the display of biological
activities of hCG, it is an urgent need to elucidate the complete
structures of the sugar chains of hCG.

We have recently used hydrazinolysis for the quantitative
release of the asparagine-linked sugar chains of Clq subcomponent
of the first component of human complement (Mizuochi et al., 1978).
This method was also successfully applied to the purified hCG for

the liberation of asparagine-linked sugar chains. This paper describes the fractionation and the structural studies of each oligosaccharide liberated from hCG.

EXPERIMENTAL PROCEDURES

Purification of HCG

One hundred milligrams of commercial hCG (3000 IU/mg) which was purchased from Mochida Pharmaceutical Co., Ltd., Tokyo, was freed from human chorionic thyroid stimulating hormone (TSH) by passing through a column of carboxymethyl cellulose which was equilibrated by 0.01 M ammonium acetate buffer, pH 6.0. The hCG in the unadsorbed fraction was further purified by the method of Ashitaka et al. (1970).

The final yield of pure hCG (specific activity = 15,000 IU/mg) was 11 mg. The preparation gave a slightly broad single band, which was stainable with both coomassie blue and with periodate-Schiff reagent, by SDS disc gel electrophoresis using 7.5% gel concentration.

Liberation of the Asparagine-linked Sugar Chains from HCG by Hydrazinolysis

Ten milligrams of the hCG was heated in 0.3 ml of anhydrous hydrazine in a sealed tube at 100°C for 20 hr. The reaction mixture was then evaporated to dryness under reduced pressure over concentrated H_2SO_4. The residue was freed from hydrazine by repeated evaporation with toluene, and dried in a dessicator over concentrated H_2SO_4 overnight. The residue was dissolved in saturated $NaHCO_3$ solution and all free primary amino groups in the residue were completely acetylated with acetic anhydride. The reaction mixture was passed through a column (6 ml) of Bio-Rad AG-50 (H^+) and the column washed with 5 bed volumes of distilled water. The eluate and washings were combined and evaporated to dryness. The residue was then dissolved in a small amount of water and spotted on a sheet of paper. The paper was developed with solvent II for two days in order to remove the degradation products from peptide moiety. The area corresponding 0-5 cm from origin was cut and oligosaccharides were recovered by elution with water.

Gel Permeation Chromatography

Bio-Gel P-4 (under 400 mesh) column chromatography was performed using the column (2 x 200 cm) equipped with water jacket. During operation the column was kept at 55°C by circulating warm water in the jacket. Differential refractometer R-403 (Waters Associated, Inc., Framingham, Mass.) was used for monitoring the standard mixture that eluted from the column. Glucose oligomers were used as standards. (In Bio-Gel P-4 column chromatography, fucose and N-acetylglucosamine residues behave as 1.2 and 2.0 glucose units, respectively.)

Paper Chromatography and Paper Electrophoresis

Descending paper chromatography was performed using ethylacetate/pyridine/acetic acid/water (5:5:1:3) and n-butanol/ethanol/water (4:1:1). High voltage paper electrophoresis was performed using pyridine/acetate buffer, pH 5.4 (pyridine/acetic acid/water, 3:1:387).

Chemicals and Enzymes

NaB^3H_4 (154 mCi/mmole) was purchased from New England Nuclear, Boston, Mass. $NaBD_4$ (98%) was purchased from Merck Co., Inc., Darmstadt, and sialidase purified from *Arthrobacter ureafaciens* was purchased from Nakarai Chemicals, Ltd., Kyoto. α-Mannosidase (Li and Li, 1972), β-galactosidase (Arakawa et al., 1974) and β-N-acetylhexosaminidase (Li and Li, 1972) were purified from jack bean meal according to the cited references. Snail β-mannosidase, *Charonia lampas* α-L-fucosidase and endo-β-N-acetylglucosaminidase D were kindly supplied by Seikagaku Kogyo Co. One unit of glycosidase was defined as the amount of the enzyme required to hydrolyze 1 μmole of the substrate per min.

Exoglycosidase Digestion of Tritium-labeled Oligosaccharides

Sugar samples (4-7 x 10^4 cpm, 2-3.5 nmole) were incubated with one of the following mixtures at 37°C for 18 hr, unless otherwise specified: β-galactosidase digestion enzyme (100 milli-unit) in 0.05 M sodium-citrate buffer, pH 4.0 (170 μl); β-N-acetylhexosaminidase digestion enzyme (100 milli-unit) in 0.05 M sodium-citrate buffer, pH 4.0 (170 μl); α-mannosidase digestion enzyme (200 milli-unit) in 0.05 M sodium-acetate buffer, pH 4.5 (170 μl); β-mannosidase digestion enzyme (75 milli-unit) in 0.05 M sodium-citrate buffer, pH 5.0 (170 μl); α-L-fucosidase digestion enzyme (50 milli-unit) in 0.05 M sodium-citrate buffer, pH 4.0 (170 μl). To all reaction mixtures 1 drop of toluene was added to inhibit bacterial growth. Reactions were terminated by heating the reaction mixture in a boiling water bath for two minutes.

Methylation Analysis

Oligosaccharide (50-100 μg) reduced with $NaBD_4$ was dissolved
in 0.1 ml of dimethylsulfoxide and methylated with 0.1 ml each of
sodium methylsulfinyl carbanion and methyliodide (Hakomori, 1964).
The permethylated sugar was recovered by extracting the reaction
mixture twice with 3 ml each of chloroform and the combined solution
was washed with 6 ml of H_2O for three times. The chloroform solution was applied to a column of silica gel (0.5 x 3 cm). The column
was washed with 6 ml of chloroform to remove the contaminating
reagents and the permethylated product was eluted from the column
with 6 ml of methanol. This procedure was performed at 25-30°C.
The solution was evaporated to dryness and the residue was mixed
thoroughly with 0.1 ml of 93% acetic acid containing 0.5 N H_2SO_4 by
stirring at room temperature for 2 hr. The mixture was then heated
at 76°C for 2 hr to hydrolize the permethylated sugar. The hydrolysate was passed through a small column (0.5 x 3 cm) of Bio-Rad
AG-3 (acetate form) and the column was washed with 5 bed volumes of
methanol. Eluate and washing were combined and evaporated to dryness.
The residue was dissolved in 0.5 ml of H_2O containing 5 mg of $NaBH_4$
and the solution was left at room temperature for 3 hr to convert
the methylated sugars to methylated alditols. The reduction was
terminated by adding 1 drop of glacial acetic acid. Methanol (3 ml)
was added and the solution was evaporated to dryness. Addition of
3 ml of methanol and evaporation was repeated two more times to
remove boric acid completely. The residue was dried over P_2O_5 in
vacuo for 1 hr. dissolved in 0.5 ml of acetic anhydride, and heated
at 100°C for 4 hr. Solvent was removed from the reaction mixture
by repeated evaporation with toluene, and the residue was dissolved
in 3 ml of chloroform. After being washed twice with 3 ml of water,
the chloroform layer was dehydrated by adding anhydrous Na_2SO_4 and
evaporated to dryness. Analysis of the partially O-methylated
alditol acetates and sialic acids was performed with a gas chromatography-mass spectrometer, model LKB 9000 (Shimazu-LKB Instrument,
Ltd.), using a glass column (3 mm x 1.0 m) of 2% OV-17 coated on
Gas-Chrom Q (80-100 mesh). The temperature was programmed from
150-260°C at a rate of 4°/min. Conditions for the mass spectrometry
were: ion source temperature, 290°C; ionizing potential, 20 eV; and
trap current, 60 μA.

Analytical Methods

Sugar composition was determined by the radioelectrophoretic
method (Takasaki and Kobata, 1978). Radioactivity was determined
with Packard Tri-Carb liquid scintillation spectrometer. Radiochromatogram scanning was performed with a Packard radiochromatogram
scanner model 7210. Radioactivity on paper was determined after
incubation of the paper pieces with 1 ml of water in the counting
vials and addition of 7 ml of scintillation fluid. Discrimination

of N-acetyl- and N-glycolylneuraminic acids were performed by the methylation analysis, as reported by Rauvala and Karkkäinen (1977).

Oligosaccharides

$Man\alpha1\rightarrow6(Man\alpha1\rightarrow3)Man\beta1\rightarrow4GlcNAc\beta1\rightarrow4(Fuc\alpha1\rightarrow6)GlcNAc_{OT}$ ($Man_3 \cdot GlcNAc \cdot Fuc \cdot GlcNAc_{OT}$)* was isolated by hydrazinolysis followed by N-acetylation and NaB^3H_4 reduction of $Man\alpha1\rightarrow6(Man\alpha1\rightarrow3)Man\beta1\rightarrow4GlcNAc\beta1\rightarrow4(Fuc\alpha1\rightarrow6)GlcNAc$ Asn peptide. The glycopeptide was obtained from bovine IgG glycopeptide by digestion with a mixture of β-galactosidase and β-N-acetylhexosaminidase.

$Man\beta1\rightarrow4GlcNAc\beta1\rightarrow4(Fuc\alpha1\rightarrow6)GlcNAc_{OT}$ was obtained by α-mannosidase digestion of $Man_3 \cdot GlcNAc \cdot Fuc \cdot GlcNAc_{OT}$. $GlcNAc\beta1\rightarrow4(Fuc\alpha1\rightarrow6)GlcNAc_{OT}$ was obtained by digesting $Man\beta1\rightarrow4GlcNAc\beta1\rightarrow4(Fuc\alpha1\rightarrow6)GlcNAc_{OT}$ with β-mannosidase. $GlcNAc\beta1\rightarrow4GlcNAc_{OT}$ was prepared by reduction of N,N'-diacetylchitobiose with NaB^3H_4. $Fuc\alpha1\rightarrow6GlcNAc_{OT}$ was prepared by NaB^3H_4 reduction of $Fuc\alpha1\rightarrow6GlcNAc$ isolated from the urine of a fucosidosis patient. Glucose oligomers were obtained by partial acid hydrolysis of dextran. $Gal\beta1\rightarrow4GlcNAc\beta1\rightarrow2Man\alpha1\rightarrow6(Gal\beta1\rightarrow4GlcNAc\beta1\rightarrow2Man\alpha1\rightarrow3)Man\beta1\rightarrow4GlcNAc_{OT}$ was obtained by sialidase digestion of a mixture of $NeuAc\alpha2\rightarrow3$ and $6Gal\beta1\rightarrow4GlcNAc\beta1\rightarrow2Man\alpha1\rightarrow6(NeuAc\alpha2\rightarrow3$ and $6Gal\beta1\rightarrow4GlcNAc\beta1\rightarrow2Man\alpha1\rightarrow3)Man\beta1\rightarrow4GlcNAc_{OT}$ isolated from urine of I-cell disease patients.

RESULTS

Liberation of the Asparagine-linked Sugar Chains of HCG

The asparagine-linked sugar chains were liberated from 10 mg of purified hCG as described in Experimental Procedures.

One tenth aliquot of the oligosaccharide fraction was reduced with 2 μmole (0.6 mCI) of NaB^3H_4 in 150 μl of 0.05 N NaOH at 30°C for 4 hr. Five milligrams of $NaBH_4$ in 50 μl of 0.05 N NaOH was added and the incubation was continued for another 2 hr to ensure the reducing reaction. The remaining 9/10 of the oligosaccharide fraction was reduced with 50 mg of $NaBD_4$ in 1.3 ml of 0.05 N NaOH under the same conditions as in the case of NaB^3H_4. The reaction was stopped by adjusting the pH of the reaction mixture to 4.0 with 1 N CH_3COOH. The mixtures were then passed through a small column (6 ml bed volume) of Bio-Rad AG 50 (H^+), and the columns were washed with 5 bed volumes of distilled water. Eluate and washings were combined and evaporated to dryness under reduced pressure. The

---

*Subscript OT indicates NaB^3H_4-reduced oligosaccharides. In the same way, OH indicates $NaBD_4$-reduced oligosaccharides. All sugars have D configuration except for fucose which has an L configuration.

residues were freed from boric acid by repeated evaporation with methanol. The residues from both NaB^3H_4 and $NaBD_4$ reductions were separately dissolved into a small amount of water and spotted on a sheet of Whatman No. 3MM paper, side by side. The paper was then subjected to paper chromatography using solvent II for two days. The area of the radioactive sample was cut and subjected to radiochromato-scanning. The major radioactive peak detected close to the origin was eluted with water. This procedure is indispensable to remove the radioactive contaminants originated from NaB^3H_4 which moved quite a distance by the chromatographic development. The yield of the radioactive oligosaccharides was 2.0×10^6 cpm. Materials which remained at the origin of the paper of deuterium labeled sample were also eluted with water. For facilitating the detection of oligosaccharides in further purification procedures, 1.8×10^5 cpm of the radioactive oligosaccharides mixture was added to the deuterium-labeled sample.

Reducing Termini of the Oligosaccharides

Aliquot (3×10^4 cpm) of the radioactive oligosaccharide was hydrolyzed in 0.4 ml of 4 N HCl at 100°C for 2 hr, and the reaction mixture was freed from acid by repeated evaporation with water. The hydrolysate was N-acetylated and analyzed by paper electrophoresis using borate buffer, as reported by Takasaki and Kobata (1978). Only N-acetylglucosaminitol was detected as a radioactive component. This result indicated that the reducing termini of all oligosaccharides released by hydrazinolysis from hCG were N-acetylglucosamine. Part of the N-acetylglycosamine residues at the reducing termini were converted to an unknown sugar which moved together with N-acetylglusaminitol in this chromatographic system. This unknown sugar which is probably formed by the side reaction of the hydrazinolysis was not detected as 1,5-O-methylated derivative of N-acetylglucosaminitol in methylation analysis (vide infra).

Fractionation of Oligosaccharides by their Anionic Charges

One half of both radioactive and deuterium-labeled samples were spotted on Whatman No. 3MM paper in series, and the paper was subjected to paper electrophoresis at pH 5.4. As shown in Figure 1A, two acidic oligosaccharide groups (A-I and A-II) were detected. The shape of each radioactive peak was very broad, indicating that both A-I and A-II were mixtures of several oligosaccharides. These two components were recovered from paper by elution with water. The yield of radioactive A-I and A-II was 4.3×10^5 cpm each. The amounts of deuterium-labeled A-I and A-II, calculated on the basis of the specific radioactivities, were 194 nmole each. When half aliquots of radioactive A-I and A-II were digested with sialidase, they were completely converted to neutral oligosaccharides (Figure

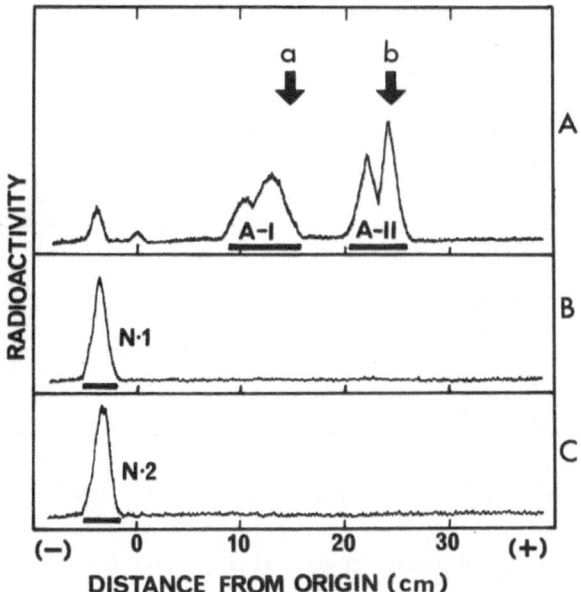

Figure 1. Radio-electrophoretogram of the oligosaccharides liberated from hCG by hydrazinolysis. After reduction with NaB^3H_4, the oligosaccharide mixture was subjected to paper electrophoresis at pH 5.4, 80 V/cm for 90 min (A). Arrows indicate the positions where standard sialyl oligosaccharides migrated: a, monosialyl lacto-N-hexaitol; b, 3'-sialyllactitol. The radioactive components in A-I and A-II of (A) were recovered, subjected to sialidase digestion (50 milli-units of sialidase in 10 µl of 0.15 M citrate-phosphate buffer, pH 5.0 for 20 hr), and again examined by paper electrophoresis. The resulting radiochromatograms are shown in (B) and (C), respectively.

1B and C). These results indicated that the acidic nature of these oligosaccharides originated in their sialic acid residues. By a shorter (5 hr) sialidase treatment in which part of the original A-I and A-II still remained, A-II gave another acidic component with the same paper electrophoretic mobility as A-I, while A-I gave only the neutral product (data not shown). These results indicated that A-II contains two sialic acid residues and A-I has one sialic acid residue. The sialic acid released from both A-I and A-II by siali-dase digestion were N-acetylneuraminic acid and no N-glycolylneura-minic acid was detected by gas chromatography (data not shown).

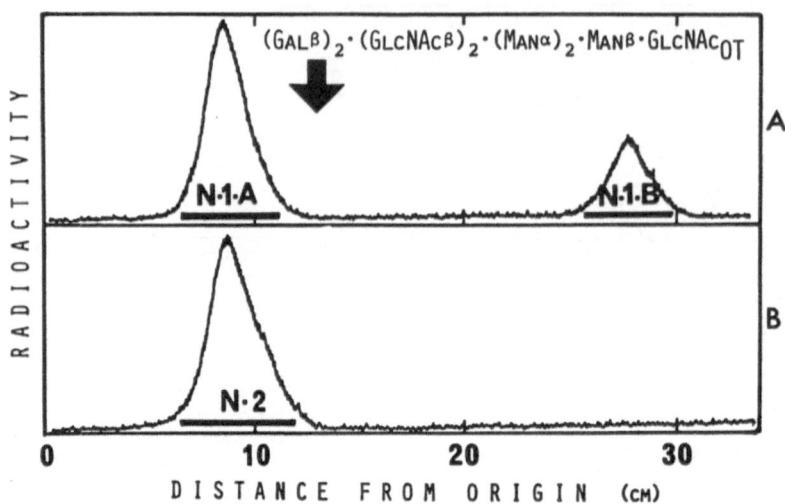

Figure 2.   The paper chromatograms of N-1 and N-2.   Peaks indicated
by bars in Figure 1B and 1C were recovered by elution with water and
subjected to paper chromatography using solvent I for 7 days.
A, fraction N-1; B, fraction N-2.   Arrow at the top indicates the
position where standard Galβ1$\rightarrow$4GlcNAcβ1$\rightarrow$2Manα1$\rightarrow$6(Galβ1$\rightarrow$4GlcNAcβ1$\rightarrow$
2Manα1$\rightarrow$3)Manβ1$\rightarrow$4GlcNAc$_{OT}$ moved.

Paper Chromatography of the Neutral Oligosaccharides N-1 and N-2

When N-1 and N-2 recovered from paper electrophoretograms (Figure
1B and 1C) were subjected to paper chromatography, N-1 gave two
radioactive peaks (Figure 2A), while N-2 gave a single radioactive
peak (Figure 2B).   These two peaks were named N-1-A and N-1-B.   N-1-A
showed the same mobility as N-2; these are smaller than authentic
Galβ1$\rightarrow$4GlcNAcβ1$\rightarrow$2Manα1$\rightarrow$6(Galβ1$\rightarrow$4GlcNAcβ1$\rightarrow$2Manα1$\rightarrow$3)Manβ1$\rightarrow$4GlcNAc$_{OT}$.
These three radioactive components were recovered from paper.
The yields of the three components were: N-1-A, 1.2 x 10^5 cpm;
N-1-B, 5.2 x 10^4 cpm; and N-2, 2.0 x 10^5 cpm.

Deutrium-labeled three oligosaccharides were also obtained by
the same process as in the case of radioactive sugars.   The amounts
recovered were: N-1-A, 53.8 nmole; N-1-B, 22.6 nmole; and N-2, 96.3
nmole.

Carbohydrate compositions of the three oligasaccharides were
determined by using deutrium-labeled samples.   Since these samples
were already reduced with NaBD, the N-acetylglucosamine residues

Table I. Monosaccharide composition of oligosaccharides N-I-A, N-I-B and N-2

Oligosaccharides	Molar ratio^a			
	Galactose	Fucose	Mannose	N-Acetylglucosamine
N-I-A	2.2	0.4	3.0	3.1 (4)
N-I-B	0.9	0	3.0	2.1 (3)
N-2	2.0	0.5	3.0	2.9 (4)

a) Values were calculated by taking the values of mannose as 3.0. Numbers in parentheses are the integers corrected for 1 mol of N-acetylglucosamine located at the reducing termini.

located at the reducing termini of three oligosaccharides could not be detected by the analysis. Therefore, the values of glucosamine in Table I were 1 mole less than the actual numbers. The corrected numbers are shown in parentheses. N-1-A and N-2 gave the same monosaccharide ratio.

Structure of Oligosaccharides N-1-A and N-2

Since these two oligosaccharides gave the same results, only the data of N-1-A will be documented below.

The Bio-Gel P-4 filtration pattern of N-1-A indicated that it was still a mixture of oligosaccharides hardly separable from each other (Figure 3A). When the radioactive N-1-A was incubated with β-galactosidase, it was completely converted to a new mixture of smaller oligosaccharides (Figure 3B). That the two new radioactive peaks eluted at the positions two glucose units smaller than the original N-1-A indicated that two galactose residues were removed from oligosaccharides in the N-1-A fraction by this enzymatic digestion.

The original N-1-A was resistant to β-N-acetylhexosaminidase treatment (data not shown), while the β-galactosidase digest liberated two N-acetylglucosamine residues by β-N-acetylhexosaminidase digestion (Figure 3C). The radioactive peak I showed the same mobility as authentic $Man_3 \cdot GlcNAc \cdot Fuc \cdot GlcNAc_{OT}$. Peaks I and II were separately collected as indicated by bars in Figure 3C. Both peaks I and II liberated two mannosyl residues by α-mannosidase digestion (Figure 3D). The product from peak I showed the same mobility as authentic $Man\beta1{\rightarrow}4GlcNAc\beta1{\rightarrow}4(Fuc\alpha1{\rightarrow}6)GlcNAc_{OT}$. When these two α-mannosidase digests were incubated with β-mannosidase, one mannose residue was released from both oligosaccharides (Figure 3E). The product of peak I series showed the same mobility as authentic $GlcNA\beta1{\rightarrow}4(Fuc\alpha1{\rightarrow}6)GlcNAc_{OT}$, and that of peak II series as authentic $GlcNAc\beta1{\rightarrow}4GlcNAc_{OT}$. These two products obtained by β-mannosidase digestion were then converted to a diitol with the same mobility as authentic $Fuc\alpha1{\rightarrow}6GlcNAc_{OT}$ and N-acetylglucosaminitol, respectively, by β-N-acetylhexosaminidase digestion (Figure 3F). α-fucosidase treatment converted the radioactive diitol to N-acetylglucosaminitol (Figure 3G). A series of the results described above indicated that N-1-A was a mixture of almost equal amounts of $(Gal\beta{\rightarrow}GlcNAc\beta{\rightarrow}Man\alpha{\rightarrow})_2Man\beta{\rightarrow}GlcNAc\beta{\rightarrow}(Fuc\alpha{\rightarrow})GlcNAc_{OT}$ and $(Gal\beta{\rightarrow}GlcNAc\beta{\rightarrow}Man\alpha{\rightarrow})_2Man\beta{\rightarrow}GlcNAc\beta{\rightarrow}GlcNAc_{OT}$, and the radioactive peak which moved faster in Figure 3A was the fucose-containing oligosaccharide. In order to determine the location of each glycosidic linkage of these two oligosaccharides, N-1-A was subjected to methylation analysis (Table II). The N-acetylglucosamines that are located at the reducing termini of oligosaccharides in N-1-A should be detected as 1,5-$\underline{O}$-methylated derivatives. Detection of 1,3,5,6-tetra-$\underline{O}$-methyl-

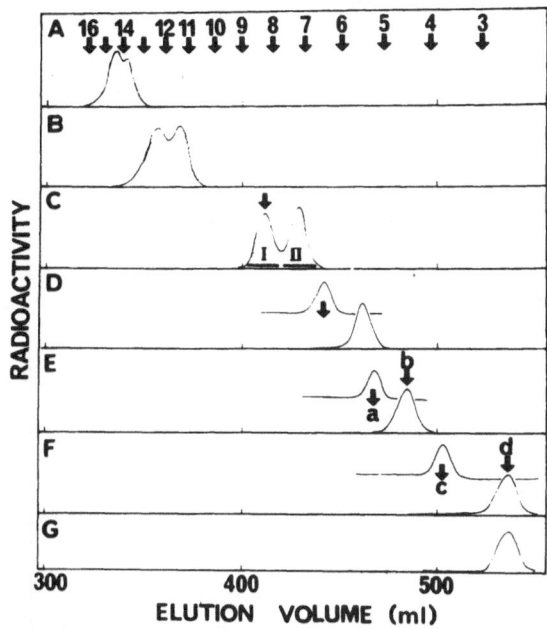

Figure 3. Sequential exoglycosidase digestion of oligosaccharide N-1-A. The radioactive sugars were subjected to Bio-Gel P-4 column chromatography and the radioactivity in each tube (3.4 ml per tube) was determined by liquid scintillation spectrometer. The arrows at the top of the figure indicate the eluting positions of glucose oligomers (numbers indicate the glucose units). A, intact oligosaccharide N-1-A; B, oligosaccharide N-1-A incubated with β-galactosidase; C, the radioactive peaks in B were digested with β-N-acetylhexosaminidase and the arrow indicates the position where authentic $Man_3 \cdot GlcNAc \cdot Fuc \cdot GlcNAc_{OT}$ eluted. In D-F, the upper radioactive patterns indicate the results of sequential exoglycosidase digestion of the peak I and the lower patterns indicate those of the peak II in C. D, the radioactive peaks in C were treated with α-mannosidase and the arrow indicates the position where authentic $Man\beta1 \rightarrow 4GlcNAc\beta1 \rightarrow 4(Fuc\alpha1 \rightarrow 6)GlcNAc_{OT}$ eluted; E, the radioactive peaks in D digested with β-mannosidase and the arrows a and b indicate the eluting positions of authentic $GlcNAc\beta1 \rightarrow 4(Fuc\alpha1 \rightarrow 6)GlcNAc_{OT}$ and $GlcNAc\beta1 \rightarrow 4GlcNAc_{OT}$, respectively; F, the radioactive peaks in E were treated with β-N-acetylhexosaminidase and the arrows c and d indicate the eluting positions of authentic $Fuc\alpha1 \rightarrow 6GlcNAc_{OT}$ and N-acetylglucosaminitol, respectively; G, the upper peak in F was digested with α-L-fucosidase.

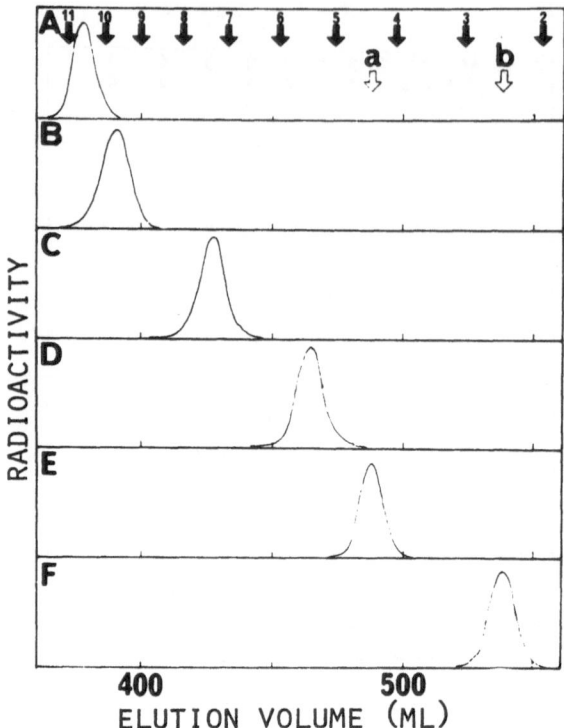

Figure 4.   Sequential exoglycosidase digestion of N-1-B.   The
radioactive oligosaccharide N-1-B and it enzymatic digestion
products were subjected to Bio-Gel P-4 column chromatographic
analysis as in the case in Figure 3.   The black arrows indicate the
eluting positions of glucose oligomers (numbers indicate the glucose
units), and white arrows a and b indicate those of standard
GlcNAcβ1→4GlcNAc$_{OT}$ and N-acetylglucosaminitol, respectively.
A, intact oligosaccharide N-1-B; B, oligosaccharide N-1-B incubated
with β-galactosidase; C, the radioactive peak in B digested with
β-N-acetylhexosaminidase; D, the radioactive peak in C digested
with α-mannosidase; E, the radioactive peak in D incubated with
β-mannosidase; F, the radioactive peak in E digested with β-N-
acetylhexosaminidase.

2-N-methylacetamido-2-deoxyglucitol acetate indicated that both
oligosaccharides in N-1-A contain N,N'-diacetylchitobiose structure at their reducing termini and the fucose-containing oligosaccharide has its fucose at the C-6 position of the proximal N-
acetylglucosamine residue.   The poor recovery (0.6 total molar
ratios of N-1-A) of the 1,5-O- methyl derivatives may reflect the

N-1-A and N-2

$Fuc\alpha 1$
$\downarrow$
6
$Gal\beta 1 \rightarrow 4GlcNAc\beta 1 \rightarrow 2Man\alpha 1$
$_6 Man\beta 1 \rightarrow 4GlcNAc\beta 1 \rightarrow 4GlcNAc_{OH}$
$Gal\beta 1 \rightarrow 4GlcNAc\beta 1 \rightarrow 2Man\alpha 1^{3}$

$Gal\beta 1 \rightarrow 4GlcNAc\beta 1 \rightarrow 2Man\alpha 1$
$_6 Man\beta 1 \rightarrow 4GlcNAc\beta 1 \rightarrow 4GlcNAc_{OH}$
$Gal\beta 1 \rightarrow 4GlcNAc\beta 1 \rightarrow 2Man\alpha 1^{3}$

N-1-B

$Man\alpha 1$
$_6 Man\beta 1 \rightarrow 4GlcNAc\beta 1 \rightarrow 4GlcNAc_{OH}$
$Gal\beta 1 \rightarrow 4GlcNAc\beta 1 \rightarrow 2Man\alpha 1^{3}$

Figure 5.   Proposed structures of the neutral oligosaccharides
(N-1-A, N-1-B, and N-2) liberated from A-1 and A-II by sialidase
digestion.

results of modification of the N-acetylglucosamine residue at the
reducing terminal by hydrazinolysis (see Discussion). In any event,
complete absence of other 1,5-O-methyl derivatives rule out the
possibility of other fucosyl linkages. All other intra-chain N-
acetylglucosamine residues should be substituted at C-4 position
because only 3,6-di-O-methyl-2-N-methylacetamido-2-deoxyglucitol
acetate was detected. By combining the data of the methylation
analysis with the sequential exoglycosidase digestion, the complete
structures of 2-oligosaccharides in N-1-A were proposed as shown in
Figure 5.

Structure of Oligosaccharide N-1-B

     One galactose was removed from N-1-B by β-galactosidase digestion
(Figure 4B). No degradation occurred when intact N-1-B was incubated
with β-N-acetylhexosaminidase, but after removal of one galactose,
one β-N-acetylhexosamine became removable by β-N-acetylhexosaminidase
digestion (Figure 4C). This product then released two mannosyl
residues after α-mannosidase digestion (Figure 4D). This radioactive
product was then converted to a diitol with the same mobility as
authentic $GlcNAc\beta 1 \rightarrow 4GlcNAc_{OT}$, releasing one mannose residue after

TABLE II: Molar ratio of alditol acetates obtained from hydrolysates of permethylated oligosaccharides.

	Acidic Oligo saccharides mixture	Molar ratio[a]			
		N-1-A	N-1-B	N-2	

Fucitol

2,3,4-Tri-O-methyl-(1,5-di-O-acetyl) | + | 0.5 | - | 0.5 |

Galactitol

2,3,4,6-Tetra-O-methyl-(1,5-di-O-acetyl) | + | 2.0 | 1.0 | 2.1 |
2,4,6-Tri-O-methyl-(1,3,5-tri-O-acetyl) | + | - | - | - |

Mannitol

2,3,4,6-Tetra-O-methyl-(1,5-di-O-acetyl) | + | - | 1.1 | - |
3,4,6-Tri-O-methyl-(1,2,5-tri-O-acetyl) | + | 2.2 | 1.0 | 1.9 |
2,4-Di-O-methyl-(1,3,5,6-tri-O-acetyl) | + | 1.0 | 1.0 | 1.0 |

2-N-Methylacetamido-2-deoxyglucitol

1,3,5,6-Tetra-O-methyl-(4-mono-O-acetyl) | + | 0.2 | 0.4 | 0.3 |
1,3,5-Tri-O-methyl-(4,6-di-O-acetyl) | + | 0.4 | - | 0.5 |
3,6-Di-O-methyl-(1,4,5-tri-O-acetyl) | + | 2.7 | 2.8 | 2.8 |

a) Values were calculated by making the values of 2,4-di-O-methylmannitol as 1.0.

β-mannosidase digestion (Figure 4E). The radioactive diitol was then converted to N-acetylglucosaminitol by β-N-acetylhexosaminidase digestion (Figure 4F). In order to confirm whether the two mannose residues released by α-mannosidase digestion were arranged in linear or parallel fashion, intact N-1-B was digested with α-mannosidase. One mannose was released by this digestion, indicating that one mannose residue occurs as a non-reducing terminal in this oligosaccharide (data not shown). These results indicate that the monosaccharide sequence and the anomeric configuration of N-1-B is Gal$\beta\rightarrow$GlcNAc$\beta\rightarrow$Man$\alpha\rightarrow$(Man$\alpha\rightarrow$)[Man$\beta\rightarrow$GlcNAcβ1$\rightarrow$4GlcNAc$_{OT}$].

The data of methylation analysis is shown in Table II. Allowing for the low yield of 1,3,5,6-tetra-$\underline{O}$-methyl-2-N-methylacetamide-2-deoxygluctitol acetates, two possible structures can be considered: Galβ1$\rightarrow$4GlcNAcβ1$\rightarrow$2Manα1$\rightarrow$3 or 6(Manα1$\rightarrow$6 or 3)Manβ1$\rightarrow$4GlcNAcβ1$\rightarrow$4GlcNAc$_{OT}$. When N-1-B (4 x 10^4 cpm) was incubated with 0.20 unit of endo-β-N-acetylglucosaminidase D in 50 μl of 0.1 M citrate-phosphate buffer, pH 6.0 at 37°C for 40 hours, no release of radioactive N-acetylglucosaminitol was observed. Under the same condition, Galβ1$\rightarrow$4GlcNAcβ1$\rightarrow$2Manα1$\rightarrow$6(Manα1$\rightarrow$3)Manβ1$\rightarrow$4GlcNAcβ1$\rightarrow$4GlcNAc$_{OT}$ obtained from Clq subcomponent of the first complement was completely hydrolyzed into Galβ1$\rightarrow$4GlcNAcβ1$\rightarrow$2Manα1$\rightarrow$6(Manα1$\rightarrow$3)Manβ1$\rightarrow$4GlcNAc and [^{3}H]N-acetylglucosaminitol (11). Therefore, the only possible structure of N-1-B is as shown in Figure 5.

The Location of N-Acetylneuraminic Acid in the Asparagine-Linked Sugar Chains of HCG

In order to obtain a rough insight of the location of N-acetylneuraminic acids in the sugar chains, the mixture of acidic oligosaccharides released from hCG by hydrazinolysis was subjected to methylation analysis. As shown in Table II, a substantial amount of 2,4,6-tri-$\underline{O}$-methylgalactitol acetate was detected together with partailly $\underline{O}$-methylated sugars obtained from oligosaccharides N-1-A, N-1-B, and N-2. No additional sugars were detected by this analysis. This result indicates that the N-acetylneuraminic acid in oligosaccharides A-I and A-II is linked at the C-3 postion of the terminal galactose.

Structures of Oligosaccharides A-I and A-II

Since A-II is a mixture of the disialyl derivatives of oligosaccharides N-2, the complete structures of the oligosaccharides in the A-II fraction should be as shown in Figure 7. A-I is a mixture of the monosialyl derivatives of N-1-A and N-1-B. Since N-1-B has only one terminal galactose residue, the structure can be proposed by assigning one N-acetylneuraminic acid residue at the C-3 position of this galactose (C in Figure 7). On the other hand, both oligo-

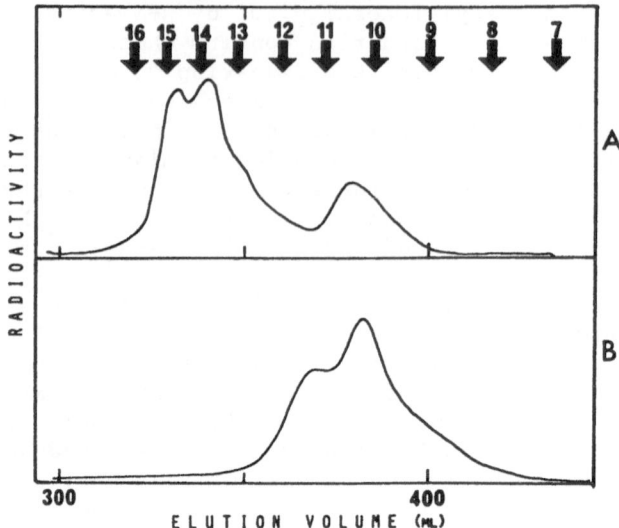

Figure 6.　　Gel permeation chromatogram of the radioactive neutral oligosaccharide mixture obtained from A-I fraction.　A, N-I fraction obtained by incubating A-I fraction (2×10^4 cpm) with 50 MU of sialidase in 10 µl of 0.15 M citrate-phosphate buffer, pH 5.0 for 20 hr; B, the racioactive neutral oligosaccharide mixture obtained by a series of exoglycosidase digestions as follows: A-I fraction (4×10^4 cpm) was incubated with a mixture of β-galactosidase (2.1 unit) and β-N-acetyl-hexosaminidase (2.4 unit) in 90 µl of 0.05 M citrate-phosphate buffer, pH 4.0 for 20 hr.　The reaction mixture was passed through a small column of Bio-Rad AG-50 (H^+) and the column was washed with three bed volumes of water.　The eluate and washing were combined and evaporated to dryness.　The residue was then incubated with 50 MU of sialidase in 0.15 M citrate-phosphate buffer, pH 5.0, for 20 hr.　Arrows at the top indicate the eluting positions of glucose oligomers (numbers indicate the glucose units).

saccharides in the N-1-A fraction have two terminal galactoses (Figure 5).　Studies were undertaken to establish which of these galactoses is substituted by N-acetylneuraminic acid.　By gel permeation chromatography, N-1 gave the elution pattern shown in Figure 6A.　However, when the radioactive A-I was pretreated with a mixture of β-galactosidase and β-N-acetylhexosaminidase and then desialized by incubation with sialidase, it gave the Bio-Gel P-4 elution pattern shown in Figure 6B.　That the two major peaks in Figure 6B eluted approximately three glucose units slower than the two major peaks in Figure 6A indicates that the Galβ→GlcNAc grouping unsubstituted by

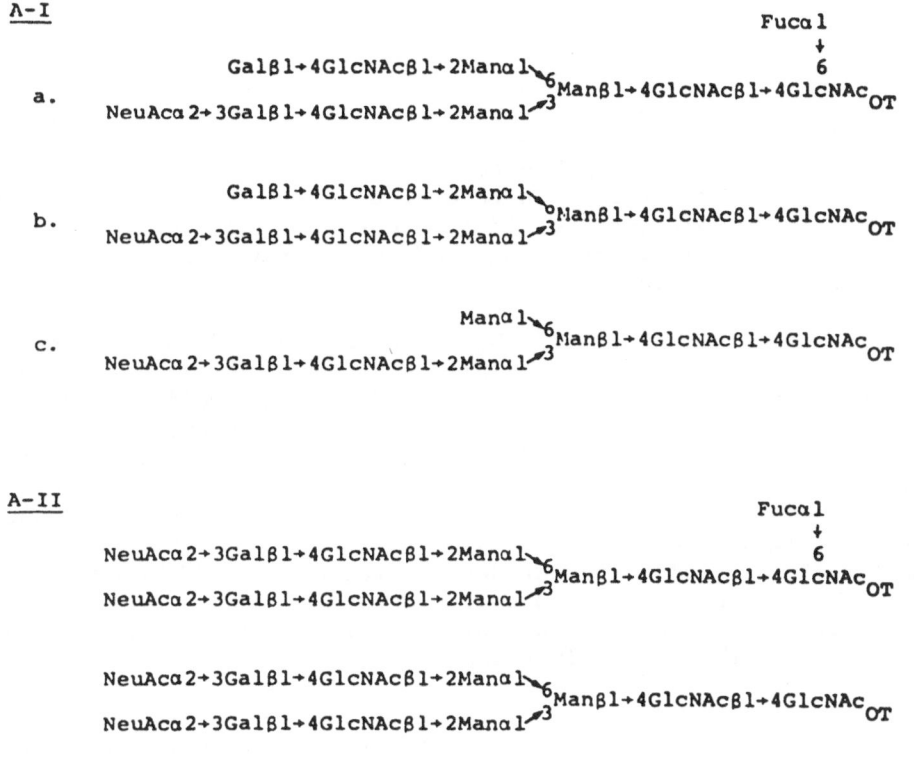

Figure 7. Proposed structures of oligosaccharides A-I and A-II.

N-acetylneuraminic acid was removed from A-I by the pretreatment with a mixture of β-galactosidase and β-N-acetylhexosaminidase. The radioactive oligosaccharides were pooled as indicated by a bar in Figure 6B and evaporated to dryness. The residue was then incubated with 0.1 unit of endo-β-N-acetylglucosaminidase D in 50 μl of 0.1 M citrate-phosphate buffer, pH 6.0, containing 20 μl of galactono-1,5-lactone at 37°C for 40 hr. The reaction mixture gave exactly the same elution pattern as Figure 6B by the gel permeation chromatography, and no release of radioactive N-acetylneuraminic acid residues in the A-I fraction are linked at the C-3 position of the galactose residue on the Manα1→3 side, protecting the Galβ1→4GlcNAc grouping from β-galactosidase and β-N-acetylhexosaminidase digestion. Therefore, the structure of the two remaining oligosaccharides in the A-1 fraction should be as shown in Figure 7, a and b.

DISCUSSION

Poor recovery of the glucosamine residue located at the reducing termini of the oligosaccharides liberated by hydrazinolysis has always been observed when the oligosaccharides are subjected to methylation study. As is clear from the data of Table II, this poor recovery is far more prominent when the N-acetylglucosamine is not substituted by fucose at C-6 position. Therefore, the side reaction which modifies the N-acetylglucosamine, if it occurs, may include the hydroxyl group at C-6 position. The nature of the side reaction product is now under investigation.

Like other glycohormones, hCG is made up with two subunits, α and β (Swaminathan and Bahl, 1970). Bahl analyzed the carbohydrate content of each subunit and found that the fucose residue is exclusively included in the β-subunit. The complete absence of fucose in the α-subunit was confirmed by Kennedy and Chaplin (1976). The fucose-containing sugar chains in Figure 7 therefore should be limited in the β-subunit. The sum total of fucose-containing sugar chains as calculated by their radioactivities is approximately 25% in moles of total oligosaccharides liberated from hCG by hydrazinolysis. Since both α- and β-subunits contain two asparagine-linked sugar chains (Swaminathan and Bahl, 1970), one of the sugar chains in the β-subunit may contain fucose.

Kennedy and Chaplin (1976) reported that the sialic acid residues in the α-subunit of hCG are a mixture of N-acetyl- and N-glycolylneuraminic acids, and that these sialic acids are linked at the C-6 position of the galactose residues in the side chain moiety. Our data indicate that all the sialic acid residues in the hCG preparation studied are N-acetylneuraminic acid and occur solely as NeuAcα2$\rightarrow$3Gal grouping. The reason for these discrepancies cannot be explained at the present time.

REFERENCES

Ashitaka, Y., Tokura, Y., Tane, M., Mochizuki, M., and Tojo, S.,1970, Studies on the biochemical propoerties of highly purified hCG, Endocrinology 87:233.

Arakawa, M., Ogata, S., Muramatsu, T., and Kobata, A., 1974, β-Galactosidases from jack bean meal and almond emulsion: Application for the enzymatic distinction of Galβ1$\rightarrow$4GlcNAc and Galβ1$\rightarrow$3GlcNAc linkages. J. Biochem. 75:707.

Bahl, O. P., 1969a, Human chorionic gonadotropin I. Purification and physicochemical properties, J. Biol. Chem. 244:567.

Bahl. O. P., 1969b, Human chorionic gonadotropin II. Nature of the carbohydrate units, J. Biol. Chem. 244:575.

Bell, J. J., Canfield, R. E., and Sciarra, J. J., 1969, Purification and characterization of human chorionic gonadotropin, Endocrinology 84:298.

Bellisario, R., Carlsen, R. B., and Bahl, O. P., 1973, Human chorionic gonadotropin: Linear amino acid sequence of the α-subunit, J. Biol. Chem. 248:6796.

Carlsen, R. B., Bahl. O. P., and Swaminathan, N., 1973, Human chorionic gonadotropin: Linear amino acid sequence of the β-subunit, J. Biol. Chem. 248:6810.

Hakomori, S., 1964, A rapid permethylation of glycolipid and polysaccharide catalyzed by methylsulfinyl carbanion in dimethyl sulfoxide, J. Biochem. 55:205.

Kennedy, J. F., and Chaplin, M. F., 1976, The structures of the carbohydrate moieties of the α-subunit of human chorionic gonadotropin, Biochem. J. 155:303.

Li, Y. T., and Li, S. C., 1972, α-Mannosidase, β-N-acetylhexosaminidase and β-galactosidase from jack bean meal, Methods Enzymol. 28:702.

Merz, W. E., Hilgenfeldt, V., Brossmer, R., and Rehberger, G., 1974, Amino acid and carbohydrate composition of human chorionic gonadotropin fractions obtained by isoelectric focusing, Hoppe-Seyler's Z. Physiol. Chem. 355:1046.

Mizuochi, T., Yonemasu, K., Yamashita, K., and Kobata, A., 1978, The asparagine-linked sugar chains of subcomponent C_{1q} of the first component of human complement, J. Biol. Chem. 253:7404.

Morgan, F. J., Birken, S., and Canfield, R. E., 1975, The amino acid sequence of human chorionic gonadotropin: The α-subunit and β-subunit, J. Biol. Chem. 250:5247.

Moyle, W. R., Bahl, O. P., and Marz L., 1975, Methylation analysis of neuraminic acids by gas chromatography-mass spectrometry, Carbohydr. Res. 56:1

Swaminathan, N., and Bahl, O. P., 1970, Dissociation and recombination of the subunits of human chorionic gonadotropin, Biochem. Biophys. Res. Commun. 40:422.

Takasaki, S., and Kobata, A., 1978, Microdetermination of sugar composition by radioisotope labeling, Methods Enzymol. 50:50.

ACKNOWLEDGEMENTS

This work was supported in part by research grants from the Scientific Research Fund (No. 237013 and 348374) of the Ministry of Education, Science and Culture of Japan, from the Mitsubishi Foundation, and from the Japan Society for the Promotion of Science (The Japan-U.S. Cooperative Science Program).

PRODUCTION AND SECRETION OF HCG AND HCG SUBUNITS BY

TROPHOBLASTIC TISSUE

Yoshihiko Ashitaka, Ryuichiro Nishimura,
Masayuki Takemori, and Shimpei Tojo

Department of Obstetrics and Gynecology,
Kobe University School of Medicine, Kobe, Japan

INTRODUCTION

Advanced techniques have brought great success in purification and characterization of glycoprotein hormones. The human glycoprotein hormones, such as luteinizing hormone (LH), follicle-stimulating hormone (FSH), thyroid-stimulating hormone (TSH), and human chorionic gonadotropin (hCG) are all composed of a protein core derived from two non-identical alpha and beta subunits, with branched carbohydrate side chains radically attached to asparagine, serines, and/or threonine. In contrast to the essentially identical or nearly identical amino acid sequence among the α-subunits, the biological properties of native hormones are greatly contributed by the β-subunit (which also carries specific antigenic sites) and are structurally unique for each species. Antisera generated to the β-subunit of hCG discriminate comparatively well between hLH and hCG, while most of those derived from intact hormones do not (Amir, 1972).

These findings have also much contributed to the studies on physiological control of glycoprotein hormone synthesis and secretion. The human placenta synthesizes and secretes both steroids and protein hormones, mainly hCG and human placental lactogen (hPL), at the same time. However, the concentrations of these hormones in maternal serum are quite different. Those of steroids and hPL reach maximum levels near term, whereas hCG peaks in the first stage of gestation. It is of interest to look for a physiological regulation mechanism of the production and secretion of hCG in the placenta.

In the present study the nature of hCG in sera and in trophoblastic tissues of normal pregnant women and patients with trophoblastic diseases has been examined. Some approaches for biosynthesis of hCG were also performed.

CHEMISTRY

Purification of HCG

In the first half of the 1970's the purification procedure of hCG employed in our laboratory required complicated steps (Ashitaka et al., 1970; Ashitaka et al., 1972). A slight modification for hCG purification has been considered by us in the latter half of the present decade: a gel filtration step on Sephadex G-50, followed by ion-exchange chromatography on CM-C, ion-exchange chromatography on DEAE Sephadex A-50, and gel filtration on Sephadex G-100.

The purified hCG (about 13,000 IU/mg by ovarian weight method) obtained was separated into subunits by 8M urea incubation, followed by chromatography on DEAE Sephadex A-50 and Sephadex G-100 gel filtration (Swaminathan and Bahl, 1970).

Immunological Characterization of HCG and HCG Subunits

Antisera of hCG subunits, as well as that of hCG, were obtained by repeated injection of these proteins into 3-month-old female white rabbits (Nihon Kurea Co., Japan) according to the small doses method of Vaitukaitis et al. (1971). In this procedure tubercle baccili supplied by Toneyama National Sanatorium and crude *Bordatella pertussis* vaccine which was a gift from E. Lilly Corp., Indiana, were utilized. Antibody titers began to increase about 45 days after the injection by B/T, and standard curves in homologous radioimmunoassay (RIA) systems resulted, as described in the next part. Antisera of hCGα and hCGβ obtained were immunologically examined by Ouchterlony immuno-diffusion technique in agar. A single precipitation band between hCGα (Kobe), Canfield's hCGα (CR-100α), hCG (Kobe) and hMG (Humegon, Organon) against anti-hCGα showed a precipitation line, while neither hCGβ (Kobe) nor hCGβ (CR-100β) formed a precipitation line with this antiserum. Anti-hCGβ reacted strongly with hCGβ (Kobe), while it did not with these hCGα and hMG at the concentrations used in this experiment (Ashitaka et al., 1974).

Homologous RIAs

Iodination of hCG and hCG subunits were prepared by the enzymatic iodination method described in detail elsewhere (Ashitaka and Koide, 1974). The average specific radioactivity of ^{125}I-hCG was 60-80 μCi/μg; hCGα, 72-88 μCi/μg; and hCGβ, 56-62 μCi/μg (Ashitaka et al., 1974a).

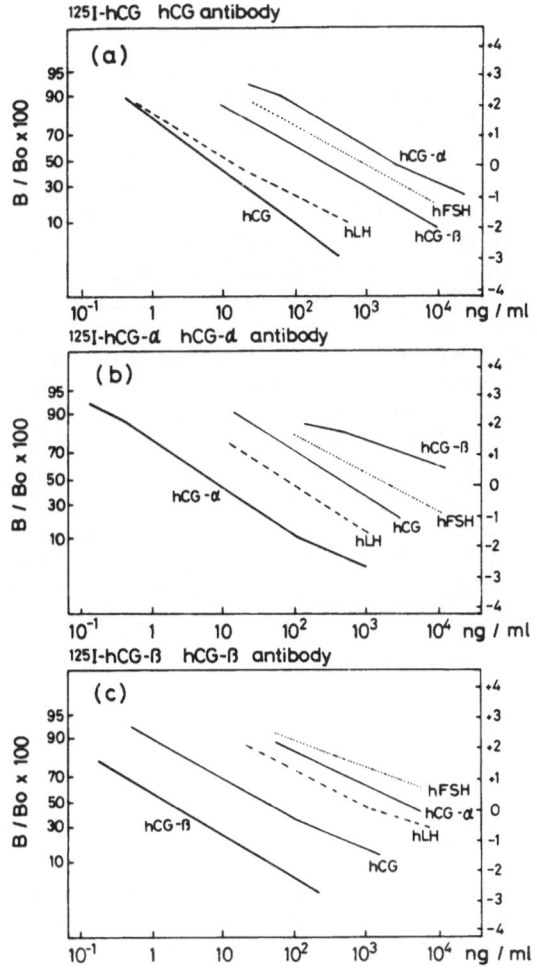

Figure 1.   Dose-response lines for hCG (Kobe-78 or CR-119), hCGα (Kobe-78), hCGβ (Kobe-78), hLH (LER-960) and hFSH (LER-1366) in each homologous system.   (a): hCG RIA   (b): hCGα RIA   (c): hCGβ RIA

All assays were carried out by the double-antibody technique (Tojo et al., 1969). HCG-Kobe, CR-117, or CR-119 was used as the reference preparation for the hCG assay. RIA results were calculated from linear regression curves (ordinate: logit scale expressed as percentage of B/T,; abscissa: log scale of antigen concentration) as described by Rodbard (1974).

Figure 1 shows the inhibition lines of native hCG, hCGα, and hCGβ in each homologous RIA system. In each system the inhibition line of non-homologous antigen started at a higher dose of homologous antigens, and amounts of these were clustered about a common area of the graph, requiring 50 to 500 times more mass for percent inhibition compared to the homologous antigens. It is generally admitted that high concentrations of hCG are found in sera and urine of normal pregnant women, especially in the first trimester. Therefore, it was estimated that large amounts of hCG interfere with the concentrations of hCG subunits obtained from homologous RIA. In hCGβ RIA, for example, 1-2% of hCG should be subtracted as the interference from the apparent value of hCGβ in order to know the real value of hCGβ. The sensitivity of hCG RIA was 0.8 ng/ml, and 50% intercept was 6.5 ng/ml. The sensitivity of hCGα was 0.5 ng/ml, and a 50% intercept was 7.0 ng/ml. The sensitivity of hCGβ was 0.2 ng/ml; a 50% intercept was 1.8 ng/ml. The within-assay coefficient of variation was 9% in hCGα and 11% in hCGβ RIA, and that for between-assay was 15% in hCGα and 20% in hCGβ RIA, for four replicate samples. Anti-hCG was used in a final dilution of 1:24,000; anti-hCGα in 1:45,000; and anti-hCGβ in 1:60,000. Bound percentages of labeled hormones to their homologous antibodies were ^{125}I-hCG:45, ^{125}I-hCGα: 75, and ^{125}I-hCGβ:30-45 at these concentrations in all RIAs.

SECRETION OF HCG AND HCG SUBUNITS

In Cases with Normal Pregnancy

Serum Concentrations. As reported already by several investigators who used hCG RIA (Dicafalusy et al., 1958; Mishell et al., 1963) and also by hCGβ RIA, which discriminates pituitary LH comparatively well (Vaitukaitis et al., 1972; Braunstein et al., 1976), the curve for serum concentration of hCG showed a peak in the 8th week of gestation, declined rapidly thereafter, and maintained a lower level until parturition. No second peak was observed. In contrast, those of subunits showed quite different manifestations. No high elevation of hCGβ was seen in the first trimester. Very low concentration and little fragmentation of hCGβ was found throughout pregnancy. The secretion pattern of hCGα has no resemblance to those of hCG and hCGβ. Secretion of hCGα rises substantially as pregnancy proceeds, reaching blood levels of several hundreds nanograms per ml in the 36th week of gestation, and declining toward parturition (Figure 2). Large amounts of hCG and hCGα, and small amounts of hCGβ in sera indicated that circulating free hCGα is not derived from spontaneous dissociation of hCG, but is directly secreted from the chorionic tissue, as discussed by Vaitukaitis (1974).

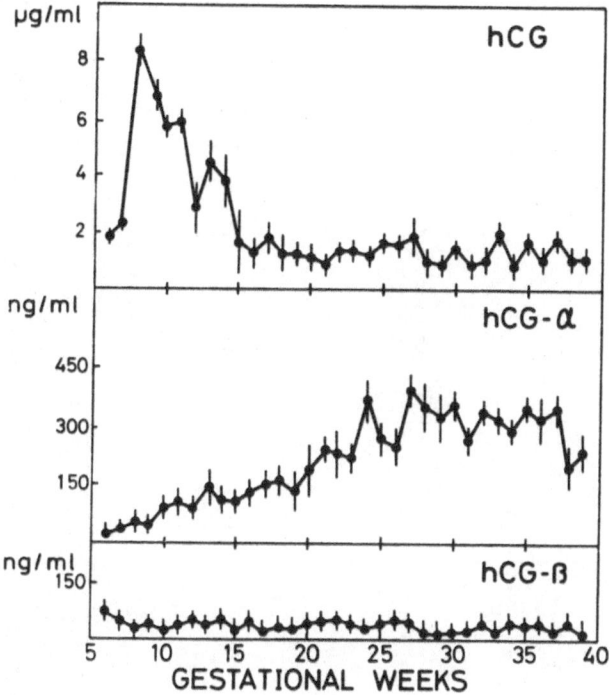

Figure 2. Serum levels of hCG and its subunits throughout pregnancy. (n = 98)

Tissue Concentrations. In view of this consideration, the tissue concentrations of these glycoproteins were examined. As shown in Table I, it was recognized that marked amounts not only of hCG, but also of its subunits, were in the chorionic tissue (Ashitaka et al., 1974b). Although absolute amounts of these glycoproteins decreased in the last two trimesters, it should be remembered that total amounts and weight of chorionic tissue become greater along the course of pregnancy. Of interest was the fact that in the term placenta the amount of hCGα was higher than that of hCG in some cases. Immuno-histochemical localization of hCG and its subunits in chorionic tissue was carried out by Hoshina et al. (1979). The tissue preparations stained both by a direct and an indirect method, showed that fluorescence was observed in the syncytiotrophoblast with a little staining in the cytotrophoblast, both with the anti-hCG and anti-hCGβ staining. With the anti-hCGα staining, on the other hand, the fluorescence was found both in the syncytio- and cytotrophoblast concurrently. Fluorescence of the latter cells was recognized as due to free α-subunit

TABLE I: Concentrations of hCG, hCGα, and hCGβ in lyophilized chorionic tissue.

	hCG	hCGα	hCGβ
8 weeks	250	711	571
10 "	10,500	552	4,113
12 "	3,720	3,770	1,030
14 "	2,590	2,790	900
17 "	1,750	1,593	600
25 "	250	675	1,016
26 weeks	5,625	1,040	undetectable
full term (a)	950	217	undetectable
full term (b)	454	858	43
full term (c)	140	339	5
full term (d)	25	108	40
full term (e)	456	134	79

(Ashitaka et al., 1974b)   ng/10 mg of powder

because the cytotrophoblast was scarcely stained with anti-hCG and anti-hCGβ. On the basis of ultrastructural findings, it would be expected that a syncytiotrophoblast which contained all the organelles might be the major site of placental hormonal synthesis including steroids and protein hormones, while cytotrophoblastic cells have an ultrastructural simplicity of which the energies are directed principally toward growth rather than synthesis. Furthermore, ultrastructural studies have also tended to confirm the origin of the syncytiotrophoblast from cytotrophoblast (Fox, 1978). Therefore, hCGα might be a structural protein rather than a functional protein.

Placental Perfusion. Up to now there have been some reports suggesting that the major detectable components in the fetal circulation were immunoreactive α-subunits of glycoprotein hormones (Hagen and McNelly. 1975). Although the origin of these subunits has not yet been determined, it is generally considered that the major source of this α-subunit is fetal pituitary gland. Therefore, we have tried to perfuse placentae obtained shortly after normal deliveries, using our organ perfusion apparatus which had been developed by Professor Tojo and Toshiba Electric Co., Japan, for the survival of utero-tubo-ovarian unit in vitro (Tojo et al., 1974b). As shown in Figure 3, along the time course of perfusion the concentrations of hCG and hCGα in the perfusate of the maternal side

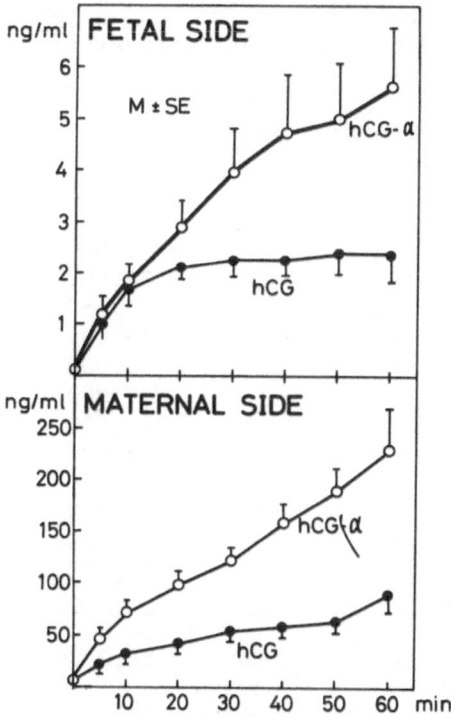

Figure 3. HCG and hCGα secretions into the fetal perfusate and into the maternal medium in term placental perfusion using an organ survival machine (n=4).

increased gradually. In the perfusate obtained between the umbilical arteries and vein the concentration of hCGα also increased, but that of hCG did not. These results clearly demonstrate that hCG produced in the placenta is not so actively shifted through the placental barrier to the fetal circulation, but immunoreactive hCGα is positively transferred to the fetus. The transferred α-subunit may be utilized in the fetus.

In Cases with Trophoblastic Diseases

In Sera and in Molar Vesicle Fluid. Samples of blood were obtained from 12 patients with hydatidiform mole which was confirmed by the evacuation of molar vesicles. Of these 12, the prognoses of four patients was histologically destructive mole (Table II). The concentrations of hCG in the sera of women with hydatidiform mole ranged from 15 µg/ml to 210 µg/ml with a mean level of 88.4±15.8 (SE)

TABLE II: Serum concentrations of hCG and hCGα measured by the respective RIAs in twelve patients with hydatidiform mole.

Case	Gestation (weeks)	hCG (ng/ml)	hCGα (ng/ml)
1	18	15,000	1,300
2	14	34,000	1,550
3*	13	97,650	640
4	14	145,000	1,050
5	20	55,000	310
6	15	99,000	1,250
7*	12	210,000	1,650
8*	14	32,000	290
9	16	75,000	220
10	12	85,000	950
11*	13	48,000	1,540
12	17	113,000	2,050

(Ashitaka et al., 1977) Mean 84,238 1,067
*patients with histolo- ±
gically destructive mole. SE 15,827 173

µg/ml. This value was significantly higher than that in sera of normal pregnant women of the corresponding gestation weeks. The concentrations of hCG did not correlate with the sequence of the patients after removal of mole. The concentrations of hCGα in sera of women with hydatidiform mole ranged from 220 to 2050 ng/ml and the mean level was 1067±137 (SE) ng/ml. There was no signifi-cant correlation between the concentrations of hCG and those of hCGα (Table III). The concentration of hCGα did not definitively reflect the clinical course of the patient after removal of mole, although Vaitukaitis and Ebersole (1976) had pointed out the positive correlation between the prognosis and the concentration of hCGα. The fluid of molar vesicles obtained at the time of evacuation contained higher amounts of hCGα than the sera of matched patients. These results were confirmed by gel filtration on Sephadex G-100 as shown in Figure 4. Vaitukaitis and Ebersole (1976) showed the presence of hCG and its subunits in the extracts of tumor tissue, serum, and urine from patients who responded to chemotherapy. In any case, we could not find detectable amounts of hCGβ.

TABLE III: The concentrations of hCG and hCGα, and hCGα/hCG ratio in serum and vesicle fluid of molar pregnancy.

Case	Molar Pregnancy Serum			Molar Vesicle Fluid		
	hCG (ng/ml)	α-subunit (ng/ml)	Ratio (%)	hCG (ng/ml)	α-subunit (ng/ml)	Ratio (%)
1	15,000	1,300	8.7	32,000	19,000	59.4
2	34,000	1,550	4.6	56,000	17,000	30.4
3	97,650	640	0.7	11,000	9,500	86.4
4	145,000	1,050	0.7	48,500	10,600	21.9
5	55,000	310	0.6	26,000	13,500	51.9
6	99,000	1,250	1.3	23,700	10,200	43.0

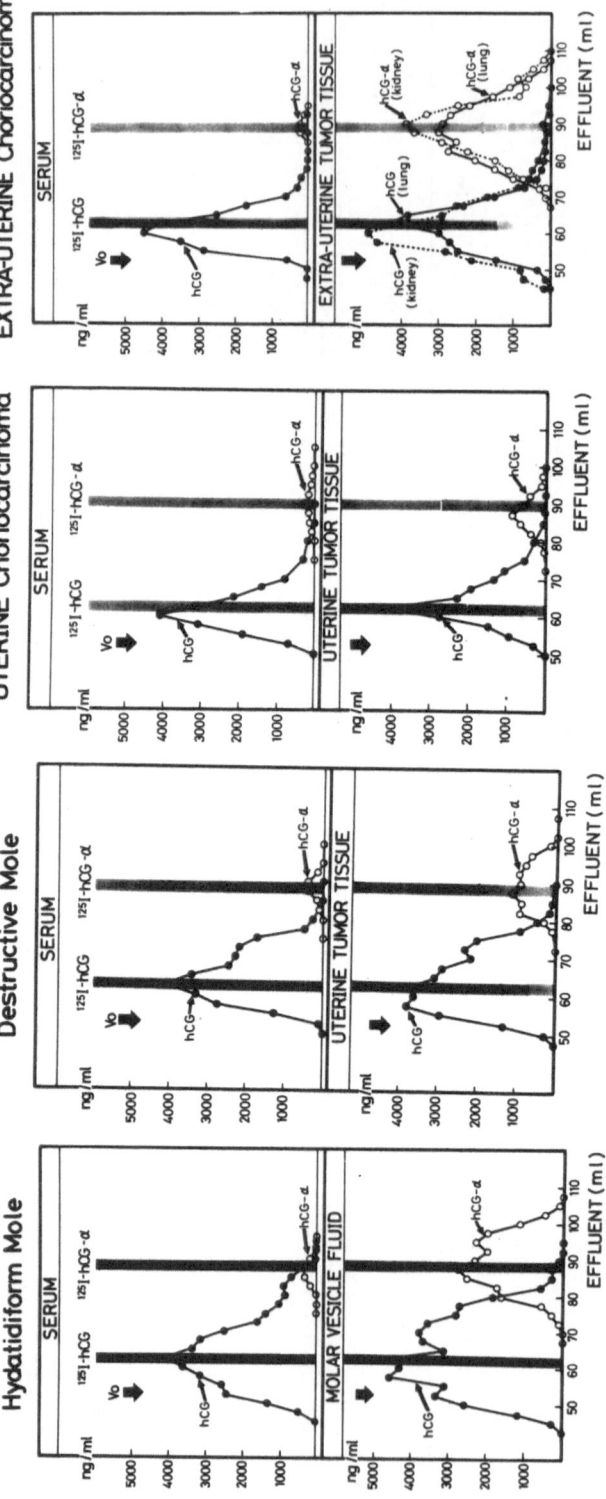

Figure 4. Elution profiles of hCG and hCGα in sera, tumor tissues, and vesicle fluid of cases with hydatidiform mole, destructive mole, and choriocarcinoma (by gel filtration on Sephadex G-100). Shaded area denotes the elution positions of ^{125}I-hCG and ^{125}I-hCGα. Column size: 15 x 900 mm; Flowrate: 12 ml/hr; Fraction tube volume: 2.5 ml; Ve/Vo: hCG (1.30), hCGα(1.73).

TABLE IV: Uptake of radioactivity in various organs of superovulated rats two hours after intravenous injection.

Samples injected	Ovary	Kidney	Liver	Serum
	(cpm/100 mg wet weight)			(cpm/100 μl)
1) [^{125}I]hCG (2.5×10^6 cpm)	$1,365,404 \pm 171,311$*	$26,719 \pm 1,914$	$2,637 \pm 132$	$18,462 \pm 1,977$
2) [^{125}I]hCG (2.5×10^6 cpm) +cold hCG (100 IU)	$34,804 \pm 8,474$	$29,788 \pm 1,900$	$3,231 \pm 383$	$34,435 \pm 6,951$
3) [^{125}I]hCG-α (1.1×10^6 cpm)	606 ± 68	$9,771 \pm 510$	456 ± 62	$1,679 \pm 83$
4) [^{125}I]hCG-β (2×10^5 cpm)	271 ± 16	$9,468 \pm 338$	106 ± 6	240 ± 28
5) [^{125}I]hCG-β (2×10^5 cpm) combined with hCG-α**	$7,911 \pm 1,120$	497 ± 37	74 ± 5	415 ± 24
6) recombined protein (2,000 cpm)***	860 ± 110	300 ± 69	470 ± 88	280 ± 55

*Standard error of mean.

**^{125}I–hCGβ incubated with hCGα (10 μg) at 37°C for 16 hr in 0.05M phosphate buffer (pH 7.4) purified through a Sephadex G-100 column.

***Immunoreactive hCGα in molar vesicle fluid incubated with ^{125}I–hCGβ, purified by the same method (n=3).

(Ashitaka et al., 1977.)

Recombination Study of HCG Subunits. Recombination study was done on the free α-subunit in fluid of molar vesicles obtained by a Sephadex G-100 gel filtration with ^{125}I-hCGβ. HCGα fractions obtained from the gel filtration were pooled and initially incubated with hCG/LH receptor fraction obtained from superovulated rat ovaries by the method of Lee and Ryan (1973). The ratio was 1 ml sample to 500 mg receptor fraction at 37°C, with 2 hr of vigorous shaking in order to minimize the hCG contamination in the α-fraction. At the end of incubation the mixture was centrifuged at 2000 x g for 20 minutes. The supernatant was reincubated with ^{125}I-hCGβ (about 10 x 10^4cpm) at 37°C for 16 hr, chilled in an ice bath, and placed on a Sephadex G-100 column. About 8 percent of the ^{125}I-hCGβ combined with this α-fraction. A newly synthesized fraction combined with ^{125}I-hCGβ was injected into the tail vein of each superovulated immature female rat (Ashitaka and Koide, 1974). The rats were sacrificed 2 hr after the injection and the ^{125}I-radioactivity of each organ was determined. As shown in Table IV, ^{125}I-hCGβ combined with α-subunit obtained from molar vesicles, ^{125}I-hCG and ^{125}I-hCGβ recombined with urinary hCGα were primarily concentrated by the ovary, while there was no significant ovarian uptake of ^{125}I-hCG subunits in vivo. In concentration by the ovary ^{125}I-hCG competed with cold hCG. Weintraub et al. (1975) reported that α-subunit harvested from a gastric carcinoid tumor incubated with hCGβ resulted in only 2% of the expected activity, and α-subunit from bronchogenic carcinoma cell line incubated with hCGβ produced no detectable activity. As discussed by Weintraub et al. (1975), ectopic α-subunits may have different physical and combination properties from those of trophoblastic origin.

Figure 5 shows a gel filtration pattern of ^{125}I-hCGβ incubated with the 105,000 supernatant of a term placental homogenate. Along the time course of incubation ^{125}I-hCGβ, when incubated with 105,000 supernatant, moves gradually to a recombination position which is identical with native ^{125}I-hCG. No big form of hCG was detected or synthesized.

Secretion Patterns of HCG and HCGα after Molar Pregnancy. The relationship between the secretory pattern of the serum hCGα and the outcome was investigated. In a case shown in Figure 6 (destructive mole) for about ten days after the evacuation of the mole, hCG and hCGα declined rapidly, and during the subsequent twenty days the hCGα level increased. On the other hand, the hCG level decreased gradually and in due time it showed a tendency to increase. This case had pulmonary metastases and was given chemotherapy postoperatively. After two courses of actinomycin-D, the serum hCG was no longer detectable. The serum hCGα had already reached undetectable levels about ten days earlier. It is interesting to note that in other cases which responded satisfactorily to chemotherapy the serum hCGα reaches undetectable levels about ten days earlier than the serum hCG. On the other hand, in cases which are resistant

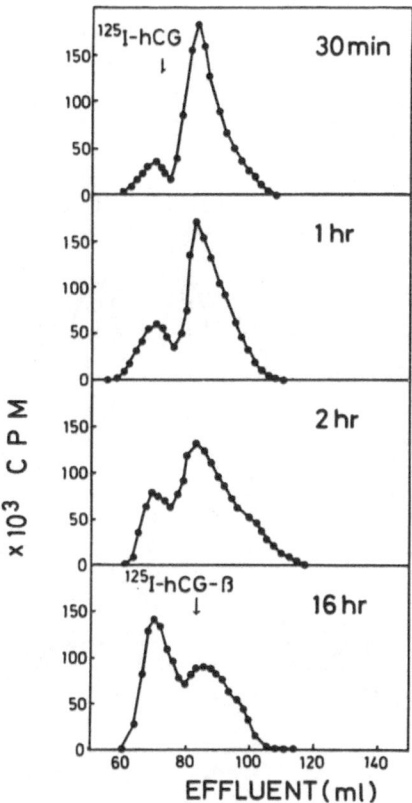

Figure 5. Gel filtration patterns of ^{125}I-hCGβ incubated with 105,000 x g supernatant of term placental homogenate. ^{125}I-hCGβ was gradually displaced to an elution position of authentic ^{125}I-hCG when incubated with the supernatant. (Ashitaka et al., 1977.)

to chemotherapy the serum hCGα is detectable almost until the time that the serum hCG becomes undetectable. In a case shown in Figure 7, choriocarcinoma, the concentration of serum hCGα was almost as high as that of hCG and the serial secretory patterns were not parallel during chemotherapy.

Response to LRF. Secretion of free subunits of glycoprotein hormones by the anterior pituitary has been demonstrated by many authors (Prentice and Ryan, 1975; Kourides et al., 1975; Kaplan et al., 1976). Bilateral oophorectomy may induce a hypergonadotropic state and free α-subunit may be secreted in higher concentration

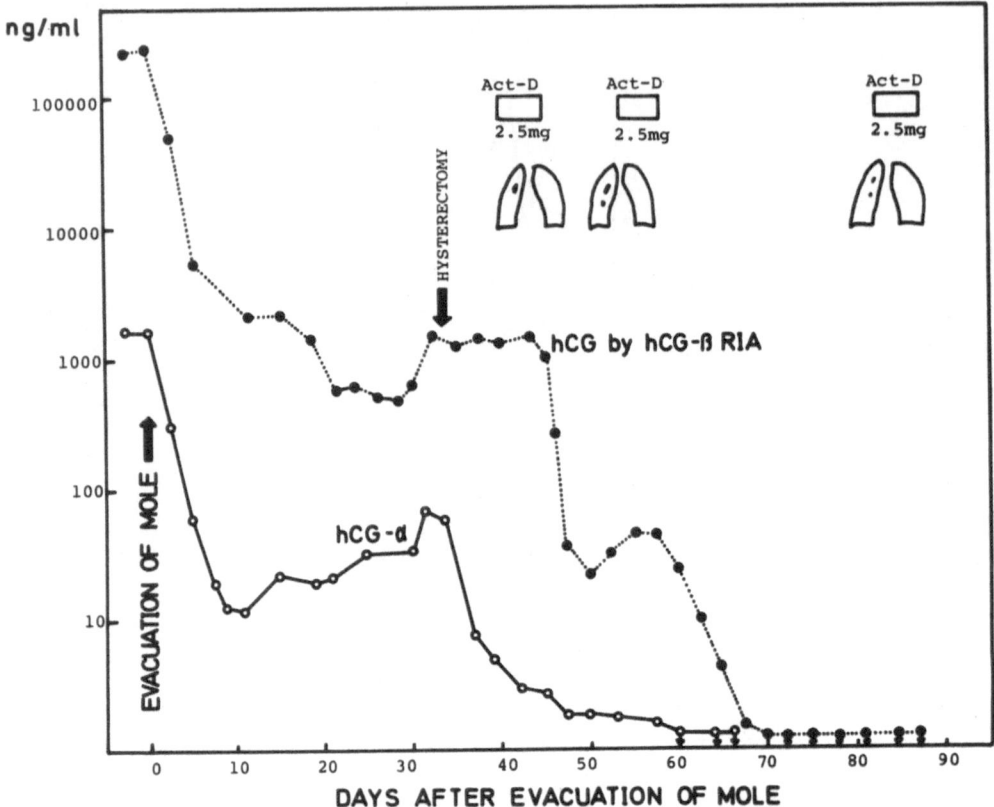

DAYS AFTER EVACUATION OF MOLE

Figure 6. Clinical course of a patient with destructive mole involving the uterus and lung, showing serum hCG and hCGα. A 30 year old woman had cervical dilatation and evacuation for hydatidiform mole. At 28 days after the evacuation procedure the levels of serum hCG stopped declining and instead started to increase gradually. From the findings of her pelvic angiography, the recurrence of trophoblastic diseases was suspected and abdominal hysterectomy was performed. The pathologic diagnosis of the excised uterine tissue was destructive mole. The chest x-ray revealed metastatic tumor shadows in the lung. After the hysterectomy, three courses of actinomycin-D chemotherapy were performed and the serum hCG levels ranged in the pituitary LH levels (less than 30 mIU/ml hCG unit).

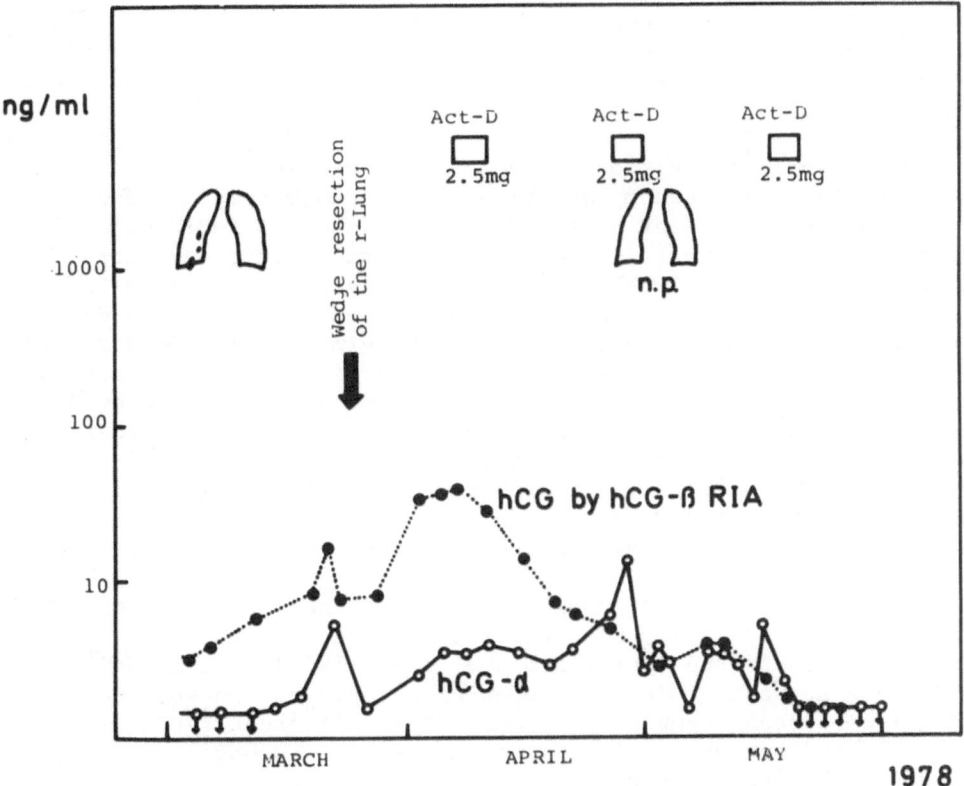

Figure 7.   Clinical course of a patient with choriocarcinoma
involving the uterus and lungs, showing serum hCG and hCGα.
A 26 year old woman was found to have a molar pregnancy in
February 1974.   Twenty days after evacuation, she had metastatic
lesions of the right lung, demonstrated by chest x-ray.   The
patient underwent hysterectomy.   She was treated post-operatively
with MTX and actinomycin-D.   In October 1975 a segmental and
wedge resection of the right lung was performed and three
tumorous lesions were removed.   Following three courses of
actinomycin-D, the concentration of hCG decreased and the chest
x-ray showed no metastatic lesion.

by the pituitary. In molar pregnancy, however, pituitary function is suppressed as in normal pregnancy (Nakano et al., 1975). Edmonds et al. (1975) showed that α-subunit of hLH was secreted by the anterior pituitary in response to luteinizing hormone-releasing factor (LRF); the peak concentration was less than 3 ng/ml. Hence, it is inconceivable that such large quantities of free α-subunit, as demonstrated in this study during molar pregnancy, are secreted by the pituitary.

A patient with choriocarcinoma showed resistance to chemotherapy after hysterectomy and bilateral oophorectomy and had continuous secretions of 50 to 100 mIU/ml (about 5 to 10 ng/ml) of hCG and 1.5 to 2.0 ng/ml of hCGα. This patient received intravenous injection of 100 μg of LRF. As shown in Figure 8, levels of LH and FSH assayed by RIA showed high values. Immunoreactive hCGα concentration showed the maximum elevation (10 ng/ml) at 15 min after the administration of LRF. Percent increase of immunoreactive hCGα was higher than those of LH and FSH. LH concentration assayed by RIA include LH and hCG. The assay could not differentiate whether immunoreactive α-subunit produced in response to LRF administration is derived from pituitary, tumor tissue, or both origins. However, the major source of α-subunit, achieving a concentration of more than 10 ng/ml in sera, must be tumor tissue.

In patients with trophoblastic disease and also with non-trophoblastic neoplasia, the secretion of hCG and its free subunits has been demonstrated (Weintraub and Rosen, 1973). Tashjian et al. (1973) demonstrated that the clones of ectopic hormone-producing cells from a bronchogenic carcinoma showed different rates of synthesis and secretion of hCG and its α- and β-subunit. The amount of one or the other subunit always exceeded that of the complete hormone molecule. Lieblich et al. (1976) found that HeLa cells derived from a carcinoma of the cervix secreted α-subunit and suggested that the α-subunit may turn out to be relatively easily de-repressed and be a more primitive protein. Ghosh and Cox (1976) showed that HeLa cells secreted hCGα and speculated the putative de-repression of an element of the genome with the synthesis of a protein normally produced only by the specialized trophoblastic cells.

It is already recognized that the measurement of hCG by hCGβ RIA using anti-hCGβ is a reliable clinical parameter for the follow-up of patients with trophoblastic diseases. In the present study, the serial levels of hCG as measured by hCGβ RIA correlated well with the clinical course of the patients undergoing chemotherapy and surgical treatment.

The levels of both hCG and hCGα paralleled the clinical course of the patients examined in this study. Moreover, the response to

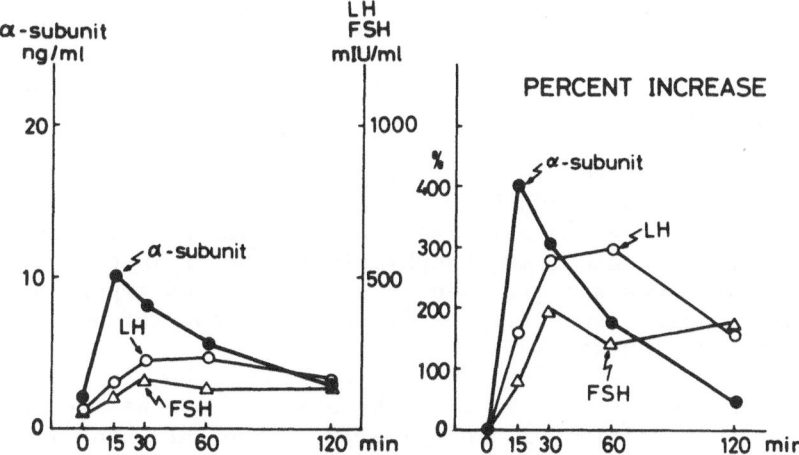

Figure 8. LRF test in a patient with choriocarcinoma.

therapies was more rapidly reflected by changes in the levels of hCGα than by hCG changes.

Based on the present study, measurements of the hCGα in blood may be a useful parameter to evaluate the efficacy of treatment in the management of trophoblastic diseases.

BIOSYNTHESIS

Since 1937, when Kido first succeeded in achieving the synthesis of hCG by chorionic tissue transplanted into the anterior chamber of the eye of a rabbit, there have been many reports of hCG synthesis by incubating placental tissue. Recently, using a CO_2 incubator, Maruo (1974) and Tojo et al. (1977) found larger forms of hCG and hCG subunits than standard hCG and subunits. Furthermore, using mRNA extracted from placental polysomes and translation in a wheat germ initiating system, Chatterjee and Munro (1977) and Boime et al. (1978) have succeeded in demonstrating α- and β-peptides of hCG. Trophoblast synthesizes and secretes two major protein hormones, hCG and human placental lactogen (hPL). Whereas hCG peaks in the 8th week of gestation, hPL reaches maximum levels in the 36th week, suggesting that the factors controlling their synthesis are quite different. HPL is considered to be synthesized at a fairly fixed rate per unit of syncytial trophoblast; a greater amount of hPL would be produced as the trophoblast differentiates and increases in mass. HCG, however, is not completely dependent on placental mass, and the synthesis of the subunits is not completely dependent on placental mass. The synthesis of the subunits is not coordinated. The greater α-levels both in sera and in third-trimester placenta might reflect an increase in placental mass similar to that seen for hPL (Boime et al., 1978).

The secretion of hCG into the medium by term placenta cells (Handweger et al., 1973) and by malignant trophoblast cells (Hussa et al., 1975) was markedly stimulated by addition of 1 mM dibutyryl cyclic AMP (dbc-AMP) and 1 mM theophyllin (alone or in combination) while that of hPL was not affected. Furthermore, an important role of divalent cations, especially Ca^{++}, on the release of hCG has been demonstrated (Hussa, 1977).

A striking observation is that the placenta synthesizes and contains large quantities of biologically active LRF which is biochemically and immunologically indistinguishable from hypothalamic LRF (Gibbons et al., 1975; Siler-Khodr and Khodr, 1978; Imakita et al., 1979). Secretion of hCG by placenta was dose-dependently stimulated in culture medium by hypothalamic extracts (Takagi, 1971) and by synthetic LRF. HPL secretion was not stimulated (Khodr and Siler-Khodr, 1978). In addition, it was found that even epidermal growth factor (EGF) with a molecular weight of about 6000 could stimulate secretion of hCG and, to a lesser extent, the secretion of free $hCG\alpha$ (Benveniste et al., 1978). High levels of EGF receptor have been detected in term placenta (O'Keefe et al., 1974).

Incubation with CO_2

As a preliminary experiment, tissue culture in a CO_2 incubator was performed. Chorionic tissue obtained at therapeutic abortion of normal pregnancy was minced into fragments of about 1 mm and cultivated in synthetic medium-199 (TCM-199) containing 100 U of penicillin and 100 ug of streptomycin per ml. No serum component was added to the medium to simplify the procedure of extraction and purification (Tojo et al., 1974; Maruo, 1976). Fifty mg of wet weight of minced placental fragments were placed on filter paper (25 mm diameter) within a glass Petri dish (70 mm diameter). Fifteen ml of culture medium per dish were then added. Incubations were performed at 37°C under a 95% O_2-5% CO_2 atmosphere. At the end of each culture, tissues and media were separated. A total of 500 mg of the cultured chorionic tissue was homogenized in 3 ml distilled water with a Pyrex tissue homogenized and centrifuged at 10,000 x g for 10 min at 4°C. As shown in Figure 9a, the secretion of hCG and $hCG\alpha$ was stimulated by adding 0.01-1.0 mM of dbc-AMP dose-dependently. The addition of 0.01-1.0 mM of dibutyryl cyclic GMP (dbc-GMP) inhibited secretion during 24 hr incubation. Various

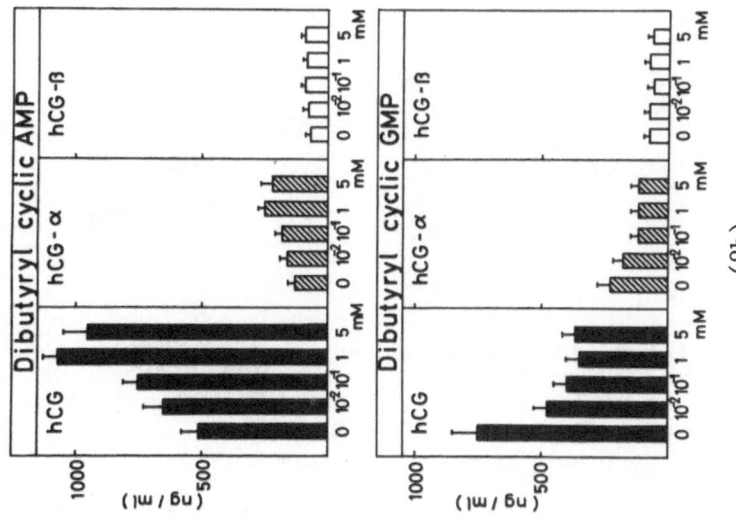

(9b)

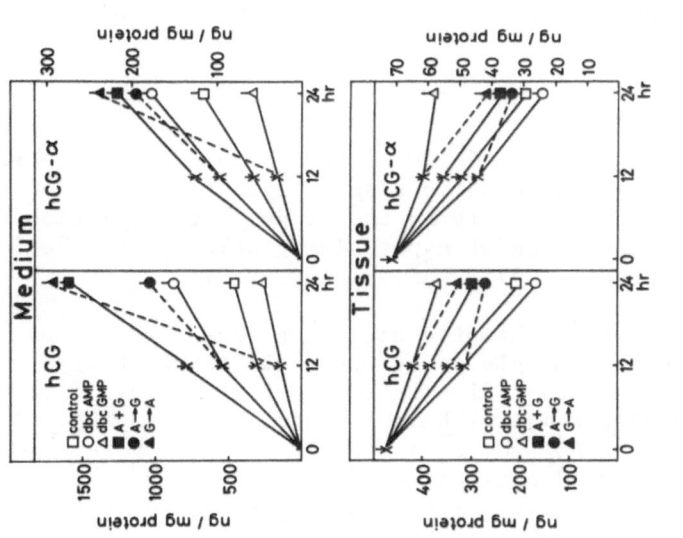

(9a)

Figure 9. The effect of dbc-AMP and dbc-GMP on hCG and hCGα secretion by trophoblastic tissue of early gestation. (9a): Influence of these agents on hCG and hCGα secretion into the media for 24 hr incubation. (9b): Effects of dbc-AMP and dbc-GMP.

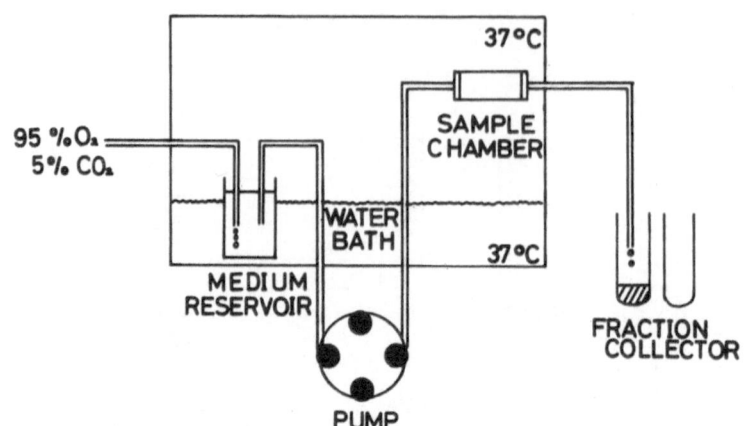

Figure 10.   Schematic diagram of the perifusion apparatus.

combinations of dbc-AMP or dbc-GMP were added to incubations of chorionic tissue. As shown in Figure 9b, combinations of 1 mM dbc-AMP stimulated the secretion of hCG and hCGα into the media, while the tissue content of these cultures were not mostly depleted, indicating that dbc-AMP stimulates the secretion and that dbc-GMP with or without dbc-AMP also stimulates the production.

Perifusion Experiment

We have followed the effects of some agents on the secretion of hCG and hCGα by trophoblastic tissue, using a perifusion system which had been utilized mainly in the study of the relationship between releasing hormones of hypothalamic origin and anterior pituitary (Dowd et al., 1975; Kao et al., 1977).

Figure 10 shows a schematic diagram of our perifusion apparatus. Krebs-Ringer-Bicarbonate-glucose (1.8 mg/ml) (KRBG) buffer, pH 7.4, was perfused at a constant flow rate of 0.2 ml/min by means of a perifusion pump with a multi-channel system (Gilson HP4). A gas mixture of 95% O_2-5% CO_2 was delivered to the medium reservoir. The effluent was forced out to the sample chamber by the pump and delivered via Teflon tubing (2.4 mm diameter). The retention capacity of the sample chamber is about 2 ml. The windows located at both ends of the chamber were sealed with Millipore filter (pore size: 0.45 m). A three-way stopcock was connected at the inlet of the sample chamber. In the chamber 100-200 mg wet weight of chorionic tissue was added. The perfusates were collected at

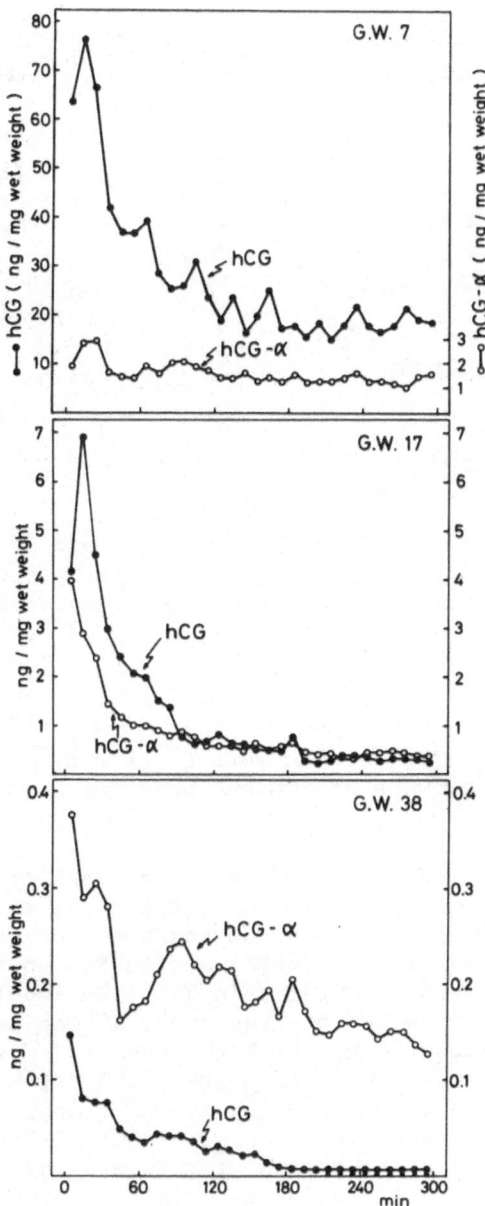

Figure 11.   Patterns of hCG and hCGα release by chorionic tissue of various gestation weeks during perifusion for up to 300 minutes.

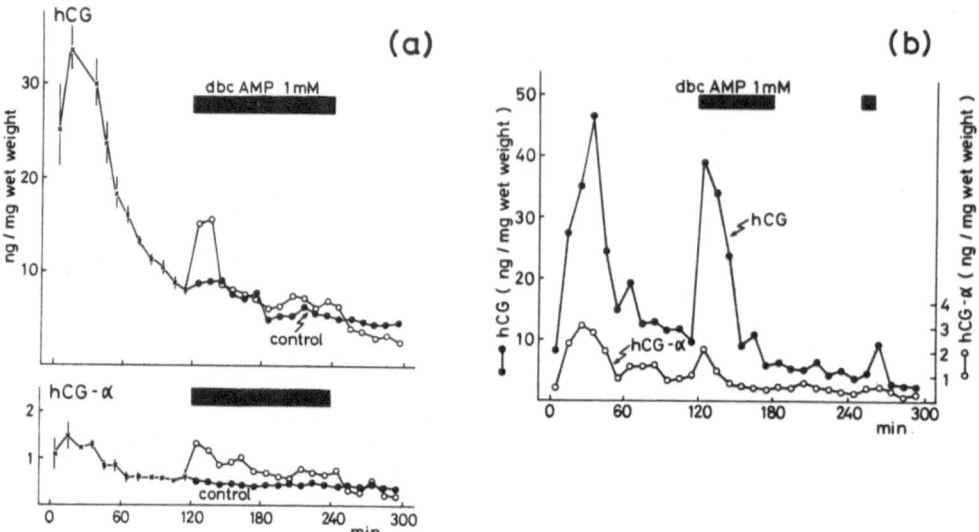

Figure 12.   Effect of dbc-AMP on the release of hCG and hCGα by chorionic tissue of early gestation. (a): by chorionic tissue of 8th week of gestation. (b): by tissue of hydatidiform mole.

10 min intervals. The results were expressed as ng/mg wet weight tissue, that is, amounts of hCG and hCGα released from 1 mg of tissue for 10 min.

As shown in Figure 11, initial high peaks of hCG and hCGα would indicate the direct release of these proteins by the trophoblast. After these peaks both hCG and hCGα concentratrations maintained low basal levels during perifusion up to 300 min. Of interest was that hCGα/hCG ratio in baseline levels was gradually increased along the course of pregnancy; it was less than 1 in the first trimester, about 1 in the 17th week, and more than 1 after the 22nd week of gestation. Of course, the total amounts of these proteins released are much greater by the trophoblast of early gestation. Present data, however, could not differentiate whether proteins in the media at baseline levels are released proteins or newly synthesized protein using materials incorporated into the trophoblastic cells in vivo.

One mM of dbc-AMP also stimulated both hCG and hCGα secretions by normal trophoblastic tissue of the 8th week of gestation (Figure 12a) and by trophoblast of hydatidiform mole (Figure 12b) in this perifusion system. Although 10 ng/ml and 100 ng/ml of synthetic

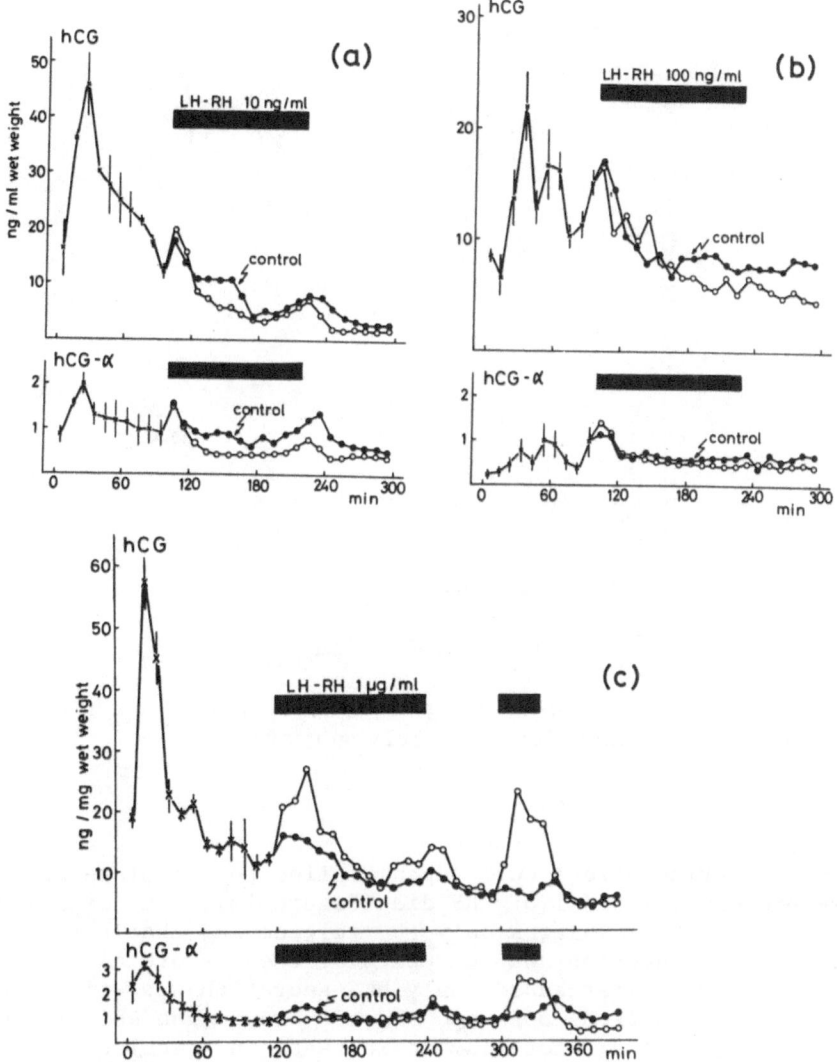

Figure 13. Effect of synthetic LRF on the release of hCG and hCGα by chorionic tissue of early gestation. The concentration of LRF perifused was 10 ng/ml in case (a); 100 ng/ml in case (b); and 1 µg/ml in case (c).

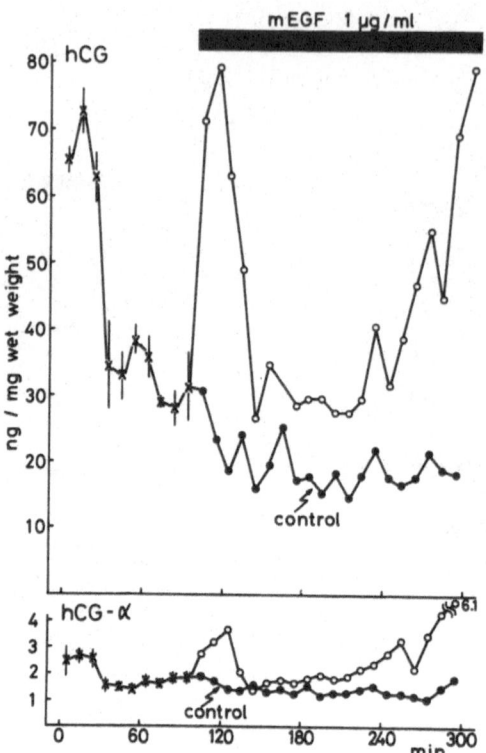

Figure 14.   Effect of EGF of mouse origin (1 µg/ml) on hCG and
hCGα secretion by trophoblast of early gestation.

LRF (Tanabe Pharmaceutical Co., Japan) failed to stimulate secretion
of these proteins, 1 µg/ml of LRF did (Figure 13). Our data indicated that dbc-AMP stimulates only the release and that LRF might
stimulate both production and secretion of these proteins. When
1 µg/ml of LRF was first added, only hCG secretion was stimulated.
With the second addition, both hCG and hCGα secretion were stimulated.
Tamada et al. (1976) did not find an increase in circulating maternal
hCG levels following the administration of 200 µg LRF. HCG secretion
was stimulated by 1600 and 3200 ng/ml (Khodr and Siler-Khodr, 1978).
As stated, a dose of 1000 ng/ml could succeed the stimulation in
vitro. Although these stimulatory doses seem unphysiological, 36.6
pg of LRF contained in 1 mg of placenta is a large amount (Siler-
Khodr and Khodr, 1978). Thus, microgram quantities of LRF might not
be unphysiological for the stimulation of the secretion of these
proteins, In addition, 1 µg/ml of EGF (Japan Chemical Research Co.,
Japan) could also stimulate the release of these proteins (Figure 14).

DISCUSSION

Both hCG and hCG subunits were found in chorionic tissue. HCGα concentrations in chorionic tissue were much higher than in sera of normal pregnant women and patients with trophoblastic diseases. In contrast to excess amounts of hCG and free hCGα, hCGβ was barely detectable in sera. It is well known that cytotrophoblast is a primitive component of the placental trophoblast. HCGα may be one of the main structural proteins of the trophoblast. Cytotrophoblast, which may have only a simple function to produce hCGα alone, may develop the capacity of synthesizing hCGβ, and to produce and release native hCG in the course of its functional differentiation.

As hCGβ may be a rate-limiting factor of hCG production in placenta (Franchimont and Reuter, 1972; Chatterjee and Munro, 1977), all hCGβ is utilized to form native hCG. HCGα may be produced in excess. Chatterjee and Munro (1977) and Boime et al. (1978) demonstrated that both α- and β-subunit of hCG were produced with mRNA extracted from placental tissue by incubation with cell-free system of ascites or wheat germ. It seems that both α- and β-subunit are produced as pre-subunits initially, and then they are transformed into native subunits by the change of pre-subunits and attachment of sugar chains (Boime et al., 1978).

Because the secretion of hCG reaches its peak at the 8th week of gestation, while the placental mass continues to grow during the course of pregnancy, it may be assumed that intracellular control mechanisms exist regulating the production and secretion of hCG. Although dbc-AMP, LRF, and EGF were used in the present study to stimulate the release of hCG and hCGα in vitro, there has as yet been no evidence that these agents exert physiological effects on hCG secretions.

REFERENCES

Amir, S. M., 1972, Dissociation of glycoprotein hormones, Acta Endocrinol. 70:21.

Ashitaka, Y., and Koide, S. S., 1974, Interaction of human chorionic gonadotropin with rat gonads, Fertil. Steril. 25:177.

Ashitaka, Y., Mochizuki, M., and Tojo, S., 1972, Purification and properties of chorionic gonadotropin from the trophoblastic tissue of hydatidiform mole, Endocrinology 90:609.

Ashitaka, Y., Nishimura, R., Endo, Y., and Tojo, S., 1974a, Subunits of human chorionic gonadotropin and their radioimmunoassays, Endocrinol. Japon. 21:429.

Ashitaka, Y., Nishimura, R., Futamura, K., and Tojo, S., 1977, Alpha-subunit of human chorionic gonadotropin in fluid of molar vesicles, Endocrinol. Japon. 24:115.

Ashitaka, Y., Nishimura, R., Ohashi, M., Futamura, K., and Tojo, S., 1974b, Serum and chorionic tissue concentrations of human chorionic gonadotropin and its subunits during pregnancy, Endocrinol. Japon. 21:429.

Ashitaka, Y., Tokura, Y., Tane, M., Mochizuki, M., and Tojo, S., 1970, Studies on the biochemical properties of highly purified HCG, Endocrinology 87:233.

Benveniste, R., Speeg, K. V., Carpenter, G., Cohen, S., Linder, J., and Rabinowita, D., 1978, Epidermal growth factor stimulates secretion of human chorionic gonadotropin by cultured human choriocarcinoma cells, J. Clin. Endocrinol. Metab. 36:1268.

Braunstein, G. D., Rasor, J., and Adler, D., 1976, Serum human chorionic gonadotropin levels throughout normal pregnancy, Am. J. Obstet. Gynecol. 126:677.

Boime, I., Landefeld, T., McQueen, S., and McWilliams, D., 1978, The biosynthesis of chorionic gonadotropin and placental lactogen in first- and third-trimester human placenta, in Structure and Function of the Gonadotropins, K. W. McKerns, ed., pp. 235-258, Plenum Press, New York.

Chatterjee, M., and Munro, H. N., 1977, Structure and biosynthesis of human placental peptide, Vitamin Hormones 35:149.

Dicafalusy, E., Nilsson, L., and Westman, A., 1958, Chorionic gonadotropin in hydatidiform moles, Acta Endocrinol. 28:137.

Dowd, A. J., Barofsky, A. L., Chaudhuri, N., Lloyd, C. W., and Weisz, J., 1975, Patterns of LH and FSH release from perifused rat pituitaries in response to infusions of hypothalamic extract, Endocrinology 96:243.

Edmonds, M., Molitch, J., Pierce, J. G., and Odell, W. D., 1975, Secretion of alpha-subunits of luteinizing hormone (LH) by the anterior pituitary, J. Clin. Endocrinol. Metab. 41:551.

Franchimont, P., and Reuter, A., 1972, Evidence of alpha and beta subunits of hCG in serum urine of pregnant women, in Protein and Polypeptide Hormones, M. Margoulies and F. Greenwood, eds., p. 381, Excerpta Medica, Amsterdam.

Fox, H., 1978, Placental Structure, in Scientific Basis of Obstetrics and Gynecology, R. R. Macdonald, ed., pp. 27-60, Churchill livingstone, Edinburgh, London and New York.

Ghosh, N. K., and Cox, R. P., 1976, Production of human chorionic gonadotropin in HeLa cell culture, Nature (London) 259:416.

Gibbons, J. M., Mitnick, M., and Chieffo, V., 1975, In vitro biosynthesis of TSH- and LH-releasing factors by the human placenta, Am. J. Obstet. Gynecol. 130:127.

Hagen, C., and McNeilly, A. S., 1975, The gonadotropic hormones and their subunits in human maternal and fetal circulation at delivery, Am. J. Obstet. Gynecol. 121:926.

Handwerger, S., Barrett, J., Tyrey, L., and Schomberg, D., 1973, Differential effect of cyclic adenosine monophosphate on the secretion of human placental lactogen and human chorionic gonadotropin, J. Clin. Endocrinol. Metab. 36:1268.

Hosina, M., Ashitaka, Y., and Tojo, S., 1979, Immunohistochemical interaction on antisera to hCG and its subunits with chorionic tissue of early gestation, Endocrinol. Japon. 26:175.

Hussa, R. O., 1977, Studies on human chorionic gonadotropin secretion: Effects of EGTA, Lanthanum, and the Ionophore A:3187, J. Clin. Endocrinol. Metab. 44:520.

Hussa, R. O., Story, M. T., and Pattillo, R. A., 1975, Regulation of human chorionic gonadotropin (hCG) secretion by serum and dibutyryl cyclic AMP in malignant trophoblast cells in vitro, J. Clin. Endocrinol. Metab. 46:69.

Imakita, T., Kumasaka, T., Suzuki, A., and Saito, M., 1979, A study on the immunoreactive luteinizing hormone-releasing hormone in villi by radioimmunoassay in the first trimester, Folia Endocrinol. Jap. 55:797.

Kao, L. W. L., Gunsalus, G. L., Williams, G. H., and Weisz, J., 1977, Response to the perifused anterior pituitaries of rats of synthetic gonadotrophin releasing hormone: A comparison with hypothalamic extract and demonstration of role for potassium in the release of luteinizing hormone and follicle-stimulating hormone, Endocrinology 101:1441.

Kaplan, S. L., Grumback, M. M., and Aubert, M. L., 1976, alpha and beta glycoprotein hormone subunits (hLH, hFSH, hCG) in the serum and pituitary of the human fetus, J. Clin. Endocrinol. Metab. 42:995.

Khodr, G. S., and Siler-Khodr, T. M., 1978, The effect of luteinizing hormone-releasing factor on human chorionic gonadotropin secretion, Fertil. Steril. 30:127.

Kourides, I. A., Weintraub, B. D., Ridgway, E. C., and Maloof, F., 1975, Pituitary secretion of free alpha and beta subunit of human thyrotropin in patients with thyroid disorders, J. Clin. Endocrinol. Metab. 40:872.

Lee, Y., and Ryan, R. F., 1973, Interaction of ovarian receptors with luteinizing hormone and human chorionic gonadotropin, Biochemistry 12:4609.

Lieblich, J. M., Weintraub, B. D., and Rosen, S. W., 1976, HeLa cell secreted alpha-subunit of glycoprotein hormones, Nature (London) 260:530.

Maruo, T., 1976, Studies on in vitro synthesis and secretion of human chorionic gonadotropin and its subunits, Endocrinol. Japon. 23:119.

Mishell, D. R., Wide, L., and Gemzell, C. A., 1963, Immunologic determination of human chorionic gonadotropin in serum, J. Clin. Endocrinol. Metab. 23:125.

Nakano, R., Akahori, T., Kotsuji, F., and Tojo, S., 1975, Follicle-stimulating hormone response to luteinizing hormone releasing hormone in patients with hydatidiform mole, Obstet. Gynecol. 46:453.

O'Keefe, E., Hollenberg, M. D., and Cuatrecasas, P., 1974, Epidermal growth factor: Characteristics of specific binding in membranes from liver, placenta, and other target tissues, Arch. Biochem.

Biophys. 164:518.

Prentice, L. G., and Ryan, R. J., 1975, LH and its subunits in human pituitary, serum, and urine, J. Clin. Endocrinol. Metab. 40:303.

Rodbard, D., 1974, Statistical quantity control and routine data processing for radioimmunoassays and immunoradiometric assays, Clin. Chem. 20:1255.

Siler-Khodr, T. M., and Khodr, G. S., 1978, Content of luteinizing hormone-releasing factor in the human placenta, Am. J. Gynecol. 130:216.

Swaminathan, B., and Bahl, O. P., 1970, Dissociation and recombination of the subunits of human chorionic gonadotropin, Biochem. Biophys. Res. Commun. 40:422.

Takagi, S., 1971, Formation and metabolism of hormones from the standpoint of fetal-maternal relationship, Nippon Sanka-Fujinka Gakkai Zasshi 23:750.

Tamada, T., Akabori, A., Konuma, S., and Araki, S., 1976, Lack of release of human chorionic gonadotropin by gonadotropin-releasing hormone, Endocrinol. Japon. 23:531.

Tojo, S., Mochizuki, M., and Maruo, T., 1974a, Chorionic gonadotropin produced from cultivated trophoblast, in Gonadotropins and Gonadal Function, N. R. Moudgal, ed., pp. 321–331, Academic Press, New York.

Tojo, S., Ashitaka, Y., Maruo, T., and Ohashi, M., 1977, Large immunologic species of human chorionic gonadotropin in placental extracts, Endocrinol. Japon. 24:351.

Tojo, S., Mochizuki, M., Tokura, Y., and Mizusawa, T., 1969, Radioimmunoassay of human chorionic gonadotropin (hCG) (in Japanese), Clin. Endocrinol. (Tokyo) 17:523.

Tojo, S., Mochizuki, M., Milami, K., Tsuchihashi, T., and Shimura, T., 1974b, In vitro perfusion of the human utero-tubo-ovarian unit, Am. J. Obstet. Gynecol. 118:119.

Vaitukaitis, J. L., 1974, Changing placental concentrations of hCG and its subunits during gestation, J. Clin. Endocrinol. Metab. 38:755.

Vaitukaitis, J. L., and Ebersole, E. R., 1976, Evidence for altered synthesis human chorionic gonadotropin in gestational trophoblast tumors, J. Clin.Endocrinol. Metab. 42:1048.

Vaitukaitis, J. L., Robbins, J. B., Nieschlag, E., and Ross, G. T., 1971, A method for producing specific antisera with small doses of immunogen, J. Clin. Endocrinol. Metab. 33:988.

Vaitukaitis, J. L., Braunstein, G. D., and Ross, G. T., 1972, A radioimmunoassay which specifically measures human chorionic gonadotropin in the presence of human luteinizing hormone, Am. J. Obstet. Gynecol. 113:751.

Weintraub, B. D., Krauth, G. K., Rosen, S. W., and Rabson, A. S., 1975, Differences between purified ectopic and normal alpha subunit of human glycoprotein hormones, J. Clin. Invest. 56:1043.

ACKNOWLEDGEMENT

We thank Dr. R. E. Canfield, Columbia University, College of Physicians and Surgeons, New York, N.Y., for hCG and hCG subunits. Human pituitary FSH and LH were gifts from NIAMDD, Bethesda, Md.

This work was partly supported by grants from the Ministry of Education, Japan (grants #348301 and #457407), and by a grant for cancer research from the Ministry of Health and Welfare of Japan.

LARGE MOLECULAR SPECIES OF HUMAN CHORIONIC GONADOTROPIN

Takeshi Maruo, Sheldon J. Segal, and S. S. Koide

Center for Biomedical Research, The Population Council
The Rockefeller University, New York, New York, U.S.A.
and
Population Sciences, The Rockefeller Foundation
New York, New York, U.S.A.

INTRODUCTION

Human chorionic gonadotropin (hCG) is a glycoprotein composed of two non-identical glycosylated subunits, designated as α and β. The α-subunit of hCG is virtually identical to pituitary glycoprotein hormones -- luteinizing hormone (LH), follicle stimulating hormone (FSH), and thyroid stimulating hormone (TSH); the β-subunit is structurally distinct and confers biologic and immunologic specificity to each of the glycoprotein hormones.

Recently, several reports have appeared demonstrating the existence of large molecular species of glycoprotein hormones: LH (Prentice and Ryan, 1975; Liu et al., 1978, 1979), FSH (Reichert and Ramsey, 1977), TSH (Erhardt, 1975; Vanhaelst and Golstein-Golaire, 1976; Erhardt and Scriba, 1977; Klug and Adelman, 1977; Kourides et al., 1978), and hCG (Vaitukaitis, 1974; Good et al., 1977; Tojo et al., 1977; Pattillo et al., 1979). Some of these reports have suggested that the large molecular species might be a biosynthetic precursor or prohormone of the respective glycoprotein hormone. Nevertheless, evidence that a large species of hCG exists in placental tissues is based on the finding that the material was eluted in fractions near the void volume upon gel filtration on Sephadex G-100. Little is known about the biochemical and physico-chemical properties of the large molecular species of hCG.

In the present study, the large species of hCG was partially purified from human placental tissue cultured in vitro with radioactive amino acid and analyzed by electrophoresis on SDS-

polyacrylamide gel. On the other hand, a possible synthesis of
the large species of hCG in a cell-free protein synthesizing system
with placental polyribosomes was examined. Evidence will be
presented in this report to show that a large molecular species of
hCG is produced by human placental tissues, but not by in vitro
incubation of placental polyribosomes in a wheat germ, cell-free
system.

PREPARATION OF LARGE MOLECULAR SPECIES OF HCG FROM HUMAN PLACENTAL
TISSUES CULTURED IN VITRO WITH [^{3}H]PROLINE

Human placental tissues were obtained from women undergoing
therapeutic abortions in the first trimester of pregnancy. Tissues
were rinsed thoroughly with ice-cold Hank's solution, and were cut
into approximately 1 mm^3 explants. The explants, with a total wet
weight of approximately 3.0g, were placed on filter papers within
a Petri dish to which 20 ml of medium "199" containing 200 μCi of
[^{3}H]proline (specific activity 115 Ci/mmol, New England Nuclear),
500 IU penicillin, and 500 μg streptomycin were added. The tissue
explants were incubated for 90 min at 37°C in an atmosphere of 95%
O_2-5% CO_2 as previously described (Maruo et al., 1974). At the end
of the incubation period, the tissues were separated from the medium,
homogenized in 0.25M sucrose containing 1 mM N-α-p-tosyl-L-lysine
chloromethyl ketone (TLCK), a potent inhibitor of proteolysis, 5
mM magnesium acetate, 50 mM NH_4Cl in 0.01M Tris-HCl buffer, pH 7.5.
The homogenate was centrifuged according to the following scheme:

Component I:	500 x g for 5 min
Component II:	10,000 x g for 20 min
Component III:	105,000 x g for 60 min
Component IV:	final soluble supernatant

Components II and III were reconstituted in 0.01M Tris-HCl buffer
(pH 7.5) containing 1 mM TLCK, sonicated, and the undissolved
material removed by centrifugation.

Aliquots of component II (secretory granules), component III
(microsomal fraction), and Component IV (post-microsomal soluble
fraction) were subjected to gel filtration on a column (2.0 x 120 cm)
of Sephadex G-100. The amounts of hCG, hCGα and hCGβ were determined
by the homologous radioimmunoassays (RIAs) for hCG, hCGα, and hCGβ,
respectively, as previously described by Maruo et al. (1979). The
cross-reactivity of hCG and hCGβ in the homologous hCGα RIA was
approximately 1.4% and 0.1%, respectively, and that of hCG and hCGα
in the homologous hCGβ RIA was approximately 9.0% and 0.1%, respectively, while that of hCGα and hCGβ in the homologous hCG RIA was
1.1% and 0.2%, respectively. The radioactivity in the fractions
immunoprecipitated with antisera to hCG, hCGα, and hCGβ was determined as described by Maruo et al. (1980).

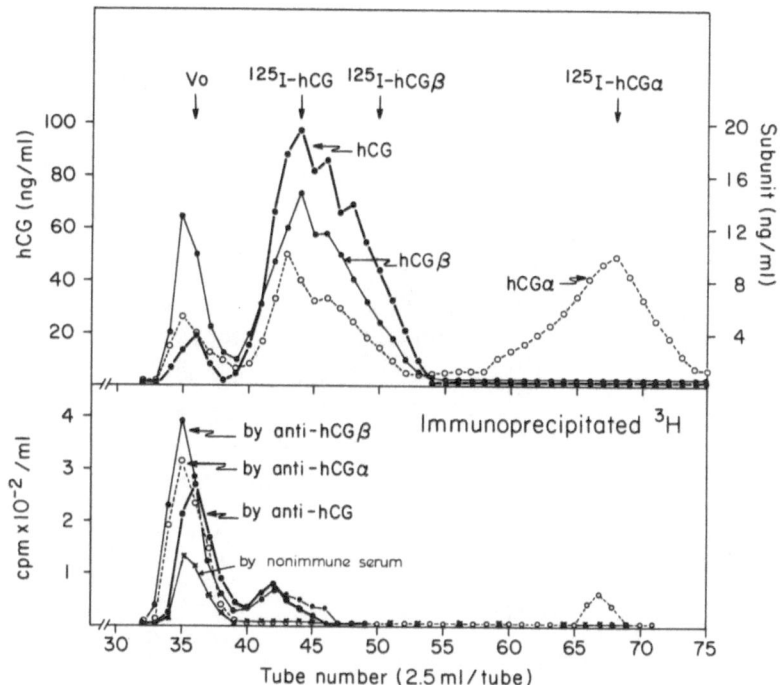

Figure 1. Sephadex G-100 elution profile of subcellular Component III of placental tissues cultured in vitro with [³H]proline. A column (2 x 120 cm) was equilibrated and eluted with 0.01 M Tris-HCl buffer (pH 7.5), 0.15 M NaCl at 4°C. Fractions of 2.5 ml were collected. V_0 represents the void volume determined by the blue dextran elution peak. The vertical arrows indicate the elution positions of [¹²⁵I]hCG, [¹²⁵I]hCGα, and [¹²⁵I]hCGβ.

The elution profiles of the microsomal (Figure 1) and post-microsomal components (Figure 2) consistently showed a small peak containing large molecular weight material. This material, emerging near the void volume, reacted with antisera to hCG, hCGα, and hCGβ, demonstrated dose-response curves parallel to those of the respective standard preparation in the three RIA systems (not shown), and possessed the highest [³H] radioactivities which were immunoprecipitated with all three antisera. Two additional peaks appeared after the void volume. The earlier peak which was RIA-positive for hCG, hCGα, and hCGβ was eluted in the region corresponding to [¹²⁵I]hCG. The later peak gave a positive reaction with only anti-hCGα, and contained [³H] radioactivity, which immunoprecipitated with anti-hCGα

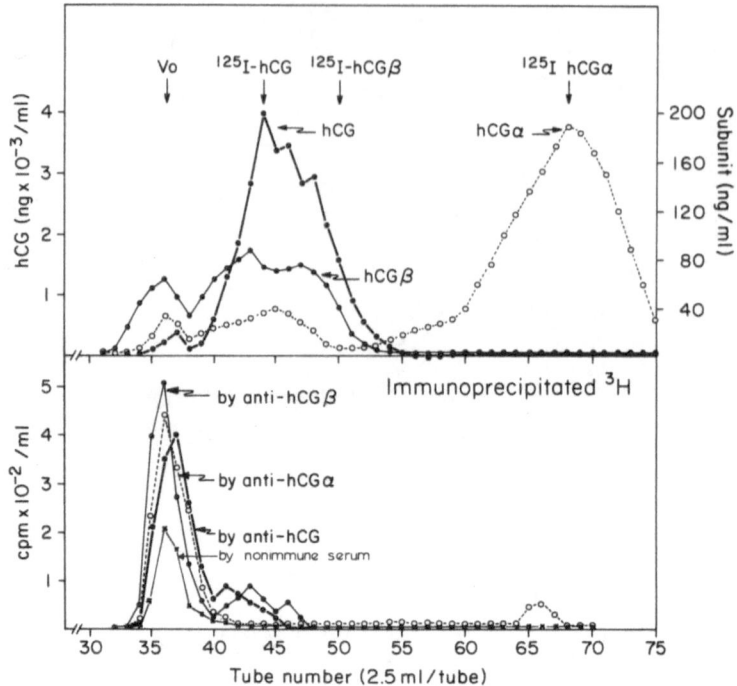

Figure 2.   Sephadex G-100 elution profile of subcellular component
IV of placental tissues cultured in vitro with [^{3}H]proline.   See
Figure 1 for description.

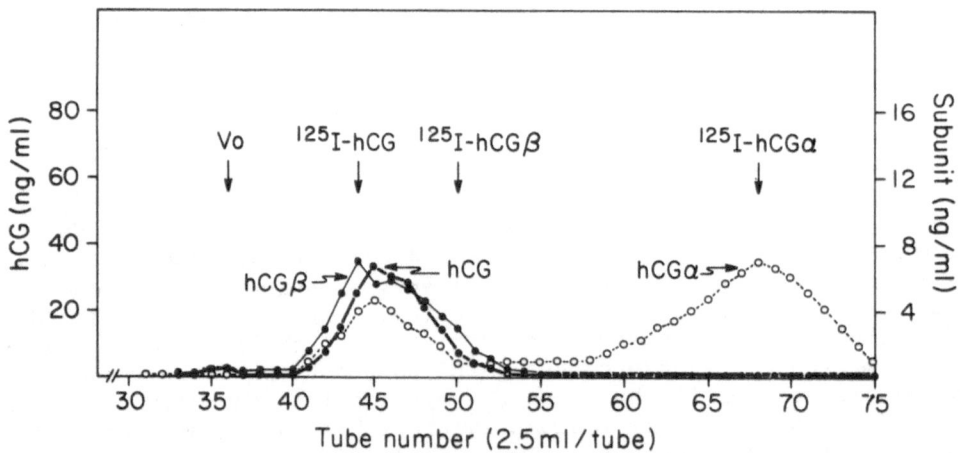

Figure 3.   Sephadex G-100 elution profile of subcellular component
II of placental tissues cultured in vitro.   Each fraction was assayed
by the homologous RIA systems for hCH, hCGα, and hCGβ.

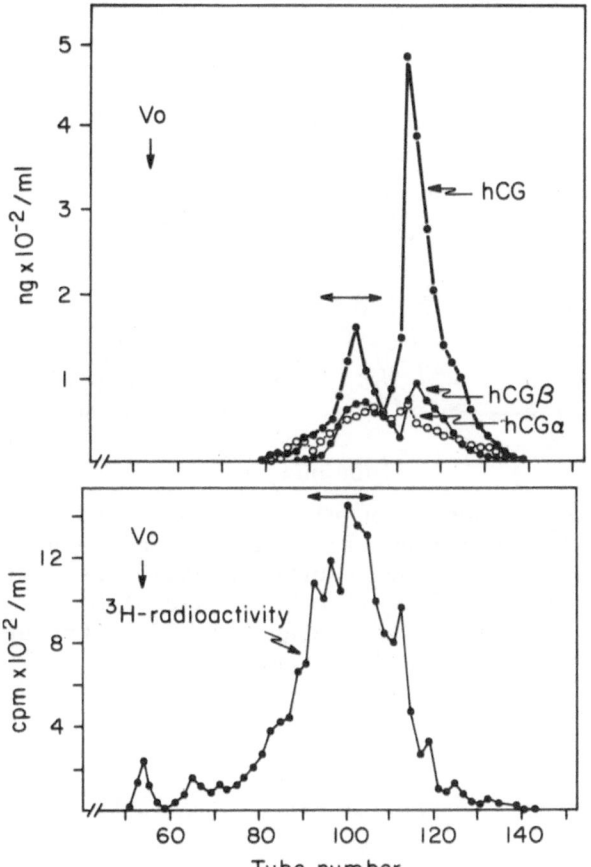

Figure 4.   Sepharose-6B elution profile of the immunoreactive hCG material of placental extracts previously obtained by gel filtration of Sephadex G-100 (see Figures 1 and 2).   A column (2 x 55 cm) was equilibrated and eluted at 4°C with 0.05M Tris-HCl buffer (pH 7.5), 0.15M NaCl.   1 ml fractions were collected. V_o represents the void volume determined by blue dextran elution peak.

serum.   Its elution position corresponded to $[^{125}I]hCG\alpha$.   It is noteworthy that at no time was free hCGβ corresponding to $[^{125}I]hCG\beta$ detected.   Furthermore, the large species material described above was not found in the secretory granules component (Figure 3).

Fractions (#33-48) (Figures 1 and 2) composed of immunoreactive hCG peaks obtained from gel filtration on Sephadex G-100 of the

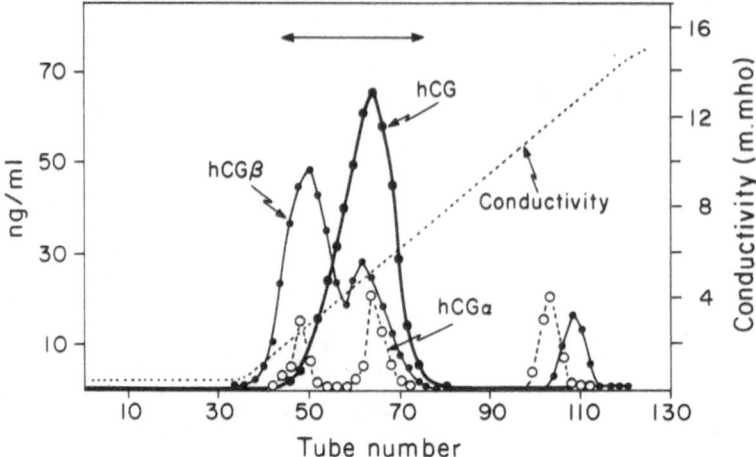

Figure 5.   DEAE-Sephadex A-50 elution profile of the fraction
containing the "large molecular species" obtained by refiltration
of Sepharose-6B column.   The adsorbed protein was eluted with a
300 ml linear gradient of 0-0.5 M NaCl in 0.01 M Tris-HCl buffer
(pH 7.4).   Each fraction was assayed for hCG, hCGα, and hCGβ by
the respective homologous RIA systems.

aliquots of microsomal and the postmicrosomal soluble components
were pooled, dialyzed, lyophilized, and refiltered through a column
(2 x 55 cm) of Sepharose-6B.   A small peak corresponding to the
large molecular weight material appeared again, followed by a major
peak corresponding to the standard form of hCG (Figure 4).   The
pattern of [^{3}H]radioactivity consisted of multiple peaks with a
prominent peak eluting at the region corresponding to the large
molecular weight material (Figure 4).

   Fractions (#88-105) containing the large molecular weight
material were pooled, dialyzed, lyophilized, and further purified
by ion exchange chromatography on a column (1.5 x 50 cm) of DEAE-
Sephadex A-50 (Figure 5).   The column was eluted with a linear
gradient of NaCl.   An early major fraction eluted at a conductivity
of 1.5 to 6.0 mmho contained material which immunoreacted with all
three antisera.   The major fraction was combined, dialyzed and
lyophilized.

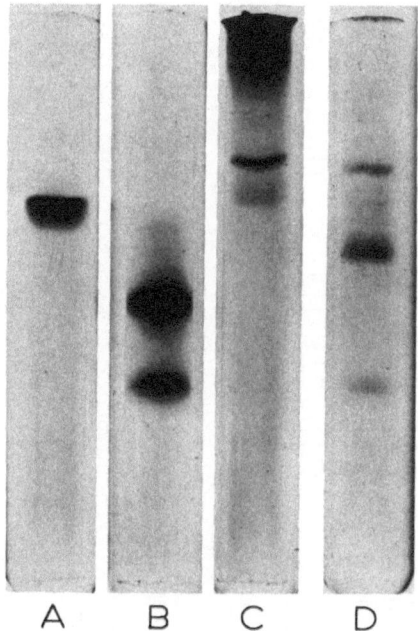

Figure 6. SDS-polyacrylamide gel electrophoresis of purified hCG (CR-119) and large molecular fraction obtained from DEAE-Sephadex A-50 chromatography. Gel A represents the elctrophoretic pattern of hCG (20μg) without 2-mercaptoethanol treatment. Gel B shows the electrophoretic pattern of hCG (20μg) after treatment with 2-mercaptoethanol. Gel C and Gel D represent electrophoretic patterns of the large molecular hCG fraction (20μg) without and with prior reduction by 2-mercaptoethanol, respectively. The migration is toward the anode at the bottom of the Figure.

SDS-POLYACRYLAMIDE GEL ELECTROPHORESIS OF THE LARGE MOLECULAR SPECIES OF HCG

The partially purified large molecular hCG material obtained from the above isolation procedure was subjected to electrophoresis in 7.5% polyacrylamide gel containing 0.1% sodium dodecyl sulfate (SDS). SDS-gel electrophoresis was performed essentially as described by Weber and Osborn (1969). Without reduction by mercaptoethanol, standard hCG (CR-119) did not dissociate into subunits, supporting the findings of Reichert and Lawson (1973) and Schlaff

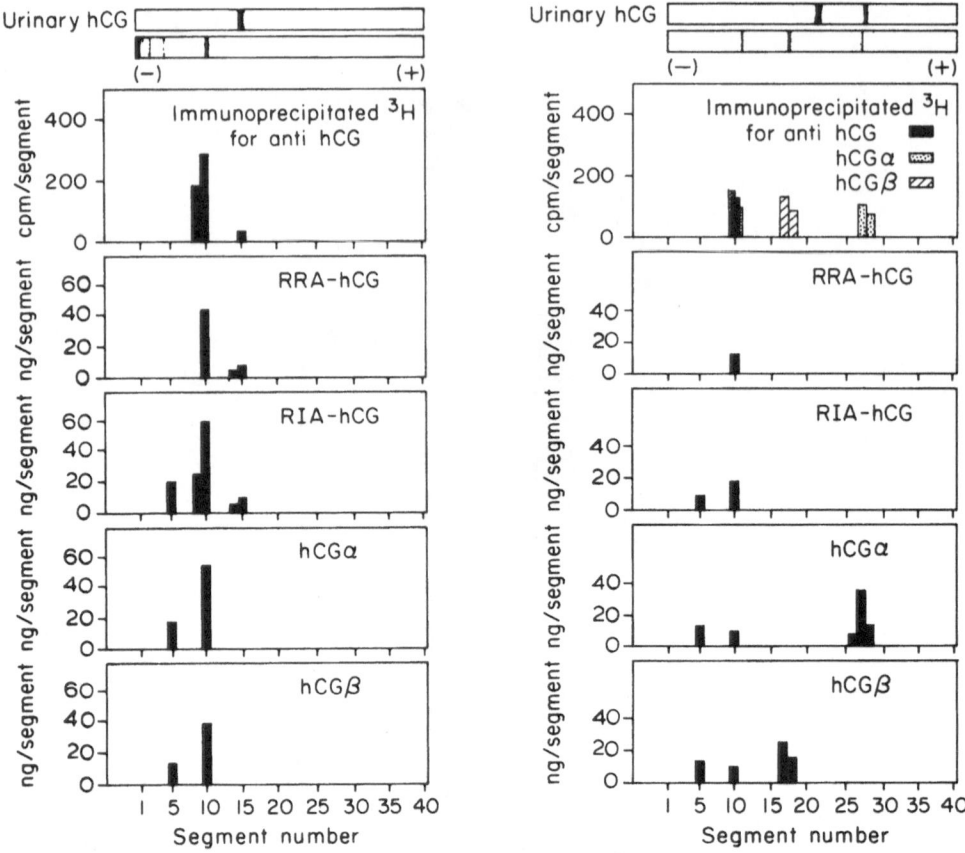

Figure 7 (left) and Figure 8 (right).   Localization of hCG, hCGα, and hCGβ activities in Gel C (7) and Gel D (8) shown in Figure 6. The gel was sliced into 2.2 mm segments.   Each segment was homogenized in P0.01 PBS (pH 7.4).   The amount of hCG and its subunits in each supernatant was determined by the homologous RIAs and RRA using bovine corpus luteum membranes.   The supernatant was also treated with anti-hCG serum, and the radioactivity in the immunoprecipitated fraction was determined.

(1976) (Figure 6A).   Under these conditions the mobility of the large molecular hCG fraction was retarded compared to standard hCG without showing any common bands between the two preparations (Figure 6C).

Upon reduction with mercaptoenthanol, standard hCG dissociated into two subunits in SDS-gel (Figure 6B) whereas the large molecular hCG fraction showed three major bands (Figure 6D): the mobility of the first band was retarded compared to standard hCG; the second band migrated between standard hCG and hCGβ, and the third band migrated slightly slower than standard hCGα.

The gels were sliced into segments of 2.2 mm thickness. Each segment was homogenized in 1 ml of 0.01M phosphate buffer (pH 7.4) and centrifuged. The supernatant was immunoprecipitated with antiserum to hCG, hCGα, or hCGβ, and the radioactivity measured. In addition, the samples were analyzed for hCG, hCGα, and hCGβ by RIAs, and its receptor binding activity measured. Segment #10 of the gel containing material not reduced with mercaptoethanol (Gel C, Figure 6) showed a coincidental peak of immunoprecipitated [^{3}H] radioactivity, and immunological activities with antisera to hCG, hCGα, and hCGβ, as well as receptor binding activity (Figure 7). On the other hand, segment #10 of the gel prepared with material after mercaptoethanol treatment (Gel D, Figure 6), contained [^{3}H]radioactivities immunoprecipitated with all three antisera and showed immunoreactivities with antisera to hCG, hCGα, and hCGβ, and slight receptor binding activity (Figure 8). In the same gel, segments 16-17 and 27-28, corresponding to the protein bands described above, showed immunoprecipitable radioactivities and immunoreactivities with antisera to hCGβ and hCGα, respectively (Figure 8). Thus, segment 10 corresponded to the large molecular weight hCG material, segments 16-17 to hCGβ and segments 27-28 to hCGα. Figure 9 shows a plot of the mobilities of several proteins of known molecular weights by electrophoresis on SDS-polyacrylamide gels. Based on these standard proteins as reference, the apparent molecular weights of hCG (CR-119), hCGα (CR-119), and hCGβ (CR-119-2) were estimated to be about 58,000, 22,000 and 36,000 daltons, respectively. Under the same conditions, the molecular weights of the material in segment 10 (reacting with all three antisera), in segment 27 (reacting with anti-hCGα), and in segment 16 (reacting with anti-hCGβ) were estimated to be about 90,000, 24,000 and 52,000 daltons, respectively. Hence, these materials analyzed by electrophoresis are somewhat larger than authentic hCG and the respective subunits.

8M-UREA TREATMENT OF THE LARGE MOLECULAR SPECIES OF HCG

Large molecular hCG species obtained from the Sepharose-6B column was dissolved in a medium containing 8M-urea in 0.04 M Tris-phosphate buffer (pH 7.5) and incubated at 37°C for two hours. The mixture was then transferred to the column of Sephadex G-100, as described above. The large molecular hCG material did not contain any free subunits when analyzed by gel filtration on Sephadex G-100 (Figure 10). Following treatment with 8M urea, a significant portion of the large molecular hCG species remained undissociated, although immunoreactive hCGα and hCGβ slightly larger than standard subunits were separated. It was noted that the remaining

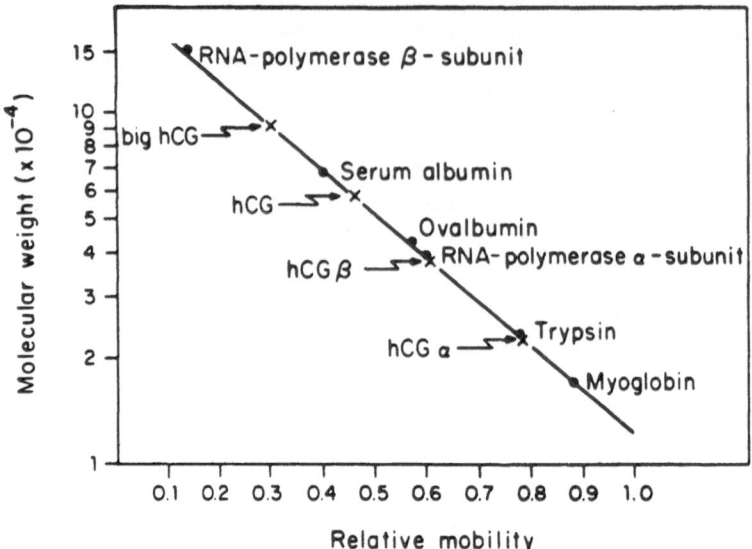

Figure 9.   Estimation of the molecular weight of the large molecular species of hCG by electrophoresis on SDS-polyacrylamide gel. The relative mobilities of several proteins of known molecular weight are plotted using bromophenol blue as reference. 7.5% gel was used containing 0.1% SDS. The marker proteins utilized were myoglobin, trypsin, and RNA-polymerase α-subunit, ovalbumin, serum albumin, and RNA-polymerase β-subunit.

undissociated material after 8M urea treatment displayed a significant loss of binding activity to corpus luteum membrane receptor, in spite of the fact that it retained its immunoreactivity (Figure 10).

CELL-FREE PROTEIN SYNTHESIZING SYSTEM WITH PLACENTAL POLYRIBOSOMES

Human placentas from eight to twelve weeks gestational period were obtained by vacuum curretage. Immediately after evacuation, the tissues were immersed in ice-cold buffer solution containing 30 mM Tris-HCl, pH 7.5, 120 mM KCl, 5 mM magnesium acetate, 5 mM 2-mercaptoethanol, 100 mM NH_4Cl, and transported to the laboratory. Placental tissues were pooled to collect 40g of placental villi.

The placental villi were separated from fetal and maternal tissues, washed in buffer to remove blood, and minced into suitable pieces with scissors. Minced tissue was homogenized with buffer

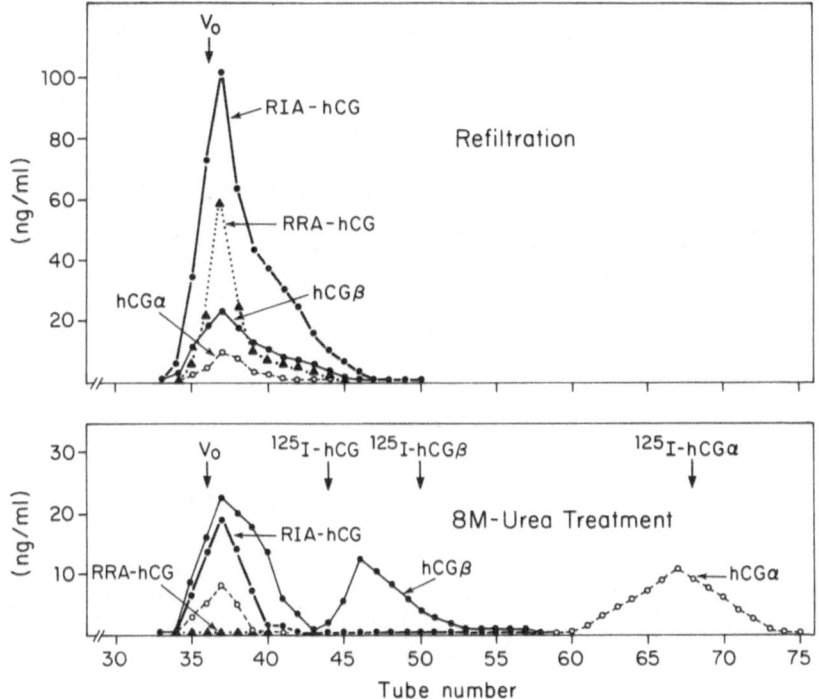

Figure 10. Gel filtration on Sephadex G-100 of the large molecular species of hCG before and after 8M-urea treatment. Upper panel shows the elution profile of untreated large molecular hCG species (1 mg). Lower panel displays the elution profile after 8M-urea treatment. Each fraction was assayed by the homologous RIA systems for hCG, hCGα, and hCGβ, and by RRA.

containing 0.5 mM EDTA. Homogenization was carried out in the cold for about 3 min with motor-driven Teflon-glass homogenizers. The homogenate was centrifuged at 8000 x g for 20 min at 4°C.

Sodium deoxycholate solution (10%) was added to the supernatant fluid to 1% concentration. Each 10 ml of suspension was layered over a discontinuous gradient made up of 2 ml of 1.30 M and 2 ml of 1.17 M sucrose solution prepared in the homogenizing buffer. The gradients were centrifuged at 200,000 x g for 4 hr at 4°C. The top layers were then aspirated and the tubes containing the pellets were rinsed gently with homogenizing buffer to remove any residual deoxycholate. The pellets were resuspended in the homogenizing buffer.

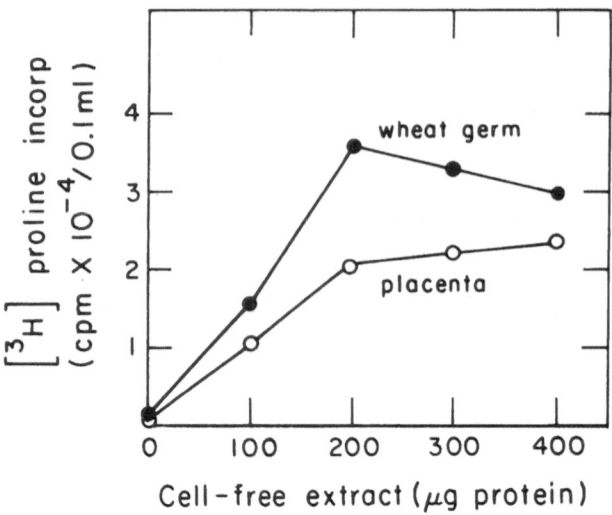

Cell-free extract (μg protein)

Figure 11. Incorporation of [^{3}H]proline by placental polyribosomes in the presence of wheat germ extract or placental cell sap. All reaction mixtures contained 50 µg polyribosomes and were incubated for 60 min at 33°C. Incorp: incorporated.

The cell-sap fraction derived from placental tissue and 30,000 x g supernatants (S-30) derived from wheat germ were prepared according to the methods of Laga et al. (1970) and Roberts and Patterson (1973), respectively. Protein was measured by the method of Lowry et al. (1951).

Protein synthesis was assayed in a final volume of 100 µl of reaction mixtures composed of 50 mM Tris-HCl, pH 7.5, 70 mM KCl, 1.5 mM $MgCl_2$, 2 mM dithiothreitol (DTT), 1 mM ATP, 1 mM GTP, 10 mM phophocreatine, 100 µg/ml of creatine phosphokinase, 40 µmoles each of 19 unlabeled amino acids and 2 µCi [^{3}H]proline (specific activity, 115 Ci/mmol, New England Nuclear), and appropriate amounts of polyribosomes and cell-free extract. Each reaction mixture was incubated for varying time periods at 33°C. After incubation, incorporation of radioactivity into trichloroacetic acid (TCA)-precipitable protein was measured.

Endogenous protein synthetic activity of the placental polyribosomes incubated with either cell-free extract derived from wheat germ or from placental tissue was capable of incorporating [^{3}H]proline. The activity with the cell-free extract from wheat germ was higher

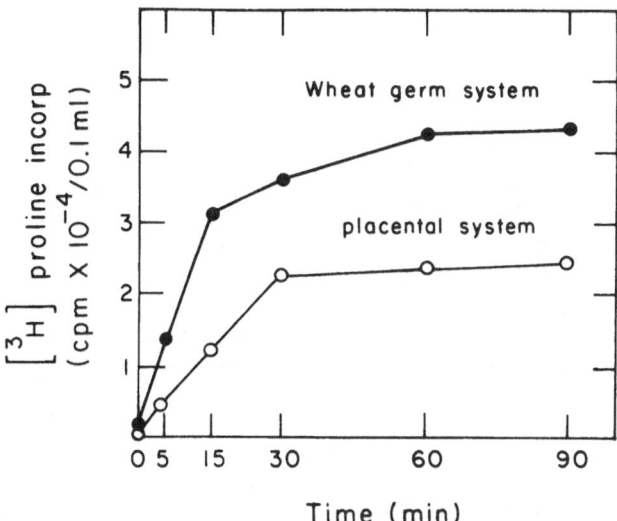

Time (min)

Figure 12. Time course of [^{3}H]proline incorporation into protein on incubation of placental polyribosomes with a wheat germ or placental cell-free system. Each reaction mixture contained 50 μg polyribosomes and wheat germ extract or placental cell sap equivalent to 200 μg of protein. Aliquots of the incubation mixture were removed at varying times indicated, and the reaction stopped by the addition of cold 10% trichloroacetic acid. Incorp: incorporated.

than that with the cell-sap from placental tissue (Figure 11). No incorporation of [^{3}H]glucosamine (18.8 Ci/mmol, New England Nuclear) was found.

The time course of incorporation of [^{3}H]proline with the wheat germ system and homologous placental system was linear for at least 15 min and for 30 min, respectively. Slight residual incorporation was observed after 60 min (Figure 12).

The amount of immunoreactive hCG, hCGα, and hCGβ produced by placental polyribosomes in a wheat germ cell-free system were determined by the respective homologous RIAs. Immunoreactivities of hCG and hCGα in the incubation mixture showed a linear increment for at least 90 min incubation, while immunoreactivity of hCGβ increased linearly only for 15 min, and gradually decreased after that time period (Figure 13).

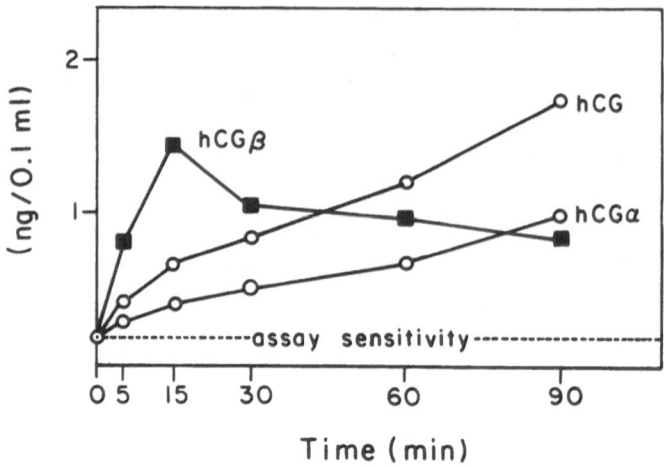

Time (min)

Figure 13.   Production of immunoreactive hCG, hCGα, and hCGβ by placental polyribosomes in a wheat germ cell-free translating system. 100 μl aliquots of the cell-free incubation mixture were removed at each incubation period and assayed for hCG, hCGα, and hCGβ by the respective homologous RIAs.

In view of the pattern of the production of immunoreactive hCG and its subunits observed, the cell-free incubation mixtures obtained after 15 min incubation and 90 min incubation of placental polyribosomes were, respectively, immunoprecipitated with antisera to hCG, hCGα, and hCGβ according to the procedures described by Palmiter (1974) with a slight modification. The resulting immunoprecipitates were dissolved in 50 μl each of a solution containing 50 mM Tris-HCl, pH 7.5, 1% SDS, 1% 2-mercaptoethanol, 10% glycerol, and 0.001% bromophenol blue, and solubilized by heating at 100°C for one min. These solutions were analyzed by electrophoresis on 7.5% polyacrylamide gels containing 0.1% SDS. After electrophoresis, the gels were sliced into 2.2mm segments and radioactivity was measured by dissolving each segment in 0.1 ml of H_2O_2 at 55°C for several hours, taking up the aqueous phase in 0.7 ml of Protosol (New England Nuclear), incubating for one hour at 55°C and counting the mixture in a liquid scintillation counter.

Figure 14 shows a radioactivity profile on SDS-polyacrylamide gel of [³H]labeled peptides synthesized on incubation of placental polyribosomes for 15 min. The material precipitated with anti-hCG serum was resolved into two major peaks of radioactivity, one being approximately 15,000 daltons in molecular weight, and the other

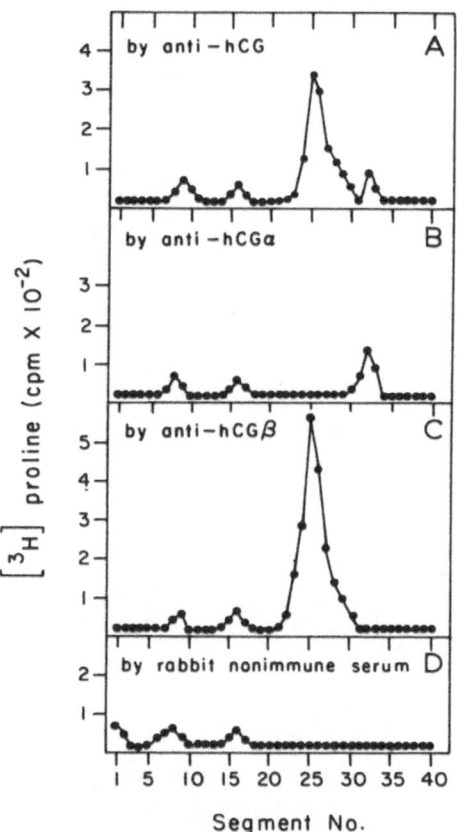

Figure 14. SDS-polyacrylamide gel analysis of $[^3H]$labeled peptides synthesized during in vitro incubation for 15 min of placental polyribosomes. Polyribosomes prepared from first trimmester placenta were incubated in the presence of wheat germ extract and $[^3H]$proline, and $[^3H]$labeled hCG and its subunits were immunoprecipitated by anti-hCG serum (panel A), anti-hCGα serum (panel B), or anti-hCGβ serum (panel C), respectively. Each immunoprecipitate was resolved on SDS gels and radioactivity was measured in gel slice. Panel D shows the profile of control experiment where non-immune serum was added to the cell-free reaction mixture.

24,000 daltons (Figure 14A). In addition, two smaller peaks were observed in the retarded region, representing non-specific radioactivities, since the material precipitated with non-immune serum also exhibited these peaks (Figure 14D). The profiles after the same incubation mixtures were treated with antisera to hCGα and hCGβ

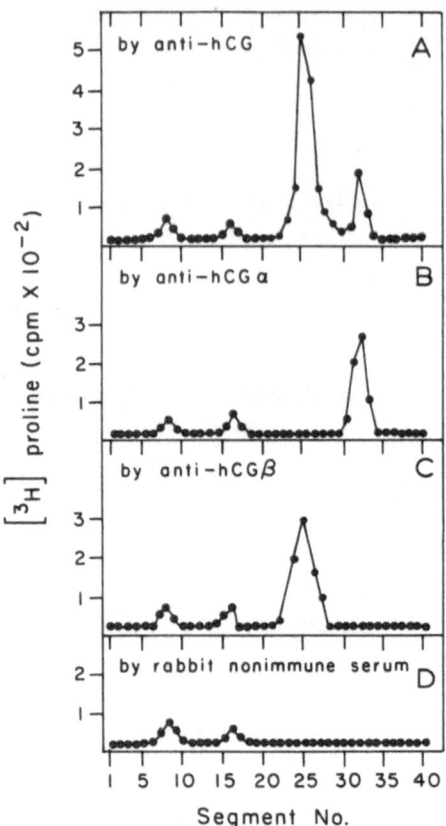

Segment No.

Figure 15. SDS-polyacrylamide gel analysis of [^{3}H]labeled peptides synthesized during in vitro incubation for 90 min of placental polyribosomes. Details are same as for Figure 14.

are shown in Figure 14B and 14C, respectively. Single sharp peaks of radioactivity corresponding to a molecular weight of 15,000 and 24,000 daltons were observed after precipitation with antisera to hCGα and hCGβ, respectively. With the wheat germ system used, glycosylation does not take place, since the addition of microsomal membranes appears to be essential to allow glycosylation in the cell-free system (Bielinska and Boime, 1978). The observed molecular weights are probably non-glycosylated subunits. Since molecular weights of protein of authentic hCGα and hCGβ correspond to 10,200 and 16,000 daltons, respectively (Bellisario et al., 1973; Carlsen et al., 1973), the apparent molecular weights of the cell-free products are greater than those of protein portions of authentic subunits, suggesting that subunits of hCG are initially synthesized as the precursor form of each subunit protein. A noteworthy finding was that the radioactivity peak obtained with anti-hCGβ serum was considerably higher than that with anti-hCGα serum. The position of radioactive peaks for α- and β-chains coincided closely with those peaks obtained with material precipitated with anti-hCG serum. These results suggest that the α- and β-subunit protein might combine at this stage to form hCG protein.

Although analysis on SDS-polyacrylamide gel of [^{3}H]labeled peptides synthesized during 90 min incubation of placental polyribosomes showed similar profiles to those obtained with the 15 min incubation mixture, the radioactive peak of the β-chain precipitated with anti-hCGβ serum was smaller compared to that observed with the 15 min incubation mixture, whereas peaks of α-chain and β-chain dissociated from the material precipitated with anti-hCG serum were higher than those observed with the 15 min incubation mixture (Figure 15).

The present results that the synthesis of the β-subunit is active at the beginning of the incubation of polyribisomes and subsequently becomes limited, supports the notion that earlier accelerated synthesis of β-subunit protein is required for the subsequent association with the newly synthesized α-subunit to form hCG. In this manner, synthesis of the β-subunit protein may be the limiting step in the production of hCG.

DISCUSSION

The present results indicate that human placental tissue contains a large molecular species of hCG which interacts with antisera to hCG, hCGα, and hCGβ and with the receptor membranes of bovine corpus luteum. On SDS-gel electrophoresis in which the reduction step with mercaptoethanol was omitted, the partially purified large species of hCG showed electrophoretic pattern similar to that of the large molecular species of FSH in pituitary extract, described by Reichert and Ramsey (1977). The exact molecular weight of the material cannot be established by this method, since the migration of glycoprotein on SDS-gel electrophoresis would not reflect the authentic molecular weight, due to the sugar moieties which tend to retard its mobility (Segrest et al., 1971). Nevertheless, the large molecular species of hCG observed on SDS-gel electrophoresis corresponded to a molecular weight of about 90,000 daltons under the same conditions.

The large species of hCG appeared to be relatively stable to treatment with 8M-urea and mercaptoethanol in the presence of SDS. Under these conditions, standard hCG readily separated into subunits, while a significant potion of the large species of hCG remained undissociated. Nevertheless, the large species of hCG appears to consist of subunits larger than standard hCG subunits, since treatment of the large species with 8M-urea and reduction with mercaptoethanol in the presence of SDS resulted in dissociating immunoreactive α and β-subunits of rather high molecular weights compared to standard hCG subunits. Furthermore, the large species of hCG possessed immunoreactivities against anti-hCGα serum and anti-hCGβ serum and interacted with the receptor membranes of bovine corpus luteum. In contrast, it is well known that free α and β subunits lack receptor binding activity (Lee and Ryan, 1973). Hence, the large molecular species of hCG might conceivably be a complex of immunoreactive α and β-subunits somewhat larger than standard hCG subunits.

The observation that [^{3}H]proline used as a radioactive marker is incorporated into the large species of hCG after 90 min incubation of the placental tissues cultured in vitro suggests that the large species of hCG may be a biosynthetic product by placental tissues. This thesis is supported by the fact that the large species of hCG was located in the microsomal component which contains elements of the protein biosynthetic system and in the postmicrosomal supernatant, but not in the secretory granules component.

Biosynthesis of large molecular species of TSH has been reported by Klug and Adelman (1977) and LH by Liu et al. (1978, 1979). It has been suggested that α and β-subunits of LH and TSH are initially synthesized as a covalently linked large precursor protein (prohormone) by Prentice and Ryan (1975) and by Klug and Adelman (1977), respectively. Accordingly, if one assumes that any glycoprotein hormone is synthesized as a prohormone, its production would be under the control of a single gene operon. However, recent studies using cell-free translation of mRNA from human placenta have identified the α and β-subunits of hCG and suggested their synthesis from separate mRNA (Landefield et al., 1976; Daniels-McQueen et al., 1978). The facts that placental polyribosomes in the wheat germ cell-free system demonstrated the synthesis of α-subunit and β-subunit proteins with apparent molecular weights of 15,000 and 24,000 daltons, respectively, and that the large molecular species of hCG was not detected in the same cell-free system, suggest that the subunits of hCG are initially synthesized as precursor forms of the subunits rather than as a covalently-linked large prohormone of hCG. Hence, in spite of the substantial incorpotation of [^{3}H]proline used as a marker into the large species of hCG by in vitro incubation of placental tissues, its physiological significance is still obscure. If the large molecular species of hCG is not an intermediary component of hCG biosynthesis, it may be a product of a post-translational modification, probably due to a modification of carbohydrate moieties.

REFERENCES

Ashitaka, Y., and Koide, S. S., 1974, Interaction of human chorionic gonadotropin with rat gonads, Fertil. Steril. 25:177.

Bellisario, R., Carlsen, R. B., and Bahl, O. P., 1973, Human chorionic gonadotropin, Linear sequence of the α-subunit, J. Biol. Chem. 248:6796.

Bielinska, M., and Boime, I., 1978, The synthesis of a glycosylated subunit of human chorionic gonadotropin in cell-free extracts derived from ascites tumor cells, Proc. Natl. Acad. Sci. U.S.A. 75:1768.

Canfield, R. E., and Morgan, F. J., 1973, Human chorionic gonadotropin, in *Methods in Investigative and Diagnostic Endocrinology*, Berson, S. A., and Yalow, R., eds., pp. 727-733, North Holland Publishing Co., Amsterdam.

Carlsen, R. B., Bahl, O. P., and Swaminatham, C. N., 1973, Human chorionic gonadotropin. Linear sequence of the β-subunit, J. Biol. Chem. 248:6810.

Daniel-McQueen, S., McWilliams, D., Birken, S., Canfield, R. E., Lanfeld, T., and Boime, I., 1978, Identification of mRNAs encoding the α and β subunits of human choriogonadotropin, J. Biol. Chem. 253:7109.

Erhardt, F. W., 1975, Isolation of a 'big'-hTSH by affinity chromatography, Acta Endocrinol. (Kbh), Suppl. 193:3.

Erhardt, F. W., and Scriba, P. C., High molecular thyrotropin from human pituitaries. Preparation and partial characterization, Acta Endocrinol. (Kbh.) 85:698.

Good, A., Ramos-Uribe, M., Ryan, R. J., and Kemper, R. D., 1977, Molecular forms of human chorionic gonadotropin in serum, urine and placental extracts, Fertil. Steril. 28:846.

Klug, T. L., and Adelman, R. C., 1977, Evidence for a large thyrotropin and its accumulation during aging in rats, Biochem. Biophys. Res. Commun. 77:1431.

Kourides, I. A., Weinbraub, B. D., and Maloof, F., 1978, Large molecular weight TSH-β. The sole immunoreactive form of TSH-in certain human sera, J. Clin. Endocrinol. Metab. 47:24.

Laga, E. M., Baliga, B. S., and Munro, H. N., 1970, Isolation and properties of polysomes from human placents, Biochem. Biophys. Acta 213:391.

Landefeld, T. D., McWilliams, D. R., and Boime, I., 1976, The cell-free synthesis of the α-subunit of human chorionic gonadotropin, Endocrinology 98:1220.

Lee, C. Y., and Ryan, R. J., 1973, Interaction of ovarian receptors with human luteinizing hormone and human chorionic gonadotropin, Biochemistry 12:4609.

Liu, T. C., Ax, R., and Jackson, G. L., 1978, Characterization of LH synthesized and released by rat pituitaries in vitro, Endocrinology Suppl. 102:104.

Liu, T. C., Ax, R., and Jackson, G. L., 1979, 'Big'LH. Possible precursor of native LH in anterior pituitary glands of rats, Biol.

Reprod. 20, Suppl. 1:43.

Lowry, O. H., Rosebrough, N. J., Fiard, A. L., and Randall, R. J., 1951, Protein measurement with the felin phenol reagent, J. Biol. Chem. 193:265.

Maruo, T., 1976, Studies on in vitro synthesis and secretion of human choriogonadotropin and its subunits, Endocrinol. Japan. 23:119.

Maruo, T., Segal, S. J., and Koide, S. S., 1978, Evidence for the in vitro biosynthesis of large molecular species of human choriogonadotropin, Endocrinology, Suppl. 102:93.

Maruo, T., Ashitaka, Y., Mochizuki, M., and Tojo, S., 1974, Chorionic gonadotropin synthesized in cultivated trophoblasts, Endocrinol. Japan. 21:499.

Maruo, T., Segal, S. J. and Koide, S. S., 1979, Studies on the apparent human chorionic gonadotropin-like factor in the crab Ovalipes ocellatus, Endocrinology 104:932.

Maruo, T., Segal, S. J., and Koide, S. S., 1980, Large molecular species of choriogonadotropin from human placental tissues. Biosynthesis and physico-chemical properties, Acta Endocrinol. (Kbh), In press.

Palmiter, R. D., 1974, Differential rates of initiation on conalbumin and ovalbumin messenger ribonucleic acid in reticulocyte lysates, J. Biol. Chem. 249:6779.

Pattillo, R. A., Hussa, R. O., Ruckert, A. C. F., Kurtz, J. W., Cade, J. M., and Rinke, M. L., 1979, Human chorionic gonadotropin in BeWo trophoblastic cells after 12 years in continuous culture. Retention of intact human chorionic gonadotropin secretion in mechanically-versus enzyme-dispersed cells, Endocrinology 105:974.

Prentice, L. G., and Ryan, R. J., 1975, LH and its subunits in human pituitary, serum and urine, J. Clin. Endocrinol. Metab. 40:303.

Reichert, L. E., and Ramsey, R. B., 1977, Evidence for the existence of a large molecular weight protein in human pituitary tissue having follicle stimulating hormone activity, J. Clin. Endocrinol. Metab. 44:545.

Roberts, B. E., and Paterson, B. M., 1973, Efficient translation of tobacco mosaic virus RNA and rabbit globin 9S RNA in a cell-free system from commercial wheat germ, Proc. Natl. Acad. Sci. U.S.A. 70:2330.

Segrest, J. P., Jackson, R. L., Andrews, E. D., and Marchesi, V. T., 1971. Human erythrocyte membrane glycoprotein. A re-evaluation of the molecular weight as determined by SDS polyacrylamide gel electrophoresis, Biochem. Biophys. Res. Commun. 44:390.

Vaitukaitis, J. L., Robbins, J. B., Nieschlag, E., and Ross, G. T., 1971, A method for producing specific antisera with small doses of immunogen, J. Clin. Endocrinol. Metab. 33:988.

Vanhaelst, L., and Golstein-Golaire, J., 1976, Gel filtration profile of immunoreactive thyrotropin and subunits of human pituitaries, J. Clin. Endocrinol. Metab.

Weber, K., and Osborn, M., 1969, The reliability of molecular weight determinations by dodecyl sulfate-polyacrylamide gel electrophoresis, J. Biol. Chem. 244:4406.

ACKNOWLEDGEMENTS

We thank Dr. Ione Kourides at the Memorial Sloan-Kettering Cancer Center for valuable suggestions about this study. We thank Dr. R. E. Canfield for the gifts of reference preparations of hCG and its subunits and Drs. Y-Y. Tsong and C-C. Chang for providing antisera to hCG, hCGα, and hCGβ. This study was performed as part of the Contraceptive Development Program of the International Committee for Contraceptive Research of the Population Council. T. Maruo was supported by a Rockefeller Foundation Fellowship Award in Reproductive Biology and Biomedical Fellowship of the Population Council, Rockefeller University, New York.

DISTRIBUTION, METABOLISM, AND EXCRETION OF

HUMAN CHORIONIC GONADOTROPIN AND ITS SUBUNITS IN MAN

Bruce C. Nisula and Robert E. Wehmann

Developmental Endocrinology Branch, National
Institute of Child Health and Human Development
National Institutes of Health, Bethesda, Maryland
and Gerontology Research Center, National Institute
on Aging, Baltimore City Hospitals, Baltimore
Maryland, U.S.A.

INTRODUCTION

It has been well established that the serum and urine of
pregnant women contain several molecules immunologically related
to, but smaller than the human chorionic gonadotropin (hCG)
molecule. A number of laboratories have reported that the most
abundant of these hCG-related molecules is one which behaves on
gel chromatography and in radioimmunoassays for the hCG alpha-
subunit (hCGα) very much like the authentic hCGα subunit (Franchimont and Reuter, 1972; Hagen and McNeilly, 1975; Vaitukaitis et al.,
1976; Good et al., 1977). Also, some workers have produced evidence
to suggest that a moiety with properties like those of the hCG beta-
subunit (hCGβ) can be found in the serum and urine of pregnancy
(Franchimont and Reuter, 1972; Good et al., 1977). The presence of
free hCG subunits, or molecules with similar immunological and
physicochemical characteristics, in normal pregnancy raises questions
concerning the origin of these hCG-related peptides. It is not known
whether they are degradation products of secreted hCH, or whether
they are secreted themselves, or whether they are degradation products of other hCG-related peptides. We have been exploring the
distribution, metabolism, and excretion of hCG and its subunits in
normal human subjects with the aim of establishing the fundamental
kinetic characteristics of these molecules, and with the aim of
assessing the extent to which the degradation of secreted hCG
accounts for the presence of hCG-related peptides in the biological
fluids of pregnancy. In this chapter, we will attempt to summarize

recent findings on the kinetics of metabolism of hCG and its subunits and to present some information concerning their disposal and degradation pathways.

PREPARATIONS OF HCG AND ITS SUBUNITS

To investigate the metabolism of hCG and its subunits in normal subjects, the purified hCG preparations are made suitable for administration by millipore filtration. Following this procedure, the hCG subunits will recombine to form biologically active hCG (Wehmann and Nisula, 1979). The same materials as those injected are used as reference preparations and radioligands in the radioimmunoassays. The purified preparations used for investigations thus far include the subunits derived from the purified hCG (CR119) preparation and the hCG purified from batch CR121. These materials were provided by the Center for Population Research, National Institute of Child Health and Human Development. The details of purification and characterization have been extensively described (Morgan et al., 1974; Canfield and Ross, 1976). We find that the purified CR119 batch of hCG is indistinguishable from the CR121 batch of hCG with respect to biologic activities and behavior in radioligand-receptor assays and radioimmunoassays. The specifics of the experimental procedures for measuring hCG and its subunits and the methods of calculation are detailed in earlier reports (Wehmann and Nisula, 1979). Measurement of hCG and its subunits in urine is usually performed after extraction by adsorption to concanavalin A covalently linked to Sepharose as outlined elsewhere (Nisula et al., 1978; Ayala et al., 1978). We use antisera generated to the intact subunits (Vaitukaitis et al., 1972) and antisera to the carboxy-terminal peptide of hCGβ (Louvet et al., 1974) to measure serum and urine levels by radioimmunoassay, and to examine immunoreactive degradation products in the fractions eluted from Sephadex G-100 columns.

Several other laboratories have studied hCG metabolism in man by injecting hCG preparations (Wide et al., 1968; Rizkallah et al., 1969; Sowers et al., 1978). It is evident that when crude commercial preparations are used, biologic methods for measurement of hCG have a distinct advantage over immunologic methods because the injected crude preparations contain immunoreactive, biologically inactive hCG-related peptides. The kinetic picture obtained of a crude hCG preparation studied by radioimmunoassay is actually a composite picture of the kinetics of the hCG and the contaminants. The more homogeneous the preparation, the better. With regard to the purified preparations used in our studies, some heterogeneity is apparent in polycrylamide gel electrophoresis. The hCGα gives two bands, and the hCGβ 5 bands (Morgan et al., 1974). These different bands probably are due to variability in the carbohydrate moieties. At present, it is unknown whether these slightly different molecular forms exhibit different kinetic behaviors.

Several laboratories have measured the decline in hCG levels after the termination of pregnancy (Midgely et al., 1968; Yen et al., 1968). Two studies concerning metabolic clearance rates of the subunits of hCG are available (Kourides et al., 1977; Wehmann and Nisula, 1979).

SINGLE INJECTION TECHNIQUE

To investigate the parameters of the metabolism of hCG and its subunits, the study design includes two different approaches, single intravenous injection and constant infusion to steady-state. The values one obtains for the clearance rates with these two techniques are generally in close agreement. Since other kinetic parameters, such as initial volume of distribution and half-lives of the components, can be determined with the single injection technique, in the present manuscript we are focusing on data generated with it. To date, we have completed the study of hCGβ and hCGα metabolism in both men and women (Wehmann and Nisula, 1979), and we have data on hCG metabolism in three men using the single injection technique. To permit the relevant comparison, the results to be presented here are for normal male subjects and are normalized to a body surface area of 1.73 square meters. However, it should be noted that the kinetic parameters of hCGβ and hCGα are the same in men and women, providing correction is made for differences in body size.

DISAPPEARANCE CURVES

Following single intravenous injection in the same dosage, hCG, hCGα, and hCGβ achieve nearly identical initial serum concentrations and their levels progressively decline thereafter (Figure I). The time course of disappearance of each molecule is non-linear when plotted on a semilogarithmic graph (Figure I). The disappearance of hCG is slowest, and that of hCGβ is slower than that of hCGα. The relative behavior of hCG, hCGβ, and hCGα which we find in human subjects is qualitatively similar to that found in rats by Braunstein et al. (1972). Of course, the absolute values of the various parameters differ by a considerable degree between the two species.

PARAMETERS OF FAST AND SLOW COMPONENTS

Each serum disappearance curve shown in Figure 1 has at least two components which are designated fast and slow. Using an exponential curve fitting program such as that of Faden and Rodbard (1975), one can derive the kinetic parameters for these curves and provide numbers to quantitate the visual impressions of Figure 1. The equation form in each case is $C = Ae^{-\alpha t} + Be^{-\beta t}$, where C is the serum concentration, t is time in minutes. A and α are the fast component

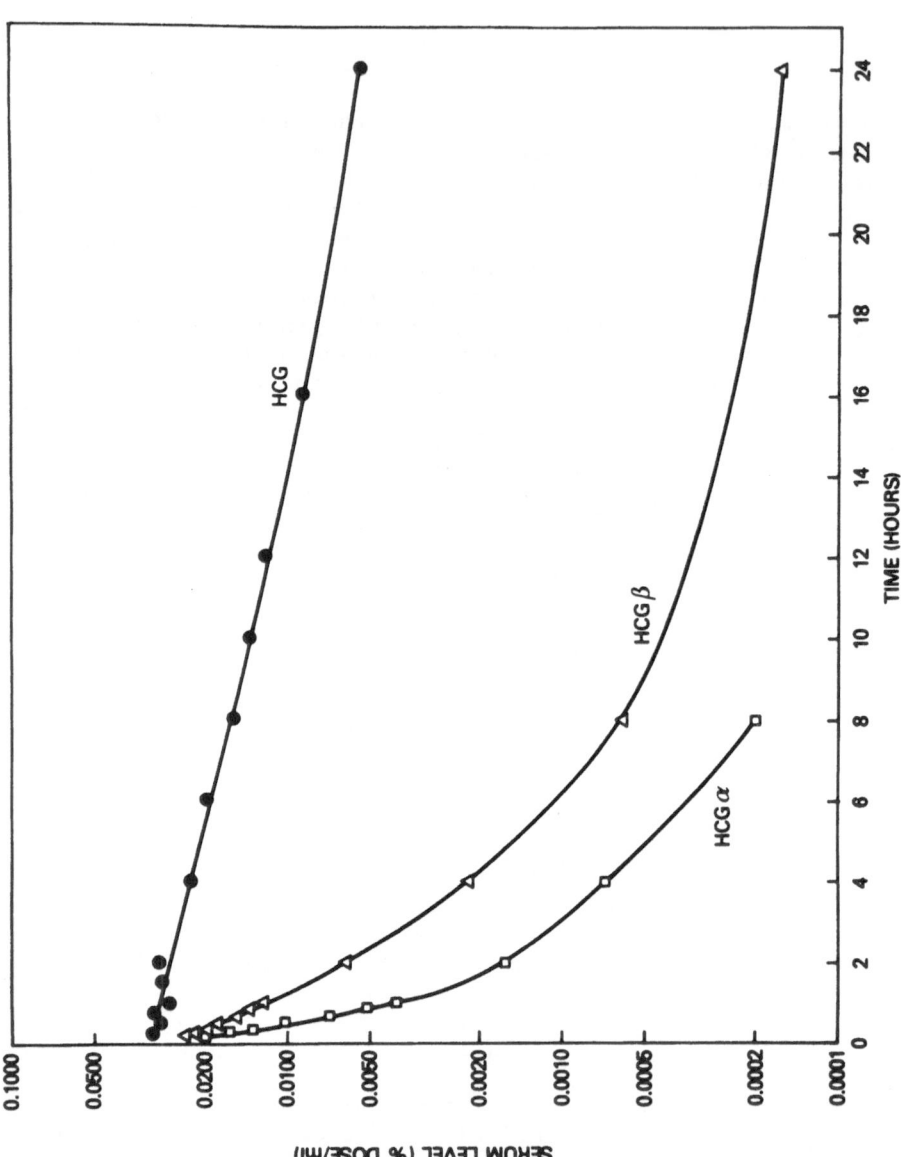

Figure 1. Comparison of the kinetics of disappearance of hCG, hCGβ, and hCGα from the serum of normal male subjects after single injection of the purified preparations. Concentrations are expressed as a percent of the injected dose per ml.

parameters, and B and β are the slow component parameters. The parameters determined for hCG, hCGβ, and hCGα are compared in Table I. The values of parameters A and B show no significant differences between the three substances, while the values of parameters α and β (not to be confused with hCGα and hCGβ) differ significantly among all three. Rizkallah et al. (1969) using a similar single injection technique, but with a commercial hCG preparation, obtained values for the hCG parameters quite different from ours. The discrepancy between the two sets of data can be accounted for by the immunoreactive contaminants in commercial hCG preparations such as free subunits. Tracer kinetic studies of the metabolism of hCG and its subunits are not available in the literature; however, it seems probable that a kinetic picture similar to that depicted in Figure I would be obtained. In support of this notion, we find that the various clearance rates calculated from the disappearance curve parameters are in agreement with those determined by constant infusion and that in the concentration range used in these studies the MCR of hCG is not dependent on serum concentration.

INITIAL VOLUMES OF DISTRIBUTION AND HALF-LIVES

From the parameters shown in Table I, one can derive the initial apparent volume of distribution of hCG, hCGβ, and hCGα and compute the half-lives of these substances in fast and slow compartments (Table II). The apparent initial volume of distribution is the same for hCG, hCGβ, and hCGα, while their half-lives in both fast and slow components differ widely. The finding that the half-lives for hCG, hCGα, and hCGβ are in similar proportion in fast and slow components suggests that the multiexponential nature of the disappearance curves is not due simply to the heterogeneity in the hormone preparations. Most other peptide hormones exhibit multiexponential disappearance curves. Contamination of the subunit preparations with intact hCG cannot account for their two-component disappearance curves, nor is there any evidence of recombination of administered subunit with endogenous complementary subunit to form intact hormones (Wehmann and Nisula, 1979).

METABOLIC CLEARANCE RATES AND RENAL CLEARANCE RATES

Calculations

To calculate the total metabolic clearance rate (MCR), one divides the dose of material administered by the integral of the equation for the serum disappearance curve as a function of time. To calculate the renal clearance rate (RCR), one does the same, but substitutes the quantity of unaltered peptide in the urine for dose and integrates over the finite time interval during which urine was

TABLE I: Kinetic parameters of the serum disappearance curves of hCG and its subunits after single intravenous injection of the purified hCG (CR119) preparation and the purified hCG (CR119) and hCG (CR119) preparations into normal men.

	Curve Parameters			
	Fast Component		Slow Component	
Preparation	A $(\%/ml)$	α (min^{-1})	B $(\%/ml)$	β (min^{-1})
CG	0.0273 ($\pm$0.0037)	0.00167 ($\pm$0.00029)	0.0046 ($\pm$0.0027)	0.00029 ($\pm$0.00012)
hCGβ	0.0220 ($\pm$0.0064)	0.0160 ($\pm$0.0038)	0.0064 ($\pm$0.0042)	0.0029 ($\pm$0.0023)
hCGα	0.0250 ($\pm$0.0088)	0.052 ($\pm$0.019)	0.0048 ($\pm$0.0038)	0.0074 ($\pm$0.0059)

Values shown are mean$\pm$SD expressed relative to a body surface area of 1.73 square meters.

TABLE II: Initial apparent volume of distribution and the half-lives of the single and slow components calculated from the serum disappearance curves of hCG and its subunits after single intravenous injection into normal men.

Preparation	Initial Volume of Distribution (ml)	Fast Component Half-life (min)	Slow Component Half-life (min)
hCG	3059 ($\pm$441)	415 ($\pm$72)	2390 ($\pm$415)
hCGβ	3601 ($\pm$974)	43 ($\pm$10)	239 ($\pm$109)
hCGα	3158 ($\pm$441)	13.4 ($\pm$5.0)	94 ($\pm$75)

Values shown are mean$\pm$SD expressed relative to a body surface area of 1.73 square meters.

collected. We are using the term renal clearance to refer to a specific pathway of disposal -- excretion into urine as unaltered material. The material is judged "unaltered" based on normal position on gel chromatography. Obviously, changes in structure which are too subtle to be detected by this method can occur and would be of interest for further work. We presume that hCG and its subunits are not only excreted by the kidney, but also degraded by the kidney. The products of such degradation might be detectable by radioimmunoassays as products in serum or urine, or they might not. To calculate the clearance rate of material via non-renal pathways (including degradation by the kidney), one subtracts the RCR from the MCR.

MCR and RCR of hCG

The MCR of hCG is 3.1 ± 0.1 ml/min (Table III), a value close to that of Wide et al. (1968) who used a bioassay method to monitor disappearance. Our value for the RCR (0.97 ml/min) agrees nicely with the mean estimate of 0.95 ml/min in pregnancy obtained by Loraine (1950). This investigator measured hCG in serum and urine using a bioassay method which was probably unaffected by any subunits or metabolites. Somewhat lower values have been obtained by other workers (Gastineau et al., 1949; Wide et al., 1968). It is of interest that Wide et al. (1968) showed that the RCR calculated from bioassay data was lower than that calculated from immunoassay data.

We find that the RCR of hCG accounts for about 30% of the total MCR with the remaining 70% being disposed of via non-renal pathways. We presume that intracellular metabolism by the liver and kidney accounts for most of the non-renal metabolism based on the studies of Braunstein et al. (1972). The sites of non-renal metabolism and disposal of the subunits in man are unknown, but may well follow qualitatively the same pathways as intact hCG, with the exception of that portion of the hCG which interacts with the gonad, of course. Although desialylation in vitro increases the MCR of exogenous hCG (Morell et al., 1971), it has not been determined whether desialylation in vivo plays a role in the disposal of endogenous hCG or its subunits.

MCR and RCR of the hCG Subunits

From the quantitative point of view, the hCG subunits are metabolized very differently from hCG. First of all, the MCR's of hCGβ and hCGα are about 10-fold and 30-fold, respectively, greater than that of hCG (Table III). Second, it is of great interest that although the MCR's of the subunit are much greater than that of hCG, their RCR's are much less. Hence, renal excretion does not account for the marked increase in metabolic disposal of the subunits.

TABLE III: Metabolic clearance rates of hCG and its subunits calculated using the equation describing serum disappearance following single intravenous injection of the purified preparations into normal men.

Preparation	Clearance Rate (ml/min)[a]		
	Total	Renal	Non-Renal
hCG	3.1	0.97	2.1
	(±0.1)	(±0.09)	(±0.1)
hCGβ	32.5	0.20	32.3
	(±5.7)	(±0.059)	(±5.7)
hCGα	85.6	0.24	85.4
	(±10.5)	(±0.042)	(±10.5)

[a] Values shown are mean±SD expressed relative to a body surface area of 1.73 square meters.

While about 30% of the hCG is excreted in urine, less than 1% of either subunit is excreted in urine (Table III). This is a consequence of hCG having both a slower MCR (more hCG available for renal clearance) and a greater RCR (of that delivered to the kidney more is cleared) than the subunits. It is important to emphasize that 99% of the disposal of hCGα and hCGβ is via pathways other than renal excretion as unaltered subunit.

Clearance Rates of Pituitary Hormone Subunits

As one would predict from their structural similarity, hCGα and the pituitary alpha-subunits exhibit similar kinetic characteristics. The MCR for hCGα determined by Kourides et al. (1977) using labeled hCGα is similar to ours for unlabeled hCGα and similar to their alpha-subunit of human thyroid-stimulating hormone. Estimates for the MCR of the alpha-subunit of human luteinizing hormone (hLHα) are not available; however, Pepperell et al. (1975) obtained an initial half-life for hLHα which is similar to our initial half-life for hCGα. This result suggests that their MCR's will also be similar.

HCG SECRETION AND SUBUNIT PRODUCTION IN PREGNANCY

Calculations Based on Metabolic Clearance Rates

It is now generally acknowledged that an hCGα-like molecule is present in both maternal serum and urine (Franchimont and Reuter, 1972; Good et al., 1977). Its level relative to hCG seems to vary considerably throughout gestation (Ashitaka et al., 1974), which is the first clue that its production may not be linked to the degradation of circulating hCG. It has not been determined whether this substance is identical with the hCGα obtained from the dissociation of native hCG; however, they exhibit similar elution patterns on Sephadex G-100 chromatography. While this hCGα could be derived from the peripheral degradation of hCG, it could have other origins as well. To calculate the production rate of hCGα in pregnancy and compare it to the secretion rate of hCG, it is necessary to assume that the hCGα material in pregnancy serum is actually authentic hCGα. Such calculations also assume that the MCR's of hCG and its subunits are unaltered during pregnancy. The amount of hCGα immuno-reactivity present in non-pregnant subjects is negligible in comparison to the amount in pregnancy. The values for relative concentrations of hCG and hCGα vary from laboratory to laboratory, possibly reflecting differences in the stage of gestation examined. A conservative approach would be to assign a molar concentration to hCGα which is 20% of that of hCG (Table IV). At these relative levels, the production rate of hCGα would be more than five-fold greater than the secretion rate of hCG in molar equivalents (Table IV). Therefore, one could account for at most only 20% of the hCGα

TABLE IV: Calculation of the secretion rate of hCG and the serum production rate of hCGα in pregnant women.

Substance	Concentration (μml/L)	Metabolic Clearance Rate (L/day)	Secretion or Production Rate	
			(μmol/day)	(mg/day)
hCG	0.025^a	4.46	0.11	4.4
hCG	0.005^a	123	0.62	9.3

^{a}Values used arbitrarily fix the molar concentration of hCGα at 20% of that of hCG. The molar ratio varies during gestation.

in pregnancy serum if all of the secreted hCG were degraded via a
pathway which resulted in the release of $hCG\alpha$ into the serum compart-
ment. It should be noted that this disparity between the $hCG\alpha$
potentially available through the metabolism of hCG and the $hCG\alpha$
apparently produced applies whether or not the $hCG\alpha$ is derived by
a mechanism which also results in the release of $hCG\beta$. Indeed,
the available data concerning $hCG\beta$ are inconsistent with the
possibility that the serum subunits are derived solely from the
dissociation of hCG. Since the MCR of $hCG\alpha$ is about 3-fold greater
than the MCR of $hCG\beta$, under circumstances in which the serum $hCG\alpha$
and $hCG\beta$ are derived from the dissociation of hCG, the production
rate of $hCG\beta$ would be the same as the production rate of $hCG\alpha$ and
the resulting serum concentration of $hCG\beta$ would be about three-fold
greater than the serum $hCG\alpha$ concentration. In fact, the concentration of $hCG\alpha$ in serum greatly exceeds that of $hCG\beta$ (Franchimont and
Reuter, 1972; Hagen and McNeilly, 1975; Vaitukaitis et al., 1976;
Good et al., 1977). To summarize, the patterns of hCG, $hCG\alpha$, and
$hCG\beta$ in pregnancy serum and urine are inconsistent with the hypothesis that they are products which arise solely from the metabolism
of hCG in the periphery.

Placental Content of $hCG\alpha$ and Secretion by Tumors

On the basis of the foregoing considerations, it seems inevi-
table to conclude that the serum $hCG\alpha$ in pregnancy is either a
direct secretory product of the placenta or a degradation product
of some molecule other than hCG. The fact that Vaitukaitis (1974)
has found an excess of $hCG\alpha$ over $hCG\beta$ subunits in placental tissue
would favor the former mechanism. Also, recently Beneviste et al.
(1979) have given evidence of secretion of an $hCG\alpha$-like molecule
by JEG choriocarcinoma cells in vitro. Other workers have reported
secretion of $hCG\alpha$-like molecules by other malignancies (Rosen and
Weintraub, 1974). Further studies of the structural and functional
properties of the $hCG\alpha$-like material in pregnancy are needed to
elucidate its relationship to the substance in placental extracts
or to the substances secreted by malignancies.

DEGRADATION OF HCG: DISCRETE $HCG\beta$-FRAGMENT IN URINE

While it is clear that one may not account entirely for the
presence of $hCG\alpha$ in pregnancy serum and urine on the basis of the
peripheral degradation of secreted hCG, a combination of direct
secretion of $hCG\alpha$ and degradation of hCG is possible. Our strategy
for studying the degradation of hCG is to give purified hCG to normal
human subjects and to examine various biologic fluids on gel chromatography for molecular species which manifest immunoreactivity in
radioimmunoassays employing antisera to $hCG\alpha$ and $hCG\beta$. Although
these studies, for the most part, are in a preliminary stage, some

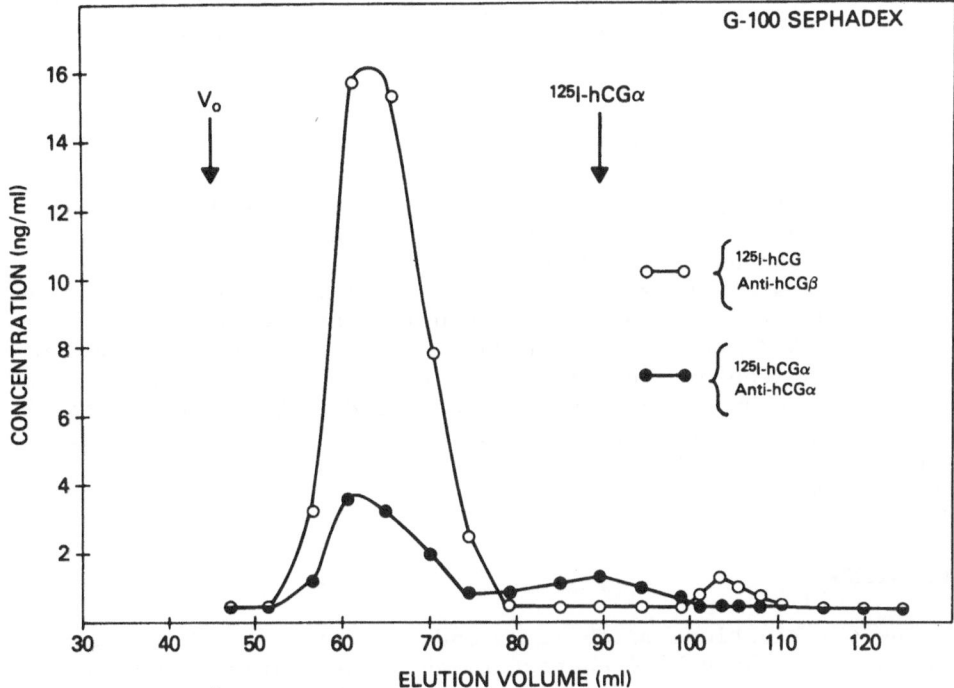

Figure 2. Gel chromatography on a G-100 column of urine obtained from a normal subject after an eight day infusion with the purified hCG (CR121) preparation. The ^{125}I-hCGα was co-chromatographed as a marker. Potency estimates with the antiserum to hCGβ and with the antiserum to hCGα were made with hCG and hCGα, respectively.

features of the data can be mentioned. Figure 2 shows the elution pattern of the urine obtained on day eight of infusion with hCG. There are two positions in the elution profile where immunoreactivity is detected with the radioimmunoassay employing antiserum to hCGβ (SB6). The position with the largest amount of immunoreactivity corresponds to the hCG molecule. Since hCGβ elutes in a position near to that of hCG, it is possible that some of the immunoreactivity in the main peak reflects hCGβ, rather than hCG. The position with the lesser amount of hCGβ immunoreactivity corresponds in molecular size to a substance smaller than hCGα. Since the urines of normal subjects, filtered in an identical manner prior to the administration of hCG, exhibit no hCGβ immunoreactivity in any of the eluted fractions, the results shown in Figure 2 clearly indicate that the hCGβ-fragment is a discrete product of the metabolism of the hCG molecule.

Where the hCGα peak is concerned, the data in Figure 2 must be interpreted equivocally. The urine of normal subjects prior to the administration of hCG contains a small amount of hCGα immunoreactivity which co-elutes on gel chromatography with ^{125}I-hCGα. Thus, some, or possibly all, of the immunoreactivity which is apparent in the hCGα position in Figure 2 may be accounted for by various endogenous proteins. On the other hand, we cannot exclude a small contribution of a putative hCGα-like degradation product derived from the degradation of injected hCG. Further work is being done to determine whether the degradation of hCG gives rise to significant quantities of its subunits. However, insofar as pregnancy is concerned, the levels of hCGα in urine reported by Franchimont and Reuter (1972) were quite substantial relative to the levels of hCG. A comparison of their results with ours suggests that only a minority of the hCGα in pregnancy could be derived from the post-secretory degradation of hCG. Thus, analysis of the degradation products of purified hCG adds support to the kinetic argument developed above.

CONCLUSIONS

The distribution, metabolism, and excretion of hCG and its subunits in man have been characterized. The initial volume of distribution is the same for hCG, hCGβ, and hCGα. Their disappearance curves fit a two-component exponential model which upon analysis reveals that in both fast and slow components the half-life of hCG is about 10-fold greater than that of hCGβ and about 30-fold greater than that of hCGα. Even though the total metabolic clearance rates of hCGβ and hCGα were approximately 10-fold and 30-fold, respectively, greater than that of hCG, their renal clearance rates were approximately 4-fold less than that of hCG. Consequently, renal excretion accounts for about 30% of the total metabolic disposal of hCG, but for less than 1% of the disposal of the subunits. Calculations indicate that the production rate of hCGα in pregnancy is more than 5-fold greater than the secretion rate of hCG and that the production rate of hCGβ is much lower than the production rate of hCGα. This suggests that little, if any, of the serum hCGα in pregnancy is derived from post-secretory metabolism of hCG. A discrete product of the degradation of hCG is evident in urine. It is a fragment of the hCGβ molecule which has an apparent molecular size smaller than that of hCGα.

REFERENCES

Ashitaka, Y., Nishimura, R., Futamura, K., Oshashi, M., and Tojo, S., 1974, Serum and chorionic tissue concentrations of human chorionic gonadotropin and its subunits during pregnancy, Endocrinol. Japon 21:547.

Ayala, A. R., Nisula, B. C., Chen, H. C., Hodgen, G. D., and Ross, G. T., Highly sensitive radioimmunoassay for human chorionic gonadotropin in human urine, J. Clin. Endocrinol. Metab. 47:767.

Beneviste, R., Lindner, J., Puett, D., and Rabin, D., 1979, Human chorionic gonadotropin α-subunit from cultured choriocarcinoma (JEG) cells: Comparison of the subunit secreted free with that prepared from secreted human chorionic gonadotropin, Endocrinology 105:581.

Braunstein, G. D., Vaitukaitis, J. S., and Ross, G. T., 1972, The in vivo behavior of human chorionic gonadotropin and its subunits after dissociation into subunits, Endocrinology 91:1030.

Canfield, R., and Ross, G. T., 1976, A new reference preparation of human chorionic gonadotropin and its subunits, Bull. WHO 54:463.

Faden, V. B., and Rodbard, D., 1975, Operating instructions and listings for new FORTRAN IV-G Program, EXPFIT, Exponential Data Processing, NICHD, NIH, Bethesda.

Franchimont, P., and Reuter, A., 1972, Evidence of α- and β-subunits hCG in serum and urine of pregnant women, in Structure-Activity Relationships of Protein and Poly-peptide Hormones, M. Margoules and F. Greenwood, eds., Excerpta Medica, The Netherlands.

Gastineau, C. F., Albert, A., and Randall, L. M., 1949, The renal clearance of gonadotropin in pregnancy, in neoplasms of the testis, and in hydatidiform mole, J. Clin. Endocrinol. Metab. 9:615.

Good, A., Ramos-Uribe, M., Ryan, R. J., and Kempers, R. D., 1977, Molecular forms of human chorionic gonadotropin in serum, urine, and placental extracts, Fertil. Steril. 28:846.

Hagen, C., and McNeilly, A. S., 1975, The gonadotropic hormones and their subunits in human maternal and fetal circulation at delivery, Am. J. Obstet. Gynecol. 121:926.

Kourides, I. A., Re, R. N., Weintraub, B. D., Ridgway, E. C., and Maloof, F., 1977, Metabolic clearance and secretion rates of subunits of human thyrotropin, J. Clin. Invest, 59:508.

Loraine, J. A., 1950, The renal clearance of chorionic gonadotropin in normal and pathological pregnancy, Quart. J. Exp. Physiol. 36:11.

Louvet, J. P., Ross, G. T., Birken, S., and Canfield, R. E., 1974, Absence of neutralizing effect of antisera to the unique region of human chorionic gonadotropin, J. Clin. Endocrinol. Metab. 39:1155.

Midgely, A. R. Jr., and Jaffe, R. B., 1968, Regulation of human gonadotropins. II. Disappearance of human chorionic gonadotropin following delivery, J. Clin. Endocrinol. Metab. 28:1712.

Morell, A. G., Gregoriadis, G., Scheinber, I. H., Hickman, J., and Ashwell, G., 1971, The role of sialic acid in determining the survival of glycoproteins in the circulation, J. Biol. Chem. 246:1461.

Morgan, F. J., Canfield, R. E., Vaitukaitis, J. L., and Ross, G. T., 1974, Properties of the subunits of human chorionic gonadotropin,

Endocrinology 94:1601.

Nisula, B. C., Ayala, A. R., Stolk, M. D., Taliadouros, G. S., and Stolk, J. M., 1978, Solid-phase group-specific adsorbants in assays for glycoproteins, in Radioimmunoassay and Related Procedueres in Medicine, vol. 1, International Atomic Energy Agency, Vienna, pp. 33–140.

Pepperell, R. J., deKretser, D. M., and Burger, H. G., 1975, Studies on the metabolic clearance rate and production rate of human luteinizing hormone and on the initial half-life of its subunits in man, J. Clin. Invest. 56:118.

Rizkallah, T., Gurpide, E., and Vande Wiele, R. L., 1969, Metabolism pf hCG in man, J. Clin. Endocrinol. Metab. 29:92.

Rosen, S. W., and Weintraub, B. D., 1974, Ectopic production of the isolated alpha subunit of the glycoprotein hormones: A quantitative marker in certain cases of cancer, N. Engl. J. Med. 290:1441.

Sowers, J. R., Pekary, A. E., Hershman, J. M., Kanter, M., and DiStefano, J., 1978, Metabolism of exogenous human chorionic gonadotropin in men, J. Endocr. 80:83.

Vaitukaitis, J. L., 1974, Changing placental concentrations of chorionic gonadotropin and its subunits during gestation, J. Clin. Endocrinol. Metab. 38:755.

Vaitukaitis, J. L., Braunstein, G. D., and Ross, G. T., 1972, A radioimmunoassay which specifically measures human chorionic gonadotropin in the presence of human luteinizing hormone, Am. J. Obstetr. Gynecol. 113:751.

Vaitukaitis, J. L., Ross, G. T., Braunstein, G. D., and Rayford, P. L., 1976, Gonadotropins and their subunits: Basic and clinical studies, Rec. Progr. Horm. Res. 32:289.

Wehmann, R. E., and Nisula, B. C., 1979, Metabolic clearance rates of the subunits of human chorionic gonadotropin in man, J. Clin. Endocrinol. Metab. 48:753.

Wide, L., Johannisson, E., Tillinger, K. G., and Diczfalusy, E., 1968, Metabolic clearance of human chorionic gonadotropin administered non-pregnant women, Acta Endocrinol. (KBH) 29:92.

Yen, S. S. C., Llerena, O., Little, B., and Pearson, O. H., 1968, Disappearance of endogenous luteinizing hormone and chorionic gonadotropin in man, J. Clin. Endocrinol. Metab. 28:1763.

IMMUNO-BIOLOGICAL STUDIES WITH BETA-SUBUNIT OF

HUMAN CHORIONIC GONADOTROPIN AND ITS SUBFRAGMENTS

S. Ramakrishnan and G. P. Talwar

Department of Biochemistry
All-India Institute of Medical Sciences
New Delhi, India

INTRODUCTION

The onset of pregnancy is associated with a number of physiological changes brought about by the hormones and other factors synthesized and secreted by the placenta. Human chorionic gonadotropin (hCG) is one of the early products of pregnancy, detectable in circulation between days 8 to 10 post-fertilization (Saxena et al., 1974; Catt et al., 1975). Experimental evidence suggests that hCG plays a crucial role in the establishment of pregnancy, as an early luteo-tropic signal extending the fuctional life of the corpus luteum (Marsh and Savard, 1966; Hanson et al., 1972; Neil and Knobil, 1972; Garner and Armstrong, 1977). In view of these properties, hCG has been identified as one of the target molecules for the immunological intervention of pregnancy.

CHOICE OF THE IMMUNOGEN

Anti-hCG antibody can be elicited by using either whole hCG, the β-subunit of hCG, chemically modified derivatives of the β-subunit, or fragments of hCGβ either obtained by enzymatic cleavage or synthesized chemically.

HCG

Antibodies generated against hCG were found to neutralize the biological activity of the exogenously administered gonadotropin in animals (Rao and Shahani, 1967; Sasamato, 1969). Its use in isoimmunizatior procedures is limited, however, since the antibodies

crossreact with other hormones like LH. FSH, and TSH (Vaitukaitis
et al., 1972b). This view is strengthened by the observations of
Stevens and Crystle (1973), in which immunization of women with
hapten—modified hCG generated crossreactive antibodies, resulting
in a reduced LH surge in these subjects.

β—Subunit of HCG

The second alternative antigen is the hormone—specific subunit
of hCG (hCGβ). Limited conformational studies carried out on hCG
and hLH indicate an overall similarity between the two gonadotropins.
Circular dichroic spectral analysis of hCG and hLH reveal an almost
identical back—bone conformation of the polypeptide chain in both
the hormones (unpublished data). However, owing to the presence of
structurally dissimilar β—subunits, it is expected that unique
conformations distinct from one another may also be present in the
two hormonal subunits. This contention is supported by several
lines of evidence. First, comparison of the amino acid sequence
reveals that hCGβ differs from hLHβ to the extent of 51 amino acid
residues (Morgan et al., 1975; Sairam et al., 1975). Thirty of these
are present in the C—terminal unique region of the hCGβ. In the
core—portion of the molecule, there are at least four places where
important substitutions have occurred and where hydrophobic amino
acid residues like Ala, Val, and Leu are substituted for Pro in
hLHβ. Such replacements are theoretically expected to cause changes
in the local conformation. Second, antibodies generated against the
β—subunit distinguish between hCG and hLH in radioimmunoassay (RIA)
system (Vaitukaitis et al., 1972a; Jacobs, 1974; Salahuddin et al.,
1976).

A differential rate of dissociation of the subunits was observed,
depending on the medium (urea or low pH). In acidic media, the
dissociation rate increased in the order hCG>hLH>oLH>bTSH>hFSH,
whereas, in urea the order was hFSH>bTSH>hCG>oLH>hLH (Aloj and Ingham,
1977). These differences suggest that in spite of extensive structural homologies, the interaction of the hormone—specific β—subunit
with the α—subunit involve different binding forces (hydrophobic or
electrostatic).

On grounds of these considerations, attempts have been made to
use hCGβ as an immunogen to elicit relatively specific anti—hCG
response. As chemically purified subunit preparations invariably
contain trace amounts of the undissociated hormone (Rayford et al.,
1972), an immunochemical processing step was introduced to obtain
hCGβ free from such contaminants (Talwar et al., 1976a). Immunochemically purified hCGβ (Pr—hCGβ) was conjugated to tetanus toxoid
(TT) as carrier. The conjugates were immunogenic in both iso- and
hetero-species (Talwar et al., 1976b, c). The duration of the
antibody response in the human was between 300 and 500 days. The

qualitative properties of antibodies produced were extensively
investigated. The antibodies were able to bind native hCG in vitro
and in vivo (Das et al., 1976; Ramakrishnan et al., 1976) and showed
a greater amount of specificity in reacting with hCG than hLH in a
variety of test systems. In the presence of anti-Pr-hCGβ-TT antibodies, the hCG-induced ovulation was blocked in mice, whereas
oLH-induced ovulation remained unaffected (Das et al., 1978). The
differential neutralization of hCG and hLH was further noticed in
Leydig cell assay system as well as in goat granulosa cell cultures
(Mohini et al., 1978). In vivo clearance studies further indicated
that circulating antibodies in rhesus monkeys neutralized the biological activity of hCG, but not of hLH, when the hormones were
injected in the late luteal phase of the cycle (Ramakrishnan et al.,
1978a). Moreover, the antibodies showed greater affinity (5 to 10
fold) for binding with hCG as compared to hLH (Shastri et al., 1978).
The neutralizing type of antibodies could have been either directed
against the biologically active site of the hormone, or alternatively,
against other determinants in the hormone, so as to prevent the
hormone from binding to the tissue receptors.

From these findings it was of interest to investigate the possible
sites involved in the biological activity of the hormone, the antigenic determinants predominantly expressed in hCGβ, and the merits
of using the C-terminal synthetic peptides to elicit specific anti-
hCG response.

BIOLOGICALLY IMPORTANT REGIONS OF HCG

The dissociation of the hormone into individual subunits results
in a large decrease in biological activity as measured by ventral
prostate weight gain assay (Canfield et al., 1971). Several investigators have in the past ascribed some intrinsic biological activity
to the β-subunit of the gonadotropins (Farmer et al., 1973; Rao and
Carman, 1973; Yang et al., 1973; Muralidhar and Moudgal, 1976).
However, the observed biological activity associated with β-subunit
was attributed by Rayford et al., (1972) and Morgan et al., (1974)
to the likely presence in trace amounts (1% to 5%) of the contaminating hCGα and undissociated hCG in the preparation; its biological
activity was assayed in the sensitive mouse Leydig cell assay system.

Does hCGβ Possess Intrinsic Biological Activity?

Total hCG, in which the subunits are in an associated state,
was highly potent and induced steroidogenesis at concentrations as
low as 0.19 fmole/tube (0.63 pM). A linear dose response was observed up to 0.96 fmole (3.19 pM). Pr-hCGβ was found to have no
biological activity at comparable concentrations. However, when
the subunit was used at higher concentrations (100-1000 fold, i.e.,

0.1 pmole to 1.0 pmole), there was a significant stimulation of testosterone production. The dose response curve had a parallel slope to that of hCG. An almost equivalent response was observed with Pr-hCGβ at 400-fold higher concentrations than hCG (Figure 1A).

To check whether the observed biological activity was indeed intrinsic to the β-subunit of hCG, two types of experiments were carried out. In one case, the native molecule was chemically denatured and then tested for its ability to stimulate Leydig cells. β-subunit of hCG has six disulfide bridges and reductive alkylation of S-S bonds results in alteration of the backbone conformation of the subunit to a completely 'random-coil' structure (unpublished data). The reduced carboxymethyl derivative of asialo hCGβ (ARCM-hCGβ) was devoid of steroidogenic activity when tested up to a concentration of 2.05 pmole/assay tube (Figure 1A).

Another approach was to use synthetic peptides conforming to the amino acid sequence of hCGβ, which would in any case be free from even ultra-trace amounts of hCG. The following five poly-peptides conforming to the sequence proposed by Morgan et al., (1975) were synthesized by Dr. Karl Folkers of the University of Texas, and supplied through the Population Council, New York: carboxyl-terminal 31 amino acid residues (115-145); carboxyl-terminal 35 amino acid residues (111-145); carboxyl-terminal 45 amino acid residues (101-145); core 18 amino acid residues (39-56); and core 33 amino acid residues (39-71).

Results shown in Figure 1B indicate that the C-terminal 31-, 35-, and 45- amino acid peptides do not possess any biological activity up to 1.0 nmole/tube (i.e., 3.33 μM), which are amounts approximately 1000-fold higher than the highest amount of Pr-hCGβ used in the studies reported in Figure 1A. It is interesting to note that the synthetic peptide conforming to the sequence of residues 39-71 stimulated the Leydig cells to produce significant amounts of testosterone. A dose-dependent response with this peptide was observed between 50-1000 pmole/tube (0.16-3.33 μM). On the other hand, peptide 39-56 did not have any steroidogenic activity at comparable concentrations.

These studies indicate that although the β-subunit of hCG has adequate information to stimulate steroidogenesis, the efficiency with which the hormonal message is transmitted is much better in the associated form with α-subunit. This could be due to the conformational changes imparted by the α-subunit to the β-subunit. It has been shown that dissociation of LH and hCG results in limited conformational changes, as indicated by the decrease in β structure and exposure of two to three tyrosine residues to the solvent medium (Garnier et al., 1974; Salesse et al., 1975; Ingham et al., 1976). The native hormone has requisite hydrophobic regions for the binding of the hydrophobic fluorescence probe 8-anilino-

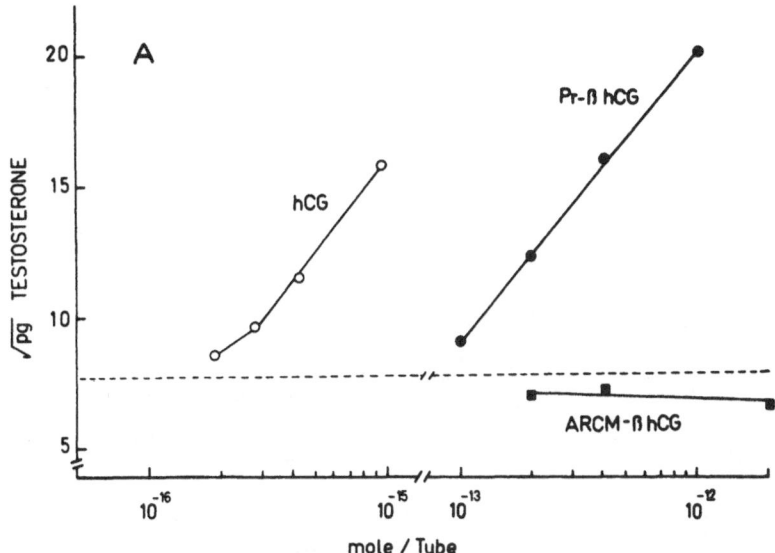

Figure 1A. Tissue receptor recognition of determinants in hCGβ. Effect of human chorionic gonadotropin (O) and immunochemically purified β-subunit of hCG (●) on testosterone production by mouse Leydig cells in vitro. The assay was according to the method reported elsewhere (Das et al., 1978). The values shown are the mean of quadruplicate determinations. Basal production of testosterone by the Leydig cells in the absence of added gonadotropic stimulus (-----). The reduced carboxymethylated derivative of asialo-hCGβ (ARCM-β-hCG) failed to stimulate steroidogenesis up to a concentration of 2 pmole/assay tube.

napthalene-1-sulphonic acid (ANS), whereas dissociation of the hormone into subunits results in the loss of this property. Association dependent active folding of the polypeptide chain was also noticed during recombination of LH (Salesse et al., 1975). Thus, it is quite probable that the new conformations produced after associations of α- and β-subunits enhance the efficiency of the determinants present in the hCGβ to interact with the tissue receptors optimally.

In the β-subunit of hCG the determinants--or at least a part of the epitopes involved in receptor recognition, which are instrumental in inducing functional response in target cells--were found to reside between residues 39 and 71. Since the peptide 39-56 could not induce steroidogenesis, it can be inferred that the sequence of

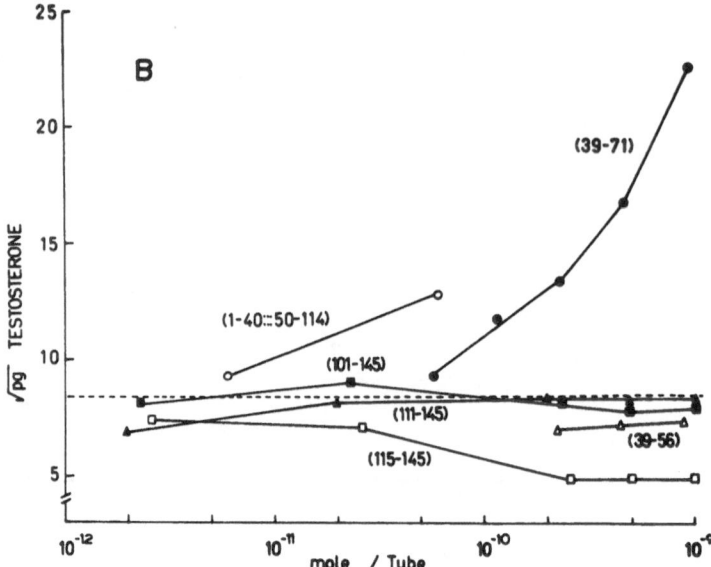

Figure 1B.   Tissue receptor recognition of determinants in hCGβ.
Effect of synthetic peptides and an enzyme-cleaved fragment of
β-subunit of hCG on testosterone production by mouse Leydig cells
in vitro: □ = C-terminal peptide 115-145; ▲ = C-terminal peptide
111-145; ■ = C-terminal peptide 101-145; △ = Core 18 amino acid
peptide 39-56; ● = core 33 amino acid peptide 39-71; ○ = thermolysin-
cleaved fragment of asialo-hCGβ in which fragment 1-40 was linked to
fragment 50-114 with disulfide bonds.
(Data from Ramakrishnan et al., 1978.)

residues between 57-71 per se, or in combination with 39-56, is
important for the biological activity. The primary sequence of
hCGβ and hLHβ indicates that in this region (51-71), except for one
amino acid substitution (Asn^{56}-Thr^{56}), the rest of the residues are
identical and could possibly indicate the conservation of biologically
active site in these two sister hormones.

The C-terminal moiety of the β-subunit of hCG is of special
interest, since the last 30 amino acid residues are not present in
the hLHβ. This part of the molecule, however, is not involved in
receptor recognition. All three C-terminal peptides (31, 35, and 45)
did not compete with the binding of ^{125}I-hCG to sheep corpus luteum
receptors up to a concentration of 537.6 μM (Figure 2). The determinants on the target cells are likely to reside in the core part of
the molecule, and not at the tail end.

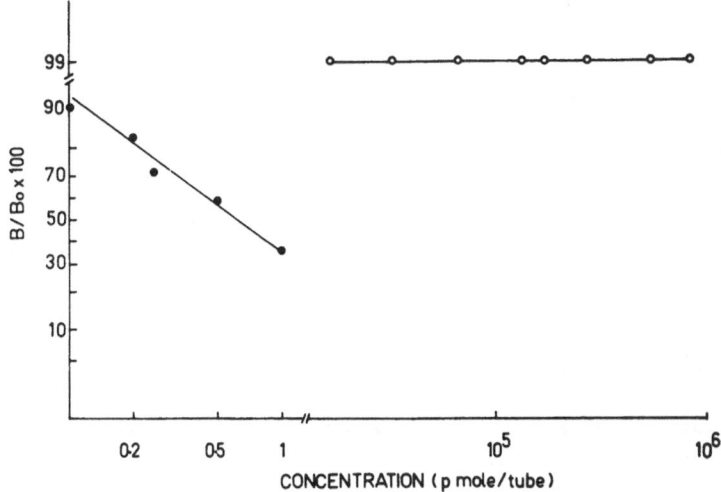

Figure 2. Competitive inhibition of ^{125}I-hCG binding corpus luteum receptors by C-terminal synthetic peptides. Homogenates of goat corpora lutea (2000 x g pellet) was used as receptor preparation. (●——●) = competitive inhibition curve obtained with hCG; (O——O) = ^{125}I-hCG binding in presence of C-terminal peptides (31-, 35-, 45-CTP).

IMMUNOLOGICAL STUDIES WITH CARBOXYL-TERMINAL SYNTHETIC PEPTIDES

Structural analyses have shown the presence of unique C-terminal sequence in hCGβ. Attempts have been made in many laboratories to utilize this region as antigens to elicit specific anti-hCG response. In our studies, we have investigated the following three C-terminal synthetic peptides: 31-amino acid residues (115-145); 35-amino acid residues (111-145); 45-amino acid residues (101-145).

The peptides were conjugated chemically to tetanus toxoid (TT), a carrier used in our earlier studies with Pr-hCGβ. The conjugates were used to immunize rabbits (10) and monkeys (8) after emulsification with complete Freund's adjuvant. The primary immunization was carried out intradermally at multiple sites. Follow-up boosters were given in alum-precipitated form, or in incomplete Freund's adjuvant at two contralateral sites intramuscularly. In several rabbits and monkeys higher doses (4-5 fold) were used to check the immunogenicity of the peptide conjugates. In spite of the higher doses and usage of highly potent adjuvants (CFA), the anti-hCG response elicited by the synthetic C-terminal peptides was poor when

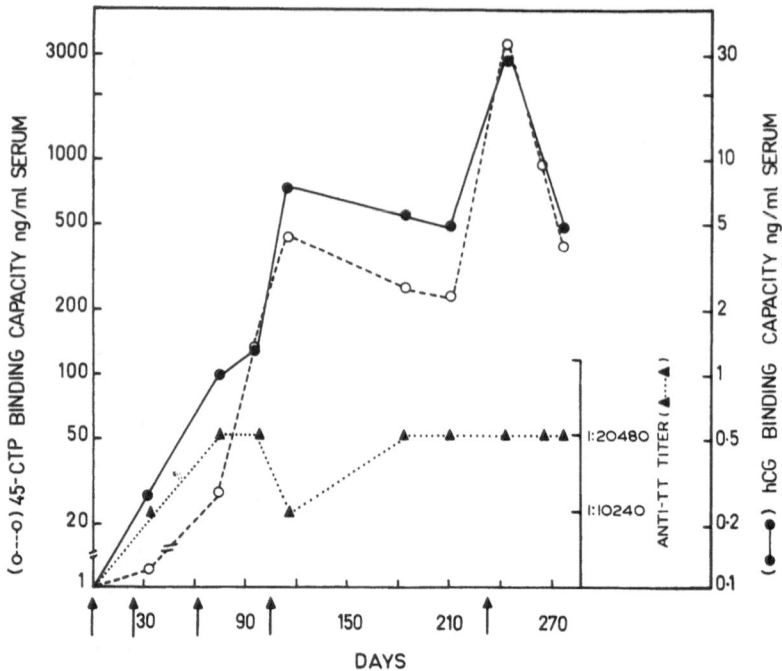

Figure 3.   Kinetics of antibody response in a rhesus monkey immunized with synthetic C-terminal 45-amino acid peptide conjugated to tetanus toxoid (TT). The first injection was given in complete Freund's adjuvant (CFA) at multiple sites intradermally. The subsequent injections were given in alum adsorbed form after emulsification with sterile sesame oil. Arrows denote the days on which injections (10 µg fragment) were given. The antibody titers (Binding capacity) were measured by radioimmunoassay using radioiodinated peptide (O----O) and hCG ($\bullet$——$\bullet$). The anti-TT titers were described by Talwar et al., (1976b). Data from Ramakrishna et al., 1979.

compared to immunization with β-subunit conjugated to TT. Only three out of eight monkeys showed any significant anti-hCG response (>1 ng hCG bound/ml serum). Figure 3 shows the kinetics of antibody response in a monkey (BB) immunized with 45-CTP-TT which had an appreciable amount of anti-hCG antibodies (29.184 ng/ml serum) when compared to other monkeys immunized with 31- and 35-CTP-TT. However, all the monkeys responded well to the carrier protein. On the other hand, a single injection of Pr-hCGβ-TT (20 µg in CFA) resulted in higher anti-hCG titers (14.20 µg ^{125}I-hCG binding/ml serum) which showed a phenomenal increase to 110.79 µg ^{125}I-hCG binding/ml serum with two booster injections (Figure 4).

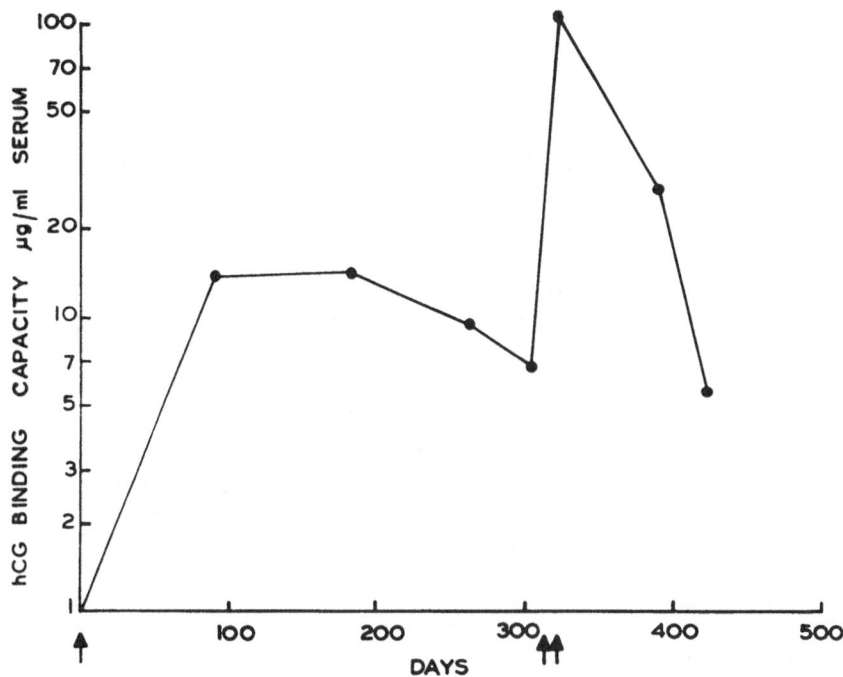

Figure 4. Kinetics of antibody response in a rhesus monkey immunized with Pr-hCGβ-TT. The conjugate (20 μg of Pr-hCGβ conjugated to tetanus toxoid) was emulsified in equal volume of complete Freund's adjuvant and injected intradermally at multiple sites. Booster injections (alum precipitate) were given on day 304 and day 310. The antibody titers were measured by RIA (Shastri et al., 1978). Data from Ramakrishnan et al., 1979.

The kinetics of antibody response against 45-CTP conjugated to tetanus toxoid is shown in Figure 3. The antibody titers were measured for binding with both ^{125}I-45-CTP and ^{125}I-hCG. Quantitatively, the sera taken at different points showed a greater binding capacity for the peptide than with the intact hCG. For example, at peak titers, the antiserum bound 3.49 μg of C-terminal peptide per ml of serum, whereas it bound only 29.18 ng of hCG (120 times lower amount). The specificity of the antiserum was checked in an homologous RIA system. HCG inhibited competitively at 0.312 pmole and at higher concentrations, although the slope was non-parallel to that obtained with the homologous antigen. HLH did not react in the system up to 1.6 pmole concentration. The other two synthetic peptides gave comparatively lower degree of inhibition in the order 31-CTP<35-CTP<45-CTP. To

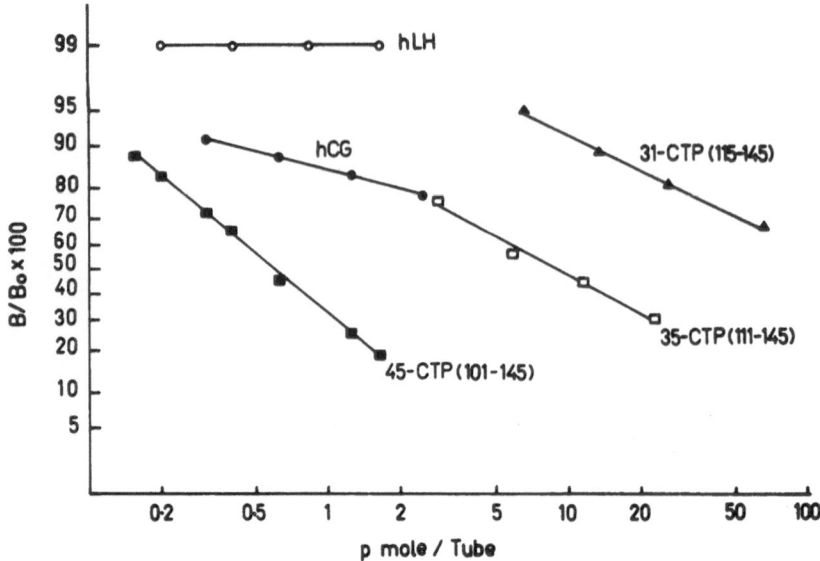

Figure 5.   Specificity of the antiserum raised in monkey against the 45-CTP-TT. Competition curves obtained in RIA system using ^{125}I-Tyr-45-CTP and anti-45-CTP-TT antiserum are shown as follows: ●——●, hCG; o——o, hLH; ▲—— ▲, 31-CTP (115-145); (□——□), 35-CTP (111-145); (■——■), 45-CTP (101-145). B = radioactivity bound to the antibodies in the presence of labeled peptide and unlabeled hormone/peptide. Bo = radioactivity bound with labeled peptide alone.

elicit a similar degree of inhibition caused by 45-CTP, an 11-fold excess of 35-CTP and 156 times higher concentration of 31-CTP were needed (Figure 5). This may be due to the fact that antibodies were generated against the conformations created by the amino acid residues added beyond 31-CTP.

Chen et al. (1976) and Matsuura et al. (1978) have shown that antisera raised against the 23-amino acid C-terminal fragment react predominantly with the 15 residues from the C-terminal end. The same antigenic determinant (last 15 residues) has been found to be expressed when the immunogen was increased in length up to 30 amino acid residues (Matsuura et al., 1979).

The hormonal specificity of these antibodies was further ascertained by carrying out direct binding studies with ^{125}I-hLH. None of the sera taken at different time periods bound any significant amount

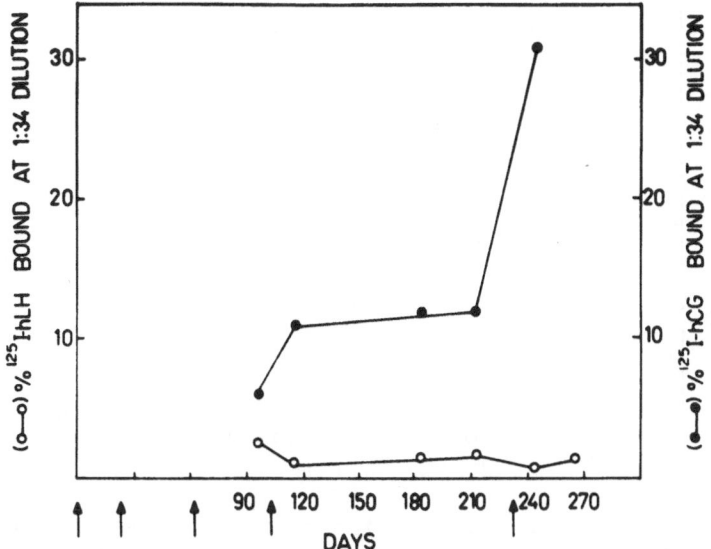

Figure 6. Differential binding of ^{125}I-hCG and ^{125}I-hLH by antibodies raised against 45-CTP-TT. Sera taken at different time points
after immunization were checked for their ability to bind ^{125}I-hCG
and ^{125}I-hLH at 1:34 dilution. The assay conditions have been
described elsewhere, except that ^{125}I-hLH was incubated with the sera
for 72 hr at 4°C. The arrows indicate the time points at which
antigen was injected. ●——●, binding of ^{125}I-hCG; O——O, binding of
^{125}I-hLH.

of ^{125}I-hLH, although the binding with ^{125}I-hCG was substantial, as
shown in Figure 6.

Biological Neutralization of HCG

The ability of anti-45-CTP antiserum to neutralize the biological
activity of hCG was checked in mouse Leydig cell assay system. HCG-
induced production of testosterone was blocked by preincubation of
the hormone with antibodies (Figure 7). This could most probably be
due to the steric hindrance caused by the binding of antibodies to
the hormone (as the biologically active site is away from the C-
terminal end), so that it could no longer bind to the tissue receptors.
Previous investigations carried out by Louvet et al. (1974) have
indicated that antibodies raised against the C-terminal 23 amino
acid residues, although bound to hCG, could not neutralize the

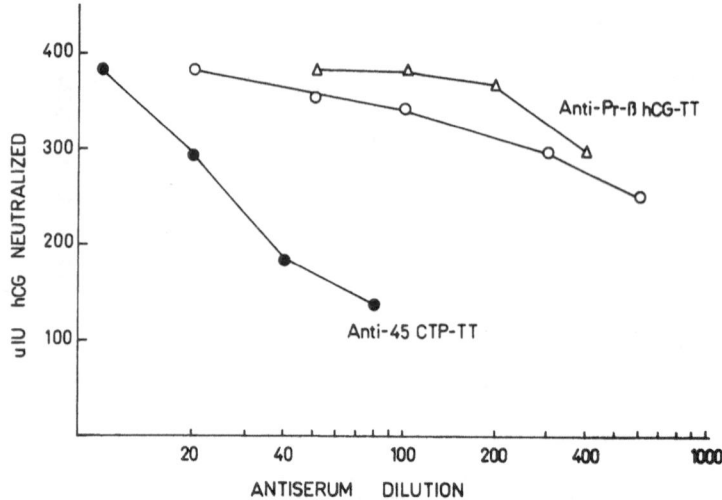

Figure 7.   Comparative neutralization of the biological activity
of hCG by anti-Pr hCGβ-TT sera in mouse Leydig cell bioassay system.
The antibody titers of the sera as measured by RIA were as follows:
O——O, anti-Pr-hCGβ-TT (117ng/ml serum); Δ——Δ, anti-Pr-hCGβ-TT
(424 ng/ml serum); ●——●, anti-45-CTP-TT (3.49 g/ml serum).

biological activity of the hormone. Antibodies against the 30-CTP
(116-145) were also unable to block the biological activity of the
hormone (Matsuura et al., 1979). However, neutralizing type of
antibodies were obtained with 35-CTP (Stevens, 1976). Thus, it is
tempting to suggest that to evoke neutralizing type of antibodies
the antigen must have residues beyond 31-CTP. With native hCGβ as
antigen, there would be a far greater probability of getting neutralizing type of antibodies. Furthermore, investigations show that the
anti-hCGβ antisera of comparable titers have a better neutralizing
capacity than anti-peptide antibodies (Figure 7). This could be
due to the difference in affinity and avidity of the two types of
sera, as well as in the valency of the antibodies.

The possible reason for the better neutralization capacity of
the anti-hCGβ antisera was checked by analyzing the number of antibody molecules binding with hCG in the two cases. The antisera
against hCGβ and the sizes of the antigen-antibody complexes thus
formed were estimated by sedimentation on sucrose density gradients.
Figure 8 shows the sedimentation profile of the two types of complexes.
Anti-hCGβ antibodies formed heavier complex (17 S) with hCG, whereas
anti-45-CTP-hCG complex had a sedimentation constant of 10.5 S.
These findings suggest that anti-hCGβ antibodies bind in 3:1 ratio

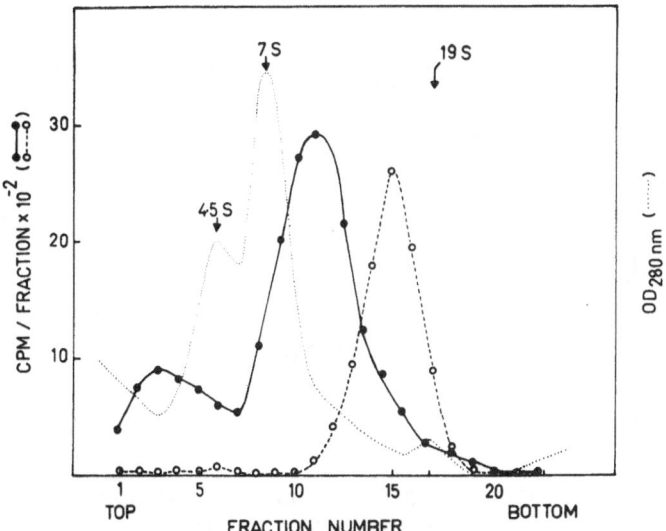

Figure 8.   Sedimentation profile of immune complexes formed by anti-Pr-hCGβ-TT and anti-45-CTP-TT with ^{125}I-hCG. The antisera were incubated with ^{125}I-hCG (20,000 cpm) for 4 hr at room temperature and 17 hr at 4°C. The mixture was run on sucrose density gradients (5-40%) for 18 hr at 105,000 g. (........) indicates the location of marker proteins by the continuous recording of absorbance at 280 nm during fractionation. (_____) shows the radioactivity of ^{125}I-hCG incubated with anti-45-CTP-TT antiserum, and (--------) indicates the radioactivity of ^{125}I-hCG incubated with anti-Pr-hCGβ antiserum. The volume of the fractions was 0.5 ml.

with hCG (multiple binding sites), whereas the anti-45-CTP bind in a ratio of 1:1 (single binding site). Thus, the larger number of immuno-determinants in hCGβ may account for the better efficacy of anti-Pr-hCGβ antibodies to neutralize the biological activity of hCG.

IMMUNORECESSIVE NATURE OF ANTIGENIC DETERMINANTS IN THE C-TERMINAL UNIQUE REGION OF HCGβ

Protein macromolecules have antigenic determinants constituted by linear sequence of amino acids and by conformations resulting from secondary and tertiary structure of the protein. In the course of our studies with Pr-hCGβ-TT it was observed that the antibodies were generated invariably against the determinants present in the core portion of the subunit and not to the linear sequence of the

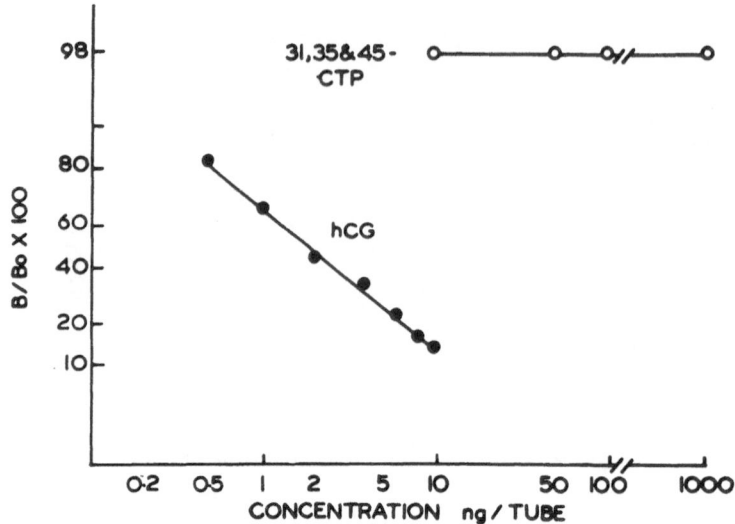

Figure 9.   Competitive inhibition of ^{125}I-hCG binding to anti-hCGβ antisera by C-terminal peptides. Five antisera raised against Pr-hCGβ-TT in monkeys were pooled and diluted appropriately for the use in RIA. ●——●, hCG inhibition curve; O——O, inhibition pattern obtained with C-terminal peptides 31-, 35-, and 45-CTP. Bo = the radioactivity bound to antibodies in the absence of any added substance. B = the antibody bound radioactivity in the presence of hormone/C-terminal peptides.

C-terminal end. The C-terminal synthetic peptides (31, 35, and 45 amino acid residues) failed to compete with ^{125}I-hCG in RIA system using pooled antisera against Pr-hCGβ-TT. Data in Figure 9 show the competitive inhibition profile obtained with hCG and the C-terminal peptides. The peptides did not show any significant competitive inhibition up to a concentration of 1 µg/assay tube. Similar observations have been made by Chen et al. (1976), and by Swaminathan and Braunstein (1978) with SB-6 antiserum.

In a parallel experiment, direct binding studies were carried out with radiolabeled 45-amino acid C-terminal peptide (CTP). Anti-hCGβ antisera collected at different time intervals from 20 monkeys and 13 baboons were checked for their ability to bind ^{125}I-45-CTP and ^{125}I-hCG. None of them bound any significant quantity (>5%) of ^{125}I-45-CTP, suggesting that anti-hCGβ antibodies are, by and large, directed against the conformation determinants present in parts of the molecule other than the unique C-terminal region. These determinants are yet to be delineated, although the preliminary studies of Swaminathan and Braunstein (1978) indicate the presence of two major antigenic determinants made up of the peptide fragments comprising residues 21 to 31 linked by a bisulfide bridge to the 104-114 segment and the 21 to 34 segment, linked to the segment from position 65-71. Further studies on these lines would pave the way for mapping of the portions of $hCG\beta$ which are highly antigenic and unique to hCG, and antibodies of which are devoid of reactivity with hLH.

CONCLUSION

Investigations were carried out on the biological and immunological properties of the β-subunit of hCG and its subfragments. Results suggest that although the overall backbone conformation of hCG and hLH is alike, the presence of specific local conformations in hCG distinct from hLH is highly indicated. It appears that immunochemically purified $hCG\beta$ (Pr-$hCG\beta$) has intrinsic but low biological activity. The possible epitopes involved in the biological activity reside in the region 39-71 of $hCG\beta$ (of which residues 57-71 are important). The C-terminal end of $hCG\beta$ is not involved in the tissue receptor recognition and is devoid of steroidogenic potency; vaccines based on the C-terminal peptides have poor immunogenicity. Antibodies raised against 45-CTP are highly specific and neutralize the biological activity of hCG, although their neutralization capacity is low as compared to antibodies of similar titre raised against the β-subunit of hCG. Immunization with $hCG\beta$ results in the expression of multiple determinants, whereas the C-terminal peptide (45-CTP) has limited (possibly one) antigenic determinant. The C-terminal determinants are not expressed in immunization with $hCG\beta$.

REFERENCES

Aloj, S. M., and Ingham, K. C., 1977, Kinetics of subunit interactions in glycoprotein hormones in *Endocrinology Proceedings Vth Intl. Congress of Endocrinology*, V. H. T. James, ed., p 108, Excerpta Medica, Amsterdam.

Canfield, R. E., Morgan, F. J., Kammerman, S., Bell, J. J., and Agasto. G. M., 1971, Studies of human chorionic gonadotropin, Rec. Progr. Horm. Res. 27:121.

Catt, K. J., Dufau, M. L., and Vaitukaitis, J. L., 1975, Appearance of hCG in pregnancy plasma following the initiation of implantation of the blastocyst, J. Clin. Endocr. Metab. 40:537.

Channing, C. P., and Kammerman, S., 1973, Effect of hCG, asialo-hCG, subunit of hCG upon luteinization of monkey granulosa cell cultures, Endocrinology 93:1035.

Chen, H. C., Hodgen, G. D., Matsuura, S., Birken, S., Canfield, R. E., and Ross, G. T., 1976, Evidence for a gonadotropin from nonpregnant subjects that has physical, immunological, and biological similarities to hCG, Proc. Natl. Acad. Sci., 73:2285.

Das, C., Salahuddin, M., and Talwar, G. P., 1976, Investigations on the ability of antisera produced by Pr-hCG -TT to neutralize the biological activity of hCG, Contraception 13:171.

Das, C., Talwar, G. P., Ramakrishnan, S., Salahuddin, M., Kumar, S., Hingorani, V., Coutinho, E., Croxatto, H., Hemminson, E., Johansson, E., Lukkainen, T., Shahani, S., Sundaram, K., Nash, H., and Segal, S. J., 1978, Discriminatory effect of anti-Pr-β-hCG-TT antibodies on the neutralization of the biological activity of placental and pituitary gonadotropins, Contraception 18:35.

Farmer, S. W., Sairam, M. R., and Papkoff, H., 1972, Stimulation of lactic acid production in vitro from prepubertal rat ovaries by gonadotropin and their subunits, Endocrinology 92:1022.

Garner, P. R., and Armstrong, D. T., 1977, The effect of human chorionic gonadotropin and estradiol-17 beta on the maintenance of the human corpus luteum of early pregnancy, Am. J. Obstet. Gynec. 128:469.

Garnier, J., Salesse, R., and Pernollet, J. C., 1974, Reversible folding of hCG at acid pH or upon combination of the alpha and beta-subunits, FEBS Letters 45:166.

Hanson, F. W., Powell, J. E., and Stevens, V. C., 1971, Effects of hCG and LH on steroid secretion and functional life of the human corpus luteum, J. Clin. Endocr. Metab. 32:21.

Ingham, K. G., Tylenda, C., and Edelhoch, H., 1976, Structural studies of hCG and its subunits using tyrosin fluorescence, Arch. Biochem. Biophys. 173:680.

Jacobs, H. S., 1974, Relation of structure and biological action of gonadotropins, J. Steroid Biochem. 5:861.

Louvet, J. P., Ross, G. T., Birken, S., and Canfield, R. E., 1974, Absence of neutralizing effect of antisera to the unique structural region of human chorionic gonadotropin, J. Clin. Endocrinol. Metab. 39:1155.

Marsh, J. M., and Savard, K., 1966, Studies on the mode of action of luteinizing hormone on steroidogenesis in the corpus luteum in vitro, J. Reprod. Fertil. (Suppl. I):113.

Matsuura, S, Chen, H. C., and Hodgen, G. D., 1978, Antibodies to the carboxyl-terminal fragment of human chorionic gonadotropin beta subunit. Characterization of antibody recognition sites using synthetic peptide analogues, Biochemistry 17:575.

Matsuura, S., Ohashi, M., Chen, H. C., and Hodgen, G. D., 1979, A hCG specific antiserum against synthetic peptide analogs to the C-terminal peptide of its beta-subunit, Endocrinology 104:396.

Mohini, P., Chapekar, T. N., Raj, A. B., Shastri, N., Dubey, S. K., and Talwar, G. P., 1978, Differences between the discriminatory activity of antisera raised against the total gonadotropins and the Pr-β-hCG-TT for neutralization of hCG and LH action, Contraception 18:59.

Morgan, F. J., Canfield, R. E., Vaitukaitis, J. L., and Ross, G. T., 1974, Properties of the subunits of human chorionic gonadotropin, Endocrinology 94:1601.

Morgan, F. J., Birken, S., and Canfield, R. E., 1975, The amino acid sequence of human chorionic gonadotropin. The alpha-subunit and beta-subunit, J. Biol. Chem. 250:5247.

Muralidhar, K., and Moudgal, N. R., 1976, Studies on rat ovarian receptors for luteotropin. Interaction with β-subunit of sheep luteotropin, Biochem. J. 160:615.

Neil, J. D., and Knobil, E., 1972, On the nature of the initial luteotropic stimulus of pregnancy in the rhesus monkey, Endocrinology 90:34.

Ramakrishnan, S., Dubey, S. K., Das, C., Salahuddin, M., Talwar, G. P., Kumar, S., and Hingorani, V., 1976, Influence of hCG and tetanus toxoid injections on the antibody titers in a subject immunized with Pr-β-hCG-TT, Contraception 13:245.

Ramakrishnan, S., Das, C., and Talwar, G. P., 1978b, Recognition of the beta-subunit of human chorionic gonadotropin and sub-determinants by target tissue receptors, Biochem. J. 176:599.

Ramakrishnan, S., Das., C., Dubey, S. K., Salahuddin, M., and Talwar, G. P., 1979, Immunogenecity of three C-terminal synthetic peptides of the β-subunit of hCG and properties of the antibodies raised against 45-amino acid C-terminal peptide, J. Reprod. Immunol. (In press).

Rao, Ch. V., and Carman, F., 1973, Stimulation of ovarian cyclic guanosine 3', 5'-monophosphate levels by the subunits of human chorionic gonadotropin, Biochem. Biophys. Res. Comm. 54:744.

Rao, S. S., and Shahani, S. K., 1961, The antigenicity of human chorionic gonadotropin, Immunology 4:1.

Rayford, P. L., Vaitukaitis, J. L., Ross, G. T., Morgan, F. J., and Canfield, R. E., 1972, Use of specific antisera to characterize biologic activity of hCG-β subunit preparations, Endocrinology 91:144.

Sairam, M. R., and Li. C. H., 1975, Human pituitary lutropin. Isolation, properties and complete amino acid sequence of the beta-subunit, Biochim. Biophys. Acta 412:70.

Salahuddin, M., Ramakrishnan, S., Dubey, S. K., and Talwar, G. P., 1976, Immunological reactivity of antibodies produced by Pr-β-hCG-TT with different hormones, Contraception 13:163.

Salesse, R., Casteing, M., Pernollet, J. C., and Garnier, J., 1975, Association dependent active folding of alpha and beta-subunits of lutropin, J. Mol. Biol. 95:485.

Sasamato, S., 1969, Inhibition of hCG-induced ovulation by anti-hCG serum in immature mice pre-treated with PMSG, J. Reprod. Fertil. 20:271.

Saxena, B. B., Hasan, S. H., Haour, F., and Gollwitzer, S. M., 1974, Radioreceptor assay of human chorionic gonadotropin: detection of early pregnancy, Science 184:793.

Shastri, N., Dubey, S. K., Vijaya Raghavan, S., Salahuddin, M., and Talwar, G. P., 1978, Differential affinity of anti-Pr-β-hCG-TT antibodies for hCG and hLH, Contraception 18:23.

Stevens, V. C., 1976, Perspectives of development of a fertility control vaccine from hormonal antigens of the trophoblast, in Development of vaccines for fertility regulation, pp. 93-110, Scriptor, Copenhagen.

Stevens, V. C., and Crystle, G. D., 1973, Effects of immunization with hapten-coupled hCG on the human menstrual cycles, Obstet. Gynec. 42:485.

Swaminathan, N., and Braunstein, G. D., 1978, Location of major antigenic sites of the beta-subunit of human chorionic gonado-tropin, Biochemistry 17:5832.

Talwar, G. P., Sharma, N. C., Dubey, S. K., Salahuddin, M., Shastri, N., and Ramakrishnan, S., 1976a, Processing of the preparations of β-subunit of human chorionic gonadotropin for minimization of crossreactivity with human lutenizing hormone, Contraception 13:131.

Talwar, G. P., Sharma, N. C., Dubey, S. K., Salahuddin, M., Das, C., Ramakrishnan, S., Kumar, S., and Hingorani, V., 1976b, Iso-immunization against human chorionic gonadotropin with conjugates of processed β-subunit of the hormone to tetanus toxoid, Proc. Natl. Acad. Sci. 73:218.

Talwar, G. P., Dubey, S. K., Salahuddin, M., and Shastri, N., 1976c, Kinetics of antibody response in animals injected with processed beta-hCG conjugated to tetanus toxoid (Pr-β-hCG-TT), Contraception 13:153.

Vaitukaitis, J. L., Braunstein, G. D., and Ross, G. T., 1972a, A radioimmunoassay which specifically measures human chorionic gonadotropin in the presence of human luteinizing hormone, Am. J. Obstet. Gynec. 113:751.

Vaitukaitis, J. L., Ross, G. T., Reichert, L. E., Jr., and Ward, D. N., 1972b, Immunologic basis for within and between species cross-reactivity of luteinizing hormone, Endocrinology 91:1337.

Yang, W. H., Sairam, M. R., and Li, C. H., 1973, The effect of ICSH and its combination with prolactin on the maintenance of pregnancy in the rat, Acta Endocr. 72:173.

ACKNOWLEDGEMENT

This work was supported by financial assistance from Family Planning Foundation of India, I.D.R.C. of Canada, and Internationa-tional Committee of Contraception Research of the Population Council, New York.

LIMITATIONS AND PROBLEMS OF HCG-SPECIFIC ANTISERA

Hao-Chia Chen, Shuji Matsuura, and Masanobu Ohashi

Endocrinology and Reproduction Research Branch
National Institute of Child Health and Human Development
National Institutes of Health, Bethesda, Maryland, U.S.A.

INTRODUCTION

Production of antisera against intact hCG, its subunits or the unique carboxyl-terminal glycopeptide of the β-subunit, and subsequent development of radioimmunoassay systems based on these antisera, have been shown to be highly valuable for basic and clinical investigations related to pregnancy, trophoblastic neoplasms, and some non-trophoblastic neoplasms. Unlike in vitro and in vivo bioassays, and radioimmunoassays using an antiserum against hCG, radioimmunoassay systems based on either a selected antiserum against the highly purified β-subunit of hCG or the carboxyl-terminal peptide of hCGβ (known as Sb6 and H93, respectively) permit differentiation of hCG from the structurally similar hLH. However, despite their advantages these hCG-specific radioimmunoassay systems have exhibited a number of limitations in practice. In the light of recent developments such as the finding of small amounts of hCG or hCG-like substances in biological fluids and non-placental tissues of normal subjects, and the use of antifertility vaccines employing hCGβ or a portion of its molecule as antigen, the necessity of understanding such limitations become apparent.

In this report, we summarize our examination of these problems based on recent studies on the binding characteristics of three representative antisera used for radioimmunoassays, namely anti-hCG (H80), anti-hCGβ (Sb6), and anti-hCGβ-COOH-peptide (H93), and on their in vivo biological neutralization capability. Special attention will be focused on detailed analyses of the H93 antiserum in comparison with similar antisera generated against synthetic peptides analogous to the unique carboxyl-terminal peptide of the hCGβ subunit.

PRODUCTION AND CHARACTERISTICS OF HCG-SPECIFIC ANTISERA

Anti-hCG Serum

Anti-hCG serum, designated H80, was generated in a rabbit immunized with a highly purified hCG preparation (Lot CR119) by the method described by Vaitukaitis et al. (1971). The titers of pooled H80 antiserum with respect to ^{125}I-hCG-CR119 and ^{125}I-hLH-LER960VI are shown in Figure 1 and Figure 2, respectively. It is evident that the H80 antiserum binds ^{125}I-hCG and ^{125}I-hLH equally well and is similar to the antiserum produced previously by Odell et al. (1967). In a radioimmunoassay system using the H80 antiserum and ^{125}I-hCG or ^{125}I-hLH, hCG and hLH were measured indiscriminately. However, it has no detectable cross-reactivity toward highly purified hFSH-LER1575 (40 IU per tube, bioassay, 2IRPHMG) and hTSH (Pierce Fraction IV, 25 ng per tube) as reported previously (Chen et al., 1976). In Table I it is shown that the H80 radioimmunoassay measured poorly both the α- and β-subunit of hCG. Taking account of the cross-reactivity attributable to the hCG contamination in these subunit preparations (0.2% in α-subunit, 0.05% in β-subunit), the hCGβ-subunit was more cross-reactive than the α-subunit in this radioimmunoassay system. Disruption of disulfide bridges in the β-subunit further lowered its cross-reactivity with ^{125}I-hCG. It appears, therefore, that the antibody recognition sites of the H80 antiserum reside across both subunits in favor of the β-subunit in which a certain conformation prevails after association with the α-subunit. Accordingly, the H80-radioimmunoassay is capable of distinguishing not only hCG/hLH from hFSH and hTSH, but also the intact hCG molecule from its two subunits.

Anti-hCGβ Serum

When rabbits are immunized with the purified β-subunit of hCG, occasionally antisera with low cross-reactivity to hLH can be obtained. The widely distributed Sb6 antiserum produced and characterized by Vaitukaitis et al. (1972) is one example. The importance and usefulness of this antiserum in establishing a radioimmunoassay system for diagnostic purposes of pregnant women and patients with neoplasms secreting hCG have been well documented (Braunstein et al., 1973; Goldstein et al., 1974; Vaitukaitis et al., 1976).

Although the Sb6-radioimmunoassay system distinguished hCG from hLH in human serum, both pituitary and urinary hLH preparations were antigenic in this system. Klein and Mishell (1977) have reported that hLH showed approximately 10% of cross-reactivity with hCG at 50% inhibition and greater cross-reactivity at lower hormone concentrations. A similar degree of hLH cross-reactivity was

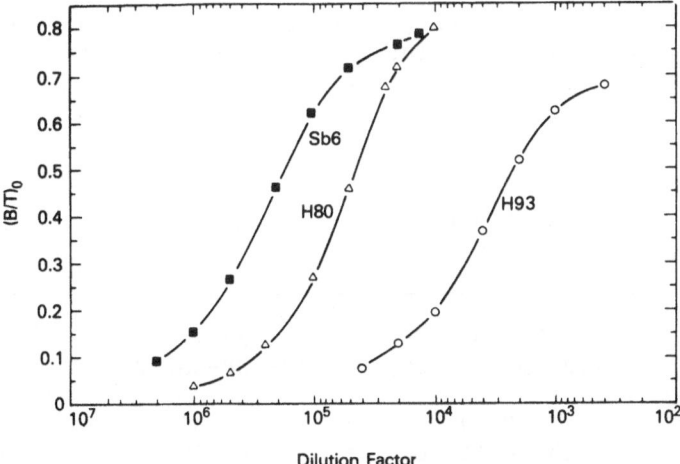

Figure 1. Binding capacity of H80, Sb6, and H93 antisera for ^{125}I-hCG (CR119). Various amounts of antisera were incubated in 0.01 M phosphate, o.15 M NaCl, and 2.5% normal rabbit serum, pH 7.8 with approximately 130 pg of ^{125}I-hCG. The fraction $(B/T)_o$ of radioiodinated hormone bound and the final dilution of antiserum are indicated on the ordinate and abscissa, respectively. Each point represents the mean of triplicate determinations.

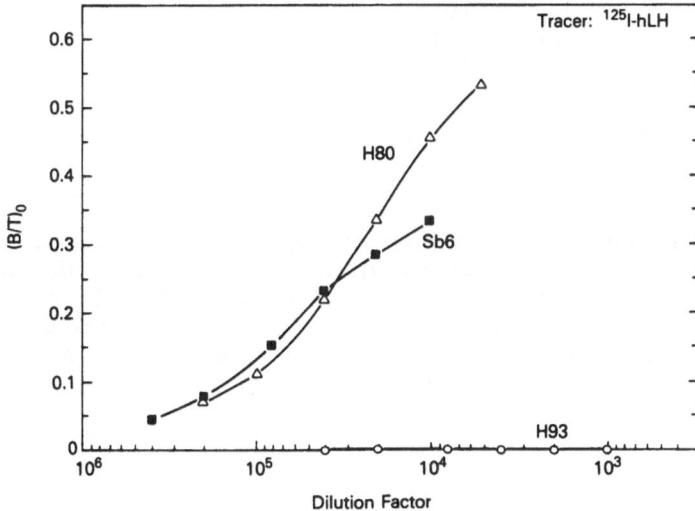

Figure 2. Binding capacity of H80, Sb6, and H93 antisera for ^{125}I-hLH (LER960VI). Except that approx. 150 pg of ^{125}I-hLH was used, other condition and expression are similar to those described in Figure 1.

TABLE I: Comparison of immunopotency of gonadotropin preparations
and the synthetic octacosapeptide in anti-hCGβ and anti-hCGβ-
carboxyl-terminal peptide radioimmunoassay systems.

Gonadotropins and Derivatives	Antiserum		
	Anti-hCG H80	Anti-hCG Sb6	Anti-hCG-CTP H93
1IRP (pituitary)^a	132.32 (122.52-143.14)	33.47 (29.28-38.52)	1.06 (0.72-1.51)
1ISTD (urinary)^a	58.67 (55.30-62.26)	36.37 (33.47-39.55)	12.45 (10.36-14.99)
NIH-LH-A1 (pituitary)^b	338.6 (313.0-366.4)	58.41 (49.35-69.47)	2.76 (2.24-3.38)
hCGα (CR119)^c	1.92×10^{-3} (1.73-2.13)	5.47×10^{-3} (5.12-5.84)	3.22×10^{-3} (2.47-4.38)
hCGβ (CR119)^c	10.71×10^{-3} (3.66-22.87)	2.52 (2.31-2.76)	1.14 (0.98-1.42)
SCM-hCGβ^c	3.4×10^{-5} (2.9-3.9)	3.95×1^{-4} (3.23-4.83)	1.18 (0.98-1.42)
C28^c (Octacosapeptide)	n.d.	n.d.	18.88 (15.90-22.53)

Numbers in parentheses are values of 95% confidence limit.
n.d.: not detectable; a: In nanograms of hCG-CR119/IU, international unit of these preparations defined individually by WHO;
b: In nanograms of hCG-CR119/IU, IU refers to 2IRP-HMG in vivo
bioactivity; c: In nanogram of hCG-CR119/nanogram of sample.

indicated by Swaminathan and Braunstein (1978). As shown in Figure
2, the Sb6 antiserum bound ^{125}I-hLH similar to H80, except that it
showed a tendency to plateau at the higher antiserum concentration.

Taken at the point of $(B/T)_o=0.25$, the amounts of antibodies that bound ^{125}I-hLH were approximately 6% of those displayed as in the case of ^{125}I-hCG shown in Figure 1. When the First International Reference Preparation of LH/FSH from human pituitary (1IRP, 69/104), the First International Standard of LH/FSH from urine of post-menopausal women (1ISTD, 70/45), and a purified human pituitary LH distributed by the National Institutes of Health for radioiodination (NIH-LH-A$_1$) were subjected to the Sb6-radioimmunoassay using ^{125}I-hCG as a tracer, two pituitary fractions, the 1IRP and NIH-LH-A$_1$, exhibited 25% and 17% of immunopotency, respectively, as revealed by the H80-radioimmunoassay shown in Table I. The urinary preparation, 1ISTD, displayed as much as 60% of its H80 immunopotency. Accordingly, these results have demonstrated that detection of immunoreactivity based on the Sb6 antiserum alone is not sufficient evidence to show the presence of hCG or hCG-like substance in concentrated biological fluids or tissue extracts. The presence of as low as 30 mIU/ml of hLH in terms of either 1IRP or 1STD immunopotency in an assay sample can display a positive cross-reactivity in this system. Although such a level is not often observed in a serum of a normal subject, a higher level is common in the kaoline-acetone extract of 24 hr urine and pituitary extracts.

Also shown in Table I, hCG and hCGβ were the most inhibitory in this Sb6-radioimmunoassay system. However, neither the synthetic octacosapeptide (C28, residues 116-145 of hCGβ) nor the reduced S-carboxy-methylated hCGβ (SCM-hCGβ) exhibited substantial cross-reactivity. Swaminathan and Braunstein (1978) have identified that the major antigenic sites of hCGβ reside in the region of residues 21-23 with a disulfide bridge connecting Cys-23 or Cys-26 with Cys-72 or Cys-110. Similarly, Birken and Canfield (1978) have shown that a thermolytic "core" protein of hCGβ, which contains regions of peptide sequences identified by Swaminathan and Braunstein (1978), cross-reacted fully in the Sb6 system. All these results are consistent with our previous finding (Chen et al., 1976) that the specificity of the Sb6 antiserum lies in the conformational characteristics of hCGβ structure, which allows distinction of hCG and hLH, and not in the region of the unique carboxyl-terminal peptide of the sequence.

It should be pointed out that the higher titer and the high binding affinity of hCG-specific antibodies in the Sb6 (Table II) and other antisera similar in characteristics, have allowed the assay to be highly sensitive and practical despite its limitation in specificity. However, it may become disputable if one tends to assume the presence of low amounts of hCG or hCG-like substances (based on assay methods employing the Sb6 antiserum in particular) when the assay sample contains a large pool of hLH, because the antiserum does not distinguish hCG from hLH fully.

TABLE II: Comparison of radioimmunoassay characteristics among anti-hCG, anti-hCGβ, and anti-hCGβ-carboxyl-terminal peptide systems.

RIA Characteristics	Antiserum		
	Anti-hCG H80	Anti-hCGβ Sb6	Anti-hCGβ-CTP H93
Slope	-0.95 ± 0.02	-1.11 ± 0.03	-0.96 ± 0.07
ED_{50} (ng/ml)	4.28 ± 0.17	6.35 ± 0.25	171.5 ± 7.7
MDD, ng/ml	0.45	0.90	19.4
$(B/B_0)_0=0.9$	(0.65 - 0.25)	(1.20 - 0.55)	(5.6 - 47.9)
Keq (M^{-1})	6.74 x 10^{10}	5.40 x 10^{10}	1.20 x 10^9
Free Energy (kcal/mole)	13.75	13.60	11.52

ED_{50} and MDD are potency (ng hCG-CR119) at $B/B_0=0.5$ and 0.9, respectively. B: cpm bound in the presence of ^{125}I-hCG and unlabeled ligand; B_0: cpm bound in the presence of ^{125}I-hCG alone. Numbers in parentheses are values of 95% confidence limit.

Anti-hCGβ-COOH-Terminal Peptide Serum

Since the β-subunit of hCG contains an extended carboxyl-terminal glycopeptide of 35 amino acid residues not presented in hLH and other glycoprotein hormones, efforts were undertaken to take advantage of this structural difference and to produce antisera against this unique portion of the hCGβ peptide in order to develop a specific assay for hCG. An antiserum, designated as H93, was generated in a rabbit immunized with a BSA conjugate of the carboxyl-terminal tricosaglycopeptide (residues 123-145) isolated after digestion of an S-carboxyl-methylated, desialylated preparation of purified hCGβ. A similar antiserum, designated H114, was also generated using a chemically synthesized N^α-acetyl-triaconta-peptide analogous to the carboxyl-terminal peptide of hCGβ (residues 116-145) conjugated to bovine thyroglobulin as immunogen.

Unlike the Sb6 antiserum, H93 antiserum did not bind ^{125}I-hLH as indicated in Figure 2. It has been demonstrated previously (Chen et al., 1976) that several of the most highly purified glycoprotein hormones (at the dose level per tube shown in parenthesis) did not cross-react with ^{125}I-hCG in the H93 radioimmunoassay system: hLH-LER960VI (23 IU, 21RPHMG), hFSH-LER1575 (40 IU, 21RPHMG), NIH pregnant mare serum gonadotropin (100 IU, 21RPHMG), and hTSH (Pierce Fraction IV, 4 µg). As shown in Table I, three hLH preparations exhibited significantly lower cross-reactivities in the H93-radioimmunoassay system than that of the Sb6 system. The differences observed in pituitary preparations between these two assays are particularly striking. Less difference was observed in the case of the urinary preparation (1ISTD). The high H93 cross-reactivity in ISTD is consistent with the estimations revealed previously in Pergonal and the Second International Reference Preparation of Human Postmenopausal Gonadotropin (21IRP-HMG) (Chen et al., 1976). All three of these urinary gonadotropins were derived from the same origin and prepared by the same procedure. Further evidence based on physico-chemical, immunological, and biological studies has led us to conclude that an hCG-like substance in pituitary and urinary extracts of normal subjects indeed is present (Chen et al., 1978). Thus, it is unlikely the observed H93 cross-reactivities in the hLH preparations (1ISTD, 1IRP, NIH-LH-A$_1$, Pergonal, and 21IRP-HMG) were results of intrinsic properties of hLH. Collectively, it is suggested that the H93 radioimmunoassay system specifically measures hCG without cross-reactivity with hLH or other glycoprotein hormones.

Although the H93 antiserum is highly specific to hCG, it also has limitations and problems. First, the carboxyl-terminal portion of hCGβ has not been highly antigenic. Based on experiments with 45 rabbits immunized with seven different antigens, we have so far recorded one rabbit which produced antibodies to reach a titer of 2×10^4 [dilution factor required to give (B/B)$_0$=0.3]. The remaining rabbits either provided no detectable amount or a titer below 5×10^3. Second, the apparent association constant ($1.2 \times 10^9 M^{-1}$) of H93 antiserum is also low as compared with those of Sb6 ($5.4 \times 10^{10} M^{-1}$) and H80 ($6.7 \times 10^{10} M^{-1}$) as listed in Table II. As a result, the sensitivity of the H93 radioimmunoassay is more than one order lower than those of Sb6 and H80. Third, the insensitivity coupled with a non-specific serum effect associated with this H93-radioimmunoassay system make it impractical to assay hCG in serum samples. Thus, the direct use of this radioimmunoassay system for diagnostic purposes in a clinical laboratory is restricted.

Because of the high specificity allowable in the H93-radioimmunoassay, the specimen can be further concentrated by simple procedures prior to assay in order to increase its sensitivity. Ayala et al. (1978) have demonstrated that the H93 assay of urinary extracts processed by the kaolin-acetone procedure followed by the concanavalin A absorption method is far more advantageous in terms of both sensitivity and specificity over the Sb6 assay in serum.

Comments

The radioimmunoassay system based on an anti-hCG serum (H80)
does not discriminate hCG from hLH and does not measure either of
its subunits. The anti-hCGβ system (Sb6) is highly useful and
practical in monitoring hCG content in serum when the amount of
hLH is low. However, it is important to be aware that variable
degrees of cross-reaction toward hLH preparations have been observed.
Accordingly, immunological methods based on the Sb6 antiserum do not
always guarantee the specific measurement of hCG. The contribution
of cross-reactivity from hLH may be significant in specimens which
contain relatively high concentrations of hLH.

The antiserum against the unique carboxyl-terminal peptide of
hCGβ (H93) provides the highest specificity among all hCG-specific
antisera. Due to its low sensitivity and the non-specific serum
effect, a sensitive and reliable measurement has to depend on how
an assay sample is prepared. Presently, urinary extracts after the
kaolin-acetone procedure or the concanavalin A absorption method
offer the most applicable approach in increasing the sensitivity
and specificity of the H93 radioimmunoassay.

LIMITATION OF ANTIGENIC SITES IN ANTISERA AGAINST THE CARBOXYL-
TERMINAL PEPTIDE OF HCGβ

Antiserum to the Tricosaglycopeptide

One approach to characterize the antigenic sites of antisera
against the carboxyl-terminal peptide of hCGβ has been studies of
the inhibition of interaction between ^{125}I-hCG and an antiserum by
a series of synthetic peptides analogous to the antigen. This
approach is particularly useful for identification of antigenic
sites in a sequence-specific antibody such as the H93 series
described previously (Matsuura et al., 1978).

As shown in Figure 3, graded amounts of a highly purified hCG
(Lot CR119) and representative synthetic peptides elongated from
the carboxyl-terminal residue, Gln, and one intermediate peptide
corresponding to residues 125-137 in the hCGβ peptide sequence
displayed dose-response curves in the H93-radioimmunoassay system.
Remarkable parallelism between lines of the synthetic peptides and
that of a highly purified hCG, especially with lengthened peptide
chains, was noted, indicating that these peptides were capable of
competing with native hCG for binding to the antibody. Figure 4
shows that the elongation of chain length from the dipeptide to
octapeptide did not increase binding activity. However, increasing
chain length from nonapeptide to the pentadecapeptide significantly
increased the cross-reactivity, which reached a plateau after the

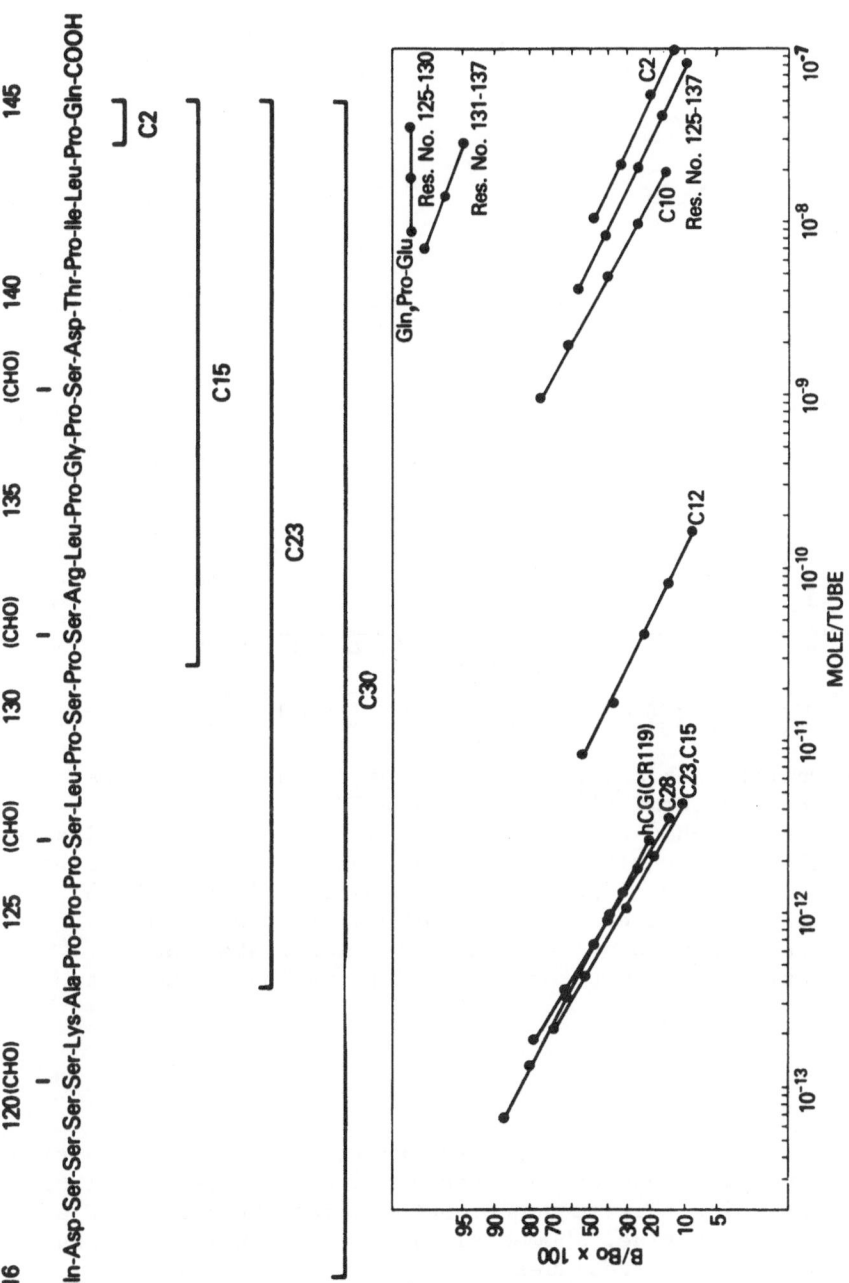

Figure 3. Dose-response curves of synthetic peptides analogous to the carboxyl-terminal sequence of hCGβ in an RIA system based on H93 antiserum. Antiserum dilution 1:8000. B = cpm bound in the presence of ^{125}I-hCG and unlabeled ligand, Bo = cpm bound in the presence of ^{125}I-hCG alone. Upper part shows a portion of the amino acid sequence of the carboxyl-terminal sequence of hCGβ. CHO represents a polysaccharide moiety which is not present in synthetic peptides. Numbers with prefix C indicate chain length elongated from the carboxyl-terminus Gln as shown.

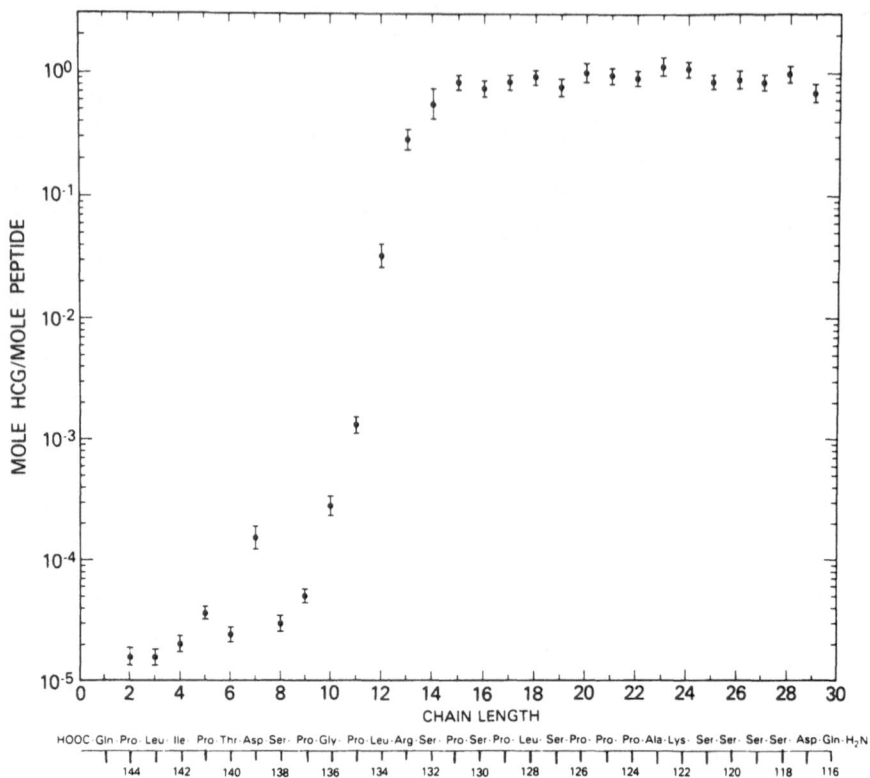

Figure 4. Competitive binding activities of synthetic peptides
analogous to the COOH-terminal sequence of hCGβ in a radioimmunoassay system with ^{125}I-hCG and H93 antiserum. The ordinate indicates
moles of unlabeled hCG required to inhibit equally ^{125}I-hCG binding
to the antiserum per mole of peptide. The abscissa is the chain
length of a peptide elongated from the carboxyl-terminus. The
sequence of corresponding peptide is shown at lower abscissa.
Values of 95% confidence limit for each point are indicated by two
horizontal bars.

pentadecapeptide. Although cross-reactivity increased most significantly over the peptide sequence Arg-Leu-Pro-Gly (residues 133-136),
two peptides containing this sequence, but lacking the last portion
of carboxyl-terminal peptide, showed significantly lower (residues
125-137) or insignificant (residues 131-137) cross-reactivity
(Figure 3). Neither Gln nor Pro-Glu was active. Based on these
data, it has been concluded that the carboxyl-terminal dipeptide
Pro-Gln is the primary antigenic site and that the segment containing

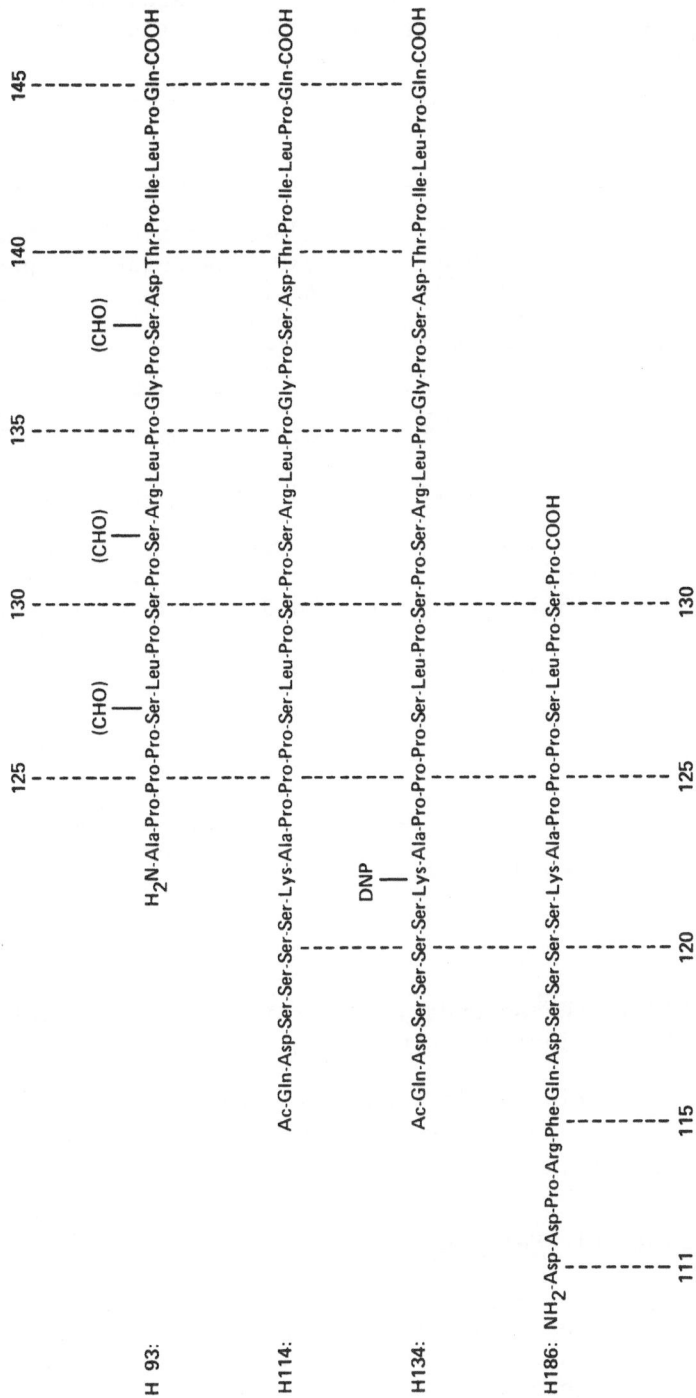

Figure 5. Amino acid sequence of antigens used to generate antisera H93, H114, H134, and H186. Ac and DNP represent acetyl- and dinitrophenyl-group, respectively, at the amino group. CHO represents the carbohydrate moiety.

TABLE III: Comparison of radioimmunoassay characteristics among systems based on antisera against synthetic peptides analogous to the carboxyl-terminal peptide of hCGβ.

Antiserum	H114	H134	H186
Antigen	N^{α}-acetyl-triaconta-**peptide** (residues 116–145)	N^{α}-acetyl-N^{ϵ}-DNP-triaconta-peptide (residues 116–145)	Heneicosa-peptide (residues 111–131)
Slope	−1.19 ± 0.05	−0.96 ± 0.05	−1.13 ± 0.01
ED_{50} (ng/ml)	199.63 ± 6.3	143.2 ± 3.1	2770.5 ± 60.85
MDD (ng/ml) $(B/B_0)_0 = 0.9$	31.5 (13.7 – 50.0)	25.1 (14.8 – 35.4)	394.95 (309.4 – 482.35)
Keq (M^{-1})	1.20×10^9	3.6×10^9	1.5×10^8
Free Energy Kcal/mole	11.52	12.41	10.36

(See Table II for footnotes.)

Arg-Leu-Pro-Gly is the secondary site which acts cooperatively with the primary site to increase cross-reactivity.

In the same series of five antisera, all displayed very similar binding characteristics and specificity toward the same series of synthetic peptides.

Antisera to Synthetic Peptides

Recently, we have generated in rabbits two antisera designated as H114 and H134. The bovine thyroglobulin conjugates of synthetic peptides whose sequence structures are illustrated in Figure 5 were used to prepare immunogens.

TABLE IV: Comparison of immunopotency of synthetic peptides in anti-hCGβ-carboxyl-terminal peptide radioimmunoassay systems.

Peptide	Antiserum		
	H93	H114 (mole hCG/ mole peptide)	H134
C2	2.40×10^{-5} $(1.80 - 3.10)$	3.98×10^{-5} $(3.14 - 4.92)$	1.22×10^{-5} $(1.02 - 1.48)$
C12	1.11×10^{-2} $(0.98 - 1.26)$	2.23×10^{-2} $(1.94 - 2.58)$	1.00×10^{-2} $(0.90 - 1.11)$
C30	0.88 $(0.79 - 0.97)$	1.55 $(1.44 - 1.68)$	0.86 $(0.80 - 0.92)$

Numbers in parentheses are values of 95% confidence limit.

Both H114 and H134 antisera showed nearly identical immuno-logical specificities and sensitivity to that of H93 when examined in a conventional RIA system. The results are summarized in Table III and Table IV. In case of the H114 antiserum, the antibody recognition sites were found to reside at the carboxyl-terminal pentadecapeptide region as described previously (Matsuura et al., 1979). Notably, synthetic dodecapeptide or longer peptide were twice as potent in inhibiting ^{125}I-hCG binding to H114 than to H134, as shown in Table IV. It is intriguing that H114 and H134 exhibited different binding affinity toward longer synthetic peptides. The two antigens which were used to generate H114 and H134 differ only at the Lys residue in which ε-amino group is dinitro-phenylated, in the case of H134. Since the DNP-peptide leaves only three carboxyl-groups permissable as sites for conjugation -- namely, Asp 117, Asp 139, and Gln 145 -- a linkage to thyroglobulin occurring at Asp 139 or Gln 145 may keep the terminal dipeptide Pro-Gln from expressing antigenicity. Indeed, results in Table IV indicated that the synthetic dipeptide (C2) was less potent in replacing hCG from the H134 serum when it was compared to two analogous antisera, H93 and H114. Perhaps the restriction existed in the first locus, Pro-Gly, lessened overall affinity despite the fact that the potentially antigenic sedond locus is free. On the other hand, two carbohydrate chains attached near the second locus (Ser-132 and Ser-138) in the case of H93 exerted hindrance for the second locus from expressing antigenicity. It appears, therefore, that cooperative action of two binding sites, namely Pro-Gln (residues 144-145) and Arg-Leu-Pro-Gly (residues 133-136) are required to elicit the maximal antigenicity as reached by the H114 antiserum.

Antigenically Inert Segment

The fact that the antigenic determinants for all antisera against the carboxyl-terminal peptides of hCGβ are limited to the pentadecapeptide is most intriguing. In our earlier report, it was considered that the NH_2-terminal region of the native antigen fragment, tricosaglycopeptide of hCGβ, was sterically hindered by its attachment to the carrier protein, thereby preventing this segment consisting of residues 123-130 from participating as an antigenic region (Matsuura et al., 1978). Alternatively, intrinsic inertness in eliciting antigenicity from this segment, not involving the carrier protein, was also considered. In order to answer this question, we have conducted studies in an attempt to delineate antigenic properties of the NH_2-terminal portion of the unique carboxyl-terminal peptide of hCGβ.

A peptide corresponding to residues 111-131 was chemically synthesized by the solid phase method and was conjugated to bovine thyroglobulin according to procedures described previously (Matsuura, 1979). An antiserum against this henicosapeptide was produced and designated as H186. The titer to achieve 30% binding of ^{125}I-hCG was only 200, as compared to 8000 for H93. The binding character-istics of H186 were determined in an ^{125}I-hCG-RIA system and compared with those of H114 and H134 as described in Table IV. The apparent association constant of the H186 antiserum toward the binding of ^{125}I-hCG is one order lower than that of either H114 or H134. Accordingly, the H186 RIA system is one order less sensitive than H93, H114, and H134 systems in assaying hCG.

Although the antigen (henicosapeptide, residues 111-131) was highly effective in displacing ^{125}I-hCG, N^α-acetyl-triacontapeptide (residues 116-145) failed to show cross-reactivity on the H186 RIA system, despite the fact that the triacontapeptide overlaps a segment (residues 116-131) with the antigen. The antigenic inert-ness of this paricular segment which constitutes the amino-terminal portion of the carboxyl-terminal peptides, explains sufficiently why antigenic determinants of all anti-hCGβ-carboxyl-terminal peptide sera are limited to the carboxyl-terminal pentadecapeptide region.

As to the antigenic sites for the H186 antiserum, the penta-peptide Asp-Asp-Pro-Arg-Phe corresponding to residues 111-115 remains as only a possibility. Circumstantial evidence based on

low titer and low affinity of the H186 antiserum toward ^{125}I–hCG
has led us to speculate that the pentapeptide sequence in the
structure of intact hCG may not be easily accessible for antibody
binding. Although more direct evidence is needed, the presence of
a disulfide bridge immediately preceding this pentapeptide supports
such speculation.

Three Possible Antigenic Sites

An approach to characterizing antisera to the unique carboxyl-
terminal region of the hCGβ subunit, using a series of synthetic
peptide analogues, has allowed us to identify peptide sequence
structures important for antigenic recognition. Two loci, namely
Pro-Gln of the carboxyl-terminal peptide and the sequence of Arg-
Leu-Pro-Gly (residues 133-136) within the pentadecapeptide, are
two dominant sites. The cooperative enhancement of these two sites
appears to provide the maximal antigenicity and the basis of high
specificity for hCG and hCGβ without cross-reactivity to hLH.

Finally, an additional antigenic site at the amino-terminal
pentapeptide (residues 111-115) within the unique carboxyl-terminal
sequence of hCGβ was identified. The accessibility of this segment
in the hCG protein molecule and its role in enhancing specificity
that distinguishes hCG from hLH is not yet clear.

NEUTRALIZATION OF GONADOTROPIC ACTIVITIES

In Vivo Neutralization

Previously, it has been demonstrated that antisera to intact
hCG and its α- and β-subunits are capable of neutralizing the
biological activity of hCG in in vivo bioassays (Nixon et al., 1971;
Hodgen et al., 1973). In contrast, antisera to the carboxyl-terminal
glycopeptide of hCGβ including H93 (Louvet et al., 1974; Chen and
Hodgen, 1976) and a similar synthetic peptide analogue, residues
116-145 (Matsuura et al., 1979) fail to neutralize the biological
activities under the same condition.

Whether this difference is due to the intrinsic activity of
the hCG/antibody complex, or to the free hCG dissociated from the
complex, is not known. Since the primary antibody recognition
sites for this unique carboxyl-terminal peptide of the hCGβ subunit
reside in the carboxyl-terminal pentadecapeptide sequence (the
sequence which is absent from hLH) it may extend outward as an
appendage to the hCG molecule. Thus, the binding of an antibody to
this biologically unessential "tail piece" might not inhibit interaction of the hormone with gonadal receptor. Consequently, the

hormone/antibody complex might retain biological activity. Alternatively, hCG may become dissociated from these low affinity antibodies in circulation and, thereby, express biological activity as free hCG. In order to resolve this question, we have compared the biological activity of hCG bound to either H93 antiserum or H80 antiserum in vitro and have examined their plasma half lives and uptake by testis in vivo.

In Vitro Studies

Two types of in vitro experiments, namely, effects of antisera on the binding of hCG to the testis receptor and on the stimulation of interstitial cell testosterone production, were conducted.

The binding of ^{125}I-hCG to rat testis homogenates in the presence of either H93 antiserum or H80 antiserum was evaluated (Figure 6). Addition of increasing amount of antiserum progressively reduced the binding of ^{125}I-hCG to the receptor. Similarly, in the presence

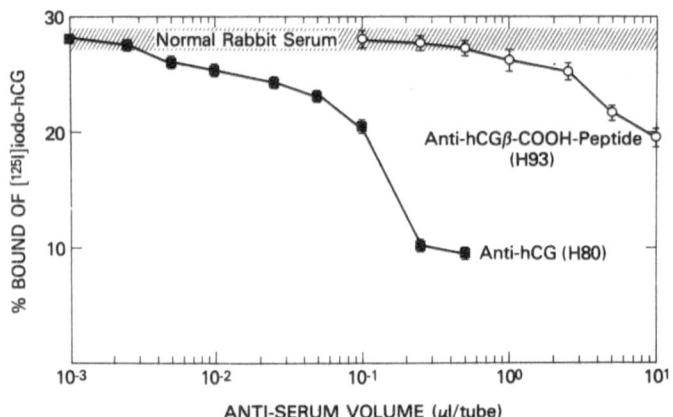

Figure 6. Effect of antisera H80 and H93 on the ^{125}I-hCG binding to the receptor. The graded amount of antisera shown on the abscissa were incubated with ^{125}I-hCG (1 x 10^5 dpm) in a total volume of 110 µl diluted with PBS (0.01 M phosphate, 0.15 M NaCl) plus 0.1% BSA, pH 714 at 37°C for 2 hr and 4°C overnight. In control tubes, the normal rabbit serum was used as a replacement for antisera. Incubation was continued at 37°C for 3 hr after adding 100 µl of rat testis homogenates (1 pair/25 ml PBS). Data are expressed as the percentages of total ^{125}I-hCG bound to the rat testis homogenates. Values represent the mean ± SD of triplicate determinations. The shaded area is the range of response from triplicate assays in the presence of normal rabbit serum at 10^{-3} and 10 µl without antisera.

of 1 ng of purified hCG, both H93 and H80 inhibited testosterone production in the rat interstitial testosterone production assay (Figure 7). Clearly, the H80 antiserum, on a volume basis, was approximately 100 times more effective in reducing these activities of hCG than the H93 antiserum, and the slopes of dose-response curves were indicative of higher affinity (50 times) of the H80 antiserum over that of H93.

In order to ascertain if the hCG/H93 complex binds to the testis receptor, the binding to testis homogenates of purified ^{125}I-antibodies (Ab$\underline{c}$) derived from the H93 antiserum, was investigated. The antibody fraction used for radioiodination was purified by affinity chromatography employing a synthetic dodecapeptide (residues 134-145) as ligand. In the presence of 0.1 ng-10 μg of unlabeled hCG, ^{125}I-Ab$\underline{c}$ failed to exhibit detectable binding to the receptor.

These results collectively indicate that the hCG/H93 complex does not bind to the receptor. Both H80 and H93 antisera inhibited

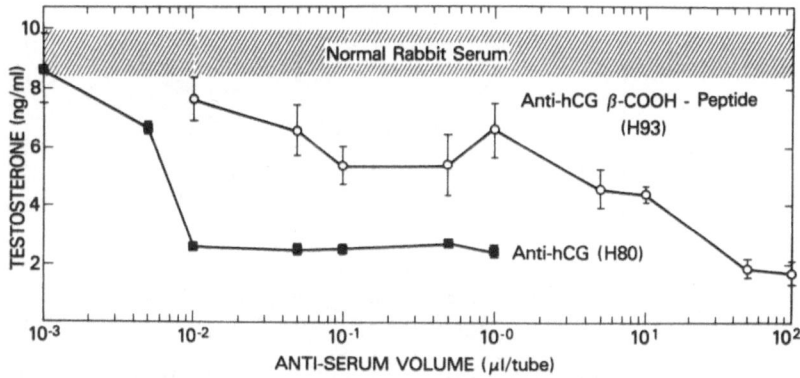

Figure 7. Effect of antisera H80 and H93 on the hCG stimulation of testosterone production in collagenase-dispersed Leydig cells. The graded amounts of antisera were incubated with 1 ng of hCG in the total volume of 100 μl diluted with the PBS-BSA buffer, pH 7.4 at 37°C for 2 hr and 4°C overnight. The rat interstitial cell testosterone production assay was carried out with a collagenase-dispersed Leydig cell population at 9×10^5 cells/tube. Data are expressed as the testosterone concentration in the incubation medium in the presence of antisera. Values represent the mean ± SD of triplicate determinations. The shaded area is the range of response from triplicate determinations in the presence of normal rabbit serum alone.

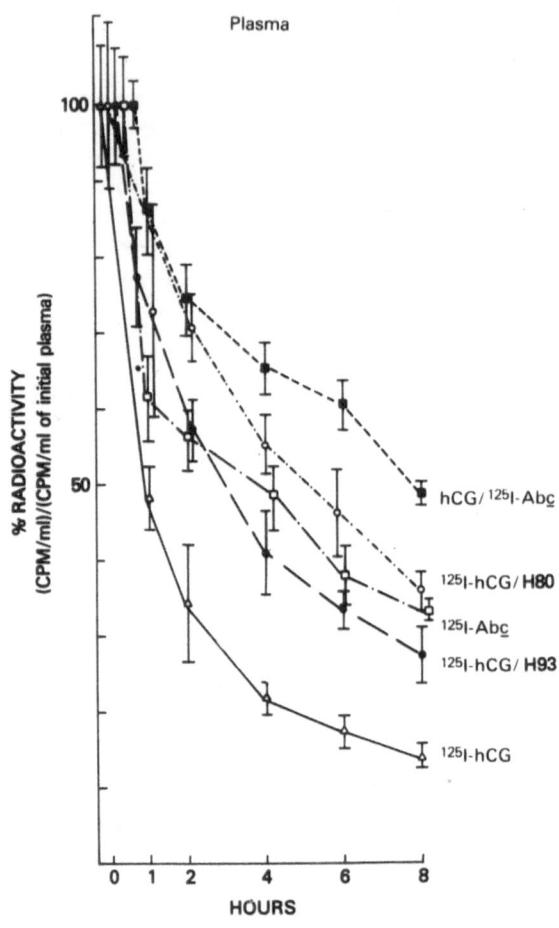

Figure 8.   Plasma half-lives of ^{125}I-hCG, ^{125}I-hCG/H93, ^{125}I-hCG/
H80, hCG/^{125}I-Abc, and ^{125}I-Abc in intact male rats (200-250 g).
Abc was purified antibodies derived from H93 antiserum. Data are
expressed as the percentages of the average radioactivities per ml
of plasma at given times using the initial plasma radioactivities
as a base. The initial plasma radioactivities were determined
from the blood withdrawn between 30 sec and 1 min after injection.
Values represent the mean ± SD from five rats.

the biological activity of hCG in vitro by forming hormone/antibodies complexes that block the normal interaction of hCG with its receptor. Despite the fact that the antigenic sites of the H93 antiserum resides at the biologically unessential carboxyl-terminal pentadeca-peptide region of $hCG\beta$, the antibodies in the H93 antiserum also mask active sites essential for hormone/receptor interaction.

In Vivo Studies

Unlike the hCG/H80 complex which showed no biological activities in both in vivo and in vitro experiments, the hCG/H93 complex, on the other hand, was active in vivo but inactive in vitro. In order to investigate this disparate effect of H93 antiserum, we carried out studies comparing plasma half-lives of these two complexes, free hCG and purified H93 antibodies (Abc) as well as their uptakes into intact adult rats. As shown in Figure 8, the plasma half-life of ^{125}I-hCG/H93 as measured by radioactivities was longer than that of ^{125}I-hCG. Also, the ^{125}hCG/H80 complex showed longer half-life than ^{125}I-hCG/H93. Furthermore, when differential labeling was applied (^{125}I-hCG/H93 versus hCG/^{125}I-Abc), the plasma half-life of hCG/^{125}I-Abc was prolonged markedly as compared with that of supposedly identical complex, ^{125}I-hCG/H93. In testis (Figure 9), the uptakes of radioactivities from ^{125}I-hCG and ^{125}I-hCG/H93 were equally high after 8 hr. In contrast, the uptakes of ^{125}I-hCG/H80, hCG/^{125}I-Abc and ^{125}I-Abc were all significantly lower. These findings suggest that dissociation of the hCG/H93 complex does occur in circulation. Further, the low apparent association constant ($1.2 \times 10^9 M^{-1}$) of hCG/H93, as compared with those of hCG/H80 ($6.7 \times 10^{10} M^{-1}$) and hCG/gonadal-receptor ($3.2 \times 10^{10} M^{-1}$, 24°C) support the present findings.

In conclusion, both hCG/H80 and hCG/H93 complexes per se are biologically inactive either in vivo or in vitro. The failure of H93 antiserum to neutralize the hCG biological activity measured by conventional in vivo assays arises from free hCG after its dissoci-ation from the antibodies during circulation, rather than the retention of intrinsic biological activity by the hCG/antibodies complex.

Clearly, in vitro bioassays alone are not sufficient to assess the antigenic responses and the contraceptive status of women receiving such immunization, because they may fail to examine the binding stability of the hormone/antibody complex in circulation. These observations are relevant to selection and evaluation of antigens used to achieve contraception by anti-hCG vaccines.

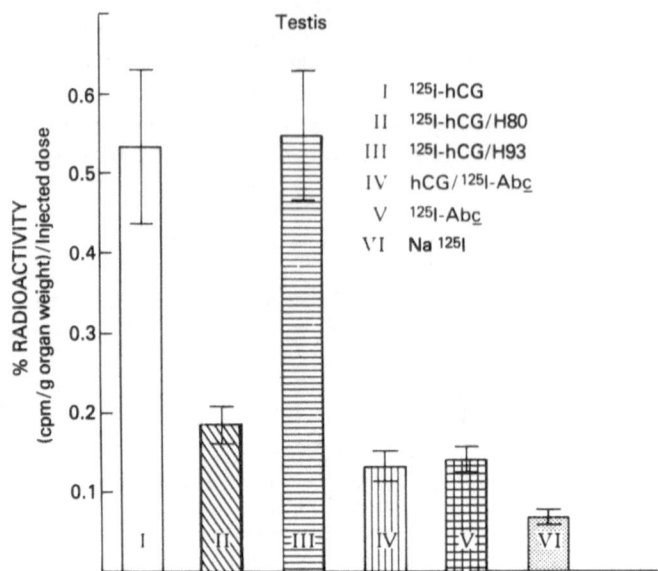

Figure 9. The testicular uptake of radioactivity from ^{125}I-hCG, ^{125}I-hCG/H93, ^{125}I-hCG/H80, hCG/^{125}I-Abc 8 hr after injection. Values represent the mean ± SD from five animals.

CONCLUSION

The RIA systems based on an anti-hCG serum (80) and anti-hCGβ serum (Sb6) are highly practical and useful for the measurement of hCG. The H80 system measures hCG and hLH indiscriminately, but not either α-subunit or β-subunit of hCG and other glycoprotein hormones. On the other hand, the Sb6 system is sensitive and specific to hCG with significantly low cross-reaction to hLH. While the Sb6 system is highly valuable in monitoring hCG and hCGβ in serum, it should not be used to distinguish hCG from hLH in urinary, pituitary, and other tissue extracts in which high contents of hLH relative to hCG might be present. Although the anti-hCGβ-carboxyl-terminal glyco-peptide serum (H93) is highly specific to hCG and hCGβ without cross-reaction with hLH, the H93 RIA system is one order less sensi-tive and has non-specific serum effects. Consequently, it cannot be used to assay hCG or hCGβ in a serum sample. In order to over-come these problems, effort to devise a simple and effective concentration method for processing biological fluids and tissues is vital. Several methods are currently available.

As to the antigenicity of the unique carboxyl-terminal peptide of the hCGβ subunit, our studies have demonstrated that it is limited to two sites at the carboxyl-pentadecapeptide region and possibly one site at the amino-terminal portion of the unique carboxyl-terminal peptide. As a result, the titer and binding affinity of the antisera against the carboxyl-terminal peptide have been low frequently. Furthermore, these antisera fail to neutralize hCG-biological activity in vivo due to free hCG dissociated from the hormone/antibodies complex in circulation.

These observations are important as to the value of strategies using either the intact molecule or fragments of the hCGβ subunit for the development of an anti-hCG antifertility vaccine. Continuing effort to understand structural and antigenic relationships is needed for the production of antisera that are specific and sensitive to hCG without the problems discussed above.

REFERENCES

Ayala, A. R., Nisula, B. C., Chen, H. C., Hodgen, G. D., and Ross, G. T., 1978, Highly sensitive radioimmunoassay for human chorionic gonadotropin in human urine, J. Clin. Endocrin. Metab. 47:767.

Birken, S., and Canfield, R. E., 1978, Structural and immunochemical properties of human choriogonadotropin, in Structure and Function of the Gonadotropins, K. W. McKerns, ed., pp. 47-80, Plenum Press, New York.

Braunstein, G. D., Vaitukaitis, J. L., Carbone, P. P., and Ross, G. T., 1973, Ectopic production of human chorionic gonadotropin by neoplasms, Ann. Intern. Med. 78:39.

Chen, H. C., and Hodgen, G. D., 1976, Primate chorionic gonadotropins: Antigenic similarities to the unique carboxyl-terminal peptide of hCGβ subunit, J. Clin. Endocrin. Metab. 43:1414.

Chen, H. C., Hodgen, G. D., Matsuura, S., Lin, L. J., Gross, E., Reichert, L. E., Jr., Birken, S., Canfield, R. E., and Ross, G. T., 1976, Evidence for a gonadtropin from nonpregnant subjects that have physical, immunological, and biological similarities to human chorionic gonadotropin, Proc. Natl. Acad. Sci. U.S.A. 73:2885.

Chen, H. C., Matsuura, S., Hodgen, G. D., and Ross, G. T., 1978, A human chorionic gonadotropin-like substance distinct from human luteinizing hormone, in Novel Aspect of Reproductive Physiology, Seventh Brooklodge Workshop on Problems of Reproductive Biology, C. H. Spilman and J. W. Wilks, eds., pp. 289-308, Spectrum Publications, Jamaica, New York.

Goldstein, D. P., Kosasa, T. S., Skarim, A. T., 1974, The clinical application of a specific radioimmunoassay for human chorionic gonadotropin in trophoblastic and nontrophoblastic tumors, Surg. Gynecol. Obstet. 138:747.

Hodgen, G. D., Nixon, W. E., Vaitukaitis, J. L., Tullner, W. W., and Ross, G. T., 1973, Neutralization of primate chorionic gonadotropin activities by antisera against the subunits of human chorionic gonadotropin in radioimmunoassay and bioassay, Endocrinology 92:705.

Klein, T. A., and Mishell, Jr., D. R., Jr., 1977, Absence of circulating chorionic gonadotropin in wearers of intrauterine contraceptive device, Am. J. Obstet. Gynecol. 129:626.

Louvet, J. P., Ross, G. T., Birken, S., and Canfield, R. E., 1974, Absence of neutralizing effect of antisera to the unique structural region of human chorionic gonadotropin, J. Clin. Endocrin. Metab. 39:1155.

Matsuura, S., Chen, H. C., and Hodgen, G. D., 1978, Antibodies to the carboxyl-terminal fragment of human chorionic gonadotropin β-dubunit: Characterization of antibody recognition sites using synthetic peptide analogues, Biochemistry 17:575.

Matsuura, S., Ohashi, M., Chen, H. C., and Hodgen, G. D., 1979, A human chorionic gonadotropin-specific antiserum against synthetic peptide analogs to the carboxyl-terminal peptide of its β-subunit, Endocrinology 104:396.

Nixon, W. E., Tullner, W. W., Rayford, P. L., and Ross, G. T., 1971, Similarity of antigenic determinants in pituitary and chorionic gonadotropins from primates, Endocrinology 88:702.

Odell, W. D., Ross, G. T., and Rayford, P. L., 1967, Radioimmunoassay for luteinizing hormone in human plasma or serum: Physiological studies, J. Clin. Invest. 46:248.

Swaminathan, N., and Braunstein, G. D., 1978, Location of major antigenic sites of the β-subunit of human chorionic gonadotropin, Biochemistry 17:5832.

Vaitukaitis, J. L., Robbins, J. B., Nieschlag, E., and Ross, G. T., 1971, A method for producing specific antisera with small doses of immunogen, J. Clin. Endocrin. Metab. 33:988.

Vaitukaitis, J. L., Braunstein, G. D., and Ross, G. T., 1972, A radioimmunoassay which specifically measures human chorionic gonadotropin in the presence of human luteinizing hormone, Am. J. Obstet. Gynecol. 113:251.

Vaitukaitis, J. L., Ross, G. T., Braunstein, G. D., and Rayford, P. L., 1976, Gonadotropins and their subunits: Basic and clinical studies, Recent Prog. Hormone Res. 32:289.

HUMAN CHORIONIC GONADOTROPIN ALPHA AND BETA SUBUNIT mRNAs:
TRANSLATABLE LEVELS DURING PREGNANCY AND MOLECULAR CLONING
OF DNA SEQUENCES COMPLEMENTARY TO HCG

Mark Boothby, Susan Daniels-McQueen, Diana
McWilliams, Maria Zernik, and Irving Boime

Department of Pharmacology and Department of
Obstetrics and Gynecology, Washington University
School of Medicine, St. Louis, Missouri, U.S.A.

INTRODUCTION

One of the important functions of the human placenta is to
produce peptide hormones during pregnancy. The major ones elabo-
rated by the trophoblast are human chorionic gonadotropin (hCG)
and human placental lactogen (hPL). The appearance of the hormones
in maternal serum during pregnancy is quite different. Whereas hCG
peaks in the first trimester, hPL reaches maximal levels near term.
Since the levels of these hormones differ during the course of
gestation, it is apparent that the factors controlling their synthesis are not the same. Thus the human placenta represents a
convenient and unique tissue for studying expression of human
hormonal genes during development.

Placental lactogen is a single non-glycosylated polypeptide
chain which shares greater than 90% homology with human growth
hormone. Chorionic gonadotropin consists of two non-identical
glycosylated subunits (alpha and beta) linked non-covalently. The
amino acid sequence of hCGα is virtually identical to that of the
α-subunits contained in human pituitary gonadotropins, as well as
in thyrotropin (Bahl, 1977). The β-subunit confers the unique
biologic action on each hormone, although there is also significant
homology between the β-subunits (Bahl, 1977). HCGβ contains an
extra 30 amino acid peptides at the carboxyl end of the molecule,
which are not found in the other β-subunits (Morgan et al., 1975).

The amounts of α- and β-subunits secreted by placenta, cultured
choriocarcinoma cells, and numerous ectopic tumors vary considerably
(Figure 1). Since the level of free α-subunit greatly exceeds that

of the β-subunit in placenta and most tumor lines, it has been suggested that synthesis of the β-subunit limits the rate of hCG production in vivo.

What features of the gonadotropin subunit and placental lactogen genes play a role in their expression during pregnancy, and in their response to tumorigenesis? To study this question, and to quantitate rates of synthesis of hPL and hCGα and β-subunit mRNAs, large amounts of pure homogeneous nucleic acid probes are required. We attempted to isolate such probes by first synthesizing complementary DNA molecules (cDNAs) to placental mRNA, and then transforming bacteria with these cDNAs attached to a suitable plasmid vector. Clones bearing hPL and hCGα cDNA sequences are reported here. Further information concerning the synthesis of hCG during pregnancy is also discussed, and the potential use of the clones to study the biology of the trophoblast is projected.

METHODS

Placental RNA was extracted and translated in wheat germ lysates as described previously (Boime et al., 1976; McQueen et al., 1978). Enrichment for hPL mRNA and for α and βhCG mRNAs, from term and first-trimester placenta respectively, was performed by oligo dT-cellulose chromatography and by sucrose gradient centrifugation (McQueen et al., 1978).

Single strand cDNA (ss cDNA) was synthesized according to the method of Buell et al. (1978). Synthesis of double strand cDNA (ds cDNA) was performed by the procedure of Wickens et al. (1978), except that reactions were stopped by phenol extraction without prior addition of an inactivation mixture. After removal of unincorporated label by passing through a Sephadex G-100 column, the ds cDNA products were analyzed by electrophoresis on non-denaturing 5% polyacrylamide gels in Tris-borate/EDTA buffer (Dingman and Peacock, 1968).

The ds cDNA product was digested with S1 nuclease to remove the hairpin loop from the 3' end of the first strand (Efstradiadis et al., 1976). Homopolymeric tracts of deoxycytidine (dC) were attached to 3' ends of the ds cDNAs with terminal deoxynucleotidyl transferase (Villa-Komaroff et al., 1978). The vector, plasmid pBR322 (Bolivar et al., 1977), was digested with the restriction endonuclease Pst1 and the 3' ends of the plasmid were similarly extended with deoxyguanosine (dG). The average lengths of the homopolymeric tails (15-30 nucleotides) were estimated by quantitating the amount of ^{3}H-dNTP incorporated in the terminal transferase reaction. The cDNA was then annealed to the vector as described (Villa-Komaroff et al., 1978) and transformed into $E.$ $Coli$ strain chi-1776 (Curtiss et al., 1977) by a modification of the method of

Enea et al.(1975). This work was conducted, in accordance with NIH Guidelines for Recombinant DNA Research, at a P3 containment level; the combination of pBR322/chi-1776 is classified EK-2.

Transformants resistant to tetracycline were transferred to nitrocellulose filters for growth, lysis, and hybridization to appropriate probes according to Grunstein and Hogness (1975). Candidates for clones bearing sequences of interest were further analyzed by restriction enzyme digestion of cleared lysates (Clewell and Helinski, 1969), treatment with RNase, and electrophoresis in non-denaturing 5% polyacrylamide gels.

Additional analysis of clones was performed by the method of Persson et al. (1979). Plasmid DNA was prepared from the clone by the method of Tilghman et al. (1979). The DNA was then linearized with the restriction enzyme Hind III or EcoRI, and 50 µg were hybridized for 18 hr at the described conditions to 250 µg total RNA (roughly equivalent to 2.5 µg poly A + RNA) from placenta. RNA hybridized to the plasmid was separated from unhybridized RNA on a column of Biogel A-50m equilibrated with 0.5 M LiCl, 1 mM EDTA, 0.1% SDS, and 10 mM Tris-HCl pH 8. Void volume fractions were pooled and concentrated by ethanol precipitation. The hybrids were then translated in a wheat germ lysate. Products were analyzed by trichloroacetic acid precipitation of the total reaction or by immunoprecipitation, as described earlier (McQueen et al., 1978).

RESULTS

Cell-free Synthesis of HCGα and β-Subunit Forms

Studies on the translation of hPL mRNA and the quantitation of this mRNA as a function of pregnancy with a cDNA have been reported previously (McWilliams et al., 1977). The following studies will deal primarily with the synthesis of hCG.

Products of the wheat germ cell-free system programmed with first-trimester RNA were immunoprecipitated with hCG subunit specific antisera (Figure 1A). The product specifically precipitated by α antiserum (Lane 2) corresponded to the product previously reported to contain authentic tryptic peptides derived from the α-subunit (Boime et al., 1978). Antiserum directed against the β-subunit precipitated a protein migrating slower than the labeled α protein (Lane 5). As expected, little if any labeled protein was observed when an identical quantity of non-immune rabbit serum was used in place of subunit-specific antisera (Lane 1).

To determine the immunologic specificity of this purification system, unlabeled purified subunits were added to reaction mixtures

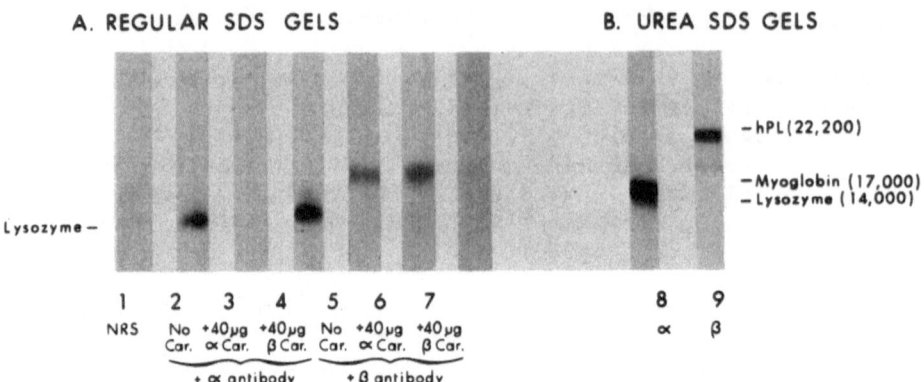

Figure 1.   A) Sodium dodecyl sulfate gel electrophoresis of [^{3}H]
proline-labeled proteins synthesized in response to first-trimester
placental RNA.   Labeled proteins synthesized in wheat germ extracts
were immunoprecipitated and the resulting immunoprecipitates were
dissolved in SDS buffer and examined on 20% SDS-polyacrylamide slab
gels.   The amounts of radioactivity applied were: Lane 1, 300 cpm;
Lane 2, 5000 cpm;   Lane 3, 2000 cpm; Lane 4, 6000 cpm; Lane 5-7,
4000 cpm.   Car., carrier, unlabeled purified subunits.   B) SDS-urea
gels of immunoprecipitated products.   The migration of hPL
(M_r=22,200), myoglobin (M_r=16,500), and lysozyme (M_r=14,000) are
shown.   The KCl and magnesium concentrations were 74 and 1.8 mM,
respectively.   The gels were subjected to fluorography (Keller et
al., 1980).   NRS, normal rabbit serum.

in an attempt to compete with labeled protein of the homologous subunit (Figure 1A).   Accordingly, 40 μg of unlabeled purified α- and
β-subunits were added simultaneously to the immunoprecipitation
reactions with subunit-specific antisera.   Unlabeled α-subunit
competed effectively with labeled pre-α (Lane 3) but had no effect
on precipitation of the labeled β-specific protein to its homologous
antiserum (Lane 6).   In contrast, addition of unlabeled β-subunit
eliminated precipitation of the labeled M_r=18,000 protein with anti-
β-subunit antisera (Lane 7), but did not inhibit precipitation of
pre-α to its homologous antiserum (Lane 4).   These results give
presumptive evidence that the two labeled proteins contain α and β
sequences.   Similar translation experiments were performed in ascites
cell-free extracts and the labeled products precipitated with subunit
specific antisera were identical to those above (data not shown).

The molecular weight of these labeled proteins was estimated using urea-SDS gels (Swank and Munkres, 1971). The labeled α- and β-subunit proteins migrated with apparent molecular weights of 14,000 and 18,000, respectively (Figure 1B). The molecular weights of the authentic α and β apoproteins are 10,500 and 15,500, respectively. In the case of the α-subunit the extra protein portion is attributed to the presence of a 24 amino acid pre- (signal) sequence (Birken et al., 1978). The larger form of the β-subunit presumably also contains a signal peptide.

The radioactive bands precipitated by antiserum to each protein were excised from the gel and solubilized with hydrogen peroxide, and the radioactivity was determined. The α- and β-subunit bands contained 4% (2600 cpm) and 1.8% (1150 cpm), respectively, of the total radioactivity incorporated into protein by the cell-free lysate (Figure 1). The native β-subunit contains three times more proline than the native α-subunit (Morgan et al., 1975; Bahl. 1977). Thus, the ratio of α- and β-subunit synthesized in the wheat germ is about 6, assuming the specific activity of the prolines incorporated was comparable.

While these data suggested that more α-subunit mRNA was present in the first-trimester population, it was possible that this difference might be related to a translation characteristic of the in vitro system. It is clear, for example, that the optimal concentrations of KCl and magnesium for the translation of a variety of mRNAs in cell-free extracts are quite different (Mathews, 1972; Tse and Taylor, 1977; Palmiter, 1973). Thus, it was possible that the differences in the amount of α- and β-subunit synthesized were related to the concentration of these salts in translation assays. Placental mRNA was translated in lysates containing [^{3}H] proline and various concentrations of KCl and magnesium. Over the range of 54 to 104 mM KCl in 10 mM increments, there was no difference in the ratio of α- to β-subunit synthesized (data not shown). However, it was observed that this ratio was markedly dependent on the magnesium concentration (Figure 2). At 1.5 mM magnesium, more of the labeled β protein was synthesized than the α-subunit. Quantitation of the labeled proteins revealed that the α and β proteins contained 0.5 to 2.3%, respectively, of the total radioactivity incorporated into protein by the cell-free lysate. Thus, considering the greater proline content in the β-subunit, the amounts of α- and β-subunits synthesized at 1.5 mM magnesium were comparable. This magnesium dependence was observed using other isotopes and was also seen in the reticulocyte lysate (data not shown). Thus, translation data cannot be used to assess quantitatively the tissue levels of the subunit mRNAs.

We had previously shown that with first-trimester RNA, four to five times more of the β protein was synthesized than with term RNA. Since we and others (Bahl, 1977; Boime et al., 1978) have suggested that the level of β mRNA constituted a rate-limiting step in the

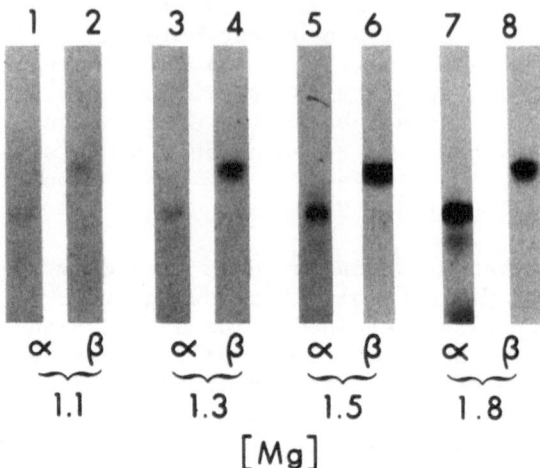

Figure 2.   Fluorograph of proteins synthesized in the presence of 74 mM KCl and varying concentrations of magnesium. The proteins were labeled with [^{3}H] proline. Equivalent amounts of protein were added to the gels.

formation of hCG in vivo, it was of interest to quantitate the translation mixtures containing different concentrations of magnesium and [^{3}H] proline were programmed with equivalent amounts of subsaturating total first-trimester and term RNAs (Figure 3). Following immunoprecipitation, quantitation of labeled protein synthesized by first-trimester and term RNA in the presence of 1.8 mM magnesium acetate was 3.5 and 0.4%, respectively, of the total radioactivity incorporated in the cell-free lysate. No significant differences were observed when the reactions were performed over the range of 54 to 104 mM KCl. Thus, approximately 8-fold less α-subunit was synthesized from term mRNA than from first-trimester RNA. No detectable synthesis of β-subunit was observed either in the presence of 1.5 mM or 1.8 mM magnesium using term RNA.

The data raise the possibility that the levels of the α- and β-subunit mRNAs are comparable and that the imbalanced ratio of the protein subunits observed in the tissue are not reflected by the steady-state mRNA levels. In this regard, Keller et al. (1980) showed that bovine pituitary RNA directed the synthesis of similar amounts of labeled proteins immunologically related to the α- and β-subunits of luteinizing hormone.

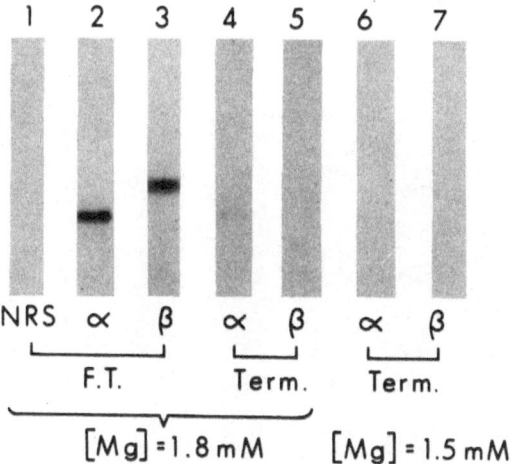

Figure 3. Fluorograph of proteins labeled with [^{3}H] proline synthesized in response to 200 µg/ml of first-trimester (F.T.) and term-placental RNA. The amounts of radioactivity applied were: Lane 1, 2000 cpm; Lane 2, 6000 cpm; Lane 3, 7000 cpm; Lanes 4 and 5, 3000 cpm; Lanes 6 and 7, 2000 cpm. The gel was exposed for 8 days. NRS, normal rabbit serum.

Cloning of Placental Complementary DNAs

From the above, it is clear that to determine directly the ratio of α- and β-subunit mRNAs requires homologous cDNA probes. To achieve this we attempted to clone cDNAs transcribed from hCGα and β-subunit mRNAs.

Our first step in the cloning process was to synthesize double stranded complementary DNAs (ds cDNA) from oligo dT purified first-trimester placental RNA enriched by sucrose gradient centrifugation. We have shown previously that each subunit is translated from separate mRNA rather than the tandem synthesis of both subunits from a single mRNA (McQueen et al., 1978). Several RNA fractions were collected from a sucrose gradient, translated in wheat germ lysates, and the products of the reaction were immunoprecipitated with subunit antisera. The fractions containing primarily α- and β-subunit mRNAs were then used as substrates for the reverse transcriptase reaction (Figure 4). Comparison of the relative cDNA band intensities generated from the gradient-enriched RNA fractions shows that the quantity of the smaller species is consistent with hCGα and that of

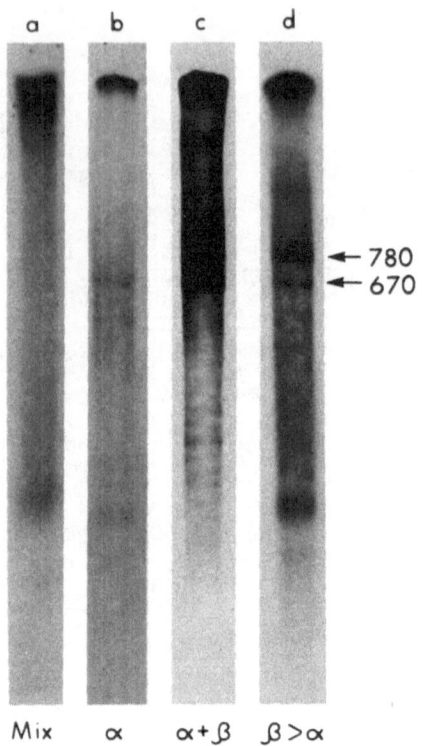

Figure 4.   Polyacrylamide gels analysis of labeled cDNAs transcribed from placental mRNA with reverse transcriptase. Lane (a) shows the products of a single strand DNA synthesis primed by total poly A-first trimester RNA with [^{32}P] dATP. Lanes (b-d) show the double strand products of reactions primed with consecutive fractions of a sucrose gradient-enriched first trimester on RNAs. The first strand was synthesized with reverse transcriptase and the second strand was transcribed with DNA polymerase, as described in Methods. The indicated sizes in nucleotide base pairs are determined from the migration of restriction fragments of known size, which were stained with ethidium bromide.

the larger band suggests an hCGβ component. Based on the migration
of ds DNA markers, we estimate that these species contain about 670
and 780 base pairs, respectively. The size of the smaller species
corresponds to the size of hCGα RNA determined by sucrose gradient
centrifugation (Landefeld et al., 1976) and by formamide gel analysis
of RNA encoding murine TSHα (Vamvakopoulos and Kourides, 1979).

Thus, we tentatively identified the 670 bp fragment as hCGα
cDNA and the 780 bp fragment as hCGβ cDNA. Since the intensity of
the two fragments is the same for several different labeled deoxy-
nucleotides, the steady-state levels of both mRNAs may be comparable
(see discussion).

Restriction Endonuclease Treatment of ds cDNAs

The above fractions of first-trimester placental RNA enriched
for hCGα and β mRNAs, as well as a fraction of term-placental RNA
enriched for hPL, were used to prime synthesis of [^{32}P] ds cDNAs.
The products were mixed with DNA derived from the plasmid pBR322.
This DNA was added as an internal marker for monitoring the efficiency of restriction digestion and to generate marker fragments for
estimating the lengths of placental cDNA fragments. The mixtures
were then mixed with restriction enzymes Hae III and Alu I, and the
products of digestion were resolved on non-denaturing polyacrylamide
gels (Figure 5). Cleavage at two sites within a species releases a
discrete fragment, so that even a rare species may show up as a
visible band (Seeburg et al., 1977). As seen in Lane c, the 670 bp
cDNA fragment generated from the fraction enriched for α-subunit mRNA
remains intact after cleavage with Hae III. In contrast, cleavage
with Alu I gives rise to several bands, and the 670 pb fragment is
not observed (Lane d). Based on band intensity, the fragments of
approximately 240, 230, and 75 bp were most likely derived from the
putative band (670 bp), since it is the major species of cDNA. The
larger intact ds cDNA (780 bp) was sensitive both to Hae III (Lane e)
and to Alu I (Lane f). Cleavage with the former generated fragments
of 145 and 135 bp, while in the latter a band of 400 was observed.

We cloned these partially characterized cDNAs as chimeric plasmids in pBR322 at its unique site for the restriction enzyme PstI
(Figure 6). After annealing cDNA to plasmid and transformation of
chi-1776, the transformants were selected by plating on tetracycline
plates, because Pst cleavage leaves intact the gene which expresses
tetracycline resistance in pBR322. Nitrocellulose filters bearing
the DNA from bacterial colonies were hybridized to ^{32}P-labeled ss
cDNA probes synthesized in reactions primed either with enriched hPL
or hCGα and β mRNAs (Figure 7). Several colonies exhibited positive
signals, and the intensities of many of the transformants varied,
depending on the probe that was used to screen them. Certain colonies

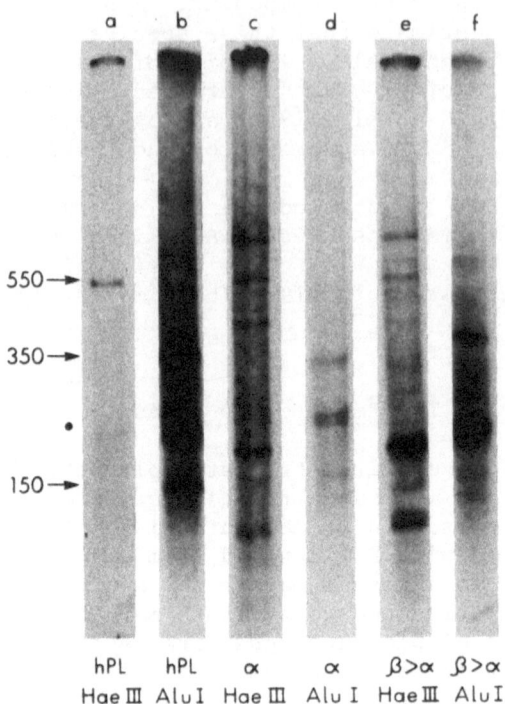

Figure 5. Autoradiograph of a polyacrylamide gel restriction, fragments derived from the ds cDNAs shown in Figure 4. HPL, α and β greater than α indicate enriched RNA fractions for hPL, hCGα and hCGβ, respectively, as determined by translational assays. The cDNAs were digested with Hae III (Lanes a, c, e) or Alu I (Lanes b, d, f) together with unlabeled pBR322 which provided standards for determination of indicated sizes.

derived from the cloning of first-trimester cDNAs elicited stronger signals when screened with a term enriched probe; we suspected these contained hPL sequences. Others hybridize better to first-trimester probe, but gave a significant signal when hybridized to term probe. Since a low, but significant, level of hCGα mRNA present in the total at term mRNA population, we suspected these corresponded to clones containing hCGα related sequences.

Plasmid DNA was isolated from colonies which displayed strong signals with the above probes, and inserted DNAs were characterized by digestion with several restriction enzymes. Because the tailing protocol used regenerates the PstI restriction recognition sequence,

CLONING STRATEGY

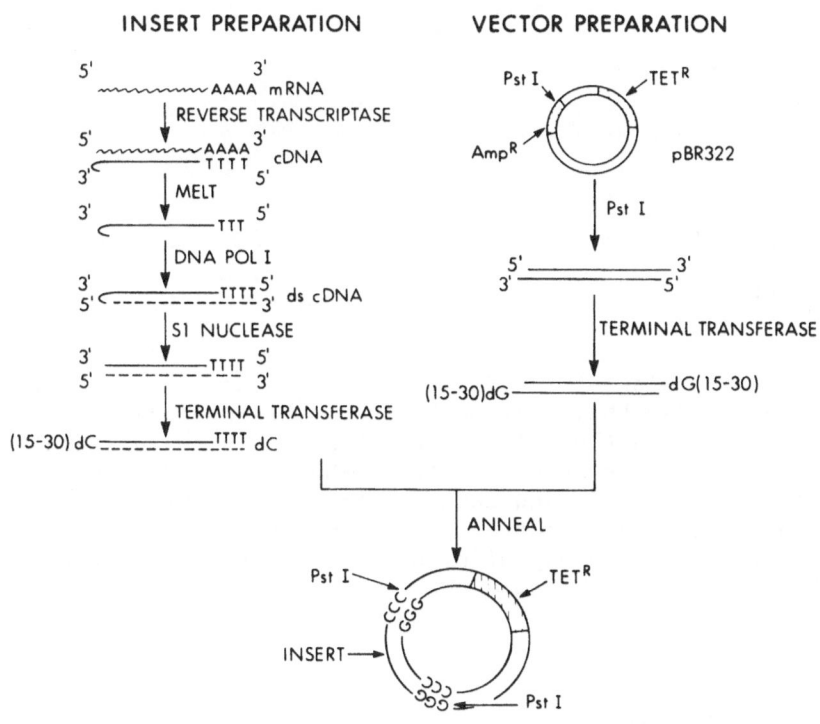

Figure 6. Schematic diagram illustrating the linking of ds cDNAs to the plasmid vector pBR322 for transfection into *E. Coli* and cloning of resultant colonies.

cleavage with this enzyme should release at least one DNA fragment which corresponds to the inserted cDNA and its G:C tails. Plasmid DNA derived from the above positive clones was digested with PstI (Figure 8). Lane a. shows that the cloned insert of pFUI contains two sites for the enzyme PstI, separated by about 170 bp. Since PstI recognizes a specific hexanucleotide sequence, i.e., it cleaves infrequently, other clones which contain two such sites with the same separation may represent independent copies of the same mRNA species. Analysis with Hae III (Lane f) shows that this clone's insert contains no site for this enzyme. However, digestion with Alu I results in a fragment doublet at about 230 bp (Lane c) seen in other clones with two PstI sites in their cDNA and similar to that released from ds cDNA (Figure 5, Lane d). All such clones hybridized well to term probe but better to first-trimester probe.

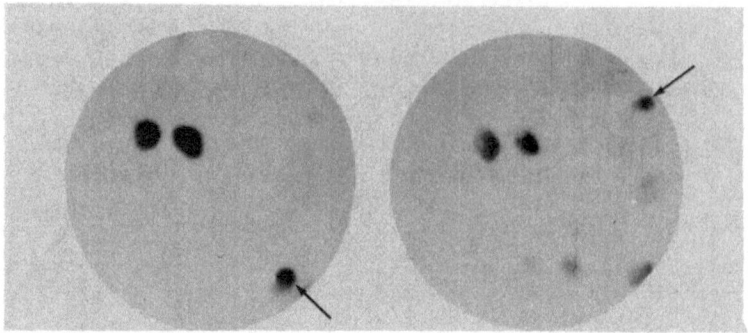

hPL Enriched cDNA $\alpha + \beta$ Enriched cDNA

Figure 7. Screening of replica filters of clones derived from first-trimester ds cDNA. Nitrocellulose filters bearing the DNA of colonies grown on the filters were lysed in situ and then hybridized to probes synthesized from mRNAs enriched on sucrose gradients for hPL or hCG sequences. The growth of the colonies on the two filters was identical. The spot at upper right on the $\alpha + \beta$ filter was the colony of plasmid pFUI; at lower right of the hPL filter was that of plasmid pPL.

It seemed likely, then, that these clones carried hCGα cDNA sequences. Restriction analysis of the clone hPL in Figure 8 was consistent with the restriction sites in hPL determined from cloning a fragment of hPL cDNA (Shine et al., 1977), and this clone hybridizes better to term probe. Therefore, it probably carries a partial hPL cDNA insert.

Of 16 clones characterized by restriction analysis of the plasmid DNA, six could be tentatively assigned to the group of hCGα containing clones based on hybridization characteristics and on the presence of PstI sites. Three more could be similarly identified as clones bearing hPL sequences. However, no clones were found whose restriction sites were consistent with those seen in the larger band of the doublet, i.e., the 780 bp putative hCGβ species. Several other colonies were observed to hybridize as intensely to first-trimester probe as the clones receiving portions of the 680 bp segment, and little (if at all) to term probe. PstI analysis showed all of these to contain small inserts (less than 200 bp).

The nature of the sequences carried by clones identified as probable hPL and hCGα species was further elucidated by a technique of mRNA selection (Figure 9; Grunstein and Hogness, 1975). Purified plasmid DNA of clones of interest was converted to its linear form

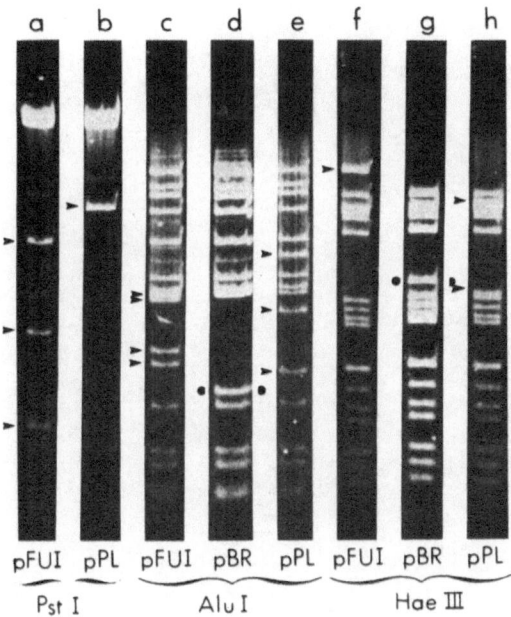

Figure 8. Restriction endonuclease analysis of suspected hCGα and hPL clones. Plasmids pFUI (an hCGα clone) and pPL (an hPL clone) were digested with endonucleases PstI (Lanes a, b), Alu I (Lanes c, e), and Hae III (Lanes f, h), and the resulting bands were compared to markers of authentic pBR322 cleaved with ALU I (lane d) and Hae III (Lane g). Digestions of crude plasmid preparations were RNAs-treated, resolved on 5% polyacrylamide gels in TBE buffer, and stained with ethidium bromide. As described in Methods, arrowheads mark bands derived from the cloned insert (in Lane c, 235, 225, 140, and 130 bp, respectively, from top to bottom); dots mark the pBR322 band which contains the PstI site (100 bp for Alu I and 267 bp for Hae III).

by digestion with Hind III or EcoRI. This DNA annealed in solution to total mRNA preparations derived from either first-trimester or term placentae under conditions which minimize formation of DNA:DNA duplexes, but allow RNA:DNA hybridization to proceed at a normal rate (Casey and Davidson, 1977). Thus, hybridization selects only those messages whose sequences are identical to those of the cloned insert. Because of this, when the RNA in hybrid form is resolved from unhybridized RNA (Perrson et al., 1979), only that species

RNA SELECTION

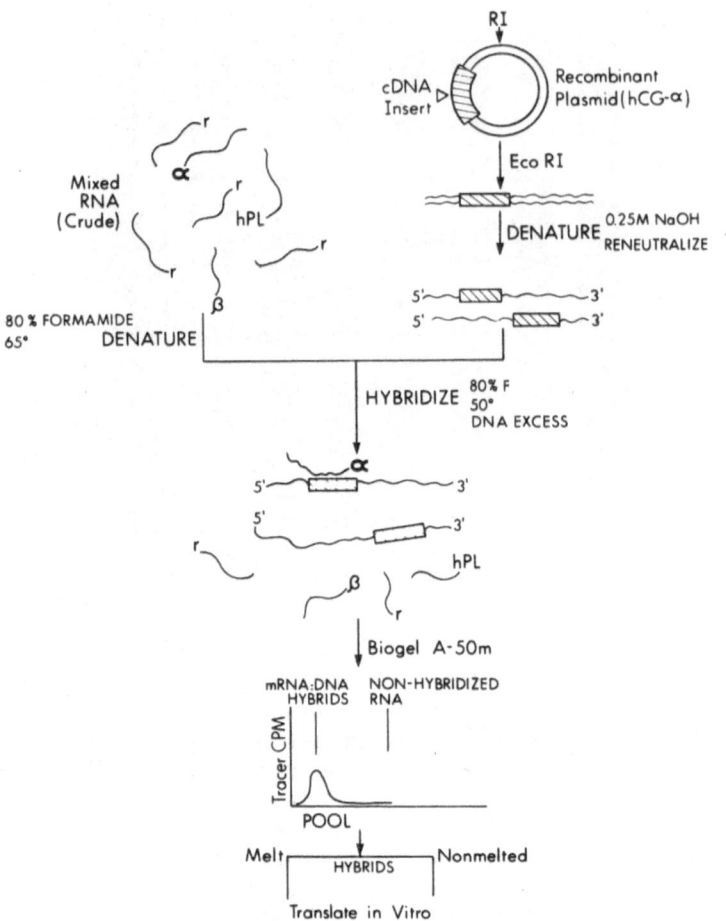

Figure 9.   Schematic diagram illustrating the technique of mRNA
selection with cloned DNA.

complementary to the insert will be selected. RNA whose translated
region is in RNA:DNA duplex form cannot be translated (Paterson et
al., 1977), but melting them should permit translation of the
selected species. The results of such an experiment with a suspected
hPL clone and putative hCGα clones are seen in Figure 10. Total
first-trimester RNA used for screening the hCG clones contained a
significant amount of translatable hPL mRNA (Lane 3). Intact hybrids
(i.e., unmelted) did not direct the synthesis of any new detectable

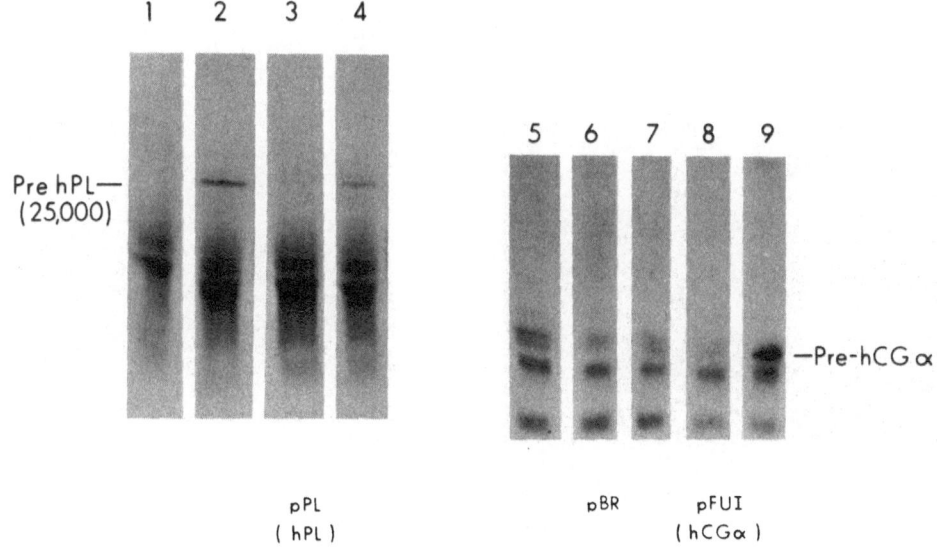

Figure 10. Autoradiograph of a sodium dodecyl sulfate electropherogram of total proteins synthesized in the presence of mRNAs isolated by clonal selection. Wheat germ translation mixture contained either [^{35}S] methionine (Lanes 1-4) or [^{35}S] cysteine (Lanes 5-9). Lane 2 indicates reaction mixtures containing first-trimester RNA and Lanes 3, 4, 6-9 contain mRNA selected from a total first-trimester RNA population by pBR322 DNA; and by DNA from clones pPL and pFUI. INT refers to intact hybrids.

proteins (Lane 8). However, when the hybrids were melted prior to translation, translational activity was unmasked and a protein co-migrating with pre-hCGα was observed (Lane 9). This protein was precipitated by hCGα-specific antiserum (Figure 11, Lane g). In the same way, no new specific protein was synthesized when intact hybrids selected from a reaction containing DNA from a putative hPL clone and term RNA were translated in the lysate (Lane 3). However, when the melted components were translated a single band co-migrating with pre-hPL (Lane 4) was seen. As expected, hybridization with pBR322 alone selects no RNA species (Lanes 6,7).

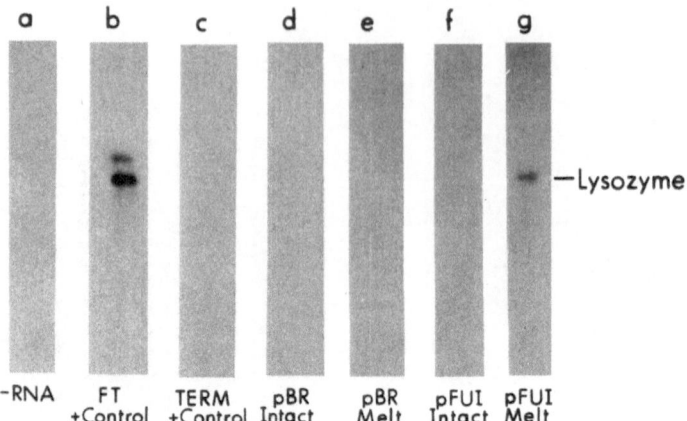

Figure 11.   Autoradiograph of an SDS-polyacrylamide gel electropherogram solution of $[^{35}S]$ cysteine labeled proteins synthesized
in wheat germ lysates in the presence of placental RNA.   Lanes b
and c contained first-trimester and term RNA, respectively, and
Lanes c-g contained RNA selected by pBR322 and pFUI DNA.   A mixture
of hCGα and β antisera was added to each sample.

DISCUSSION

     Using a sensitive immunoprecipitation technique, we have
identified the mRNAs encoding the α- and β-subunits of hCG.   It is
not clear from the data presented if the level of β-subunit mRNA
constitutes a rate-limiting step in the expression of hCG in vivo.
Although translation of placental RNA at the magnesium optimum for
each subunit resulted in the synthesis of more α- than β-subunit
protein, the difference may be related to the decreased efficiency
of translation at the lower magnesium concentrations.

     Chin et al. (1978) showed that RNA derived from a murine TSH-
secreting tumor directed the synthesis of a protein which contained
tryptic peptides that were observed in the authentic α-subunit.
Moreover, a protein was identified that based on its apparent molecular weight could correspond to the β-subunit.   The ratio of these
two synthesized subunits was significantly altered by the magnesium
concentration.   Furthermore, Keller et al. (1980) showed that,
depending on salt concentration, bovine pituitary RNA directed the
synthesis of similar amounts of labeled proteins immunologically
related to the α- and β-subunits of luteinizing hormone.   These

results suggest that each subunit mRNA has unique secondary structural features, as has been proposed by others for observed salt-dependent discrimination of particular mRNAs from a total RNA population. It seems possible, then, that the imbalance of subunit levels in the placenta does not parallel the concentration of the mRNAs in the tissue, i.e., the steady state quantity of the β-subunit mRNA may not be rate limiting in the expression of intact hormone in vivo. For example, the level of β mRNA may in fact be less than that of the α-subunit mRNA, but its rate of initiation is much greater than that of mRNA. In any case, it is now unclear whether the unbalanced tissue levels of the hCG subunits result from differences in: (1) ratio of mRNAs, (2) translation rate, or (3) the degradation of the completed peptide chains.

Several investigators have shown that in placenta and pituitary the tissue level of free α-subunit greatly exceeded the β-subunit (Bahl, 1977; Boime et al., 1978). Perhaps, as suggested by Chatterjee and Munro (1977), the greater amount of α-subunit in placenta may simply reflect a requirement for this subunit in the formation of other placental hormones. The lack of coordinated production of hCG subunits has also been seen in a variety of ectopic tumors and un-differentiated cell-lines (Bahl, 1977). While the formation of an hCGβ-related protein has been observed in some of these tissues, the most frequent observation has been that the α-subunit is synthesized in much larger amounts than β. The α-subunit of hCG and the pituitary hormones, luteinizing hormone, follicle-stimulating hormone, and thyroid-stimulating hormone have very similar amino acid sequences; it is the β-subunit which imparts the biological specificity unique to each hormone. Thus, synthesis of the β-subunit may reflect an expression of cellular differentiation.

As proposed earlier (Boime et al., 1978; Hoshina et al., 1978), it is conceivable that the syncytiotrophoblast, which is the hall-mark of placental differentiation, is the source of the β-subunit, while the relatively undifferentiated cytotrophoblast cell is the site of synthesis for the α-subunit. We would further suggest that the synthesis of the β-subunit is induced in cellular intermediates that are formed during the recruitment phase (when cytotrophoblasts coalesce and are converted to syncytium). Intact hormone formed by subunit combination could thus arise only once recruitment had started. Therefore, hCG would be a product of a specific phase of trophoblast differentiation. This hypothesis is consistent with the recent findings of Hoshina et al. (1978), who showed by immuno-histochemical methods the presence of β-subunit in the syncytial layer and the presence of the α-subunit in cytotrophoblast cells, as well as in the syncytial layer. Since morphologically individual cells in cultured lines elaborate the α-subunit, there is no a priori reason to believe that the syncytial state is necessary for hCGα synthesis.

TOTAL PRODUCTS

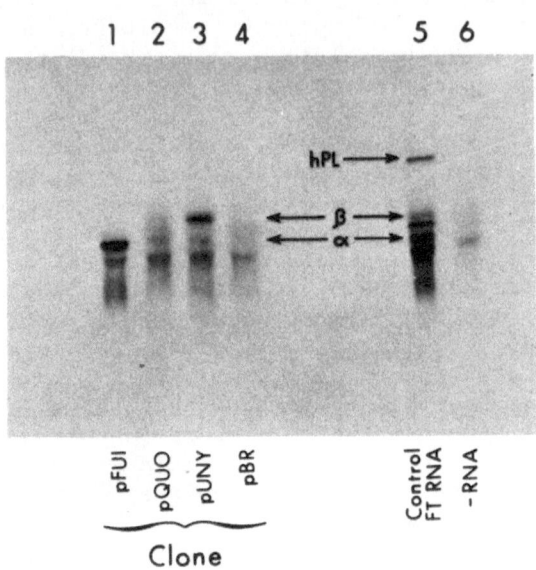

Figure 12.   Autofluorograph of an SDS-polyacrylamide electropherogram of [^{3}H] leucine-labeled proteins synthesized in wheat germ
lysates programmed by first-trimester placental RNA (lane 5) or by
RNAs selected by hybridization to the indicated plasmids (lanes 1-4).
The migration of pre-hPL, pre-hCGα, and pre-hCGβ are indicated by
hPL, α, and β, respectively. They were determined by immunoprecipitation of the products synthesized in translation mixtures containing
placental RNA electrophoresed in the same gel. Plasmids pQUO and
pUNY have small inserts which were detected in the screening of
bacterial colonies using first-trimester cDNA probes. These colonies
did not give a positive signal when they were screened with term-
derived cDNA probes.

IMMUNOPRECIPITATIONS

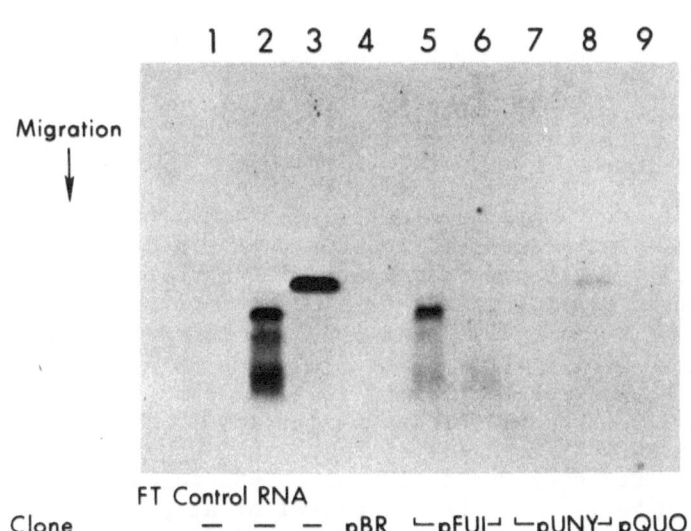

Figure 13. Immunoprecipitation of [^{3}H] leucine-labeled products synthesized in the presence of RNAs selected by placental clones. Wheat germ translation products were resolved on a 20% SDS polyacrylamide gel. Lanes 1-3 represent immunoprecipitates of first-trimester RNA products by non-immune serum (NRS, lane 1), and by hCGα (lane 2) and hCGβ (lane 3) antisera. Lanes 5-9 are immuno-precipitated products directed by plasmid selected RNAs. Lane 4: pBR-selected RNA, products precipitated by hCGβ antiserum. Lanes 5 and 6: pFUI-selected RNA, with anti-hCGα and anti-hCGβ, respectively. Lanes 7 and 8: pUNY-selected RNA, with anti-hCGα and anti-hCGβ, respecitvely. Lane 9: pQUO-selected RNA, with hCGβ antiserum.

It is clear from the above discussion that cloned probes of hCGα and β genes will be invaluable for testing the above points. We are currently characterizing several placental clones for the presence of an hCGβ insert. These cloned hCGα and β inserts will permit us (1) to assess the ratio of subunit mRNAs during pregnancy directly; (2) to determine directly by cytological hybridization techniques the cellular distribution of the α and β mRNAs in the trophoblast; and (3) to study the organization of their genes.

ADDENDUM

Several of the clones with small inserts which hybridized exclusively to first-trimester probe were screened by an RNA selection technique similar to the one discussed previously. Ten micrograms of nicked, denatured plasmid in a cleared lysate partially purified by the method of Birnboim and Doly (1979) were bound to nitrocellulose after boiling 10 min in 25 mM Tris pH 8, 1 mM EDTA, treating 20 min with 0.5 M NaOH, and reneutralizing to final conditions of 7x SSC, 0.2 M Tris pH 7.5 (standard saline citrate: 0.15 M NaCl, 0.015 M NaCitrate = 1x SSC). These filters were then hybridized to 500 μg of crude first-trimester RNA in 200 μl of 65% formamide, 10 mM PIPES (pH 6.4), 0.4 M NaCl, 0.2% SDS (Ricciardi et al., 1979). Non-hybridized RNA was removed by 10 washes at 65°C with 1x SSC, 0.05% SDS, 2 at 65°C with 0.2x SSC, and one at 65°C with 10 mM Tris pH 7.5, 5 mM NaCl, 2 mM EDTA. RNA was eluted and prepared for translation using 10 μg of wheat germ tRNA as carrier according to Ricciardi et al. (1979). The DNA of one such clone (pUNY) specifically selected only one message, whose translation product (Figure 12, lane 3) co-migrated with pre-hCHβ and was immunoprecipitated with hCGβ subunit antisera (Figure 13, lane 8). Analysis of total translation products showed that the RNA selected by the clone bearing the hCGα insert (pFUI) directed the synthesis of pre-hCGα (Figure 12, lane 2). Synthesis of pre-hCGα or pre-hCGβ was not observed with RNA selected by pBR322 (lane 4). Antisera against hCGα precipitated no translation products corresponding to pUNY (lane 7). Products selected by the hCGα clone pFUI, while immunoprecipitable by hCGα antisera (Figure 13, lane 5), were not immunoprecipitated by hCGβ antisera (lane 6). Another plasmid detected only by first-trimester cDNA probe in hybridizations to replicas of bacterial colonies, pQUO, showed a different array of translation products (Figure 12, lane 2). None of these was immunoprecipitable by hCGβ antisera (Figure 13, lane 9). We therefore believe that this clone (pUNY) represents a specific and pure probe for hCGβ message and gene, even though its insert bears only 90 bp of cDNA sequence (data not shown).

REFERENCES

Bahl, O., 1977, Human chorionic gonadotropin, its receptor and mechanism of action, Fed. Proc. 36:2119.

Birken, S., Fetherston, J., Desmond, J., Canfield, R., and Boime, I., 1978, Partial amino acid sequence of the preprotein form of the site of subsequent proteolytic cleavage, Biochem. Biophys. Res. Comm. 85:1247.

Birnboim, J., and Doly, J., 1979, Nucl. Acid Res. 7:1513.

Boime, I., Landefeld, T., McQueen, S., and McWilliams, D., 1978, The biosynthesis of chorionic gonadotropin and placental lactogen in first- and third-trimester human placenta, in *Structure and Function of the Gonadotropins*, McKerns, ed., Plenum Press, New York.

Boime, I., McWilliams, D., Szczesna, E., and Camel, M., 1976, Synthesis of human placental lactogen as a function of gestation, J. Biol. Chem. 251:820.

Bolivar, F., Rodrigues, R., Greene, P., Betlach, M., Heynecker, H., and Boyer, H., 1977, Construction and characterization of new cloning vehicles. II. A multipurpose cloning system, Gene 2:95.

Buell, G., Wickens, M., Payvar, F., and Schimke, R., 1978, Synthesis of full length cDNAs from four partially purified oviduct mRNAs, J. Biol. Chem. 253:2471.

Casey, T., and Davidson, N., 1977, Rates of formation and thermal stabilities of RNA:DNA and DNA:DNA duplexes in high concentrations of formamide, Nucl. Acids Res. 4:1539.

Chatterjee, M., and Munro, H., 1977, Changing ratio of human chorionic gonadotropin subunits synthesized by early and full-term placental polyribosomes, Biochem. Biophys. Res. Comm. 77:426.

Chin, W., Habener, J., Kieffer, J., and Maloof, F., 1978, Cell-free translation of the mRNA coding for the α subunit of thyroid stimulating hormone, J. Biol. Chem. 253:7985.

Clewell, D., and Helsinki, D., 1969, Supercoiled circular DNA-protein complex in *E. coli*: purification and induced conversion to an open circular form, Proc. Nat. Acad. Sci. (USA) 62:1159.

Curtiss, R., Pereira, O., Hsu, J., Hull, S., Clarke, J., Maturin, L., Goldschmidt, R., Moody, R., Inove, M., and Alexander, L., 1977, in *Recombinant Molecules: Impact on Science and Society. Proceedings of the 10th Miles Symposium*, pp. 45-56, R. Beers and E. G. Bassett, eds., Raven Press, New York.

Dingman, C., and Peacock, A., 1968, Analytical studies on nuclear ribonucleic acid using polyacrylamide electrophoresis, Biochemistry 7:659.

Efstradiadis, A., Kafatos, F., Maxam, A., and Maniatis, T., 1976, Enzymatic in vitro synthesis of globin genes, Cell 7:279.

Enea, V., Rovis, G., and Zinder, N., 1975, Genetic studies with heteroduplex DNA of bacteriophage f-1, J. Mol. Biol. 98:112.

Grunstein, M., and Hogness, D., 1975, Colony hybridization: A method for the isolation of cloned DNAs that contain a specific gene,

Proc. Nat. Acad. Sci. (USA) 72:3961.

Hoshina, M., Ashitaka, Y., Yamashita, S., and Tojo, S., 1978, Immune histochemical interaction of antisera to hCG and its subunits with chorionic tissue of early gestation, Acta Obstet. Gynaec. (Japan) 30:187.

Keller, D., Fetherston, J., and Boime, I., 1980, Isolation of mRNA from bovine pituitary: The cell-free synthesis of the alpha and beta subunits of luteotropin, European J. Biochem., in press.

Landefeld, T., McWilliams, D., and Boime, I., 1976, The isolation of mRNA encoding the alpha subunit of human chorionic gonadotropin, Biochem. Biophys. Res. Comm. 72:381.

Mathews, M., 1972, Further studies on the translation of globin RNA and encephalomycarditis virus RNA in a cell-free system from Krebs II ascites cells, Biochim. Biophys. Acta 272:108.

McQueen, S., McWilliams, D., Birken, S., Canfield, R., Landefeld, T., and Boime, I., 1978, Identification of mRNAs encoding the α and β subunits of human choriogonadotropin, J. Biol. Chem. 253:7109.

McWilliams, D., Callahan, R., and Boime, I., 1977, Human placental lactogen mRNA and its structural genes during pregnancy: Quantitation with a complementary DNA, Proc. Nat. Acad. Sci. (USA) 74:1024.

Morgan, F., Birken, S., and Canfield, R., 1975, The amino acid sequence of human chorionic gonadotropin, J. Biol. Chem. 250:5247.

Palmiter, R. D., 1973, Ovalbumin messenger ribonucleic acid translation comparable rates of polypeptide initiation and elongation on ovalbumin and globin messenger ribonucleic acid in rabbit reticulocyte lysate, J. Biol. Chem. 248:2095.

Paterson, B., Roberts, B., and Kuff, E., 1977, Structural gene identification and mapping by DNA in RNA hybrid-arrested cell-free translation, Proc. Nat. Acad. Sci.(USA) 74:4370.

Persson, H., Perricaudet, M., Tolum, A., Philipson, L., and Pettersson, U., 1979, Purification of RNA-DNA hybrids by exclusion chromatography, J. Biol. Chem. 254:7999.

Ricciardi, R. P., Miller, J. S., and Roberts, B. E., 1979, Proc. Nat. Acad. Sci. (USA) 76:4927.

Seeburg, P., Shine, J., Martial, J., Ullrich, A., Baxter, J., and Goodman, H., 1977, Nucleotide sequence of part of the gene for human chorionic somatomammotropin. Purification of DNA complementary to predominant mRNA species, Cell 12:157.

Shine, J., Seeburg, P., Martial, J., Baxter, J., and Goodman, H., 1977, Construction and analysis of recombinant DNA for human chorionic somatomammotropin, Nature 270:494.

Swank, R. T., and Munkres, K., 1971, Molecular weight analysis of oligopeptides by electrophoresis in polyacrylamide gel with sodium dodecyl sulfate, Anal. Biochem. 39:462.

Tilghman, S., Kioussis, D., Gorin, M., Ruiz, J., and Ingram, R., 1979, The presence of intervening sequences in the α-fetoprotein gene of the mouse, J. Biol. Chem. 254:7393.

Vamvakopoulos, N., and Kourides, I., 1979, Identification of separate mRNAs encoding the α and β subunits of thyrotropin, Proc. Nat. Acad. Sci. (USA) 76:3809.

Villa-Komaroff, L., Efstradiadis, A., Broome, S., Lomedico, P., Tizard, R., Naber, S., Chick, W., and Gilbert, W., 1978, A bacterial clone synthesizing proinsulin, Proc. Nat. Acad. Sci. (USA) 75:3727.

Wickens, M., Buell, G., and Schimke, R., 1978, Synthesis of double-stranded DNA complementary to lysozyme, ovomucoid, and ovalbumin mRNAs, J. Biol. Chem. 253:2483.

ACKNOWLEDGEMENT

The authors are indebted to Drs. Dimitri Kioussis and Shirley Tilghman for their help in recombinant DNA technology. This work was supported by a grant from the Public Health Service (HD-13481). M. B. was supported by a Public Health Service Grant (T32-GM07200) as part of the Medical Scientist Training Program. I. B. is a recipient of a Research Career Development Award (AM-00174) from the National Institutes of Health.

HUMAN CHORIONIC GONADOTROPIN: STUDIES ON THE MECHANISM OF SECRETION

R. Folman, J. Ilan, N. de Groot, and A. A. Hochberg

Institute for Life Sciences, Department of Biological
Chemistry, The Hebrew University, Jerusalem, Israel
and
Department of Reproductive Biology, Case Western
Reserve University, Cleveland, Ohio, U.S.A.

INTRODUCTION

Human chorionic gonadotropin (hCG) is a major protein of the
first-trimester placenta. It is a glycoprotein composed of two
non-identical subunits (Bahl, 1969); one of them (the α subunit) is
in common with the α subunit of the pituitary hormones FSH, LH and
TSH (Liao, 1970). Its presence in the serum is already detectable
four days after fertilization and its concentration reaches a peak
level (Brody, 1962) during the 8th-11th week of pregnancy. Considerable individual variations exist in peak values and peak times.

The serum level of hCG drops rapidly after the first trimester
and remains at a more or less constant value until delivery (about
10% of the peak value). High levels of hCG occur in all trophoblastic carcinomas and hCG is ectopically synthesized by a variety
of tumor tissues (Braunstein et al., 1973). Recently, it has been
reported that low levels of hCG or hCG-like substances are normally
present in several human tissues (Yoshimoto et al., 1979). On the
basis of these findings, it has been proposed that the production
of the HCG peptide backbones may be a common property of many pro-
liferating tissues (Borkowski and Muquardt, 1979). However, the
degree of glycosylation may differ from tissue to tissue. Fully
glycosylated hCG, which has the highest in vivo biological activity,
is produced by the placenta.

The control of hCG synthesis and secretion is not clear. Proteins destined for export are synthesized on rough endoplasmic
membrane-bound ribosomes (Redman, 1968), nearly always as precursor

proteins with an N-terminal hydrophobic signal peptide (Milstein et al., 1972). The glycosylation of the peptide chains occurs biochemically and topographically in several stages (Schacter, 1974).

Protein secretion can be regulated by chemical and neurological signals. Proteins which are secreted discontinuously (such as pancreatic zymogens) are packed in zymogen granules and are released into the blood stream after the cell has received an appropriate signal (Palade, 1975). However, some other proteins such as serum albumin seem to be secreted continuously (Peters, 1975), and normally serum albumin never accumulates in the cell of its synthesis.

In the work presented here, we have studied some aspects of the relationship between the synthesis and the secretion of hCG by the first-trimester placenta.

METHODS

First-trimester placental tissue was obtained from therapeutic abortions, transported in 0.9% NaCl, and processed within 30 min. Tissues slices were incubated in Krebs Ringer bicarbonate buffer, pH = 7.4, containing 10 μCi of radioactive substrate. The incubation was carried out in a shaker bath at 37°C, in an atmosphere of 95% O_2 and 5% CO_2. All long-term incubations (longer than 8 hr) were done by using organ culture technique.

For organ culture, placental explants were placed in petri dishes containing 2 ml of culture medium [M-199 (Biolab, Israel); 20mM Hepes; 0.75% Bovine Serum Albumin fraction V: 10 μCi of radioactive substrate, penicillin, streptomycin, and mycostatin].

The incubation was carried out in an atmosphere of air/5% CO_2 at 37°C. Culture medium was replaced every 24 hr.

After incubation, the tissues was separated from the medium by centrifugation and homogenized in 0.25M sucrose containing Tris buffer (Tris-HCl pH = 7.4, 50mM; KCl 25mM; $MgCl_2$ 10mM; NH_4Cl 100mM; EDTA 0.5mM). Subcellular fractions were isolated from the homogenate according to Gal et al. (1977). Radioactivity of the hot 5% TCA insoluble material was determined according to Bollum (1965). Protein was determined according to Lowry et al. (1951). RNA was determined according to Bloemendal et al. (1967). The hCG content of the tissue homogenate and the medium was determined by using the double antibody precipitation technique. SDS gel electrophoresis was done according to Laemmli (1970).

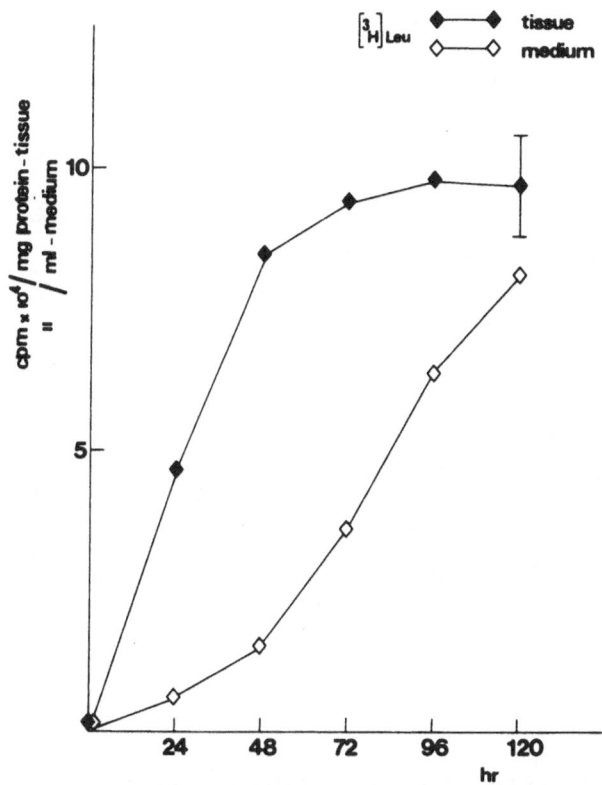

Figure 1. Protein synthesis and secretion by first-trimester placental tissue in organ culture. Protein was not determined in the medium because of the presence of high levels of BSA.

RESULTS AND DISCUSSION

We have used both tissue slices and organ culture techniques in studying the synthesis and secretion of human chorionic gonadotropin. Tissue slices effectively synthesize and secrete proteins only for approximately 10 hr of incubation, but tissue in organ culture continues protein synthesis and secretion for at least 96 hr (Figure 1). However, proteins are much faster labeled in tissue slices than in organ culture, probably as a result of faster penetration of nutrients into the cells. Therefore, the use of tissue slices enabled us to do short-time experiments. For example, protein is secreted for at least 96 hr by the placental tissue in organ culture (Figure 1), but the results obtained using tissue slices

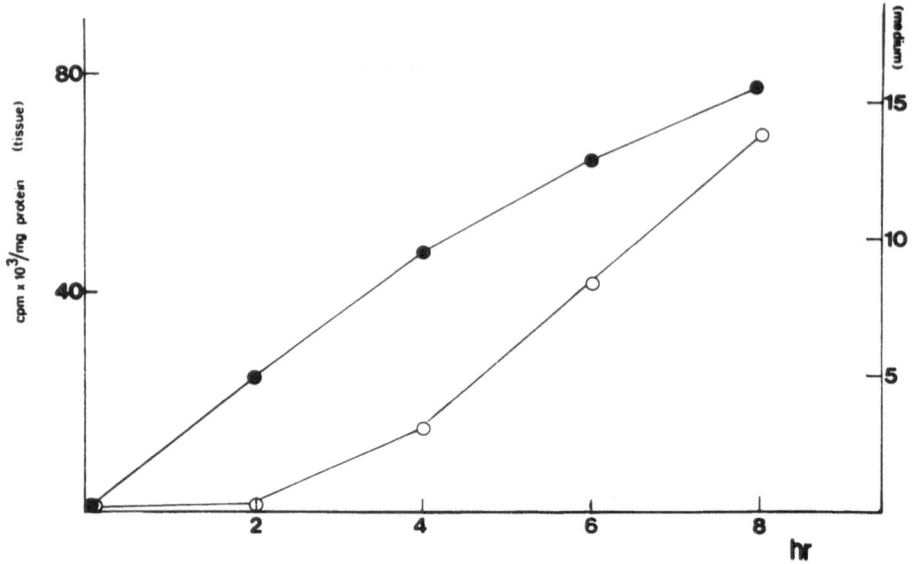

Figure 2.   Protein synthesis by and protein secretion from human placental tissue slice.   ●——●: tissue slices;   o——o: medium; substrate: [^{3}H]leucine.

clearly show that there is a lag period of two hours between the radioactive pulse and the appearance of radioactive protein in the medium (Figure 2).

The placentas used in these experiments (Figure 1 and 2) were from 8-11 weeks of pregnancy. The results shown are averages of at least 100 individual experiments. We found only rather small differences between the amino acid incorporation activities of all those placentas. In nearly all the determinations the deviation was not more than 5% of the values shown. However, the deviations tended to increase with incubation time, and after 120 hr of incubation, they were up to ±10% of the average values.

The two hours needed for the appearance of radioactive proteins in the medium is the sum of the time needed for the completion of chain elongation and for the processing of the peptide chain backbone (glycosylation) during and after peptide chain elongation and the transport of the protein from the site of its synthesis to the site of secretion. The same lag period was observed by measuring the synthesis and secretion of radioactive hot TCA insoluble material labeled by [^{3}H]glucosamine (Figure 3). Glucosamine can be incorporated as N-acetylglucosamine or as sialic acid into the carbohydrate

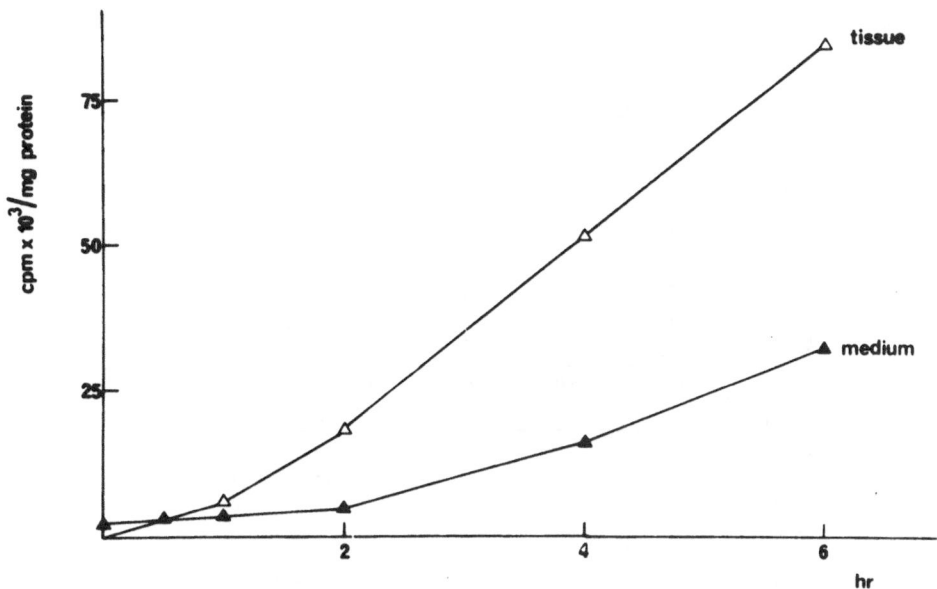

Figure 3. The rate of synthesis and secretion of glycoprotein by the tissue slices. [^{3}H]glucosamine was used as substrate.

moiety of glycoproteins such as hCG. Therefore, it seems likely that the lag period observed is due to events occurring after glycosylation. This lag period was also observed when the secretion of newly synthesized radioactive hCG was followed by the highly specific precipitation reaction with antiserum (Folman et al., 1979).

From the results shown one can calculate that approximately 5% of the hot TCA insoluble material appeared in the medium (tissue slices - 6 hr), but at least 30% of the glucosamine labeled material is secreted during the same time period. The corresponding numbers were 10% and 30% for organ cultures after 120 hr of incubation. Therefore, it is clear that glycoproteins which include hCG are preferentially secreted from the tissue slices.

In organ cultures hCG is secreted for at least 96 hr. However, the rate of secretion linearly decreases during the time of incubation (Figure 4). We have measured the hCG content of the placental tissue in organ culture by radioimmunoassay (Figure 4). The intracellular concentration of hCG does not change significantly during the 120 hr of incubation. The same results were obtained when the homogenizing medium contained a detergent (deoxycholate, Triton X-100, or a mix of both). The amount of hCG synthesized during the

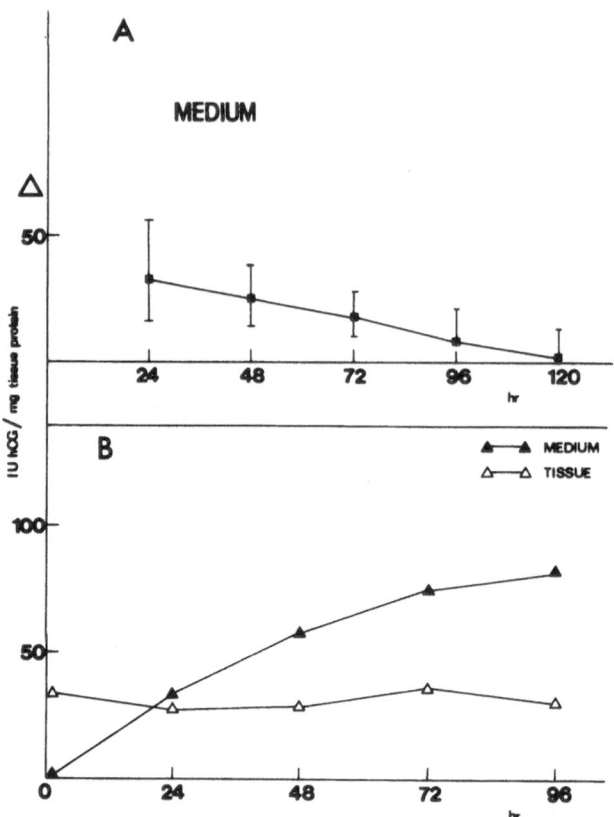

Figure 4.   (A) Rate of hCG secretion. Results are expressed as
IU hCG secreted per 24 hr intervals. (B) hCG concentration of the
tissue and the medium as a function of incubation time. The
concentration of hCG in the medium is expressed as IU hCG/mg
protein of the secreting tissue.

incubation period is twice that of the tissue hCG content. There
seems to be a direct relationship between the placental intracellular
concentration of hCG and the capacity of the placental tissue to
synthesize and secrete hCG. The values shown in Figure 4 are the
average of those obtained from placentas of the 8th-11th week of
pregnancy. However, we also investigated early pregnancy placentas
(5th-6th week). They had a much lower hCG concentration, some not
higher than 6 IU/mg tissue protein. The overall rate of hCG secretion and -- and as the intracellular concentration of hCG remains
constant, also of hCG synthesis -- by organ cultures from these
placentas, calculated as hCG secreted (synthesized) per mg tissue

protein was much lower and proportional to the tissue hCG concentration. It has to be stressed that the specific amino acid incorporation activities of those early pregnancy placentas were independent of the placental age and therefore bear no relationship to their hCG concentration. It seems likely that hCG intracellular concentration, hCG synthesizing capacity and secretion are an expression of its mRNA concentration. The relationship between hCG concentration (in the maternal serum) and the cytoplasmic mRNA concentration has already been pointed out by Chatterjee et al. (1976) and by Daniels-McQueen et al. (1978). In organ culture experiments protein synthesis is dependent on continuous RNA synthesis. Low actinomycin D concentrations in the medium (0.2 µg/ml) inhibited both RNA and protein synthesis completely (results not shown).

If we incubated tissue slices with radioactive amino acids and followed the specific radioactivities of the different fractions as a function of time, we obtained the following results. After a short-time incubation ($\sim$1 min), the specific radioactivity (Figure 5A) of the rough membrane was three times higher than that of the smooth membrane. After a longer incubation period (Figure 5B) the specific activity of the smooth membrane fraction exceeded that of the rough membrane by a factor of 1.5. This ratio, or even a higher one, was also obtained from results of an organ culture experiment. The specific activity of the free polyribosomal fraction was much lower. Radioactive proteins with electrophoretic mobilities identical to that of α and β hCG were detected on SDS gel electrophoretograms of rough and smooth membrane fractions. Also radioactive α and β hCG subunits could be identified in these fractions by direct specific antibody precipitation reactions. These results support the notion that both hCG subunits are synthesized on the rough endoplasmic reticulum bound ribosomes.

The subcellular distribution of hCG between different fractions is shown in Table I. Around 30% of the cellular content of hCG was found in the post-microsomal supernatant. It is possible that the hCG content of the post-microsomal supernatant is partly due to leakage of hCG from the endoplasmic reticulum components during the preparation of the subcellular fractions.

In order to investigate the relationship between the rate of total protein synthesis and that of hCG, and their respective secretion rates, we have used protein synthesis inhibitors and investigated the effects of these substances on total protein and on hCG secretion. Puromycin seems to be a convenient substance to work with. Not only can puromycin cause a practically 100% inhibition of protein synthesis (in both tissue slices and organ culture), but it can be easily removed from the cells by simply washing the tissue with medium. Cycloheximide was as effective as puromycin in

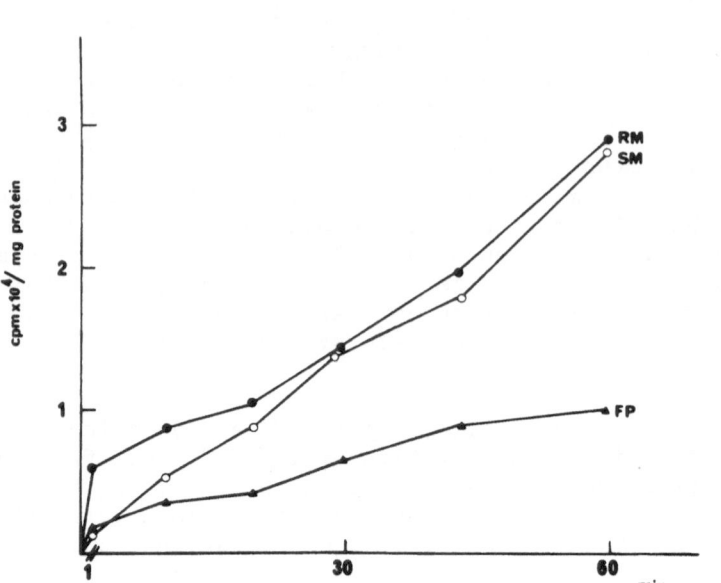

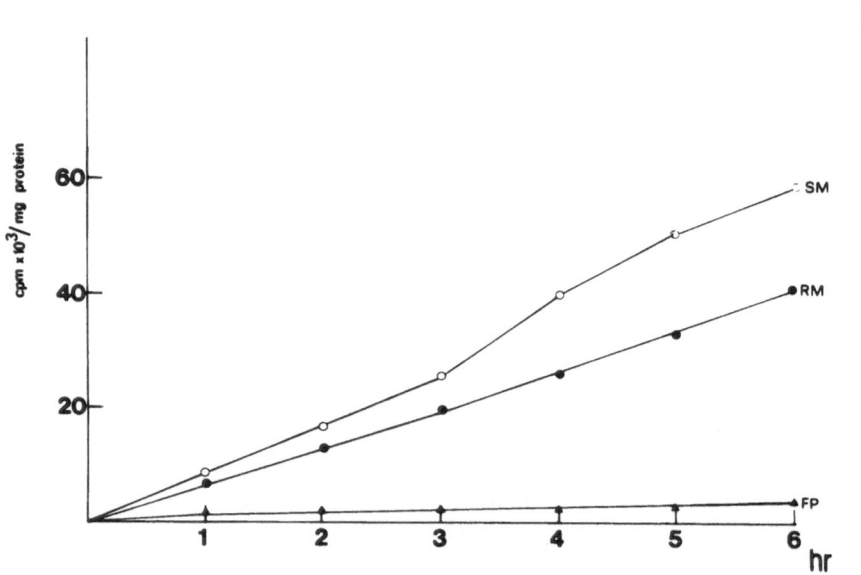

Figure 5. (A) and (B): The specific activity of labeled proteins in subcellular fractions isolated from tissue slices labeled in vitro. [^{3}H]leucine was used as substrate. RM = rough membrane; SM = smooth membrane; FP = free polyribosomes.

TABLE I: The distribution of hCG between subcellular fractions from first-trimester placenta.

Fraction	I.U. hCG/mg Protein	% of Total Content
Rough membrane	45.0	44.0
Smooth membrane	21.0	22.6
Free polyribosomes	0.1	<0.1
Post-microsomal supernatant	19.0	33.4

protein synthesis inhibition, but it was rather difficult to remove this inhibitor from the tissue. Aurine tricarboxylic acid (ATA) and fusidic acid inhibited the protein synthesis to a much smaller extent. The inhibition of protein synthesis by puromycin and cyclohexamide is instantaneous (Figure 6A). The sudden drop in radioactive TCA insoluble material in the tissue slices may be due to a rapid breakdown of peptidylpuromycin and of immature peptides released by abortive termination. The secretion of protein continues for 1.5-2 hr after the addition of the inhibitor before it completely stops (Figure 6B). After removal of puromycin from the tissue, protein synthesis and secretion were resumed (Figure 7).

We also measured hCG concentration in the tissue and in the medium in an organ culture experiment in which puromycin was added at different times. The secretion of hCG into the medium was stopped upon the addition of puromycin (Figure 8).

The relative constant level of hCG throughout the incubation period in the presence of puromycin is a very interesting phenomenon, because proteins synthesized during the incubation period are partly broken down. This breakdown seems to be independent of protein synthesis. This can be concluded from experiments in which after labeling the proteins of the organ culture, radioactive amino acids were omitted from the medium and the fate of the newly synthesized labeled proteins was followed (Figure 9). The rate of the protein degradation seems to be a linear function of the time the organ

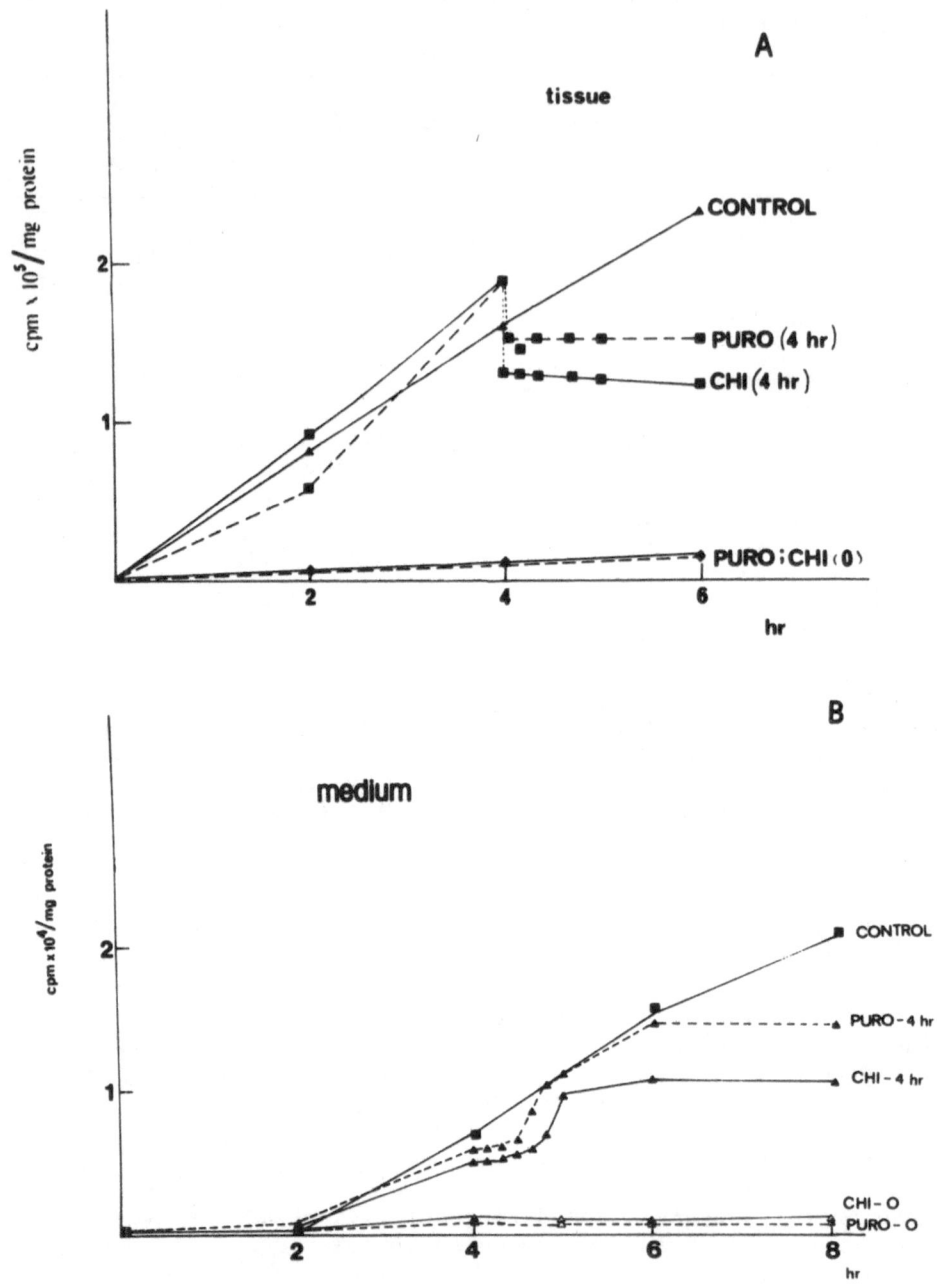

Figure 6.   The effect of protein synthesis inhibitors on the synthesis (A) and the secretion (B) of proteins by tissue slices. Inhibitors were added at zero time or after 4 hr of incubation. [^{3}H]leucine was used as substrate.

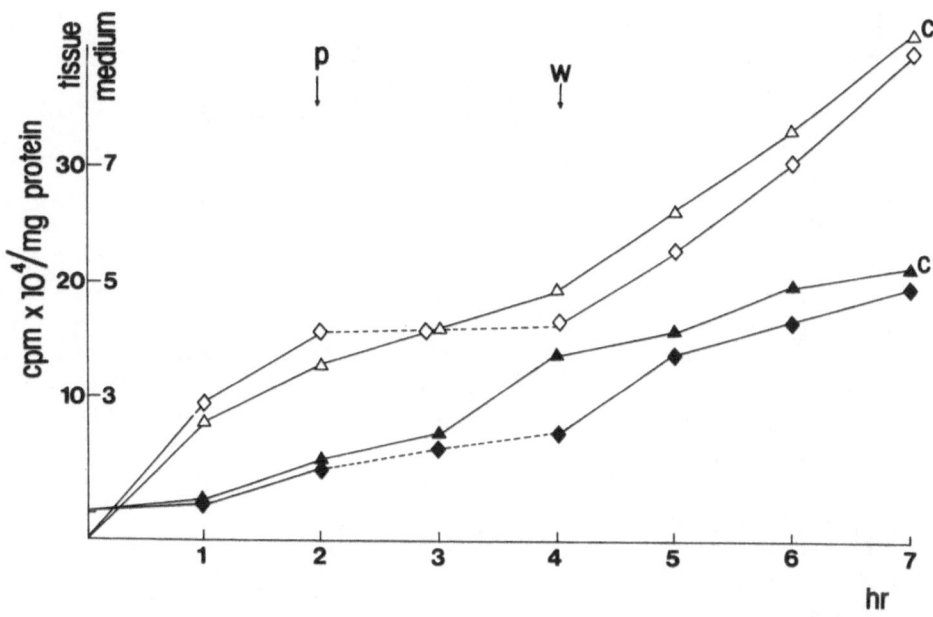

Figure 7.   Synthesis and secretion of proteins after removal of puromycin by washing.

$\triangle$ = tissue, control
$\diamond$ = tissue, puromycin added
$\blacktriangle$ = medium, control
$\blacklozenge$ = medium, puromycin added
$[^3H]$leucine was used as substrate.

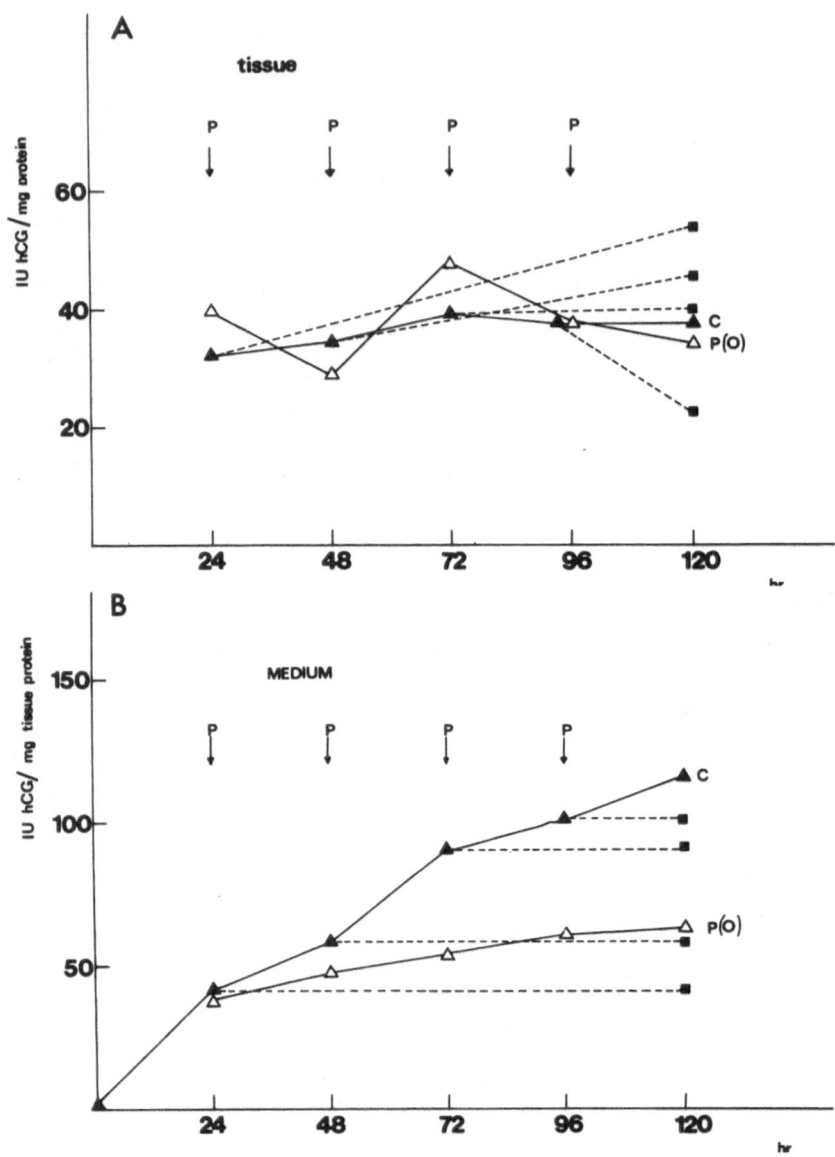

Figure 8. The effect of puromycin on the hCG concentration of placental tissue (A) and of the incubation medium (B). Puromycin (0.1mM final concentration) added as indicated by arrows: ▲——▲; C: control; ▲----■: puromycin added as indicated; △——△P(0): puromycin present from zero time.

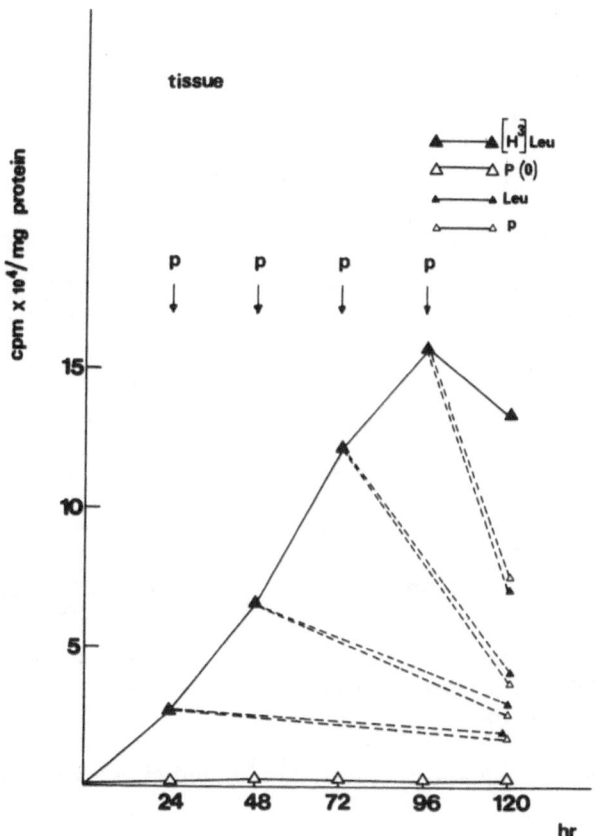

Figure 9.   Degradation of newly synthesized proteins in placental tissue as a function of the culture age.   Puromycin added as indicated by arrows.

▲———▲   = $[^3H]$leucine, control

△———△P(0) = radioactive medium containing 0.1mM puromycin during the entire incubation period

▲----▲   = leucine medium replaced by non-radioactive medium

△----△   = puromycin medium replaced by non-radioactive medium containing 0.1mM puromycin

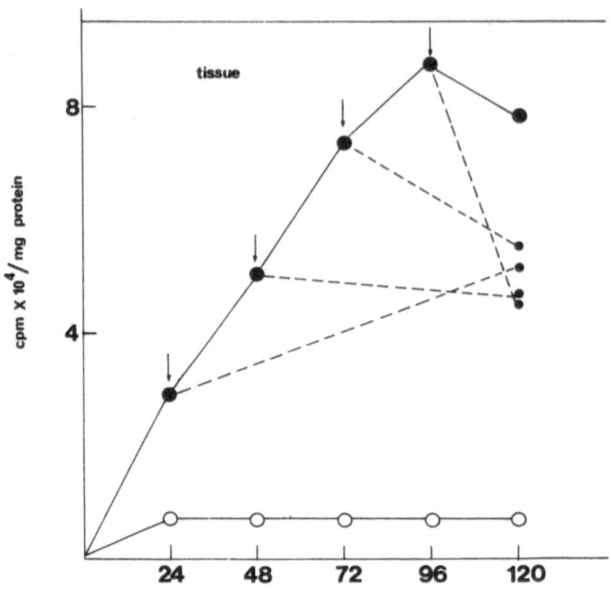

Figure 10. The effect of puromycin on the amount of newly synthesized glycoproteins in placental tissue. Puromycin added as indicated by arrows.

●——● = control;   o——o = puromycin added at zero time.

culture was incubated. The same rate of protein degradation was observed when, after labeling the proteins of the tissue, protein synthesis was stopped by the addition of puromycin (Figure 9). As the concentration of hCG in the tissue does not change significantly after incubation in the presence of puromycin, it can be concluded that hCG is a relatively metabolic stable protein. This supposition is strengthened by the results shown in Figure 10. Glycoproteins were labeled by glucosamine and to some of the incubation mixtures puromycin was added at different times. It is clear from the results that glycoproteins are broken down, but the degree of their degradation is smaller than that of proteins in general (Figure 9).

The synthesis and secretion of proteins labeled by glucosamine in organ culture in the presence of 2-deoxyglucose is shown in Figure 11. The synthesis is completely inhibited after 48 hr and partly inhibited before that time. However, when we measured the secretion of hCG by the organ cultures under the same conditions, hCG secretion was not inhibited at all. It was also not inhibited

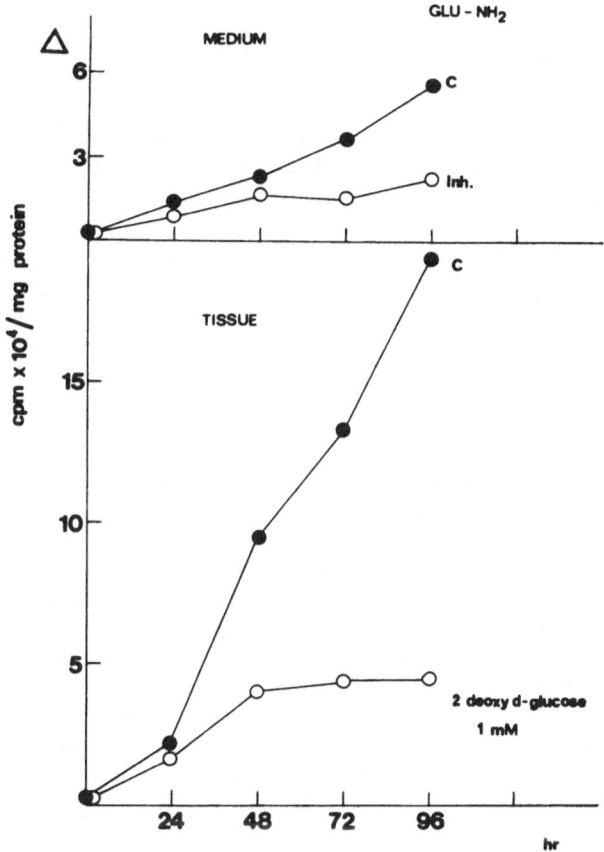

Figure 11. The effect of 2-deoxyglucose on the synthesis and secretion of glycoproteins by placental tissue. C = control; inh = inhibition by deoxy-glucose.

in an experiment where a considerable hCG secretion continued until the end of the incubation period (120 hr). These results can be explained by assuming that either glycosylation is not obligatory for secretion or that the glycosylation of hCG is not inhibited by the 2-deoxyglucose. This matter is presently under investigation.

The most important conclusion to be drawn from our results is the close relationship between hCG synthesis and secretion. HCG secretion continues only to a very limited extent after protein synthesis is stopped. The intracellular level of hCG is still close to its normal level the moment secretion comes to a standstill, and is resumed immediately upon renewal of protein synthesis. Therefore, initiation and termination of hCG secretion occur at closely the same intracellular hCG level. It is thus likely that the intracellular level of hCG does not regulate the secretion rate of this hormone, but it is the active synthesis of hCG (or a factor -- or factors -- closely related to the synthesis of hCG such as the corresponding mRNA) which has a decisive influence on the regulation of hCG secretion.

It seems likely from our results that glycosylation is not obligatory for the secretion of hCG.

SUMMARY

HCG synthesis and secretion by first-trimester placenta was studied by tissue slices and organ culture techniques.

Placental tissue in vitro synthesizes and secretes proteins including hCG. Protein synthesis is inhibited by actinomycin D. In tissue slices there is a 2 hr lag period between the incorporation of labeled amino acids into proteins and the appearance of radioactive proteins, including hCG, in the medium. During long-term incubations (120 hr) the hCG content of the tissue remains constant. However, the rate of hCG synthesis and secretion drops continuously during the incubation. The secretion of proteins in general continues, however, undiminished during the incubation period.

Newly synthesized α and β subunits could be detected in the rough membrane fraction by electrophoretic and immunological methods, indicating that both subunits are synthesized on bound ribosomes. Puromycin inhibits protein synthesis and secretion including that of hCG. Both synthesis and secretion are renewed upon removal of puromycin. Secretion of hCG seems to be directly connected to hCG synthesis.

The capacity of the placental tissue to synthesize and secrete hCG is proportional to its hCG content.

Protein degradation increases during the incubation (organ cultures). Glycoproteins, including hCG, are relatively resistant to degradation.

Upon introduction of 2-deoxyglucose, secretion of hCG takes place at a normal rate in organ cultures where glycosylation of proteins is severely inhibited.

REFERENCES

Bahl, O. P., 1969, Human chorionic gonadotropin, J. Biol. Chem. 244:567.

Bloemendal, H., Bont, W. S., de Vries, M., Benedetti, E. L., 1967, Isolation and properties of polyribosomes and fragments of the endoplasmic reticulum from rat liver, Biochem. J. 103:177.

Bollum, F. J., 1965, Filter paper disk techniques for assaying radioactive macromolecules, in Procedures in Nucleic Acid Research, G. L. Cantoni and D. R. Davies, eds., p. 296, Harper and Row, New York.

Borkowski, A., and Muquardt, C., 1979, Human chorionic gonadotropin in the plasma of normal, nonpregnant subjects, N. Engl. J. Med., 301:298.

Braunstein, G. D., Vaitukaitis, J. L., Carbone, P. P., and Ross, G. T., 1973, Ectopic production of human chorionic gonadotropin by neoplasms, Ann. Intern. Med. 78:39.

Brody, S., and Carlström, G., 1962, Immunoassay of human chorionic gonadotropin in normal and pathological pregnancies, J. Clin. Endocrinol. Metab. 22:564.

Chatterjee, M., Baliga, B. S., and Munro, H. N., 1976, Synthesis of human placental lactogen and human chorionic gonadotropin by polyribosomes and messengers RNAs from early and full term placentas, J. Biol. Chem. 251:2945.

Daniels-McQueen, S., McWilliams, D., Birken, S., Canfield, R., Landefeld, T., and Boime, I., 1978, Identification of mRNAs encoding the α and β subunits of human choriogonadotropin, J. Biol. Chem. 253:7109.

Folman, R., Ilan, J., Shiklosh, J., De Groot, N., and Hochberg, A. A., 1979, The synthesis and secretion of human chorionic gonadotropin by tissue slices from first trimester placentas, Molec. Biol. Rep. 5(3):175.

Gal, A. L., Folman, R., Czosnek, H. H., Shiklosh, J., De Groot, N., and Hochberg, A. A., 1977, The in vitro reconstitution of rough endoplasmic reticulum membrane derived from human placenta, Life Sci. 21:779.

Laemmli, U. K., 1970, Cleavage of structural proteins during the assembly of the head of bacteriophage T_4, Nature 227:680.

Liao, T. H., and Pierce, J. G., 1970, The presence of a common type of subunit in bovine thyroid-stimulating and luteinizing hormones, J. Biol. Chem. 245:3275.

Lowry, O. H., Rosebrough, N. J., Farr, A. L., and Randall, R. J., 1951, Protein measurement with the folin phenol reagent, J. Biol. Chem. 193:265.

Milstein, C., Brownlee, G., Harrison, T., and Mathews, M., 1972, A possible precursor of immunoglobulin light chain, Nature New Biol. 239:117.

Palade, G., 1975, Intracellular aspects of the process of protein synthesis, Science 189:347.

Peters, T., Jr., 1975, Serum albumin, in *Plasma Protein*, F. W. Putnam, ed., Vol. 1:133, Academic Press, New York.

Redman, C. M., 1968, The synthesis of serum proteins on attached rather than free ribosomes of rat liver, Biochem. Biophys. Res. Commun. 31:845.

Schachter, H., 1974, The subcellular sites of glycosylation, Biochem. Soc. Symp. printed in Great Britain 40:57.

Yoshimoto, Y., Wolfsen, A. R., Hirose, F., and Odell, W. D., 1979, Human chorionic gonadotropin-like material: presence in normal human tissues, Am. J. Obstet. Gynecol. 134:729.

ACKNOWLEDGEMENTS

This work was supported by grant No. GA PS 7901 from the Rockefeller Foundation, New York, U.S.A.

We thank Mrs. T. Schnedier for her excellent technical assistance.

SYNTHESIS, PROCESSING, AND SECRETION OF HUMAN

CHORIONIC GONADOTROPIN SUBUNITS BY CULTURED HUMAN CELLS

Raymond W. Ruddon, Charlotte A. Hanson,
Albert H. Bryan, and Carmen Anderson

Biological Markers Program, National Cancer Institute-
Frederick Cancer Research Center
Frederick, Maryland, U.S.A.

INTRODUCTION

Human chorionic gonadotropin (hCG) is produced eutopically
(i.e., as part of the expected repertoire of gene products) by
trophoblastic malignant cells, and ectopically by other human cancer
cells, including carcinomas of the lung, breast, ovary, testis, and
gastrointestinal tract, as well as by certain lymphomas and melanomas
(Vaitukaitis et al., 1976). The clinical prevalence of hCG-producing
tumors appears to be greater than would be predicted by the incidence
of elevated hCG levels in the blood of cancer patients. For example,
Hattori et al. (1978) have reported that 10% of plasma samples from
patients with various cancers were positive for hCG, whereas 42% of
the patients had tumors that contained hCG. Grieve et al. (1978)
have found that 8% of patients with operable breast cancer (Stages
I & II) had detectable hCG-α in the serum, but hCG-α was identified
in 42% of the primary mammary carcinomas examined. These data suggest that diagnostic acuity could be increased for hCG as a cancer
marker if the mechanisms controlling the secretion of hCG subunits
from cancer cells could be established. We have begun to examine
the synthesis, processing, and secretion of hCG subunits by a number
of cultured human cell lines previously shown to be producers of one
or both hCG subunits (Ruddon et al., 1979a). To date, we have shown
that hCG-α producing cell lines contain 15,000 mol. wt. and 18,000
mol. wt. (by SDS-PAGE, i.e., sodium dodecyl sulfate-polyacrylamide
gel electrophoresis) precursors of α-subunit and secrete "mature"
alpha of 22,000 mol. wt. and that hCG-β producing lines contain 18,000
mol. wt. and 24,000 mol. wt. precursors of β-subunit and secrete
"mature" beta of 34,000 mol. wt. (Ruddon et al., 1979b and 1980).

The present manuscript describes further work on the characterization of the intracellular and extracellular forms of hCG subunits
produced by cultured human cells.

MATERIALS AND METHODS

Cell Culture Lines

JAR choriocarcinoma cells, obtained from Dr. Roland Pattillo,
Medical College of Wisconsin (Pattillo et al., 1971), were grown
in Dulbecco's modified Eagle's medium with 10% fetal bovine serum.
ChaGo bronchogenic carcinoma cells, obtained from Dr. Alan Rabson,
National Cancer Institute (Rabson et al., 1973), were grown in RPMI
1640 medium with 20% fetal bovine serum.

Radioactive Labeling and Preparation of Cell Lysates

Late log or early confluent cultures, grown in 60 or 100 mm
diameter Petri dishes, were incubated at 37°C for various times
with the following radioactively labeled substrates: 100 µCi/ml of
[^{35}S]methionine (500-900 Ci/mmole, New England Nuclear Corp.) in
methionine-free medium; 200 µCi/ml D-[6-^{3}H]glucosamine (20 Ci/mmole,
Amersham/Searle Corp.) in glucose-free medium, or 200 µCi/ml D-[1-^{3}H]
mannose (5 Ci/mmole, Amersham/Searle Corp.). In some experiments,
the radioactivity was "chased" by removing the labeling medium,
washing the cells three times with complete medium, and incubating
for various times in the presence of complete medium. Tunicamycin
(obtained from the Developmental Therapeutics Program, National
Cancer Institute) was added to some culture plates 16 hr prior to
a radioactive pulse. After pulsing, the medium was removed, and the
cells were washed with phosphate-buffered saline solution (0.01 M
sodium phosphate-containing 0.14 M NaCl, pH 7.2) and lysed by adding
2 to 5 ml of phosphate-buffered saline containing 1.0% Triton X-100,
0.5% sodium deoxycholate, and 0.1% sodium dodecyl sulfate (lysis
buffer) and shearing the cells with a 21-gauge needle. Culture
medium was brought to the same concentration of lysis buffer by the
addition of a concentrated solution. Cell lysates were clarified
at 100,000 g for 1 hr at 0°C. The 100,000 g pellet contained no
detectable hCG subunits as determined by SDS-PAGE followed by
fluorography (vide infra) and was discarded. Cell lysates and media
were stored at -70°C until analyzed.

Immunoprecipitation and SDS-PAGE

Detection of hCG-specific polypeptides in cell lysates and media
was performed with rabbit antisera directed against complete hCG,

hCG-α, hCG-β, or the carboxyl terminal 15 amino acids of hCG-β (Ruddon et al., 1980). Serum from nonimmunized rabbits was used as a control. Cell lysates or media were incubated with immune or nonimmune rabbit serum (1/5000 final dilution) at 4°C for 16 hr. Immune complexes were precipitated by the addition of Protein A Sepharose CL-4B (Pharmacia) followed by mixing for 2 hr at 4°C and centrifugation at 1000 g for 15 min. The immunoprecipitates were washed three times in lysis buffer, dissolved in electrophoresis buffer containing 0.062 M Tris-HCl (pH 6.7), 1% SDS, 10% glycerol, and a 2.5 mercaptoethanol, heated at 100°C for 5 min, and layered on 5 to 20% linear gradient gels prepared by the method of Laemmli (1970). Electrophoresis was carried out for 16 hr at 35 V in a BioRad Model 220 slab gel apparatus. Radioactivity was visualized by the flourographic method of Bonner and Laskey (1974). Two-dimensional gels were performed by the method of O'Farrell (1975). The following ^{14}C-labeled molecular weight standards (New England Nuclear Corp.) were employed: phosphorylase B (92,500), bovine serum albumin (69,000), ovalbumin (46,000), carbonic anhydrase (30,000), and cytochrome C (12,300).

Digestion with Endoglycosidase H or Neuraminidase

Clarified cell lysates (100,000 g for 60 min) were immunoprecipitated with anti-α or anti-β as described above. The immunoprecipitates were washed twice with lysis buffer and once in distilled water, resuspended in 1 ml of 0.1 M sodium citrate (pH 5.3), and 0.05 units of endoglycosidase H (Miles Laboratories, Inc.) which had been pretreated with 2 mM PMSF for 30 min at 0°C to inhibit residual protease activity, were added to one-half of the suspension. The other half was used as the control. The samples were then incubated with shaking for 24 hr at 37°C. For neuraminidase digestion, the samples were suspended in a buffer (pH 4.9) containing 0.05 M sodium acetate, 2 mM $CaCl_2$, and 0.2 mM EDTA; 0.04 units of neuraminidase (Miles Laboratories, Inc.) were added, and the samples were incubated for 24 hr. After 24 hr of incubation, the samples were centrifuged at 1000 g for 10 min and the supernatants were removed. The pellets were washed once with distilled water and then dissolved in electrophoresis buffer and electrophoresed as described above.

RESULTS AND DISCUSSION

Gonadotropin Production by Human Cell Lines

We have previously reported the characterization of a number of human cell lines and their production of "oncodevelopmental" markers (Neuwald et al., 1979). Among the cell lines studied, approximately 35% produced hCG-α, hCG-β, or both subunits (Ruddon et al., 1980). The 21 cell lines that were found to produce one

TABLE I: Gonadotropin-producing human cell lines.

Cell Line	Tissue of Origin	hCG-α		hCG-β		hLH-β		hFSH-β		hTSH-β	
		Cells	Medium	Cells	Medium	Cells	Medium	Cells	Medium	Cells	Medium
HS0587	Normal Intestine	ND[a]	70[b]	ND	ND	ND	ND	ND	ND	ND	ND
HS0775	Normal Liver	ND	27[b]	ND	ND	ND	ND	ND	ND	ND	ND
HS0593	Normal Breast	ND	91[b]	ND	ND	–[c]	ND	–	ND	–	ND
BCT	Breast carcinoma	1.4	20[b]	ND	ND	–	ND	–	ND	–	ND
ZR-75-1	Breast carcinoma	10	33	ND	ND	–	ND	–	ND	–	ND
MCF-7	Breast carcinoma	ND	10	ND	ND	1.0	ND	ND	ND	ND	ND
BT-20[d]	Breast carcinoma	37	304	ND	ND	ND	ND	ND	ND	ND	ND
ZR-75-31	Breast carcinoma	16	ND	ND	ND	–	ND	–	ND	–	ND
496 (A1Ab)	Breast carcinoma	ND	ND	0.2	ND	ND	ND	ND	ND	ND	ND
ChaGo	Bronchogenic carcinoma	52	2920	ND	ND	ND	ND	ND	ND	ND	ND
HeLa S$_3$	Cervical carcinoma	ND	50	ND	ND	0.3	ND	ND	ND	ND	ND
HS01C1	Renal adenocarcinoma	ND	134	ND	ND	–	–	–	–	–	–
IMR-32	Neuroblastoma	31	ND	ND	ND	ND	ND	ND	ND	ND	ND
HS0852 T[e]	Melanoma	ND	ND	ND	6[b]	ND	ND	ND	ND	ND	ND
HS0695 T	Melanoma	ND	ND	ND	0.7[b]	–	–	–	–	–	–
A375	Melanoma	ND	ND	ND	0.1[b]	0.2	ND	0.4	ND	ND	ND
CBT	Glioblastoma multiforme	ND	ND	26	273	4.0	91	ND	ND	ND	ND

TABLE I (continued): Gonadotropin-producing human cell lines.

Cell Line	Tissue of Origin	$hCG-\alpha$		$hCG-\beta$		$hLH-\beta$		$hFSH-\beta$		$hTSH-\beta$	
		Cells	Medium	Cells	Medium	Cells	Medium	Cells	Medium	Cells	Medium
SV80	SV40 transformed fibroblast	ND	ND	0.9	24[b]	ND	ND	0.6	ND	ND	ND
WI-38 VA_{13}	SV40 transformed fibroblast	ND	ND	ND	26	ND	ND	ND	ND	ND	ND
JAR	Choriocarcinoma	10	380	13	350	3	60	ND	ND	ND	ND
BeWo	Choriocarcinoma	25	844	1.7	82	ND	2	ND	ND	ND	ND

The concentration of hormone subunits was determined in cell lysates or media by radioimmunoassay as previously described (Ruddon et al., 1979a). Antisera used were developed to the individual subunits in each case. Cells were harvested in log phase of growth. Medium was collected for RIA 24 hr after refeeding unless otherwise indicated. Values are expressed as ng/mg cellular protein for the cells and ng/mg cellular protein secreted in 24 hr (or 48 hr) for the medium (data from Ruddon et al., 1979a, with permission).

[a] ND, not detectable, indicating that the amount of subunit was <0.1 $ng/10^6$ cells.

[b] 48 hr secretion into medium.

[c] —, not analyzed.

[d] Possible HeLa variant based on karyology and G6PD isoenzyme analysis.

[e] Identified as primarily "normal," not tumor cells, by karyology.

or both hCG subunits are listed in Table I. A number of lines produce significant amounts of free alpha subunit. On the other hand, some cell lines produce hCG-β but no detectable free alpha subunit. It should be noted that the antiserum to hCG-α used in these radioimmunoassays (RIA's) was specific for free alpha subunit, whereas the anti-beta serum did not discriminate entirely between free beta and intact hCG (Ruddon et al., 1979a). In all lines that synthesize free alpha, the production of alpha subunit is in excess of the beta subunits of all the related glycoprotein hormones. Thus, there is an apparent "overproduction" of alpha subunit in these cells. Although most of the alpha producing lines secrete alpha subunit into the medium, two lines appear to retain it intracellularly (ZR-75-31 and IMR-32). A few of the lines contain and/or secrete detectable amounts of hLH-β, human luteinizing hormone-beta (MCF-7, HeLa S_3, A375, CBT, JAR, and BeWo) or hFSH-β, human follicle-stimulating hormone-beta (A375 and SV80). None of the lines examined contain or secrete detectable amounts of human thyroid stimulating hormone-beta (hTSH-β).

Evidence for the Presence of Intracellular Precursors of hCG Subunits in JAR and ChaGo Cells

We have begun to examine by pulse-chase techniques the synthesis, processing, and secretion of hCG subunits by the hCG-producing lines listed in Table I. Some of the experiments characterizing these processes in JAR and ChaGo cells will be described in detail here.

JAR choriocarcinoma cells (Pattillo et al., 1971) synthesize and secrete both hCG subunits, although there is an excess production of free alpha subunit by these cells. Figure 1 illustrates the forms of the hCG subunits synthesized in these cells. In this experiment JAR cells were pulsed for 1 hr with [^{35}S]methionine, and the cell lysates were then immunoprecipitated with anti-hCG, anti-alpha, or anti-C-terminal beta. Anti-hCG precipitates bands at 24,000, 18,000, and 15,000 mol wt (Lane 1). Anti-alpha precipitates polypeptides of 24,000 and 18,000 mol wt (Lane 3). Immunoprecipitation of the 18,000 and 15,000 mol wt bands by anti-alpha is inhibited by excess placental alpha (Lane 5) but not by excess beta subunit (Lane 8), whereas immunoprecipitation of the 24,000 and 18,000 mol wt polypeptides by anti-C-terminal beta is blocked by excess beta subunit (Lane 9) but not by excess alpha subunit (Lane 6). Nonimmune serum does not precipitate any of these bands (Ruddon et al., 1979b and 1980). Using [^{35}S]methionine as the labeled precursor, only small amounts of "mature" alpha (22,000 mol wt) and beta (34,000 mol wt) were detected intracellularly in these experiments, as previously reported (Ruddon et al., 1979b, 1980). However, with [^{3}H] glucosamine as the labeled tracer, it is clear that mature subunits are formed in JAR cells (Figure 2). The reason for the difference in detectability of the various subunit forms with different labeled

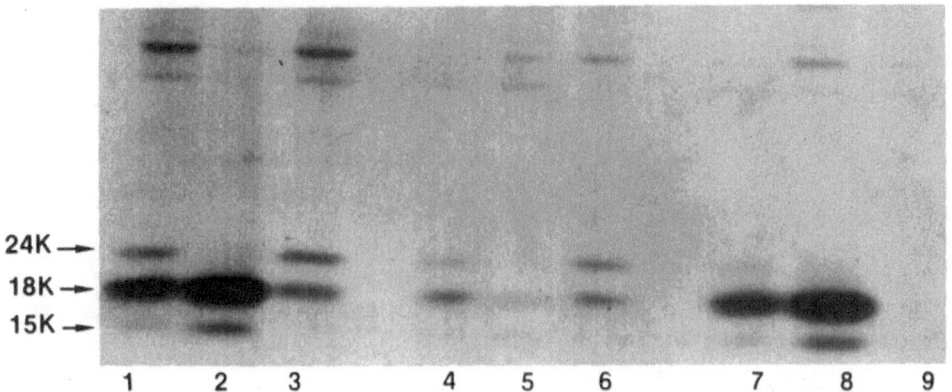

Figure 1.   Identification of putative hCG-α and hCG-β precursors
in JAR cells by competition with excess unlabeled placental hCG-α
and hCG-β.   JAR cells were pulsed for 1 hr with [^{35}S]methionine
(100 µCi/ml).   Immediately before immunprecipitation, excess unlabeled
placental hCG-α (260 pmol/ml) or hCG-β (140 pmol/ml) was added to the
clarified cell lysates (this was approximately a 100-fold excess
based on RIA of cell lysates for hCG-α and hCG-β).   Arrows indicate
the migration of the 24,000, 18,000, and 15,000 mol. wt. precursors.
Lanes 1-3, controls: 1, anti-hCG; 2, anti-α; 3, anti-C-terminal β.
Lanes 4-6: same sequence of antisera + excess α.   Lane 7-9: same
sequence of antisera + excess β.   (From Ruddon et al., 1980, with
permission.)

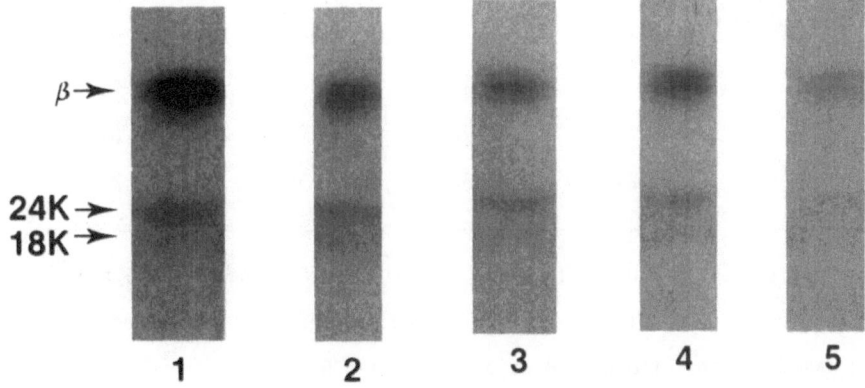

Figure 2.   Incorporation of [^{3}H]glucosamine into precursor and mature
forms of hCG-β in JAR cells.   Cells were pulsed 1 hr with 200 µCi/ml
of [^{3}H]glucosamine, washed 3 times with complete medium, and chased
30, 60, 120, and 240 min in the presence of complete medium.   Cell
lysates were immunoprecipitated with anti-β.   Arrows indicated migration of mature β (which migrates identically to placental hCG-β
standard) and the 24,000 and 18,000 mol. wt. precursors of β-subunit.
Lanes: 1, 0 min-; 2, 30 min-; 3, 60 min-; 4, 120 min-; 5, 240 min-chase.

TABLE II: Intracellular vs. extracellular hCG during pulse-chase experiments with JAR cells.

Label	Chase Time (min)	DPM Immunoprecipitated		
		Cells	Medium	Total
[^{35}S]methionine (1 hr pulse)	0	41,800	—	41,800
	30	31,400	7,250	38,650
	60	29,200	7,500	36,700
	120	21,100	10,875	31,975
	240	23,800	11,250	35,050
[^{3}H]fucose (1 hr pulse)	0	880	—	880
	15	520	250	770
	30	330	390	720
	120	270	740	1,010
	240	290	910	1,200

JAR cells were pulsed for 1 hr with [^{35}S]methionine (100 μCi/ml) or [^{3}H]fucose (100 μCi/ml) and then chased for the times indicated. All immunoprecipitations were done with anti-hCG.

substrates is most likely due to the relative amounts of each residue in the subunits. There are three methionine residues in alpha, and only one in beta, whereas there are eight glucosamines in each of the "mature" subunits (there would only be four gluco-samines in the putative precursors, vide infra).

The kinetics of secretion of the α-subunit by JAR cells are depicted in Figure 3. JAR cells were pulsed for 15 min with [^{35}S] methionine, chased for 15, 30, 60, 120, and 240 min, and the cell lysates and media were immunoprecipitated with anti-alpha. Both the 18,000 and 15,000 mol. wt. forms of alpha are apparent in the 15 min pulse and 15 to 60 min chase samples (Lane 1-4). By 30 min into the chase, a diffuse band that corresponds to secreted alpha is detectable intracellularly, and by 120 min of chase both the precursor forms and mature alpha have decreased dramatically in the cells. However, there is a corresponding increase in the amount of secreted alpha as the chase progresses (Lanes 7-9).

These results are not due to an intracellular protease activity that might be generating the lower molecule weight forms of the subunits because i) addition of the protease inhibitor PMSF to cell lysates or incubation of clarified cell lysates for 24 hr at 37°C does not alter the SDS-PAGE banding patterns seen with anti-α or anti-β immunoprecipitation, ii) the migration of ^{125}I-labeled hCG-α and hCG-β standards is not altered by addition to cell lysates that are then carried through the standard immunoprecipitation procedure, and iii) the total DPM immunoprecipitated does not change significantly during pulse-chase experiments (Table I).

Kinetics similar to those seen with JAR cells are observed for the processing of α-subunit in ChaGo, a cell line derived from a bronchogenic carcinoma (Rabson et al., 1973) that secretes primarily α-subunit (Table I). Figure 4 shows the results of a pulse-chase experiment in which ChaGo cells were pulsed for 5 min with [^{35}S] methionine and then chased for 5, 10, 15, 30, 60, and 120 min. Both cell lysates and media were immunoprecipitated with anti-α. As with JAR cells, the 18,000 and 15,000 mol. wt. forms of alpha is blocked by excess placental alpha, but not by excess beta (data not shown). By 120 min, mature alpha is clearly detectable in the medium (Lane 12). Thus, the same intracellular precursors of α-subunit are present in both ChaGo and JAR cells and the kinetics of secretion are similar. However, detectable amounts of α-subunit are present in the 1 hr-chase medium of JAR cells, whereas alpha is not detectable in the medium from ChaGo cultures until 2 hr initiation of the chase.

Figure 3.   Pulse-chase labeling of hCG-α subunit in JAR cells.
Cells were pulsed 15 min with [^{35}S]methionine (100 µCi/ml), washed
3 times with complete medium, and chased 15, 30, 60, 120, or 240
min in the presence of complete medium.   Cell lysates and media
were immunoprecipitated with anti-α.   Arrows indicate the migration
of secreted α-subunit (which migrates identically to placental hCG-α
standard) and the 18,000 and 15,000 mol. wt. precursors.   Lanes
1-6, cells: 1, 0 min-; 2, 15 min-; 3, 30 min-; 4, 60 min-; 5, 120
min-; 6, 240 min-chase.   Lanes 7-9, media: 7, 60 min-; 8, 120 min-;
9, 240 min-chase.   Lane 10: molecular weight standards.   (From
Ruddon et al., 1980, with permission.)

Figure 4.   Pulse-chase labeling of hCG-α subunit in ChaGo cells.
Cells were pulsed for 5 min with [^{35}S]methionine (100 µCi/ml) and
chased for 5, 10, 15, 30, 60, and 120 min.   Cell lysates and media
were immunoprecipitated with anti-α.   Arrows indicate the migration
of secreted α and the 18,000 and 15,000 mol. wt. precursors.
Lanes: 1, cells, 0 chase; 2, cells, 5 min chase; 3, cells, 10 min
chase; 4, medium, 10 min chase; 5, cells, 15 min chase; 6, medium,
15 min chase; 7, cells, 30 min chase; 8, medium, 30 min chase;
9, cells, 60 min chase; 10, medium, 60 min chase; 11, cells, 120
min chase; 13, molecular weight standards.

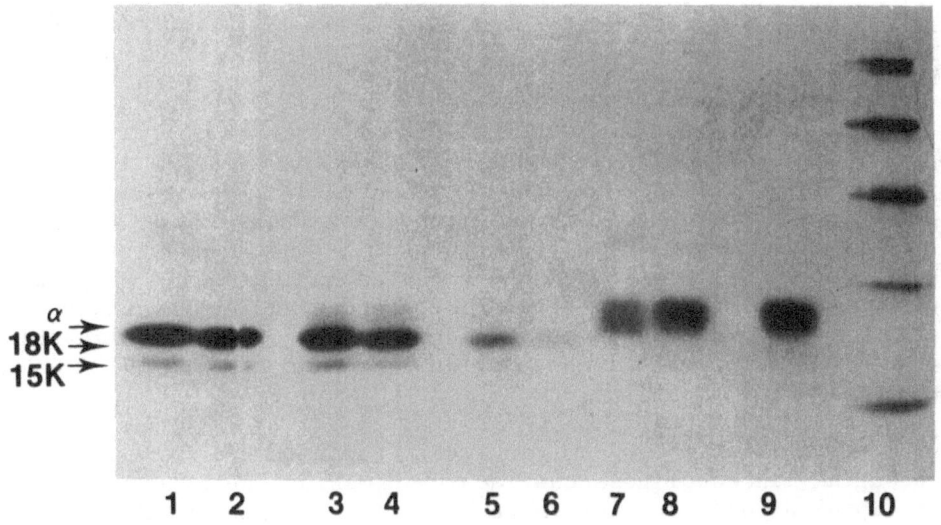

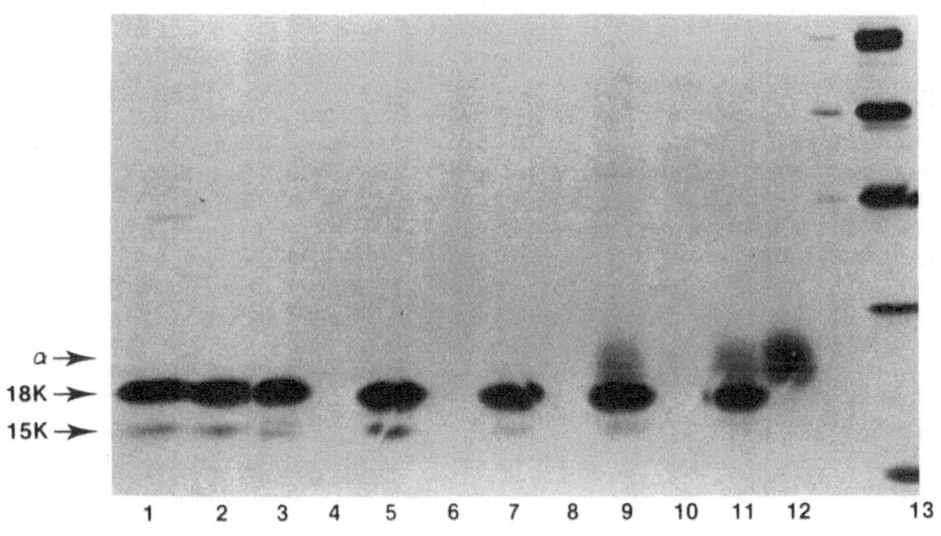

Figure 4.

Characterization of the Intracellular Forms of hCG Subunits in JAR Cells

Both the α- and β-subunits of hCG contain two asparagine-linked oligosaccharaide chains (Kessler et al., 1979b). In addition, beta has four serine-linked oligosaccharaide chains (Kessler et al., 1979a). From what is known about the synthesis, processing, and secretion of other secretory glycoproteins, it is likely that the glycosylated intracellular precursors of α- and β-subunits contain "high mannose" asparagine-linked oligosaccharide chains which are subsequently processed by removal of glucose and extra mannose residues and further modified by addition of terminal stalic acid containing "complex" oligosaccharides (Robbins et al., 1977; Tabas et al., 1978).

The antibiotic tunicamycin, which inhibits the formation of asparagine-linked oligosaccharides by blocking the synthesis of the lipid-carbohydrate carrier complex involved in the formation of asparagine-linked N-glycosidic bonds (Struck and Lennarz, 1977), and endoglycosidase H (endo H), an enzyme that cleaves high-mannose oligosaccharide units from asparagine residues of the polypeptide backbone (Tarentino and Maley, 1974), are very useful tools to study the processing of glycoproteins. We have employed these tools to characterize the intracellular forms of the hCG subunits.

Cultures of JAR cells, some of which were pretreated with tunicamycin (5 µg/ml) for 16 hr, were pulsed with [^{35}S]methionine for 1 hr, lysed, immunoprecipitated with anti-alpha, and then incubated for 24 hr in the presence or absence of endo H (Figure 5). The 18,000 and 15,000 mol. wt. alpha-specific bands are seen in the control samples incubated for 24 hr without endo H (Lane 1). After 24 hr of incubation with the enzyme, the 18,000 mol. wt. band disappears, there is a relative increase in the 15,000 mol. wt. band, and a new band appears at 12,000 mol. wt. (Lane 2). In the cells pretreated with tunicamycin, only the 12,000 mol. wt. band is specifically immunoprecipitated by anti-alpha (Lane 3), and incubation with endo H does not change the migration of this band (Lane 4). In addition, double-label experiments with [^{3}H]mannose and [^{35}S]methionine indicate that the mannose/methionine ratio in the 18K band is twice that of the 15K band and that the 12K band contains no incorporated [^{3}H]mannose (data not shown). Taken together, these data suggest that the 18,000 mol. wt. form of alpha contains one high mannose core, and that the 12,000 mol. wt. form is the apoprotein of the α-subunit. Identical data have been obtained for the α-subunit of ChaGo cells (not shown).

Similar results were observed for the β-subunit in control and tunicamycin-treated JAR cells (Figure 6). In this experiment, JAR cells were pulsed for 1 hr with [^{35}S]methionine after incubation for 16 hr with or without 5 µg/ml tunicamycin, lysed, and immuno-

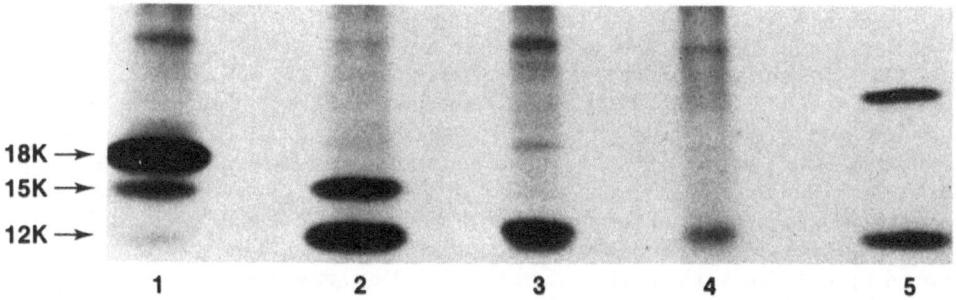

Figure 5. Effect of tunicamycin treatment and endoglycosidase H digestion on hCG-α precursors synthesized in JAR cells. Cells were incubated for 16 hr without or with tunicamycin (5 μg/ml) and then pulsed for 1 hr with [^{35}S]methionine, lysed, and immunoprecipitated with anti-α. The immunoprecipitates were incubated for 24 hr with or without endoglycosidase H (0.05 units/ml). Lanes: 1, control; 2, control + endo H; 3, tunicamycin-treated; 4, tunicamycin treated + endo H; 5, molecular weight standards.

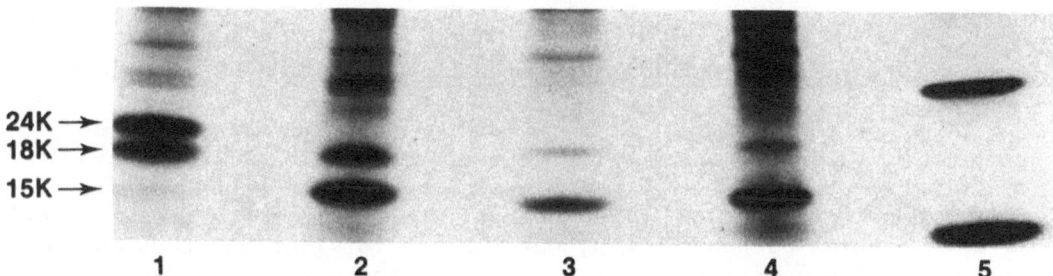

Figure 6. Effect of tunicamycin treatment and endoglycosidase H digestion on hCG-β precursors synthesized in JAR cells. Experimental procedures and sequence of the lanes were the same as for Figure 5 except that the cell lysates were immunoprecipitated with Anti-C terminal-β.

precipitated with anti-C-terminal-β. The immunoprecipitates were then incubated for 24 hr with or without endo H. The control sample has both the 24,000 and 18,000 mol. wt. beta precursor bands (Lane 1). Incubation with endo H removes the 24K band and produces a new band at 15K (Lane 3). After pretreatment with tunicamycin, the major band immunoprecipitated by anti-beta also migrates at 15,000 mol. wt. (Lane 3), the expected molecular weight of the beta apoprotein (Daniels-McQueen et al., 1978). Incubation of the anti-beta immunoprecipitate from tunicamycin-treated cells with endo H does not shift the molecular weight of the major band (Lane 4), supporting the idea that the 15,000 mol. wt. represents the beta apoprotein.

Partial Sequence of the NH_2-Termini of the 18,000 Mol. Wt. Alpha and Beta Precursors

The partial amino acid sequences of the NH_2-termini of the 18,000 mol. wt. alpha and beta precursors have been determined (Table III). Although this represents only a preliminary evaluation, it appears that the 18,000 mol. wt. alpha precursor seen in JAR cells does not contain the "signal" sequence and that it has the same NH_2-terminal sequence as placental alpha. Since the 18,000 mol. wt. form of alpha is the first one to appear during pulse-labeling of JAR cells and is seen as early as 5 min after initiation of a pulse (Ruddon et al., 1979 b), it is the moiety most likely to contain the signal peptide. That it does not indicates that the signal peptide has been cleaved very rapidly, before sufficient radioactivity has been incorporated to detect α-subunit precursors. The partial sequence of the 18,000 mol. wt. beta precursor supports the conclusion that it is different from the 18,000 mol. wt. material immunoprecipitated by anti-α, and also suggests that the signal sequence has been clipped before we are able to detect labeled beta in JAR cells.

Heterogeneity of hCG Subunits Secreted by JAR Cells

The secreted forms of both α- and β-subunits are a heterogeneous mixture of molecules that appear to contain different types of carbohydrate chains. Figure 7 shows the results of an experiment in which cultures of JAR cells, some of which were pretreated for 16 hr with 5 µg/ml of tunicamycin, were pulsed for 1 hr and then chased for 4 hr. The 4 hr chase medium was collected and immunoprecipitated by anti-α or anti-β. The immunoprecipitates were then incubated for 24 hr with or without endo H. The 4 hr-chase medium from untreated JAR cells contains a diffuse band of mature alpha (Lane 1), as seen previously (Figures 3 and 4). The tunicamycin-treated cells secrete the 12,000 mol. wt. form of alpha (Lane 2) seen intracellularly in tunicamycin-treated cells (Figure 5). Endo H partially digests the

TABLE III: NH_2-terminal sequences of hCG subunits.

Subunit or precursor	Amino acid residue 1 2 3 4 5 6 7 8 9 10 11 12	References
Pre-alpha:	Met-Asp-Tyr-Tyr-Arg-Lys-Tyr-Ala-Ala-Ile-Phe-Leu	Birken et al., 1978; Fiddes and Goodman, 1979
Alpha:	Ala-Pro-Asp-Val-Gln-Asp-Cys-Pro-Glu-Cys-Thr-Leu	Morgan et al., 1975; Fiddes and Goodman, 1979
18,000 mol.wt. alpha precursor:	X -Pro- X - X - X - X -Pro- X - X - X -Leu	Perini et al., 1979
Beta:	Ser-Lys-Glu-Pro-Leu-Arg-Pro-Arg-Cys-Arg-Pro-Ile	Morgan et al., 1975
18,000 mol.wt. beta precursor:	X - X - X -Pro-Leu- X -Pro- X - X - X - X - X	Perini et al., 1979

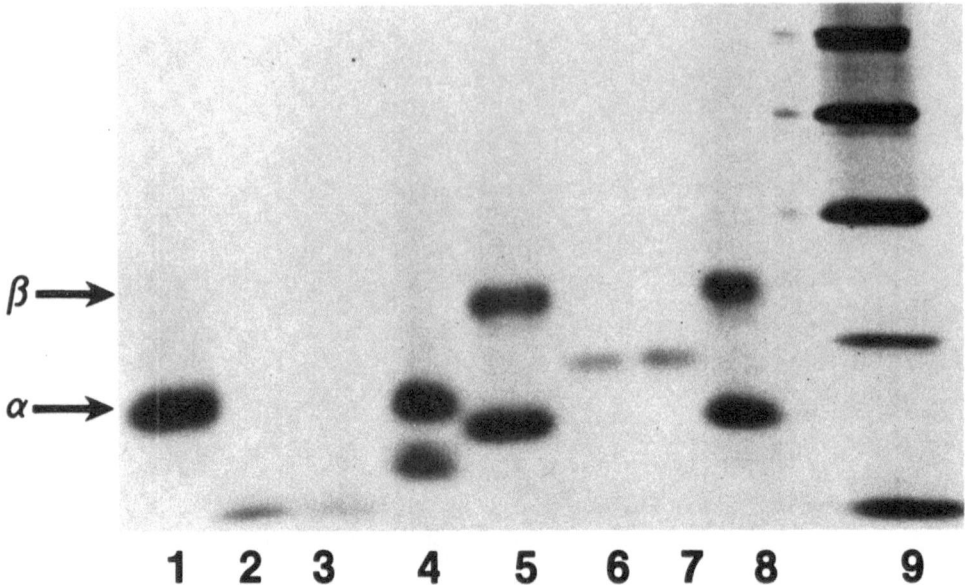

Figure 7. Effect of tunicamycin and endoglycosidase H on hCG subunits secreted by JAR cells. Cells were incubated for 16 hr with or without 5 µg/ml tunicamycin, and then pulsed for 1 hr with [^{35}S]methionine and chased for 4 hr. The 4 hr chase medium was immunoprecipitated with anti-α or anti-β and incubated for 24 hr with or without endo H. Arrows indicate the migration of "mature" α- and β-subunits. Lanes 1-4, secreted α: 1, control, no endo H; 2, tunicamycin-treated, no endo H; 3, tunicamycin-treated + endo H; 4, control + endo H. Lanes 5-8, secreted β: 5, control, no endo H; 6, tunicamycin-treated, no endo H; 7, tunicamycin-treated + endo H; 8, control + endo H. Lane 9: molecular weight standards.

α-subunit secreted by untreated cells to produce a band at 15,000 mol. wt. (Lane 4), suggesting that the α-subunit secreted by JAR cells is a mixture of molecules, some of which contain "simple" high-mannose oligosaccharides. Anti-β immunoprecipitates two bands from the chase medium, one at 34,000 mol. wt. that migrates like placental beta and a lower molecular band that migrates at about 20,000 mol. wt. (Lane 5). Neither of these is digested by endo H (Lane 8), and only the high molecular weight form is digested by neuraminidase (Figure 8). These data suggest that beta is also secreted as a mixture of molecules containing different carbohydrate chians. The lack of digestability of the lower molecular weight form of beta suggests that it has been partially processed by removal of mannose residues to the point where it is no longer a substrate

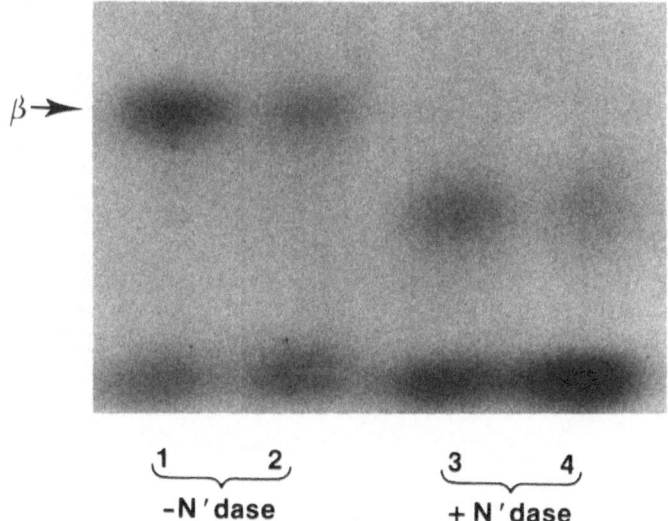

Figure 8. Effect of neuraminidase on β-subunit secreted by JAR cells. Cells were pulsed for 1 hr with [^{35}S]methionine and chased for 4 hr. Chase medium was immunoprecipitated with anti-β or anti-C-terminal-β and incubated for 24 hr with or without neuraminidase. Arrow indicated the migration of "mature" beta. Lanes 1 and 2, no neuraminidase: 1, anti-β; 2, anti-C-terminal-β. Lanes 3 and 4, with neuraminidase: 3, anti-β; 4, anti-C-terminal-β.

for endo H (Tarentino et al., 1974). It is of interest that β-subunit secreted by tunicamycin-treated cells migrates (with or without endo H digestion) between the high and low molecular weight forms of secreted beta (Figure 7, Lanes 6 and 7), suggesting that the addition of serine-linked oligosaccharides occurs even though the addition of asparagine-linked oligosaccharides has been inhibited.

The heterogeneity of the α-subunit secreted by JAR cells is more clearly seen by two-dimensional gel electrophoresis (Figure 9). The heterogeneity is primarily due to charge differences. Five distinct spots appear on the gel, which is what one would predict if all the heterogeneity were due to differences in sialylation, since there are four sialic acid residues in alpha (Kessler et al., 1979b). Pretreatment with neuraminidase completely removes the heterogeneity (Figure 10), supporting this conclusion.

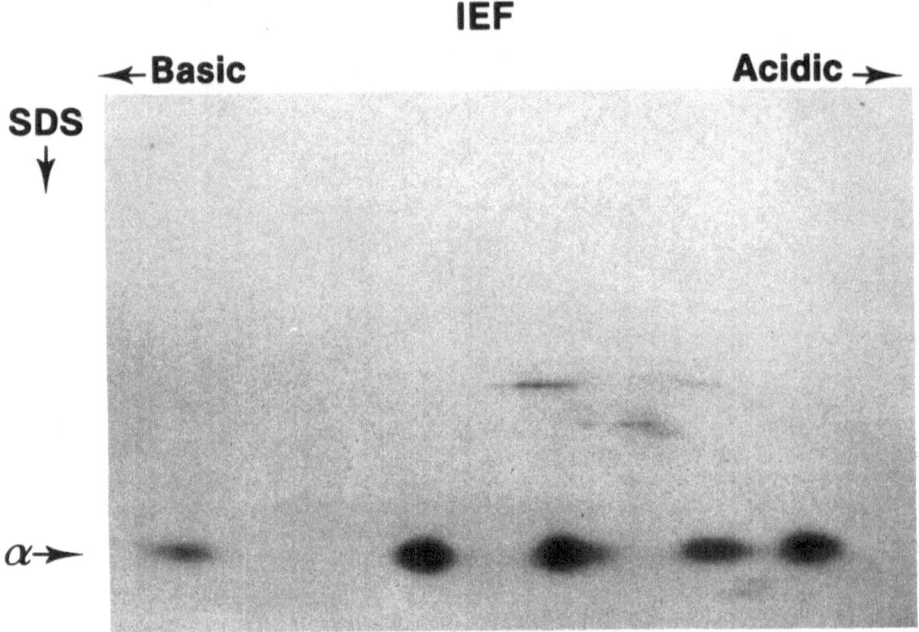

Figure 9.   Two-dimensional gel electrophoresis of hCG-α secreted
by JAR cells.   Cells were pulsed for 1 hr with [^{35}S]methionine and
chased for 4 hr.   Chase medium was immunoprecipitated with anti-α
and analyzed by two-dimensional gel electrophoresis, with isoelectric
focusing in the first dimension and SDS-PAGE in the second dimension,
by the method of O'Farrell (1975).   The pH gradient for the isoelectric focusing was 5.3 to 7.2.

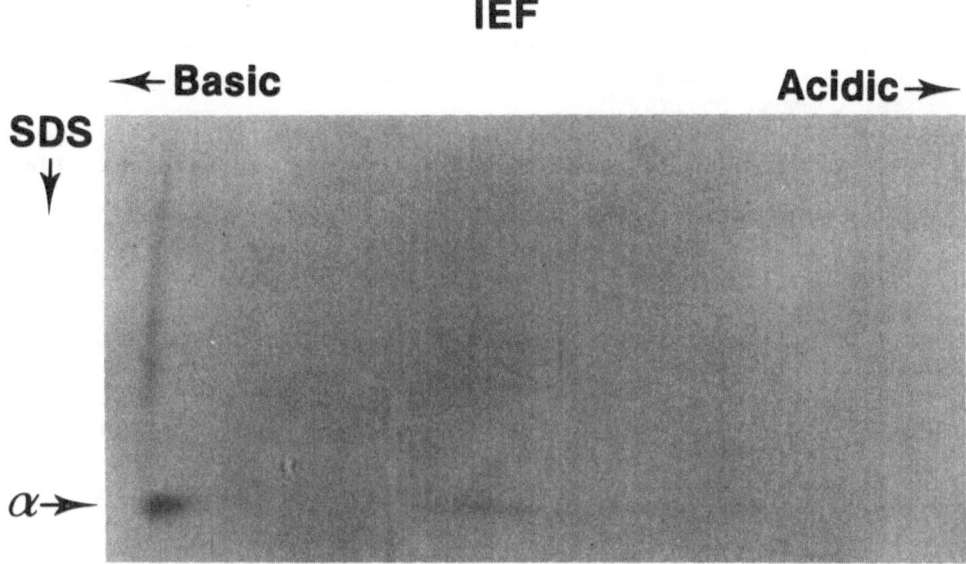

Figure 10. Effect of neuraminidase digestion on heterogeneity of hCG-α secreted by JAR cells. Experimental procedures were as described in the legend to Figure 9, except that the immunoprecipitates were digested with neuraminidase (0.04 units) for 24 hr prior to electrophoresis.

CONCLUSIONS

Pulse and pulse-chase experiments with cultured human cell lines that produce hCG subunits indicate that high-mannose oligosaccharide containing precursors of hCG-α and hCG-β, with half-lives $\geq$ 1 hr, are present in these cells. The intracellular precursors of alpha have apparent molecular weights of 15,000 and 18,000 by SDS-PAGE, and the precursors of beta are 18,000 and 24,000 mol. wt. The relatively long half-lives of the intracellular precursors of the hCG subunits suggest that there is a rate-limiting step in the processing pathway for hCG subunits and that once the mature forms of the subunits are generated, secretion occurs rapidly. The precursors of α-subunit appear to be the same in JAR choriocarcinoma and ChaGo bronchogenic carcinoma cells. The α- and β-subunits secreted by JAR cells are heterogeneous and appear to be a mixture of glycoproteins with "simple" high-mannose and "complex" sialic acid-containing oligosaccharides.

REFERENCES

Birken, S., Fetherston, J., Desmond, J., Canfield, R., and Boime, I., 1978, Partial amino acid sequence of the preprotein form of the alpha subunit of human choriogonadotropin and identification of the site of subsequent proteolytic cleavage, Biochem. Biophys. Res. Commun. 85:1247.

Bonner, W. M., and Laskey, R. A., 1974, A film detection method for tritium-lebelled proteins and nucleic acids in polyacrylamide gels, Eur. J. Biochem. 46:83.

Daniels-McQueen, S., McWilliams, D., Birken, S., Canfield, R., Landefeld, T., and Boime, I., 1978, Identification of mRNAs encoding the α and β subunits of human choriogonadotropin, J. Biol. Chem. 253:7109.

Fiddes, J. C., and Goodman, H. M., 1979, Isolation, cloning, and sequence analysis of the cDNA for the α-subunit of human chorionic gonadotropin, Nature 281:351.

Grieve, R. J., Woods, K. L., Cove, D. H., Smith, S. C., Leonard, J., and Howell, A., 1978, Synthesis and release of specific protein products by human mammary tumour cells in vitro, Br. J. Cancer 38:199.

Hattori, M., Fukase, M., Yoshimi, H., Matsukura, S., and Imura, H., 1978, Ectopic production of human chorionic gonadotropin in malignant tumors, Cancer 42:2328.

Kessler, M. J., Mise, T., Ghai, R. D., and Bahl, O. P., 1979a, Structure and location of the O-glycosidic carbohydrate units of human chorionic gonadotropin, J. Biol. Chem. 254:7909.

Kessler, M. J., Reddy, M. S., Shah, R. H., and Bahl, O. P., 1979b, Structures of N-glycosidic carbohydrate units of human chorionic gonadotropin, J. Biol. Chem. 254:7901.

Laemmli, U. K., 1970, Cleavage of structural proteins during the assembly of the head of bacteriophage T_4, Nature 227:680.

Morgan, F. J., Birken, S., and Canfield, R. E., 1975, The amino acid sequence of human chorionic gonadotropin: The α and β subunit, J. Biol. Chem. 250:5247.

Neuwald, P. D., Anderson, C., Salivar, W. O., Aldenderfer, P. H., Dermody, W. C., Weintraub, P. D., Rosen, S. W., Nelson-Rees, W. A., and Ruddon, R. W., 1980, Expression of oncodevelopmental gene products by human tumor cells in culture, J. Natl. Cancer Inst. 64:447.

O'Farrell, P. H., 1975, High resolution two-dimensional electrophoresis of proteins, J. Biol. Chem. 250:4007.

Pattillo, R. A., Ruckert, A., Hussa, R., Bernstein, R., and Delfs, E., 1971, The JAR cell line - continuous human multihormone production and controls, In Vitro 6:398.

Perini, F., Hanson, C. A., Bryan, A. H., and Ruddon, R. W., Partial sequence of the NH_2-termini of hCG precursors in cultural human cells. In preparation.

Rabson, A. S., Rosen, S. W., Tashjian, A. H., Jr., and Weintraub, B. D., 1973, Production of human chorionic gonadotropin in vitro by a cell line derived from a carcinoma of the lung, J. Natl. Cancer Inst. 50:669.

Robbins, P. W., Hubbard, S. C., Turco, S. J., and Wirth, D. F., 1977, Proposal for a common oligosaccharide intermediate in the synthesis of membrane glycoproteins, Cell 12:893.

Ruddon, R. W., Anderson, C., Meade, K. S., Aldenderfer, P. H., and Neuwald, P. D., 1979a, Content of gonadotropins in cultured human malignant cells and effects of sodium butyrate treatment on gonadotropin secretion by HeLa cells, Cancer Res. 39:3885.

Ruddon, R. W., Hanson, C. A., and Addison, N. J., 1979b, Synthesis and processing of human chorionic gonadotropin subunits in cultured choriocarcinoma cells, Proc. Natl. Acad. Sci., U.S.A. 76:5143.

Ruddon, R. W., Hanson, C. A., Bryan, A. H., Putterman, G. J., White, E. L., Perini, F., Meade, K. S., and Aldenderfer, P. H., 1980, Synthesis and secretion of human chorionic gonadotropin subunits by cultured human malignant cells, J. Biol. Chem. 255:1000.

Struck, D. K., and Lennarz, W. J., 1977, Evidence for the participation of saccharide-lipids in the synthesis of the oligosaccharide chain of ovalbumin, J. Biol. Chem. 252:1007.

Tabas, I., Schlesinger, S., and Kornfeld, S., 1978, Processing of high mannose oligosaccharides to form complex type oligosaccharides on the newly synthesized polypeptides of the vesicular stomatitis virus G protein and the IgG heavy chain, J. Biol. Chem. 253:716.

Tarentino, A. L., and Maley, F., 1974, Purification and properties of an endo-β-N-acetylflucosaminidase from *Streptomyces griseus*, J. Biol. Chem. 249:811.

Tarentino, A. L., Plummer, T. H., Jr., and Maley, F., 1974, The release of intact oligosaccharides from specific glycoproteins by endo-β-N-acetylglucosaminidase H, J. Biol. Chem. 249:818.

Vaitukaitis, J. L., Ross, G. T., Braunstein, G. D., and Rayford, P. L., 1976, Gonadotropins and their subunits: Basic and clinical studies, Recent Prog. Horm. Res. 32:289.

ACKNOWLEDGEMENTS

The authors thank Helen Beck and Jo Ann Tichnell for their help in preparation of the manuscript. This research was supported by the National Cancer Institute under Contract No. N01-CO-75380 with Litton Bionetics, Inc.

REGULATION OF HUMAN CHORIONIC GONADOTROPIN SYNTHESIS

IN PLACENTA, CHORIOCARCINOMA, AND NON-PLACENTAL TUMORS

Janice Yang Chou

Pregnancy Research Branch, National Institute
of Child Health and Human Development, National
Institutes of Health, Bethesda, Maryland, U.S.A.

INTRODUCTION

The genes coding for human chorionic gonadotropin (hCG) constitute a particularly valuable system for exploration of the molecular events underlying changes in gene expression during both fetal development and tumorigenesis. HCG is a glycoprotein tropic hormone consisting of two dissimilar, non-covalently linked polypeptide subunits: α (hCGα) and β (hCGβ) (Morgan and Canfield, 1971). This peptide hormone is normally synthesized by the placental syncytiotrophoblasts (Midgley and Pierce, 1962; Dreskin et al., 1970). However, ectopic synthesis of hCG and its subunits has been demonstrated in many nontrophoblastic tumors and tumor-derived cell lines (Tashjian et al., 1973; Rosen and Weintraub, 1974; Rosen et al., 1975; Ghosh and Cox, 1976; Chou et al., 1976; Lieblich et al., 1976). The appearance of these proteins in nontrophoblastic tumors indicates a radical change in the control mechanism for the synthesis of these proteins after transformation (Rosen et al., 1975).

HCG and its subunits are synthesized eutopically by placental cells and choriocarcinoma cells (malignant cells derived from the cancer of the placental trophoblasts), and ectopically by many nontrophoblastic tumor cells. The control mechanism for the synthesis in various types of cells may differ, however, and may correlate with the origin and physiological states of the cells. To understand the regulation of the synthesis of these proteins in normal and neoplastic cells, it is necessary to have a valid control system in which to study placental functions. Placental explants and primary cultures are difficult to establish and cannot be maintained for a long time in tissue culture. Since human tumors and tumor-derived cell lines are capable of producing "eutopic" proteins, which are

317

synthesized normally by the tissue from which the tumor originated (Pattillo and Gey, 1968; Kohler et al., 1969; Kohler and Bridson, 1971), cultured choriocarcinoma cells have been used to study placental functions. However, abnormally high levels of hCG have been routinely observed in choriocarcinoma patients (Vaitukaitis et al., 1976). These cells, therefore, would not be expected to control the synthesis of hCG as does the placenta in vivo. We have established stable cloned human placental cell lines by the transformation of normal placental cells with the A mutants of simian virus 40 (SV40 tsA mutants) that are temperature-sensitive (ts) in the gene required for maintenance of transformation (Chou, 1978a; Chou, 1978b; Chou, 1979). The expression of differentiated functions in these placental cells can be controlled by changing the growth temperature. The tsA-transformed cells behave like transformed cells at the permissive temperature (33°C) and like nontransformed differentiated cells at the restrictive temperature (40°C). Studies were undertaken to delineate the control mechanism for the synthesis of hCG and hCGα in tsA-transformed placental cells (grown at 33°C and 40°C), choriocarcinoma cells, and nontrophoblastic tumor cells. The control mechanism was most readily apparent when cells were exposed to agents that affect cellular differentiation. In these studies, the agents were sodium butyrate, 5-bromo-2'-deoxyuridine (BrdUrd), and adenosine cyclic nucleotides. Our data suggest that the synthesis of hCG in choriocarcinoma cells and of hCGα in nontrophoblastic tumor cells may be regulated abnormally.

CELL LINES AND METHODS OF CULTURE

Cloned choriocarcinoma cells, JEG-3 (Kohler and Bridson, 1971) and Reid (Kohler, P. O., unpublished results), were grown in Ham's F-12 medium. The uncloned choriocarcinoma line, BeWo (Pattillo and Gey, 1968), the pulmonary carcinoma line, ChaGo (Tashjian et al., 1973), the three HeLa lines (a carcinoma of the cervix; Gey et al., 1952), HeLa CCL2, HeLa S$_3$, and HeLa 65, and the SV40 tsA mutant-transformed human placental cells were grown in α-modified minimal essential medium (αMEM). ChaGo was obtained from Dr. S. W. Rosen; HeLa CCL2 and HeLa S$_3$ (HeLa CCL 2.2) were obatined from the American Type Culture Collection; and HeLa 65 was obtained from Dr. G. Melnykovych. Choriocarcinoma cells and nontrophoblastic tumor cells were grown at 37°C in medium supplemented with 10% fetal bovine serum, streptomycin (100 μg/ml) and penicillin (100 U/ml). Media and serum were obtained from Flow Laboratories, McLean, Virginia.

ESTABLISHMENT AND TRANSFORMATION OF HUMAN PLACENTAL CELLS

Nontransformed human first-trimester (SP) and term placental (TP) cells were obtained by collagenase (0.1%, Worthington Biochemical Co., Freehold, NJ) digestion of human first-trimester or term placentas. The primary SP or TP cells were grown at 37°C in αMEM supplemented with 10% fetal bovine serum (αMEM-10). Primary SP cells and secondary TP cells (passage 2) were infected with a temperature-sensitive A mutant (tsA) of SV40 (multiplicity of infection = 5-10). Medium supplemented with 4% fetal bovine serum (αMEM-4) was then added to the infected flask, and the cells were incubated at 33°C. After 24 hr of incubation, the cells were subcultured at various densitites. Medium (αMEM-4) was replaced twice weekly. Clones were identifiable after 4-5 weeks and were selected and purified by growing in low-serum medium (MEM-4) at low cell density. Seven independent transformants were established from the same first-trimester placenta, and more than 30 transformants were established from the same term placenta. Cultures of SP or TP cells were transformed by viral mutants A255, A30, or A209. Mutants tsA255, tsA30, and tsA209 are independent isolates of the SV40 A gene (Tegtmeyer and Ozer, 1971; Tegtmeyer, 1972; Chou and Martin, 1974). The A function of SV40 is required for the maintenance of the transformed phenotype (Brugge and Butel, 1975; Martin and Chou, 1975; Osborn and Weber, 1975; Tegtmeyer, 1975). The transformed cell lines are identified by their SP or TP origin, the transforming virus, and their isolation number. The transformed lines were thus designated: SPA255-23, SPA255-26, SPA255-27, TPA30-1, TPA30-6, and TPA209-9.

The SV40-transformed cell lines had chromosome numbers from the near diploid to the near tetraploid range. The glucose-6-phosphate dehydrogenase in these SV40-transformed placental cell lines was of the B type, as demonstrated by Cellogel electrophoresis (Rittazzi et al., 1971).

These transformed placental cells shed SV40; anti-SV40 serum (1%; Flow Laboratories) was therefore routinely added to the culture media to inhibit plaque formation.

In nearly 100% of the cells in all lines, T-antigen was clearly localized within the nucleus, as revealed by the immunofluorescence technique.

Growth Properties

Nontransformed SP or TP cells grew at nearly the same rate at 33°C or 40°C, and stopped growing at low saturation densities. The SV40-transformed first-trimester or term placental cells proliferated in culture, formed multilayered sheets, and grew to high cell densities at the permissive temperature (33°C; Figure 1). At the non-permissive temperature (40°C), the transformed cells behaved like normal placental cells; they grew slowly and to lower saturation densities. When cultures in the mid-exponential phase were shifted from 33°C to 40°C, growth of the tsA-mutant transformed cells was inhibited within 24 hr (Figure 1). When cultures grown at 40°C for

three days were shifted to 33°C, an increase in the growth rate
was seen in the tsA-transformed cell lines after a 24-48 hr lag.

Cloning efficiencies and overgrowth of normal cell layers were
temperature-sensitive for the tsA-transformed placental cells. At
40°C, colony formation was markedly inhibited and these tsA-transformed cells could not overgrow normal placental monolayers. These
cells therefore have the advantage of behaving like normal cells
(at 40°C), but not the disadvantages of primary placental cells,
which dedifferentiate in culture.

Induction of the Synthesis of hCG and hCGα in SV40 tsA-Transformed
Placental Cells at the Restrictive Temperature

HCG and hCGα are synthesized throughout gestation by the normal
placenta. The precise rates of synthesis by first-trimester and
term placenta, however, have not been determined. Secondary SP and
TP cells synthesize no detectable hCG at either temperature. Measurable amount of hCGα, however, were synthesized by these nontransformed SP and TP cells, and more hCGα was synthesized at 40°C
than at 33°C. The tsA-transformed SP or TP cell lines synthesized
hCG and hCGα, as demonstrated by radioimmunoassays with antisera to
hCGβ and hCGα (Figure 2). The anti-hCGα serum measures hCGα, and
the anti-hCGβ serum measures both hCGβ and hCG. The tsA-transformed
first-trimester and term placental cells synthesized low levels of
hCG and hCGα at the permissive temperature (33°C). At the restrictive temperature (40°C), the transformed phenotype is lost, and the
levels of these proteins are stimulated (Figure 2).

Over 90% of the hCGα and hCG plus hCGβ in the culture medium
was adsorbed to a column of Con A-Sepharose (concanavalin-A Sepharose;
Figure 3A). The immunoreactive proteins synthesized by these cells
are, therefore, glycoproteins, as are urinary hCG and its subunits.
The glycoproteins eluted from the Con A-Sepharose column were
measured by hCG receptor-binding activity by the radioreceptor
assay (Figure 4A). The slope of the dose-response curve for the
material eluted from Con A-Sepharose was indistinguishable from that
for urinary hCG. The receptor-active material, hCG, represented
only 20% of the hCG plus hCGβ estimated by the radioimmunoassay.

The hCGα and hCG plus hCGβ eluted from Con A-Sepharose were
subjected to gel filtration on a Sephadex G-100 column (Figure 3B).
The majority of the hCG plus hCGβ immunoreactive material co-eluted
with hCGβ. The hCGβ produced by the transformants was heterogeneous
in size; the main hCGβ peak eluted slightly behind the purified
urinary hCGβ. The hCGα produced by the transformants was also
heterogeneous in size; the main peak, however, co-eluted with urinary
hCGα. In addition to the hCGα in the main peak, hCGα-immunoreactive

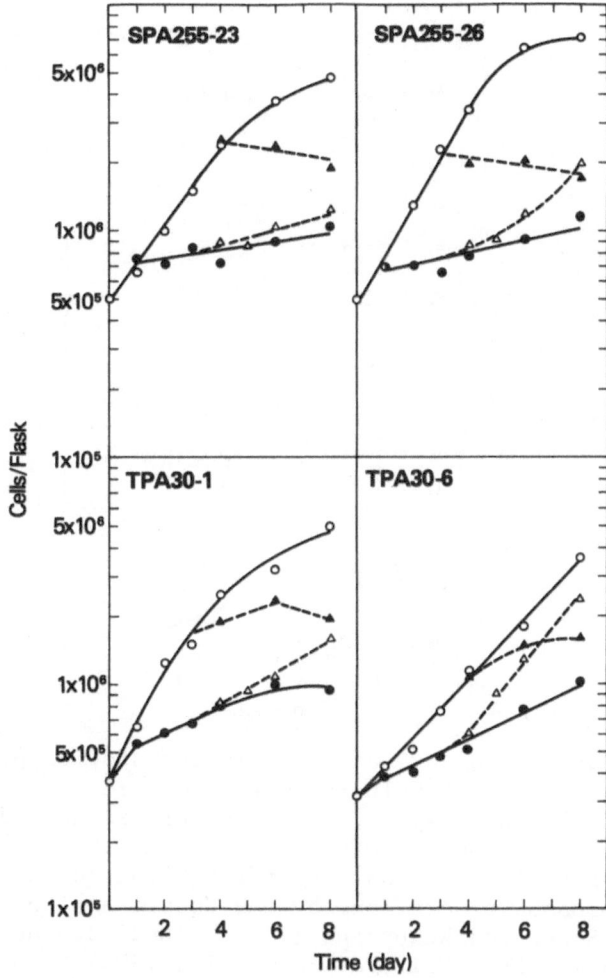

Figure 1. Growth of transformed cells at permissive (33°C) and restrictive (40°C) temperature. Cells were grown in αMEM-10 and medium was changed every other day. After three days, some of the cultures were shifted from 40°C to 33°C, or from 33°C to 40°C. Cells were counted with a Celloscope 112TH (Paricle Data, Inc., Elmhurst, Ill.). 0 = 33°C; ● = 40°C; Δ = cultures shifted from 40°C to 33°C; ▲ = cultures shifted from 33°C to 40°C.

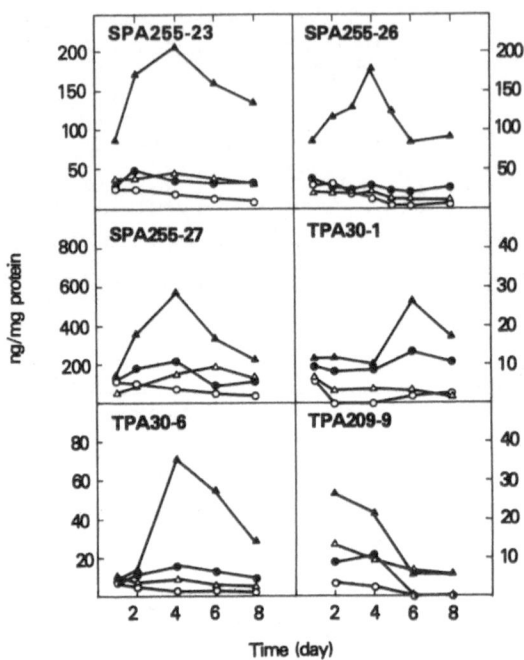

Figure 2.   Synthesis of hCG and hCGα in transformed placental cells
grown at 33°C and 40°C.   Cultures were grown in αMEM-10.   Beginning
one day after plating (day 0), cultures were incubated at 33°C or
40°C.   Medium was changed every two days.   At the indicated times,
medium from each flask was assayed for hCG and for hCGα separately.
All radioimmunoassays were done by the double-antibody technique
described by Rosen and Weintraub (1974).   Antisera used were:
anti-hCGβ serum (Sb6) (Vaitukaitis et al., 1972), and anti-hCGα
serum (CA3) (Chou et al., 1977).   Purified preparations of hCG
(CR119, 11,600 IU/mg, ventral prostate weight assay, Second
International Standard hCG), and of hCGα (CR117) were radioiodinated
and used as standards and tracers.   hCG (CR119) had 1-3% cross-
reactivity in the hCGα assay; hCGα had 0.02-0.05% crossreactivity
in the hCG assay.   Complete medium not exposed to cells had no
detectable hCG, hCGβ, or hCGα.   Antisera, standard hCG, hCGβ, and
hCGα were kindly provided by K. Catt, G. Hodgen, and H. Chen.
0 = hCG, 33°C;   ● = hCG, 40°C;   Δ = hCGα, 33°C;   ▲ = hCGα, 40°C.

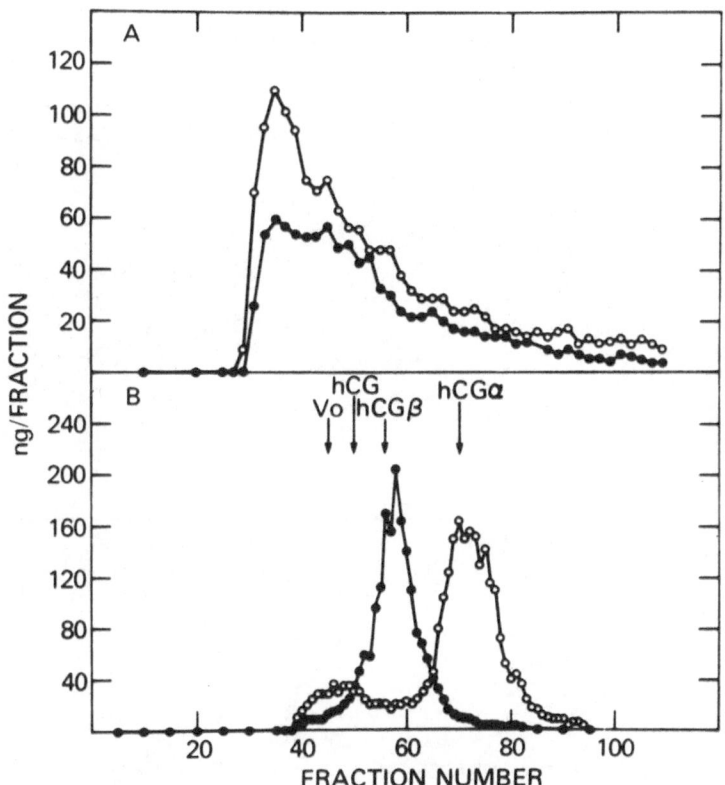

Figure 3. (A) Con A-Sepharose column chromatography of hCG in culture media from SPA255-27 cells. HCG and its subunits were purified from culture medium with Con A-Sepharose (Pharmacia, Sweden) that had been equilibrated with Dulbeco's balanced salt solution supplemented with 1mM $MgCl_2$, and 1 mM $MnCl_2$. The medium plus Con A-Sepharose was stirred overnight at 4°C and was poured into a 2.4 x 20 cm column. The column was washed with phosphate-buffered saline and the bound proteins were eluted with phosphate-buffered saline containing 0.5 M methyl-α-D-glucopyranoside. (B) Sephadex G-100 chromatographic patterns of hCG produced by SPA255-27 cells. Fractions 27-90 from the Con A-Sepharose column were pooled, concentrated, and applied to the Sephadex G-100 column (1.5 x 125 cm) equilibrated with phosphate-buffered saline at 4°C. The arrow marked V_O indicates the void volume. The migration positions of hCG, hCGβ, and hCGα in this column were determined separately and are indicated by the respective arrows. 0 = hCGα; ● = hCG plus hCGβ.

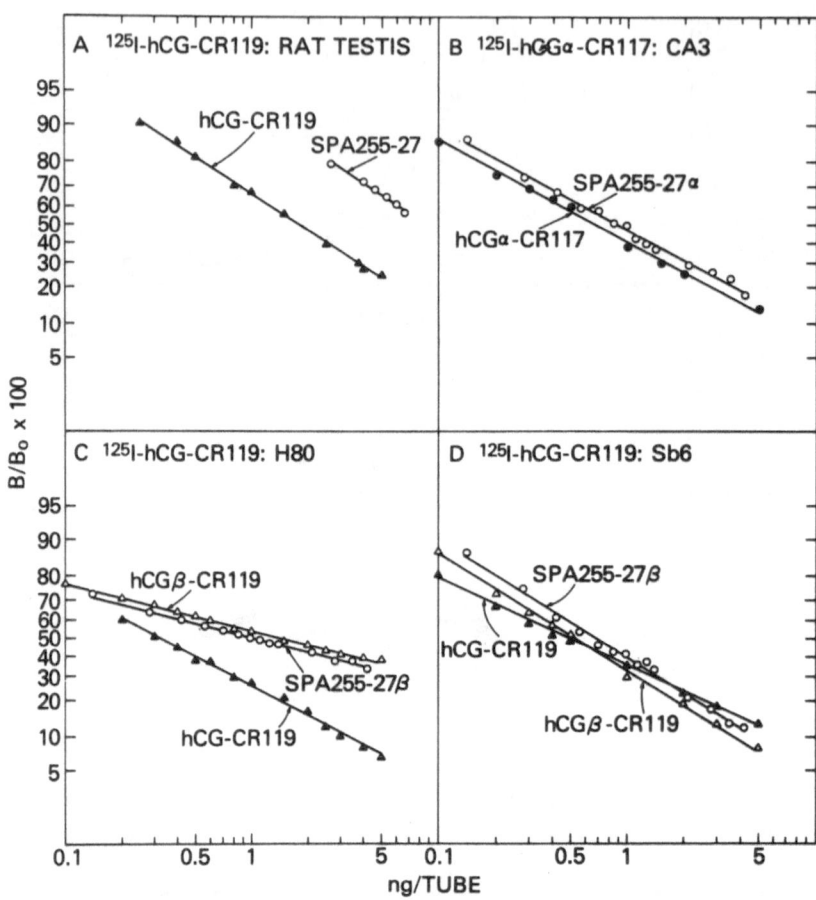

Figure 4. Dose-response curves of hCG, hCGα and hCGβ synthesized by the transformed placental cells in a radioreceptor assay or in a radioimmunoassay system. The radioreceptor assay for hCG was performed by the method of Catt et al. (1972), with a crude rat testis homogenate as the source of receptor. Anti-hCG serum (H80) (Chen et al., 1976) was kindly provided by H. Chen.

material appeared also as a broad peak in the void volume of the column. The nature of this material is not known; it is, however, possible that it represents the precursor of hCGα.

The immunological determinants of the proteins synthesized by the transformed placental cells were compared with the urinary hCG and its subunits (Figure 4). The slope of dose-response curve for the hCGα purified form SPA255-27 medium was indistinguishable from that for urinary hCGα (Figure 4B). The slopes of dose-response curves for the hCGα-like material in unfractionated media from all other transformants were also indistinguishable from that for urinary hCGα. The dose-response curve for hCGβ purified from SPA255-27 medium paralleled the inhibition line of urinary hCGβ in the presence of either anti-hCG-antiserum H80 (Figure 4C) or anti-hCGβ-antiserum Sb6 (Figure 4D). The dose-response curve for the purified hCGβ did not parallel the inhibition line of native hCG.

Increase of Alkaline Phosphatase Activity in SV40 tsA-Transformed Placental Cells at the Restrictive Temperature

Placental alkaline phosphatase is synthesized by trophoblastic cells: one form of the enzyme is characteristic of term placenta, and the second form is characteristic of first-trimester placenta (Fishman et al., 1976; Sakiyama et al., 1979). These two phosphatases differ in their physiochemical and immunological properties (Sakiyama et al., 1979). The first-trimester enzyme can be inactivated by anti-serum to liver alkaline phosphatase, but not by antiserum to the term placental enzyme. The reverse is true for the term-placental alkaline phosphatase. The specific enzyme activities in term and first-trimester placenta are approximately 1000 and 1 nmole P_i released/min/mg protein, respectively.

Alkaline phosphatase activity in tsA-mutant transformed cells grown at 33°C was lower than that in term placenta (Figure 5). Phosphatase activity in these cells was greatly increased at 40°C.

The alkaline phosphatases synthesized by the tsA-transformed first-trimester and term placental cells were not inactivated by antiserum to term placental alkaline phosphatase, but were inactivated by antiserum to liver alkaline phosphatase. Therefore, only first-trimester placental alkaline phosphatase was induced in these placental cells.

The alkaline phosphatase activities in tsA-transformed term placental lines grown at 40°C were considerably higher than those of tsA-transformed first-trimester placental lines. The alkaline phosphatase activities of term and first-trimester placental cells were proportional to the activities of this enzyme in vivo in placentas at these two stages of gestation.

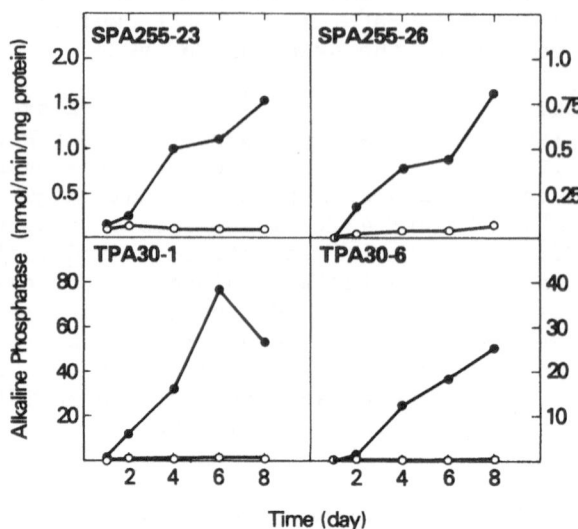

Time (day)

Figure 5.   Alkaline phosphatase activities in transformed placental cells grown at 33°C and 40°C. Cultures were grown in MEM-10 beginning one day after plating (day 0). Medium was changed every two days. Cells were harvested by scraping with a rubber policeman. The pellet was suspended in buffer (0.01 M Tris-HCl, pH 7.4, 0.15 M KCl) and the cells were ruptured by sonication (Raytheon Magneto-strictive Oscillator, Model DF-101, 250-W, 10 kHz, Raytheon Company, Manchester, N.H.) for 2 min at maximal power. The sonicates were centrifuged at 10,000 x g for 15 min; the supernatant solutions were used immediately for measurement of alkaline phosphatase. Alkaline phosphatase activity was measured by the release of p-nitrophenol from p-nitrophenyl phosphate at pH 10.7 and 37°C (Edlow et al., 1975). Protein was determined by the method of Lowry et al. (1951).

Summary and Comments

A model system has been developed by the transformation of normal human placental cells with temperature-sensitive A mutants of SV40. At the permissive temperature (33°C), these cells behave like transformed cells permitting propagation and cloning. At the restrictive temperature (40°C), however, the transformed phenotype is lost and these cells regain their normal trophoblastic behavior: they do not form clones, do not overgrow a nontransformed placental monolayer, and morphologically appear nontransformed. Likewise, with respect to hCG, hCGα, and placental alkaline phosphatase, the tsA-transformed placental cells behave like transformed (dedifferentiated) cells at the permissive temperature and like normal trophoblastic cellas at the restrictive temperature.

The glycoproteins hCG, hCGα, and hCGβ made by the transformed cells were indistinguishable from the urinary glycoproteins hCG, hCGα, and hCGβ by gel chromatography and immunological reactivity. The alkaline phosphatases produced by the first-trimester and term-placental transformants were, however, the same as the first-trimester placental enzyme. The proteins made by the transformed cells therefore appear to be authentic placental proteins. This model system should prove advantageous in further study of gene regulation and cellular differentiation, since both the malignant and normal states may be studied with the same clone of cells.

The availability of the tsA-transformed placental cells enables us to compare the effect of sodium butyrate, 5-bromo-2'-deoxyuridine (BrdUrd), and adenosine cyclic nucleotides on the synthesis of hCG and hCGα by transformed placental cells, choriocarcinoma cells, and nontrophoblastic tumor cells.

EFFECT OF SODIUM BUTYRATE ON THE SYNTHESIS OF HCG AND HCGα

Butyric acid, a four carbon fatty acid, occurs naturally in the body. In mammalian cells, sodium butyrate inhibits histone deacetylation (Candido et al., 1978; Sealy and Chalkley, 1978; Boffa et al., 1978; Vidali et al., 1978), inhibits cell proliferation, and induces morphological changes (Ginsburg et al., 1973; Altenburg et al., 1976; Henneberry and Fishman, 1976; Prasad and Sinha, 1976). In addition to inducing alkaline phophatase activity (Griffen et al., 1974; Chou and Robinson, 1977b), sodium butyrate increases the production of adenylate cyclase (Prasad and Sinha, 1976) and sialyltransferase (Fishman et al., 1974). This fatty acid suppresses the neoplastic state of Syrian hamster cells (Leavitt et al., 1978) and causes Friend erythroleukemic cells to synthesize globin (Leader and Leader, 1975). We tested the effects of sodium butyrate on the synthesis of hCGα and hCG in the various types of hCG-producing human cell lines, since this compound had been shown to induce hCG synthesis in certain HeLa cells (Ghosh and Cox, 1976).

In the absence of inducer, both choriocarcinoma cells (JEG-3, Reid, and BeWo) and nontrophoblastic tumor cells (HeLa CCL2, HeLa S_3 and ChaGo) produced hCGα. The trophoblastic tumor cell lines produced hCGα at roughly comparable rates (Figure 6), but the nontrophoblastic tumor cell lines produced hCGα at widely differing rates (Figure 7). The basal production of complete hCG by the nontrophoblastic tumor cell lines was quite small compared with its production by the choriocarcinoma cell lines. Sodium butyrate has strikingly different effects on the two classes of tumor cells: it

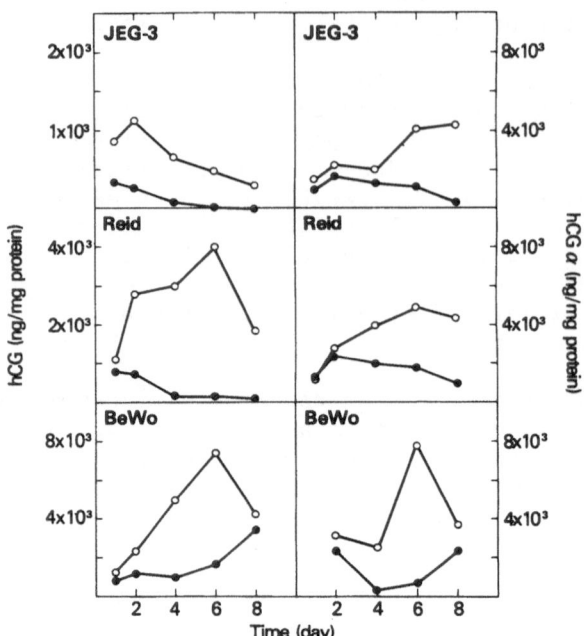

Figure 6.   Effect of sodium butyrate on the synthesis of hCG and hCGα in choriocarcinoma cells. Cultures were grown at 37°C and media were replaced every two days. At the indicated time, the media from two flasks were separately assayed for hCG and hCGα. The average values are reported here. 0 = control; ● = 2 mM sodium butyrate.

induces synthesis of hCGα and hCG in the nontrophoblastic tumor cells, but represses the synthesis in the trophoblastic cells (Figures 6 and 7). Because sodium butyrate has differential effects on synthesis of hCGα and hCG, sodium butyrate might be more toxic for the choriocarcinoma cells than the nontrophoblastic tumor cells. This is unlikely, however, for two reasons. Sodium butyrate inhibited the incorporation of uridine and leucine at roughly the same degree in JEG-3 amd HeLa S_3 cells. Although sodium butyrate slightly enhanced the incorporation of thymidine in JEG-3 cells but transiently inhibited the incorporation in HeLa S_3 cells, the long term effects seemed to be the same for both types of tumor cells (Chou et al., 1977). The placental isoenzyme of alkaline phosphatase was induced by this compound in all cell lines examined (Griffin et al., 1974; Chou et al., 1977).

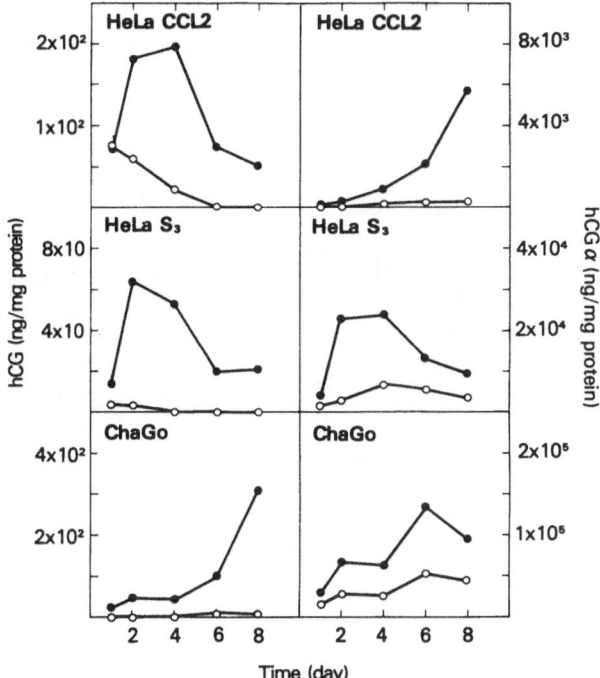

Figure 7. Effect of sodium butyrate on the synthesis of hCG and hCGα in nontrophoblastic tumor cells. The culture conditions were the same as in Figure 6. 0 = control; ● = 2 mM sodium butyrate.

The regulation of the synthesis of hCG and hCGα by sodium butyrate in the tsA-transformed human placental cells was studied both at the permissive temperature (33°C) and at the restrictive temperature (40°C). In the presence of sodium butyrate at 33°C, the synthesis of hCG, as well as hCGα, was strongly induced in the tsA-transformed first-trimester (SPA255-26; Figure 8) and term (TP30-6; Figure 9) placental cells. At 40°C, hCG synthesis was also induced by sodium butyrate, although to a lesser extent than at 33°C. HCGα synthesis, on the other hand, was inhibited by sodium butyrate at 40°C. Similar results were obtained with either term or first-trimester transformants, although the inhibition was more evident in the first-trimester transformants. Therefore, in the presence of sodium butyrate, the regulation of hCG synthesis in choriocarcinoma cells and the regulation of hCGα synthesis in nontrophoblastic tumor cells differ from the regulation in the tsA-transformed placental cells grown at the restrictive temperature.

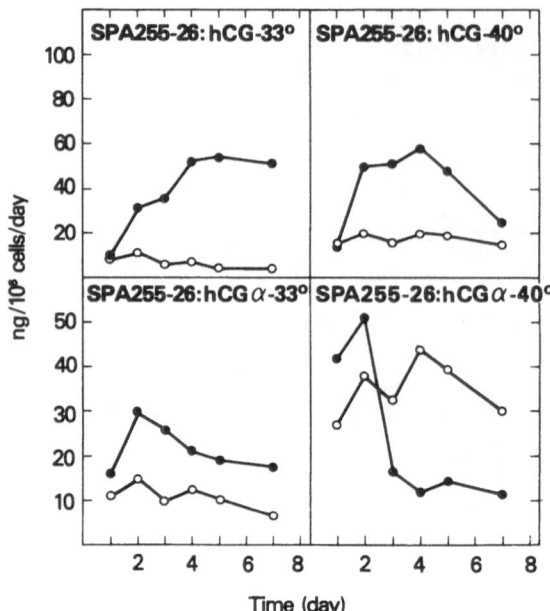

Figure 8. Effect of sodium butyrate on the synthesis of hCG and hCGα in SPA255-26 cells grown at 33°C and 40°C. Cultures were grown in the absence or presence of sodium butyrate and were incubated at 33°C or 40°C. Medium was changed every day. At the indicated times, the media from two flasks were assayed separately for hCG and hCGα. The average values are reported here. 0 = control; ● = 2 mM sodium butyrate.

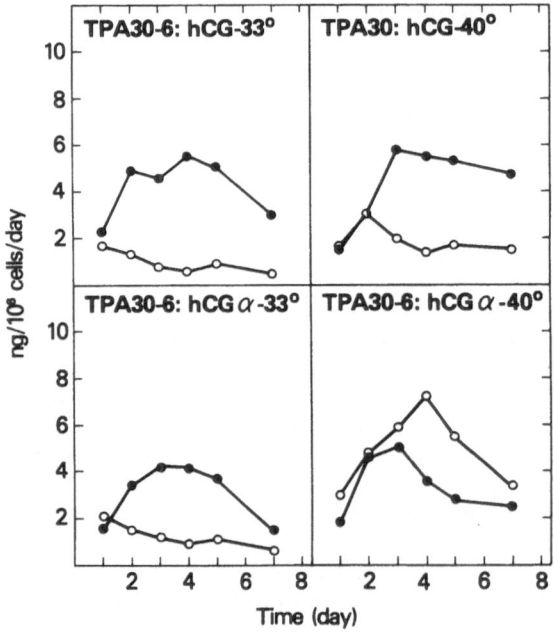

Figure 9. Effect of sodium butyrate on the synthesis of hCG and hCGα in TPA30-6 cells grown at 33°C and 40°C. The culture conditions were the same as in Figure 8. 0 = control; ● = 2 mM sodium butyrate.

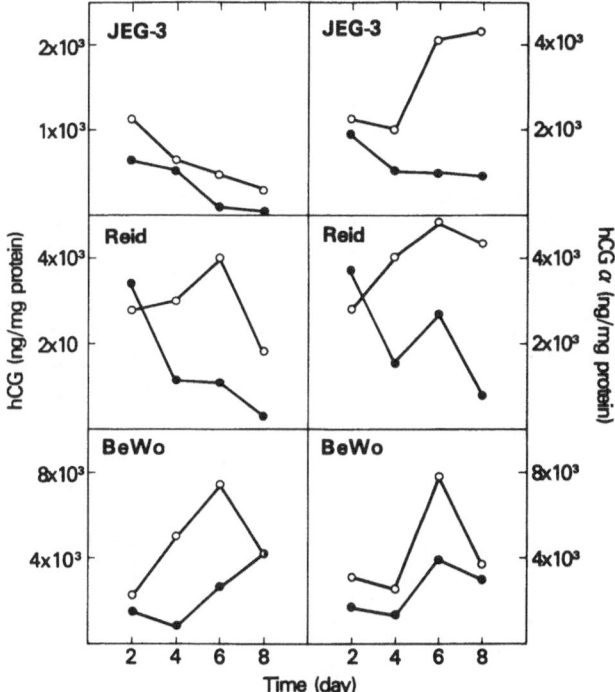

Figure 10. Effect of BrdUrd on the synthesis of hCG and hCGα in choriocarcinoma cells. Cultures were grown at 37°C and media were changed every two days. At the indicated times, the media from two flasks were separately assayed for hCG and hCGα. The average values are reported here. 0 = control; ● = 10/ μg/ml of BrdUrd.

EFFECT OF BRDURD ON THE SYNTHESIS OF HCG AND HCGα

5-Bromo-2'-deoxyuridine (BrdUrd) is incorporated readily into DNA in place of thymidine both in vivo and in vitro. Studies of *lac* represser binding to synthetic DNA and BrdUrd-substituted *lac* operator led Lin and Riggs (1971; 1972) to conclude that the replacement of the 5-methyl group of thymidine with a bromine atom results in tighter binding of this regulatory protein to DNA. BrdUrd selectively blocks the expression of differentiated functions without greatly affecting other cellular processes such as division and growth (Bischoff and Holtzer, 1970; Mayne et al., 1971; Stellwagen and Tamkins. 1971). This analogue causes loss of the tumorigenic properties of melanoma cells coincident with loss of capacity to synthesize melanin (Salagi and Bruce, 1970). BrdUrd also has been reported to induce provirus, to activate the release

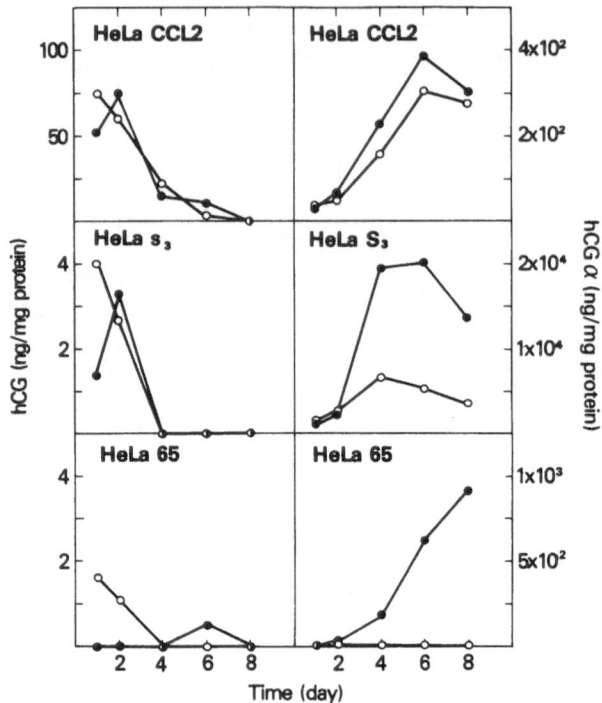

Figure 11.   Effect of BrdUrd on the synthesis of hCG and hCGα in nontrophoblastic tumor cells. The culture conditions were the same as in Figure 10.   0 = control; ● = 10 μg/ml of Brd Urd.

of virus in a variety of virus-transformed cells (Lowy et al., 1971; Aaronsen et al., 1971), and to induce alkaline phosphatase in mammalian cells (Koyama and Ono, 1972; Edlow et al., 1975; Chou and Robinson, 1977a).

In the presence of BrdUrd, synthesis of hCG and hCGα was inhibited in choriocarcinoma cell lines (Figure 10). The effect of BRDUrd on hCG synthesis usually paralleled its effects on hCGα synthesis in these cells. In contrast to its inhibitory effects in choriocarcinoma cells, BrdUrd induced hCGα synthesis in nontrophoblastic tumor cell lines (Figure 11). In the absence of inducer, very little hCG was synthesized by any of the nontrophoblastic tumor cell lines. BrdUrd did not affect the synthesis of complete hCG in any of the nontrophoblastic tumor cells (Figure 11). The different responses of trophoblastic versus nontrophoblastic tumor cells to BrdUrd suggest that the regulation of the synthesis of hCG and hCGα differs in the two types of tumor cells.

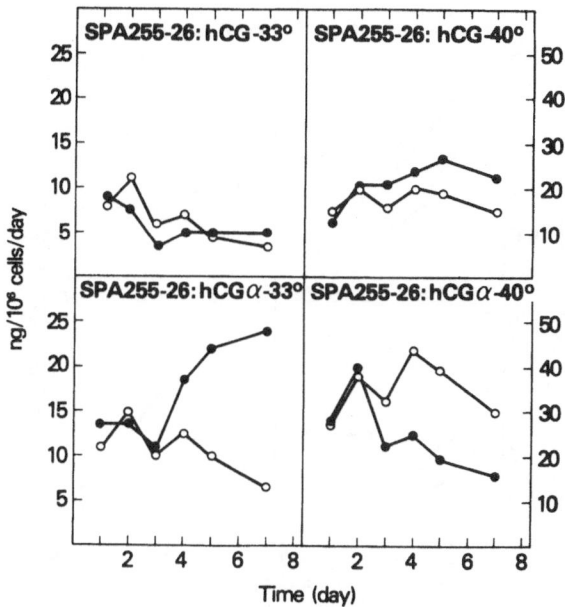

Figure 12. Effect of BrdUrd on the synthesis of hCG and hCGα in SPA255-26 cells grown at 33°C and 40°C. Cultures were grown in the absence and in the presence of BrdUrd and were incubated at 33°C and 40°C. Medium was changed every day. At the indicated times the media from two flasks were assayed separately for hCG and hCGα. The average values are reported here. 0 = control; ● = 10 µg/ml of BrdUrd.

The differential effects of BrdUrd on synthesis of hCG and hCGα are not due to BrdUrd-induced cytotoxicity. Growth of choriocarcinoma cells with BrdUrd inhibited the rate of RNA, DNA, and protein synthesis only slightly (Chou and Robinson, 1977a). Furthermore, BrdUrd has been shown to stimulate placental alkaline phophatase activity in choriocarcinoma cells and HeLa cells (Edlow et al., 1975; Bulmer et al., 1976; Chou and Robinson, 1977a).

Regulation of the synthesis of hCG and hCGα by BrdUrd in the tsA-transformed human placental cells was also studied both at 33°C and at 40°C. In the presence of BrdUrd at 33°C, synthesis of hCG was not induced in transformed first-trimester placental cells (SPA255-26; Figure 12), but was induced in transformed term placental cells (TPA30-6; Figure 13). At 33°C hCGα synthesis was induced by BrdUrd in both SPA255-26 and TPA30-6 cells.

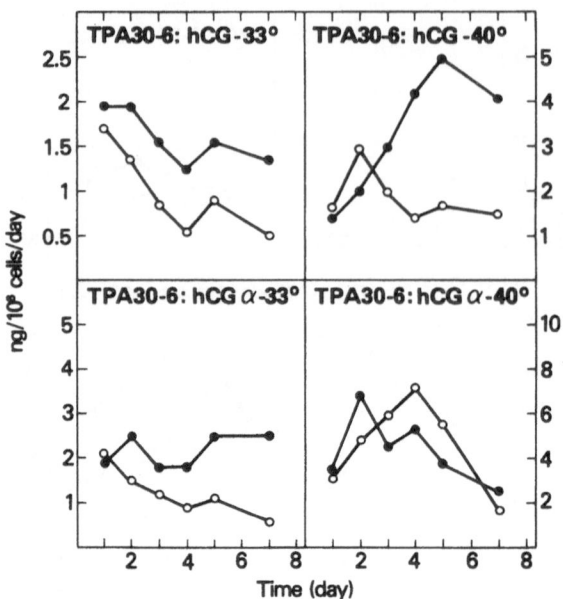

Figure 13. Effect of BrdUrd on the synthesis of hCG and hCGα in TPA30-6 cells grown at 33°C and 40°C. The culture conditions were the same as in Figure 12. 0 = control; ● = 10 µg/ml of BrdUrd.

In the presence of BrdUrd at 40°C, hCG synthesis was induced in both transformed first-trimester and term placental cells (Figures 12 and 13). HCGα synthesis in the transformed cells at 40°C was inhibited by BrdUrd.

Data presented here further corroborate the finding that the regulation of the synthesis of hCG in choriocarcinoma cells and the regulation of the synthesis of hCGα in nontrophoblastic tumor cells differ from the regulation in the tsA-transformed placental cells grown at the restrictive temperature.

EFFECT OF ADENOSINE CYCLIC NUCLEOTIDES ON THE SYNTHESIS OF HCG AND HCGα

It has been demonstrated that hCG secretion in malignant tro-phoblastic cells can be induced by dibutyryl cyclic AMP (Bt$_2$cAMP; Story et al., 1974; Hussa et al., 1975). We have extended these observations and demonstrated that synthesis of the α subunit of hCG, like synthesis of the complete hormone, is also induced by

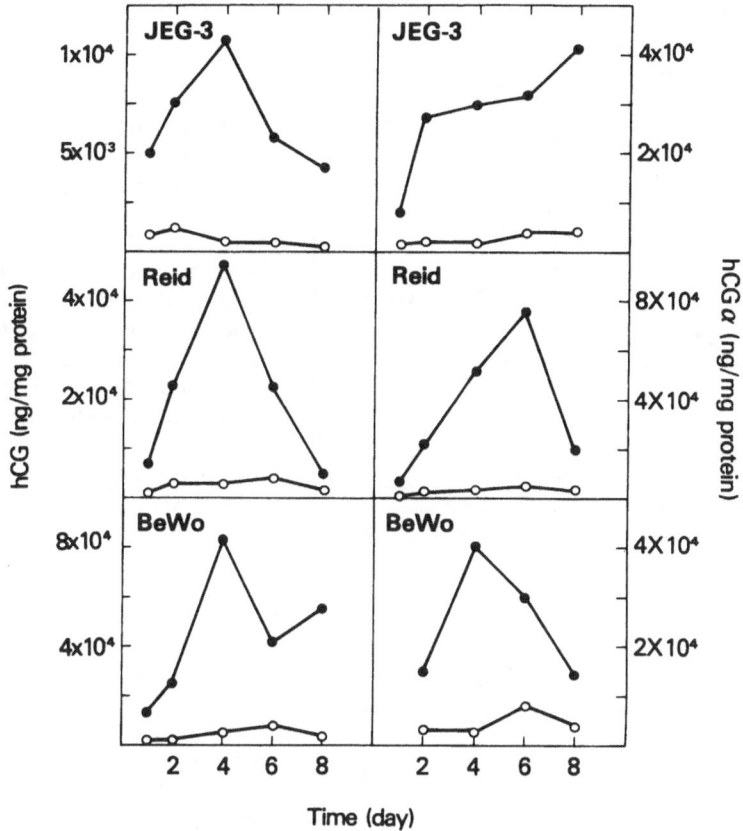

Figure 14.   Effect of Bt_2cAMP on the synthesis of hCG and $hCG\alpha$ in choriocarcinoma cells. Cultures were grown at 37°C and media were changed every two days. At the indicated times, the media from two flasks were separately assayed for hCG and $hCG\alpha$. The average values are reported here. 0 = control; ● = s mM Bt_2cAMP.

Bt_2cAMP (Figure 14). Since butyric acid cleaved from Bt_2cAMP affects the synthesis of hCG and $hCG\alpha$ in choriocarcinoma cells, nontrophoblastic tumor cells, and transformed placental cells (Chou et al., 1977; Hussa et al., 1978), 8BrcAMP was employed in experiments performed subsequently.

8BrcAMP, like Bt_2cAMP, induced the synthesis of hCG as well as $hCG\alpha$ in JEG-3 choriocarcinoma cells (Figure 15). The synthesis of hCG was decreased and the synthesis of $hCG\alpha$ was increased during growth of uninduced JEG cells in culture (Figure 15). The ratio of

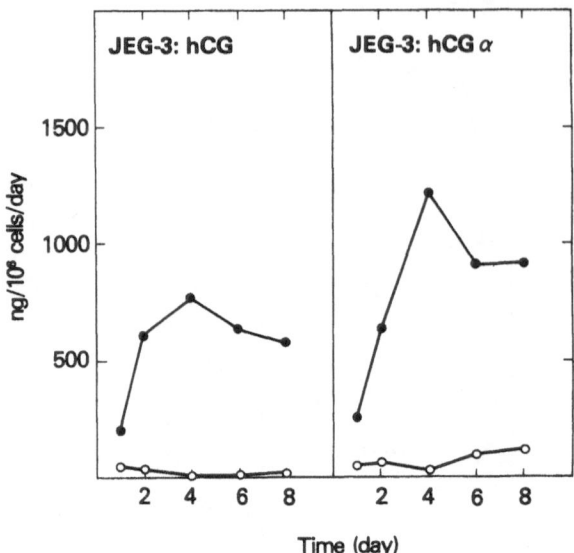

Figure 15. Effect of 8BrcAMP on the synthesis of hCG and hCGα in JEG-3 choriocarcinoma cells. Cultures were grown in the absence and presence of 8BrcAMP and medium was changed every day. At the indicated times, the media from two flasks were assayed separately for hCG and hCGα. The average values are reported here. 0 = control; ● = 1 mM 8BrcAMP.

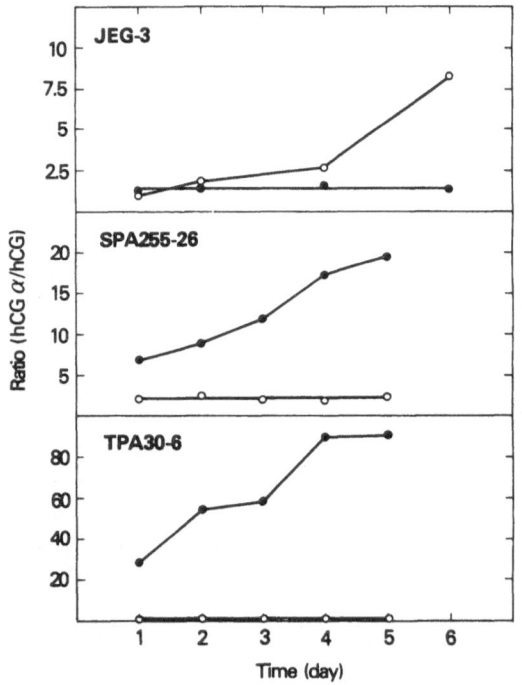

Figure 16. Effect of 8BrcAMP on the relative amounts of hCGα and hCG synthesized by JEG-3 choriocarcinoma cells, SPA255-26 cells, and TPA30-6 cells. The experimental conditions were the same as in Figures 15, 17, and 18. 0 = control; ● = 1 mM 8 BrcAMP.

TABLE I: Effect of 8BrcAMP on the synthesis of hCG and hCGα in HeLa S_3 cells.

Addition	hCG	hCGα
	ng/mg protein	
None	1.3	11,660
8BrcAMP	4.7	10,633

Cultures were exposed to 8BrcAMP for three days with no medium change. HCG and hCGα in the media were determined by radioimmunoassay.

hCGα to hCG in these cells, therefore, increased with growth (Figure 16). In the presence of 8BrcAMP, however, the levels of hCGα and hCG were maintained at nearly a constant ratio regardless of the growth stage of the cells (Figures 15 and 16). Growth of JEG-3 cells in the presence of 8BrcAMP, therefore, prevented these cells from synthesizing excess amounts of hCGα. 8BrcAMP, on the other hand, slightly induced the synthesis of hCG, but did not affect the synthesis of hCGα in HeLa S_3 nontrophoblastic tumor cells (Table I).

In the tsA-transformed first-trimester and term placental cells, 8BrcAMP induced hCGα synthesis at 33°C as well as at 40°C (Figures 17 and 18). At 33°C, hCG synthesis in the transformed placental cells was slightly induced by 8BrcAMP (Figures 17 and 18). At 40°C 8BrcAMP inhibited the synthesis of hCG after two or more days exposure. The decline in hCG synthesis at 40°C might have resulted from 8BrcAMP-induced cytotoxicity. On the other hand, in the same culture, hCGα synthesis was greatly induced by 8BrcAMP at 40°C.

The difference between choriocarcinoma cells and the tsA-transformed placental cells was more evident when the data were expressed as the ratio of hCGα to hCG (Figure 16). In the presence of 8BrcAMP, the ratio of hCGα to hCG (as compared with the control uninduced cultures) in the tsA-transformed placental cells increased, whereas the ratio decreased in choriocarcinoma cells.

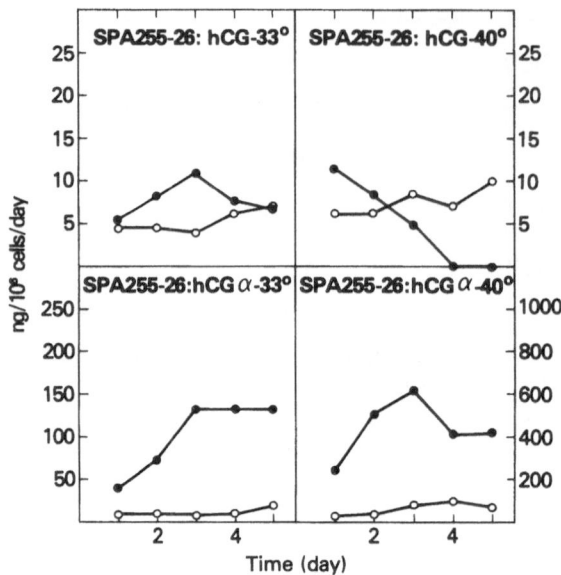

Figure 17. Effect of 8BrcAMP on the synthesis of hCG and hCGα in SPA255-26 cells grown at 33°C and 40°C. Cultures were grown in the absence and presence of 8BrcAMP, and were incubated at 33°C or 40°C. Medium was changed every day. At the indicated times, the media from two flasks were assayed separately for hCG and hCGα. The average values are reported here. ● = control; O = 1 mM 8BrcAMP.

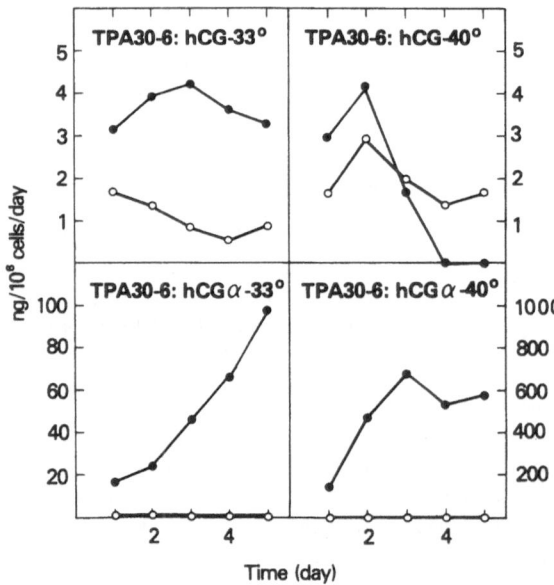

Figure 18. Effect of 8BrcAMP on the synthesis of hCG and hCGα in TPA30-6 cells grown at 33°C and 40°C. The culture conditions were the same as in Figure 17. O = control; ● = 1 mM 8BrcAMP.

GENERAL DISCUSSION

The available evidence suggests that the tsA-transformed human placental cells grown at the restrictive temperature more closely approximate normal placenta than do choriocarcinoma cells. First, hCG synthesis in choriocarcinoma patients may be regulated abnormally, leading to the very high levels of hCG observed in many of these patients (Vaitukaitis et al., 1976). Second, the transformed placental cells described here are induced by a tsA mutant of SV40; the A function of SV40 is required for the maintenance of the transformed phenotype in these cells. These cells can assume either a normal (at 40°C) or a transformed (at 33°C) phenotype. Third, the preservation of the original diploid chromosome number in many of these lines indicates that these cells are closer to normal placental cells than are the aneuploid choriocarcinoma cells. Fourth, SV40-transformed first-trimester placental cells synthesize more hCG plus hCGβ but have lower alkaline phosphatase activity than do the transformed term placental cells. The amounts of hCG plus hCGβ synthesized by the tsA-transformed first-trimester and term placental cells and their corresponding alkaline phosphatase activities were proportional to the amounts of these proteins synthesized in vivo by placentas at their respective periods of gestation. Therefore, transformation of the placental cells by SV40 may not have interfered with the normal control mechanisms for the synthesis of hCG and of alkaline phosphatase.

In conclusion, the tsA-transformed placental cells and choriocarcinoma cells regulate hCG synthesis differently and the tsA-transformed placental cells and nontrophoblastic tumor cells regulated hCG synthesis differently. Since the tsA-transformed placental cells grown at 40°C appear to be a better model system for normal placenta than are choriocarcinoma cells, the synthesis of hCG in choriocarcinoma cells and of hCGα in nontrophoblastic tumor cells may be regulated abnormally.

The nontrophoblastic tumor cells studied were mainly hCGα producers; these nontrophoblastic tumor cells synthesize abnormally high levels of hCGα (Tashjian et al., 1973; Rosen and Weintraub, 1974; Rosen et al., 1975; Leiblich et al., 1976; Chou 1978c). Additional nontrophoblastic tumor cells, especially the hCG (or hCGβ) producers should be investigated. It is possible that synthesis of hCG may be regulated abnormally in these cells.

REFERENCES

Aaronsen, S. A., Todaro, G. J., and Scolnick, E. M., 1971, Induction of murine c-type viruses from clonal lines of virus-free BALB/3T3 cells, Science 174:157.

Altenburg, B. C., Via, D. P., and Steiner, S. H., 1976, Modification of the phenotype of murine sarcoma virus-transformed cells by sodium butyrate, Exptl. Cell. Res. 102:223.

Bischoff, R., and Holtzer, H., 1970, Inhibition of myoblast fusion after one round of DNA synthesis in 5-bromodeoxyuridine, J. Cell Biol. 44:134.

Boffa, L. C., Vidali, G., Mann, R. S., and Allfrey, V. G., 1978, Suppression of histone deacetylation in vivo and in vitro by sodium butyrate, J. Biol. Chem. 253:3364.

Brugge, J. S., and Butel, J. S., 1975, Role of the simian virus 40 gene A function in maintenance of transformation, J. Virol. 15:619.

Bulmer, D., Stocco, D., and Morrow, J., 1976, Bromodeoxyuridine induced variations in the level of alkaline phosphatase in several heteroploid cell lines, J. Cell Physiol. 87:357.

Candido, E. P. M., Reeves, R., and Davie, J. R., 1978, Sodium butyrate inhibits histone deacetylation in cultured cells, Cell 14:105.

Catt, K. J., Ketelslegers, J. M., and Dufau, M. L., 1976, Receptors for gonadotrophic hormones, in Methods in Receptor Research, M. Blacher, ed., pp. 175-250, Part 1, Marcel Dekker, Inc., New York and Basel.

Chen, H. C., Hodgen, G. D., Matsura, S., Lin, L. J., Gross, E., Reichert, L. E., Jr., Birken, S., Canfield, R. E., and Ross, G. T., 1976, Evidence for a gonadotropin from nonpregnant subjects that has physical, immunological, and biological similarities to human chorionic gonadotropin, Proc. Natl. Acad. Sci. U.S.A. 73:2885.

Chou, J. Y., 1978a, Human placental cells transformed by tsA mutants of simian virus 40: A model system for the study of placental functions, Proc. Natl. Acad. Sci. U.S.A. 75:1409.

Chou, J. Y., 1978b, Establishment of Clonal human placental cells synthesizing human choriogonadotropin, Proc. Natl. Acad. Sci. U.S.A. 75:1854.

Chou, J. Y., 1978c, Regulation of the synthesis of human chorionic gonadotropin by strains of HeLa cells in culture, In Vitro 14:775.

Chou, J. Y., 1979, Gene regulation in placenta: A model system using human placental cells transformed by tsA mutants of simian virus 40, in Carcinoma-Embryonic Proteins, Frank-Gunter Lehmann, ed., Volume 2, pp. 643-650, Elsevier/North-Holland.

Chou, J. Y., and Martin, R. G., 1974, Complementation analysis of simian virus 40 mutants, J. Virol. 13:1101.

Chou, J. Y., and Robinson, J. C., 1977a, Induction of placental alkaline phosphatase in choriocarcinoma cells by 5-bromo-2'-deoxyuridine, In Vitro 13:450.

Chou, J. Y., and Robinson, J. C., 1977b, Induction of alkaline phosphatase in choriocarcinoma cells by 1-β-arabinofuranosylcytosine, mitomycin C, phleomycin and cyclic nucleotides, J. Cell. Physiol. 92:221.

Chou, J. Y., Weintraub, B. D., Rosen, S. W., WhangPeng, J., Sussman, H. H., Haughom, J. R., and Robinson, J. C., 1976, Synthesis of alpha subunit of human chorionic gonadotropin by presumptive HeLa cells, In Vitro 12:589.

Chou, J. Y., Robinson, J. C., and Wang, S. S., 1977, Effects of sodium butyrate on synthesis of human chorionic gonadotropin in trophoblastic and nontrophoblastic tumors, Nature 268:543.

Chou, J. Y., Wang, S. S., Robinson, J. C., 1978, Regulation of the synthesis of human chorionic gonadotrophin by 5-bromo-2'-deoxy-uridine and dibutyryl cyclic AMP in trophoblastic and nontropho-blastic tumor cells, J. Clin. Endocrinol. Metab. 47:46.

Dreskin, R. B., Spicer, S. S., and Greene, W. B., 1970, Ultrastruc-tural localization of chorionic gonadotropin in human term placenta, J. Histochem. Cytochem. 18:862.

Edlow, J. B., Ota, T., Relacion, J., Kohler, P. O., and Robinson, J. C., 1975, Enzymes of normal and malignant trophoblast: phosphoglucomutase, hexokinase, lactate dehydrogenase, and alkaline phophatase, Am. J. Obstet. Gynecol. 121:674.

Fishman, P. H., Simmons, J. L., Brady, R. O., and Freese, E., 1974, Induction of glycolipid biosynthesis by sodium butyrate in HeLa cells, Biochem. Biophys. Res. Commun. 59:292.

Fishman, L., Miyayama, H., Driscoll, S. G., and Fishman, W. H., 1976, Developmental phase-specific alkaline phosphatase isoenzymes of human placenta and their occurrence in human cancer, Cancer Res. 36:2268.

Gey, G. O., Coffman, W. D., and Kubieck, M. T., 1952, Tissue culture studies of the proliferative capacity of cervical carcinoma and normal epithelium, Cancer Res. 12:264.

Ghosh, N. K., and Cox, R. P., 1976, Production of human chorionic gonadotropin in HeLa cell cultures, Nature 259:416.

Ginsburg, E., Salomon, D., Sreevalsan, T., and Freese, E., 1973, Growth inhibition and morphological changes caused by lipophilic acid in mammalian cells, Proc. Natl. Acad. Sci. U.S.A. 70:2457.

Griffen, M. J., Price, G. H., and Bazzell, K. L., 1974, A study of adenosine 3':5'-cyclic monophosphate, sodium butyrate and cor-tisol as inducers of HeLa alklaine phophatase, Arch. Biochem. Biophys. 164:619.

Henneberry, R. C., and Fishman, P. H., 1976, Morphological and bio-chemical differentiation in HeLa cells, Exptl. Cell Res. 103:55.

Hussa, R. O., Story, M. T., and Pattillo, R. A., 1975, Regulation of human chorionic gonadotrophin (hCG) secretion by serum and cibu-tyryl cyclic AMP in malignant trophoblast cells in vitro, J. Clin. Endocrinol. Metab. 40:401.

Hussa, R. O., Pattillo, R. A., Ruckert, A. C. F., and Scheuerman, K. W., 1978, Effects of butyrate and dibutyryl cyclic AMP on hCG-secreting trophoblastic and non-trophoblastic cells, J. Clin. Endocrinol. Metab. 46:69.

Kohler, P. O., and Bridson, W. E., 1971, Isolation of hormone-produ-cing lines of human choriocarcinoma, J. Clin. Endocrinol. Metab. 32:683.

Kohler, P. O., Bridson, W. E., Rayford, P. L., and Kohler, S. E., 1969, Hormone production by human pituitary adenomas in culture, Metabolism 18:782.

Koyama, H., and Ono, T., 1972, Further studies on the induction of alkaline phophatase by 5-bromodeoxyuridine in a hybrid line between mouse and Chinese hamster in culture, Biochem. Biophys. Acta 264:497.

Leavitt, J., Barrett, J. C., Crawford, B. D., and Ts'o, P. O. P., 1978, Butyric acid suppression of the in vitro neoplastic state of Syrian hamster cells, Nature 271:262.

Leder, A., and Leder, P., 1975, Butyric acid, a potent inducer of erythroid differentiation in cultured erythroleukemic cells, Cell 5:319.

Lieblich, J. M., Weintraub, B. D., Rosen, S. W., Chou, J. Y., and Robinson, J. C., 1976, HeLa cells secrete α subunit of glyco-protein tropic hormones, Nature 260:530.

Lin, S. Y., and Riggs, A. D., 1971, Lac repressor binding to operator analogues: Comparison of poly[d(A-T)], poly[d(A-BrU)], and poly [d(A-U)], Biochem. Biophys. Res. Commun. 45:1542.

Lin, S. Y., and Riggs, A. D., 1972, Lac operator analogues: bromo-deoxyuridine substitution in the lac operator affects the rate of dissociation of the lac repressor, Proc. Natl. Acad. Sci. U.S.A. 69:2574.

Lowry, O.H., Rosebrough, N. J., Farr, A. L., and Randall, R. J.,1951, Protein measurement with the Folin reagent, J. Biol. Chem. 193:265.

Lowy, D. R., Rowe, W. P., Teich, N., and Hartley, J. W., 1971, Murine leukemia virus: high-frequency activation in vitro by 5-iodo-deoxyuridine and 5-bromodeoxyuridine, Science 174:155.

Martin, R. G., and Chou, J. Y., 1975, Simian virus 40 function required for the establishment and maintenance of malignant transformation, J. Virol. 15:599.

Mayne, R., Sanger, J. W., and Holtzer, H., 1971, Inhibition of muco-polysaccharide synthesis by 5-bromodeoxyuridine in cultures of chick amion cells, Dev. Biol. 25:547.

Midgley, A. R., Jr., and Pierce, G. B., 1962, Immunohistochemical localization of human chorionic gonadotropin, J. Exp. Med. 115:289.

Morgan, F. C., and Canfield, R. E., 1971, Nature of the subunits of human chorionic gonadotropin, Endocrinology 88:1045.

Osborn, M., and Weber, K., 1975, Simian virus 40 gene A function and the maintenance of transformation, J. Virol. 15:636.

Pattillo, R. A., and Gey, G. O., 1968, The establishment of a cell line of human hormone-synthesizing trophoblastic cells in vitro, Cancer Res. 28:1236.

Prasad, K. N.., and Sinha, P. K., 1976, Effect of sodium butyrate on mammalian cells in culture: A review , In Vitro ;2:125.

Rittazzi, M. C., Corash, L. M., and Piomelli, S., 1971, G6PD deficiency in chronic hemolysis: four new mutants. Relationship between clinical syndrome and enzyme kinetics, Blood 38:205.

Rosen, S. W., and Weintraub, B. D., 1974, Ectopic production of the isolated alpha subunit of the glycoprotein hormones: a quantitative marker in certain causes of cancer, N. Engl. J. Med. 290:1441.

Rosen, S. W., Weintraub, B. D., Vaitukaitis, J. L., Sussman, H. H., Hershman, J. M., and Muggia, F. M., 1975, Placental proteins and their subunits as tumor markers, Ann. Intern. Med. 82:71.

Sakiyama, T., Robinson, J. C., and Chou, J. Y., 1979, Characterization of alkaline phophatase from human first trimester placentas, J. Biol. Chem. 254:935.

Salagi, S., and Bruce, S. A., 1970, Suppression of malignancy and differentiation in melanotic melanoma cells, Proc. Natl. Acad. Sci. U.S.A. 66:72.

Sealy, L., and Chalkley, R., 1978, The effect of sodium butyrate on histone modification, Cell 14:115.

Stellwagen, R. H., and Tomkins, G. M., 1971, Preferential inhibition by 5-bromodeoxyuridine of the synthesis of tyrosine aminotransferase in hepatoma cell cultures, J. Mol. Biol. 56:167.

Story, M. T., Hussa, R. O., and Pattillo, R. A., 1974, Independent dibutyryl cyclic adenosine monophosphate stimulation of human chorionic gonadotropin and estrogen secretion by malignant trophoblast cell in vitro, J. Clin. Endocrinol. Metab. 39:877.

Tashjian, A. H., Jr., Weintraub, B. D., Barowsky, N. J., Tabson, A. S., and Rosen, S. W., 1973, Subunits of human chorionic gonadotropin: unbalanced synthesis and secretion by clonal cell strains derived from a bronchogenic carcinoma, Proc. Natl. Acad. Sci. U.S.A. 70:1419.

Tegtmeyer, P., 1972, Simian virus 40 deoxyribonucleic acid synthesis: the viral replicon, J. Virol. 10:591.

Tegtmeyer, P., 1975, Function of simian virus 40 gene A transforming infection, J. Virol. 15:613.

Tegtmeyer, P., and Ozer, H. L., 1971, Temperature-sensitive mutants of simian virus 40: infection of permissive cells, J. Virol. 8:516.

Vaitukaitis, J. L., Braunstein, G. D., and Ross, G. T., 1972, A radioimmunoassay which specifically measures human chorionic gonadotropin in the presence of human luteinizing hormone, Am. J. Obstet. Gynecol. 113:751.

Vaitukaitus, J. L., Ross, G. T., Braunstein, G. D., and Rayford, P. L., 1976, Gonadotropins and their subunits: basic and clinical studies, Recent Prog. Horm. Res. 32:289.

Vidali, G., Boffa, L. C., Bradbury, E. M., and Allfrey, V. G., 1978, Butyrate suppression of histone deacetylation leads to accumulation of multiacetylated forms of histones H3 and H4 and increased DNase I sensitivity of the associated DNA sequences, Proc. Natl. Acad. Sci. U.S.A. 75:2239.

ACKNOWLEDGEMENT

I thank Dr. C. Edwards for helpful suggestions. Certain preparations of hCG and its subunits were generously provided through the Center for Population Research of the National Institute of Child Health and Human Development, National Institutes of Health. This work was supported in part by the National Institute of Child Health and Development Contract NO1-HD-6-2864.

THE INTERACTION OF THE LH/HCG RECEPTOR

WITH ADENYLATE CYCLASE IN THE RAT OVARY

Yoram Salomon, Elhanan Ezra, Abraham Nimrod,
Yehudith Amir-Zaltsman, and Hans R. Lindner

Department of Hormone Research
The Weizmann Institute of Science
Rehovot, Israel

INTRODUCTION

The response of the gonads to luteinizing hormone (LH) and the related human chorionic gonadotropin (hCG) appears to depend on stimulation of the membrane-bound enzyme, adenylate cyclase (AC), (Lamprecht et al., 1973; Koch et al., 1974; Lindner et al., 1974; Marsh, 1976; Birnbaumer et al., 1976; Catt and Dufau, 1976; Hunzicker-Dunn and Birnbaumer, 1976; Mintz et al., 1978; Bramley and Ryan, 1978a). A wide variety of hormones share this dependence of their action on cyclase mediation. The mechanism by which adenylate cyclase responds to hormones has therefore attracted intensive investigation in recent years. Some of these studies made use of membrane preparations or cells from rat liver (Pohl et al., 1971; Rodbell et al., 1971; Birnbaumer, 1973; Londos et al., 1974; Salomon et al., 1974; Rodbell et al., 1975), in which the enzyme is sensitive to glucagon; from fat tissue (Rodbell et al., 1970; Harwood et al., 1973; Rodbell, 1975), in which the enzyme is sensitive to several hormones such as epinephrine, glucagon, adrenocorticotropic hormone (ACTH), secretin, and LH; or from gonadal tissues (Birnbaumer et al., 1976; Mintz et al., 1978; Harwood et al., 1978; Bramley and Ryan, 1978b; Dufau et al., 1978; Catt et al., 1979), in which the enzyme is sensitive to gonadotropins. Other investigators have chosen the catecholamine-sensitive AC of the turkey erythrocytes (Aurbach et al., 1975; Orly and Schramm, 1976; Cassell and Selinger, 1978), frog erythrocytes (Lefkowitz and Williams, 1978), pigeon erythrocytes (Pfeuffer, 1977), or of S_{49} lymphoma cell lines (Insel et al., 1976; Ross et al., 1978) for detailed analysis. It emerged that the different enzyme preparations show many points of similarity in their properties, despite the widely differing chemical nature of

the hormones to which they respond. The collective findings of
these studies have thus contributed substantially to our understanding of the LH/hCG-stimulable ovarian enzyme system.

The following hypothesis can now be formulated regarding the
steps that lead to hormonal activation of AC (see Figure 11):
Initially, the hormone is believed to bind to a specific receptor
molecule on the outer surface of the cell membrane. It is postulated
that the receptor hormone complex accelerates an exchange process
(Cassel and Selinger, 1978) which charges the inactive, GDP-containing
regulatory subunit of the enzyme (G/F) with GTP (Sternweis and Gilman,
1979). The GTP-containing G/F protein now stimulates adenylate
cyclase, accelerating the reaction by which 3'5' cyclic adenosine
monophosphate (cyclic AMP) is formed from ATP. This process, which
presumably occurs on the inner face of the cell membrane, is terminated by hydrolysis of the bound GTP (Cassel et al., 1977).

Changes in receptor density on the cell surface is one way in
which the cell may control its response to hormones. Obviously, no
response to particular hormones is anticipated in the complete
absence of the appropriate receptors. Indeed, cell variants lacking
ACTH receptors (Schimmer, 1972) or catecholamine receptors (Sternweis
and Gilman, 1979) have been shown to contain AC, but to be refractory
to stimulation by the respective hormones. Simian virus-40 infection
of rat granulosa cells led to selective elimination of LH receptors,
but response of the cells to isoproterenol and PGE_2 was unimpaired
(Zaltzman, Vogel and Salomon, unpublished). Selective inactivation
of hormone receptors by chemical agents (Tolkovsky and Levitzki, 1978;
Salomon and Azulai, 1979) or by high intensity light (Azulai and
Salomon, 1979) reduced the response of AC to the hormone, but did not
affect hormone-independent AC activity. Likewise, down regulation of
receptors as a result of prolonged exposure of cells or tissues to
hormones is associated with desensitization of the cyclase (Lefkowitz
and Williams, 1978; Tell et al., 1978; Catt, 1979).

It has been shown that responsiveness of AC to hormones can be
deficient at stages of development in which catalytic activity is
already expressed (Rosen and Rosen, 1968; Robison et al., 1970;
Perkins, 1973; Lamprecht et al., 1973; Salomon et al., 1977). In
the ovary, FSH induces the appearance of LH receptors in follicular
granulosa cells (Richards and Midgley, 1976). This process, as
demonstrated below, is paralleled by an increase in the response of
AC molecules (Salomon et al., 1977; Salomon, 1978; Amir and Salomon,
1980). Changes in receptor density may primarily serve long-term
control of the sensitivity to hormones, as this process is relatively
slow compared to the rapid response of AC to hormonal stimulation.

Short-term control of cellular responsiveness to hormones may
be provided by modulation of the process which couples the hormone
receptor to AC. The development of a transient refractory state

towards certain hormones has been observed in several cell types upon continued stimulation (Lamprecht et al., 1977; Su et al., 1979; Catt et al., 1979). This unresponsive state seems not to be associated with a change in receptor density. Similar observations made in isolated membrane preparations of ovarian origin confirm that reduction in response of AC to LH/hCG may occur with no changes in receptor number. We will present evidence below that this process requires the presence of GTP (Ezra and Salomon, 1979; Ezra et al., 1979; Ezra and Salomon, 1980).

Several features of the control of ovarian AC are discussed in other chapters of this book, therefore, we have chosen to confine our discussion to two aspects of the mechanism that modulates cellular response to hormones--namely, the ontogeny of the LH/hCG-sensitive AC in the rat ovary during follicular maturation and the process by which the responsiveness of purified rat ovarian plasma membranes to LH/hCG is gradually attenuated in the presence of GTP.

INDUCTION OF RESPONSIVENESS TO LH IN THE RAT OVARY

The maturation of the Graafian follicle is associated with the appearance of receptors for LH on granulosa cells (GC) (Channing and Tsafriri, 1977), a process which prepares the follicle for the subsequent action of the ovulatory LH-surge (Richards and Midgley, 1976). We have shown that in the normal cycling rat the LH/hCG-receptor content of granulosa cells increases gradually from 500 receptor sites/cell on the morning of metestrus to reach peak levels (25,000 sites/cell) two days later, on the evening of proestrus (Nimrod et al., 1977a). These findings are consistent with observations in the porcine ovary in which LH/hCG receptor concentration was found to increase with follicle size (Channing and Kammerman, 1974; Lee, 1976; Bockaert et al., 1976).

Follicular development can be induced in ovaries of immature rats devoid of corpora lutea by administration of pregnant mare serum gonadotropin (PMSG). This treatment results in massive synchronized follicular growth (20-40 follicles/ovary). The fully mature follicles which develop 48 hr after administration of PMSG will respond normally and ovulate in response to treatment with hCG (Baker and Neal, 1970). To determine the response of AC to LH in relation to follicular maturation, we compared ovarian AC activity of rats treated for 48 hr with PMSG (5-15 IU/rat) and of untreated rats.

As shown in Figure 1, the specific activity of the LH-sensitive enzyme increased with increasing dose of PMSG. The increase could be observed under assay conditions in which the enzyme was stimulated by LH alone or by LH in combination with GTP. The activation ratio (Activity in the presence of LH/basal activity), which is a measure

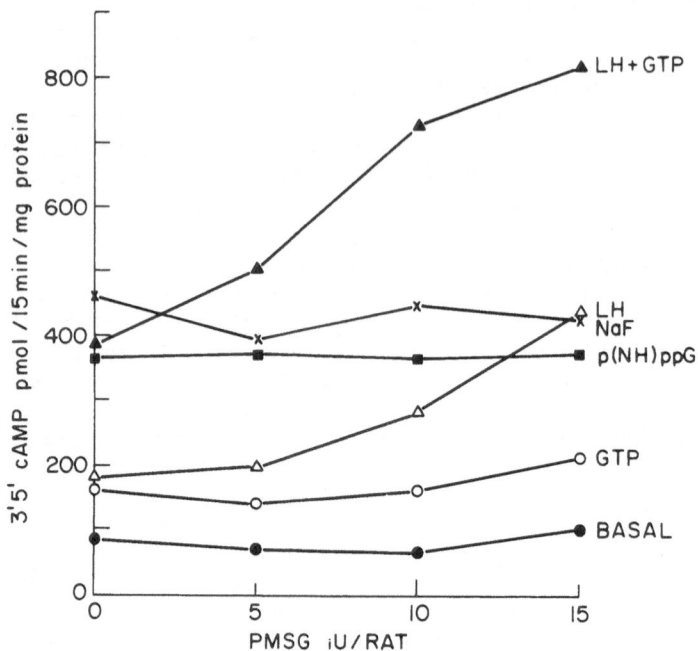

Figure 1.   PMSG-induced augmentation of LH-responsive adenylate
cyclase.   Four groups of 3 rats were injected with 0, 5, 10, or 15
IU PMSG in 0.2 ml saline between 11:00 to 12:00 a.m. Forty-eight hr
later the rats were killed by cervical dislocation.   Ovaries were
collected and homogenized (100 mg wet wt./ml) in 0.25 M sucrose
containing 1 mM dithiothreitol.   Homogenates were filtered through
Japanese silk screen and divided into 100 μl lots, which were quickly
frozen in liquid nitrogen.   Adenylate cyclase assays (Salomon, 1979)
were carried out in the absence (basal) or in the presence of the
stimulants GTP 10 μM,   p(NH)ppG 10 μM, NaF 10 mM, ovine LH (LH) 0.1
μM (NIH-LH-S-18, assuming M.W. 30,000) or of LH+GTP at the above
concentrations.   Incubations were for 15 min at 30°C (Salomon et al.,
1977; by permission of J. Cyclic Nucl. Res.).

of hormone responsiveness, increased after treatment with 15 IU/rat
of PMSG from 2 to 4.   In contrast, PMSG treatment did not change the
specific activity of hormone independent enzyme determined in the
absence of stimulants (basal) or in the presence of NaF, GTP, or
guanosine 5'-(β,γ-imido)triphosphate [p(NH)ppG].

A selective increase in the response of AC to LH in ovarian
homogenates was first noted 36 hr after injection of PMSG (15 IU/rat)

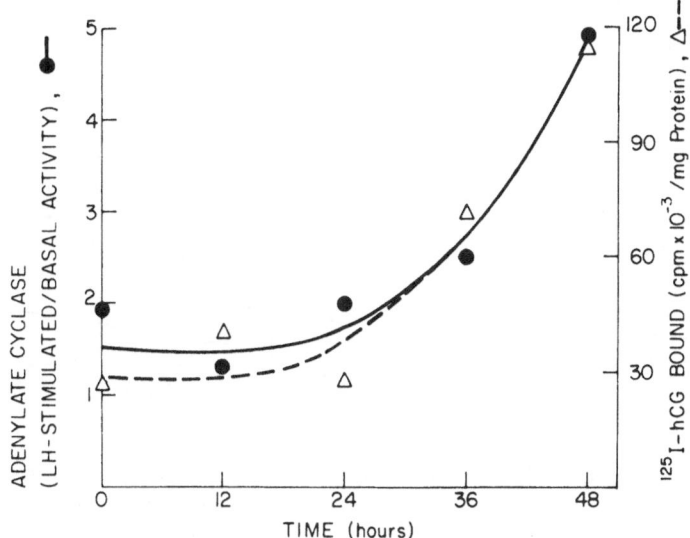

Figure 2. Effect of PMSG on the binding of ^{125}I-hCG and on the responsiveness of adenylate cyclase to LH. Four groups of 4 rats each were treated with PMSG (15 IU/rat). The control (untreated) group received saline only and was sacrificed at time zero. Homogenates were prepared at the time indicated and adenylate cyclase assays were performed as described in legend to Figure 1. Binding of ^{125}I-hCG (highly purified, 12,700 IU/mg, Serono, Rome) was determined by millipore filtration (Mintz et al., 1978; by permission of J. Cyclic Nucl. Res.)

(Salomon et al., 1977; Salomon, 1978). The observed increase in the activation ratio from 1.5 to 5 was paralleled by a 4-fold increase in the number of ^{125}I-hCG binding sites (Figure 2). This suggests that responsiveness of AC during follicular maturation is determined by receptor density in the cell membrane. Total ovarian protein increased 3-fold within this period, while total receptor population increased 9- to 12-fold. By contrast, the specific activities of mitochondrial, microsomal, and plasma membrane marker enzymes (succinate-cytochrome-C-reductase, glucose-6-phosphatase, or 5'-nucleotidase, respectively) did not change significantly after PMSG treatment (Salomon et al., 1977).

In purified ovarian plasma membrane preparations (Mintz et al., 1978) from untreated and PMSG-treated rat ovaries, the specific activity of NaF-stimulated (Salomon et al., 1977; Salomon, 1978), and p(NH)ppG-stimulated AC activities were essentially the same

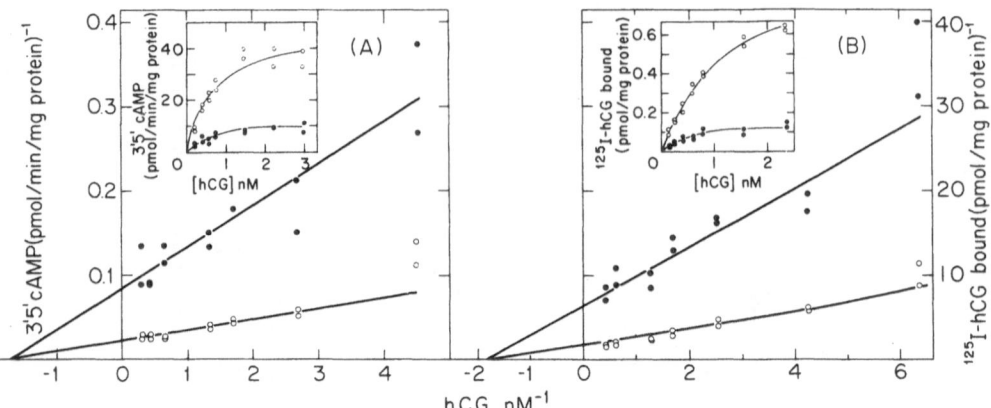

Figure 3. Binding of ^{125}I-hCG and adenylate cyclase activity in ovarian plasma membranes purified from ovaries of PMSG-treated and untreated rats. Plasma membranes from PMSG-treated (O) and from untreated (●) rats were purified according to Mintz et al. (1978). Adenylate cyclase activity (A) was determined at varying hCG concentrations in the presence of GTP (10 μM). The reaction was initiated by addition of membranes. ^{125}I-hCG binding (B) was determined at the concentrations indicated (Salomon et al., 1977). Shown is the hCG-stimulable activity after subtraction of the basal adenylate cyclase activity, which was 13 (O) or 12 (O) pmole cyclic AMP/min/mg protein, respectively. K_d, K_a and the maximal number of hormone binding sites were determined according to Lineweaver and Burk (1934). Linear regressions were fitted by the least square method.

(Amir-Zaltsman and Salomon, 1980). However, the activity of AC at saturating hCG concentrations was nearly four times higher in membranes from PMSG-treated rat ovaries than in those from untreated rats (Figure 3A). This increased response of AC was accompanied by a 6-fold increase in the number of hCG receptor sites (Figure 3B). By contrast, treatment with PMSG did not affect the affinity of the receptor for hCG: half maximal stimulation of AC by hCG was achieved at 0.66±0.2 nM and the K_d for hCG binding was 1.2±0.1 and 0.53 nM in PMSG-treated and untreated membrane preparations, respectively. Thus, the kinetic properties of the newly formed receptors are indistinguishable from those of the pre-existing ones.

The induction of LH-receptors during follicular maturation is believed to result from the action of pituitary FSH in the course of the normal estrus cycle or from the FSH-like activity of PMSG in the superstimulated immature rat ovaries. The involvement of FSH in this process was first reported by Zeleznik et al. (1974), who demonstrated that LH-receptors were induced in granulosa cells derived from preantral follicles by FSH adminstration.

Injection of FSH to immature hypophysectomized estrogen-treated rats also induced the appearance of LH-receptors in granulosa cells. Pretreatment of such rats with estrogen alone stimulated the growth of a large number of preantral follicles containing granulosa cells that are devoid of LH-receptors (Zeleznik et al., 1974; Richards and Midgley, 1976).

We have used this model system to show that both LH-receptor density and responsiveness of the granulosa cells to LH can be induced in vitro by exposing explanted ovarian fragments to FSH in organ culture (Nimrod et al., 1977b). As shown in Figure 4, exposure to FSH of the cultured explants resulted in a nearly 5-fold increase of hCG binding (from 0.38 ± 0.03 to 1.86 ± 0.22 pmole/10^6 cells) within 96 hr. These in vitro observations strengthen the evidence for the concept of heterologous receptor induction proposed on the grounds of in vivo experiments by Richards and Midgley (1976).

The appearance of LH/hCG binding sites after 96 hr of culture in the presence of FSH was accompanied by a 5- to 6-fold increase in LH-stimulable cyclic AMP accumulation in the cultured cells. By contrast, granulosa cells derived from control follicles, cultured in the absence of FSH, showed a slight decrease in LH/hCG-receptor density and consequently responded poorly to an LH challenge of cyclic AMP production.

The evidence presented suggests that the quantity of LH-receptors and the activity of LH-sensitive AC in the cell membrane are under separate control (Salomon, 1978). Furthermore, increasing the ratio of receptor to AC leads to an increased response of the cell to a challenge by the respective hormone. Thus, the initially unresponsive granulosa cells, which contain no LH-receptors, gradually acquire the ability to respond to circulating LH as their receptor content increases.

DESENSITIZATION OF RAT OVARIAN LH/HCG-STIMULABLE ADENYLATE CYCLASE IN CELL-FREE PREPARATIONS

Rat ovarian follicles have been shown to become desensitized to LH, FSH, and PGE_2 in organ culture (Lamprecht et al., 1973, 1977; Zor et al., 1976). On exposure for an extended period to one of these hormones, the follicles developed refractoriness to the homologous hormone only and responsiveness to the other two remained unimpaired. We have proposed that this desensitization of ovarian

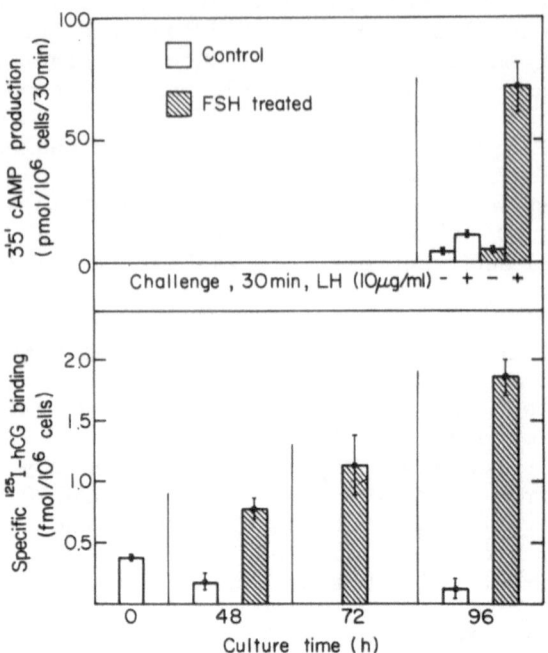

Figure 4.   In vitro induction of hCG binding sites and of LH-stimulable cyclic AMP production by FSH in granulosa cell (CG) during organ culture of ovaries from Hx-DES rats. Lower panel: specific binding of ^{125}I-hCG to GC isolated from follicles cultured with (shaded bars) or without (open bars) 0.5 µg/ml FSH for the times specified. Upper panel: cyclic AMP accumulation in GC obtained from follicles precultured for 96 hr in the presence (shaded bars) or absence (open bars) of FSH. Subsequently, GC were incubated for 30 min with (+) or without (-) LH (10 µg/ml) in the presence of isobutyl methylxanthine (IBMX). The bars and vertical brackets represent the means ± SEM of three incubation samples.

cells to gonadotropins and prostaglandins is due to uncoupling of the hormone receptor from the adenylate cyclase (Lamprecht et al., 1977; Lindner, 1979; Ezra and Salomon, 1980).

An adenylate cyclase preparation is defined as uncoupled when the following three criteria have been met: (1) It responds poorly, or not at all, to addition of hormones under assay conditions which normally yield response in a control preparation; (2) hormone *independent* activity of the enzyme (i.e., stimulation by NaF) is

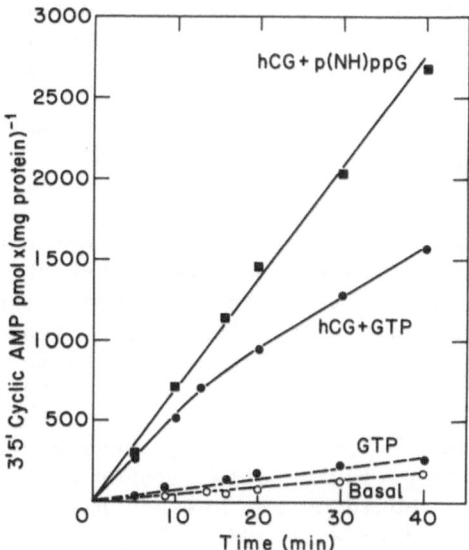

Figure 5. Stimulation of ovarian adenylate cyclase by hCG and guanosine nucleotides. Adenylate cyclase activity (Salomon, 1979) was determined in the absence of stimulants (basal activity) and in the presence of GTP, hCG+GTP, and hCG+p(NH)ppG. Incubation time was 10 min at 30°C. All other details were described elsewhere (Ezra and Salomon, 1980).

similar to that of a fully responsive control preparation; (3) binding of the hormone to the membrane preparation is unimpaired. In the case of the LH-sensitive AC, we have demonstrated that all three criteria for definition of uncoupling have been met (Lamprecht et al., 1977). Further studies of the desensitizing process have been performed in cell-free systems, using a purified rat ovarian plasma membrane preparation (Mintz et al., 1978) derived from ovaries of PMSG-treated rats, as described earlier (Salomon et al., 1977).

Under standard assay conditions (Salomon, 1979), adenylate cyclase activity in this membrane preparation is stimulated only 2-fold by hCG or GTP when each agent is added on its own (Mintz et al., 1978), but up to 15-fold by the combined action of hCG and GTP or p(NH)ppG (Figure 5). While the stimulatory effect of the hormone is sustained for up to 40 min in the presence of p(NH)ppG, a rapid decline in enzyme activity occurs 10-15 min after the onset of the reaction when GTP is the co-factor used. A similar interaction was observed earlier using LH and GTP (Ezra et al., 1979; Ezra and

Salomon, 1980). Further experiments excluded the possibilities that the decline in reaction rate was due to destruction of GTP to an extent that would render its concentration limiting or that it resulted from accumulation of an inhibitor of AC in the incubation medium. Additional studies also demonstrated that desensitization ensued only in the presence of both LH and GTP (Ezra and Salomon, 1980).

While the desensitized state is only expressed in the presence of LH+GTP, the possibility was considered that the desensitizing process may be induced by either one of these reagents on its own. However, it was found that adenylate cyclase remained fully responsive to GTP or p(NH)ppG after prolonged incubation with LH only. Addition of GTP 20-30 min after initiation of the reaction in the presence of LH stimulated enzyme activity to values similar to the initial rates observed in controls stimulated concomitantly with LH+GTP, though this activity remained linear for only 5-6 min after addition of GTP. It should be emphasized that in the control assay system in which GTP and LH were added simultaneously at zero time, activity had declined by 60% within 10 min. Addition of p(NH)ppG induced a sustained increase in adenylate cyclase activity when added 20-30 min after initiation of the reaction in the presence of LH alone. In plasma membranes preincubated with GTP for 30 min, adenylate cyclase was fully stimulated by subsequent addition of LH to the system, the activity generated being simlar to the initial rate observed when LH+GTP were added simultaneously at zero time. Thus, the response to a combined challenge by LH+GTP was fully preserved, despite the prolonged exposure of the membranes to either one of these ligands alone (Ezra and Salomon, 1980).

The poorly responsive state of the enzyme persisted after the membranes were washed free of the incubation medium and challenged with fresh hormone + GTP (Table I). Untreated membranes responded to challenge by GTP or LH+GTP with a 3-fold and 18-fold increase in AC activity, respectively. Membranes preincubated for 10 min with LH+GTP showed a similar response. However, following 40 min of preincubation, 50% of the response to LH+GTP was lost, despite the addition of GTP on its own to pretreated membrane preparations results probably from partial retention of LH by the washed membranes, the response to the residual hormone being dependent on an adequate supply of GTP.

To examine whether the enzyme was inactivated during preincubation with LH+GTP, the response of the desensitized enzyme to NaF was tested (Figure 6). Membrane preparations were preincubated for 10 min (control) or 40 min with LH+GTP and activity of AC was subsequently determined in the washed membranes in the presence of LH+GTP, LH+p(NH)ppG, or NaF. While the response of the membrane preparation to either LH+GTP or LH+p(NH)ppG declined by nearly 50%, the response to NaF remained unchanged (p>0.05) (Figure 6). The

TABLE I: Desensitization of ovarian plasma membranes by preincubation with LH and GTP.

Preincubation \ Challenge	Adenylate cyclase activity pmol/min/mg protein		
	No additions		LH + GTP
No additions	3.8 ± 0.8	10.5 ± 1.6	69.9 ± 0.5
GTP + LH (10 min)	11.6 ± 0.3	64.9 ± 2.1	66.2 ± 2.9
GTP + LH (40 min)	7.4 ± 1.1	30 ± 1.5	30.3 ± 1.0

For experimental details see legend to Figure 6.

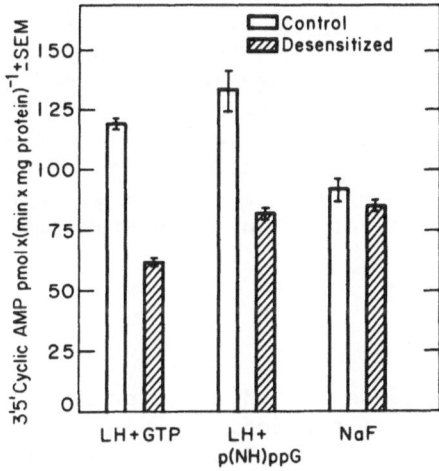

Figure 6. Stimulation of adenylate cyclase by LH + GTP, LH + p(NH)ppG, and NaF in desensitized and control membrane preparations. Control membranes were incubated for 10 min at 30°C with LH (0.1 μM) and GTP (10 μM) in 25 mM tris acetate (pH 715), 510 mM Mg acetate, 0.5 mM ATP, 50 μM cyclic AMP, 1.0 mM dithiothreitol, 510 mM creatine phosphate, and 50 U/ml creatine kinase. For desensitization, membrane preparations were incubated under the same conditions for 40 min. After the incubation, membrane suspensions were chilled and centrifuged 90 min at 90,000 x g. The resulting pellets were suspended in an ice cold solution containing 10 mM tris (pH 7.5) containing 1.0 mM DTT and immediately assayed for adenylate cyclase activity (Salomon, 1979) in the presence of LH 0.1 μM + GTP 10 μM or LH + p(NH)ppG 10 M or NaF 10 mM under standard assay conditions (10 min, 30°C).

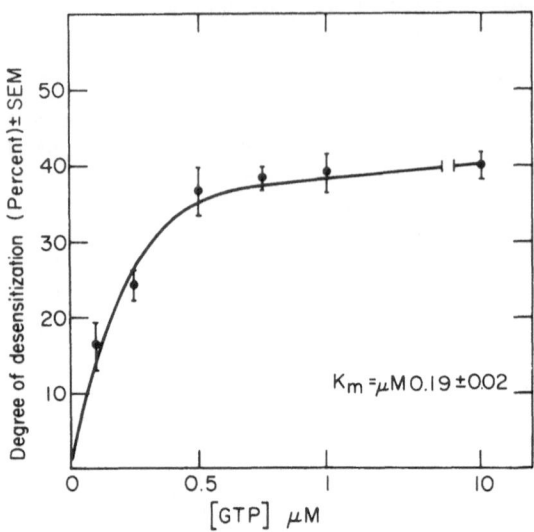

Figure 7. Desensitization of rat ovarian adenylate cyclase by LH at various GTP concentrations. Control and desensitized ovarian membranes were prepared as described in legend to Figure 6. LH concentration during the preincubation step (40 min) was kept constant (0.1 μM) and GTP concentration was varied within the range indicated. Membranes were subsequently washed and assayed for response to LH + GTP, as described in Figure 6. Results are expressed as percent activity of a control preparation preincubated for only 10 min.

results of the experiments described thus far satisfy the first two of the criteria listed above for defining the AC of desensitized membranes as uncoupled. These results also exclude the possibility that desensitization results from excessive activity of the "turn-off" GTPase, since the desensitized enzyme fails to respond to LH, even in the presence of p(NH)ppG, which is largely resistant to hydrolysis by turn-off GTPase (Salomon and Rodbell, 1975; Cassel and Selinger, 1977).

The induction of the desensitized state in the presence of saturating LH (10 μM) was dose-dependent with respect to GTP (Figure 7). Half maximal desensitization was obtained at 0.19±0.02 μM GTP (=K_m), a value identical with the activation constant obtained for the stimulation of ovarian AC by GTP (Mintz et al., 1978). Likewise, the degree of desensitization was dose-dependent with respect to LH concentrations (0.2 - 50 nM) (Figure 8). However, the concentration of LH required for half maximal desensitization was about ten times

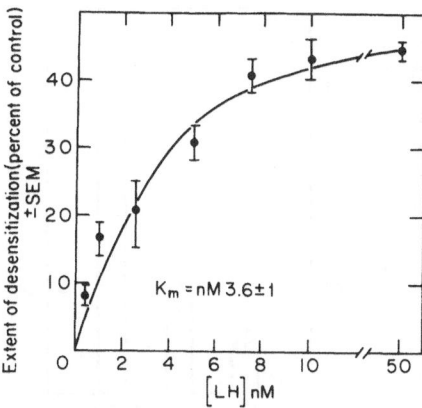

Figure 8. LH-induced desensitization of ovarian adenylate cyclase: dose dependence. Control and desensitized ovarian plasma membranes were prepared as described in Figures 6 and 7, except that LH concentration in the preincubation step was varied, as indicated, and GTP concentration was kept at 10 μM. AC assay was performed with saturating LH + GTP as in experiments in Figures 6 and 7.

greater than that required to stimulate AC by this hormone (Mintz et al., 1978), a finding in agreement with observations by Bockaert et al. (1976).

LH alone was ineffective in inducing the desensitized state in the presence of 0.5 mM ATP which is routinely utilized throughout the assay and preincubation steps (Ezra and Salomon, 1980). We substituted adenosine 5'-(β,γ-imido)triphosphate [p(NH)ppA], 0.5 mM for ATP in the preincubation step to test the effect of GTP in the absence of any other phosphorylating tri-phosphonucleotide and to compare the relative effectiveness of GTP and ATP. Preincubation was carried out for 40 min in the presence of LH alone, LH + 1 μM ATP or LH + 1 μM GTP and AC activity was determined on the washed membrane in the presence of LH + GTP with [α^{32}P]ATP as substrate (Figure 9). Preincubation in the presence of LH alone reduced AC activity (in response to subsequent stimulation by LH + GTP) by about 10%. The addition of 1 μM ATP, together with LH, in the preincubation step further reduced AC activity by 8%. However, preincubation of ovarian plasma membrane in the presence of LH + GTP (1 μM) induced a reduction in AC activity by more than 60%. Further experiments revealed that neither CTP nor ITP can substitute for GTP in this process. Experiments also indicated that continuous catalytic activity by AC is not needed for the development of the desensitized state. Desensitization ensued when ATP or p(NH)ppA, which are substrates for the enzyme, were replaced during the preincubation step by either 0.5 mM CTP or adenosine 5'-(α,β-

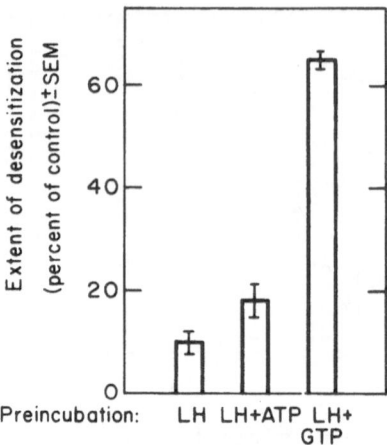

Figure 9.   Specificity of the GTP effect on LH-induced desensitization of rat ovarian adenylate cyclase. Control and desensitized
ovarian plasma membranes were prepared as described in Figures 6
and 8, except that p(NH)ppA (0.5 mM) was substituted for ATP (0.5
mM) and either ATP 1 μM or GTP 1 μM were used in combination with
LH to induce desensitization. AC activity of the washed membranes
was assayed in the presence of LH and GTP at saturating concentrations with $[\alpha^{32}P]ATP$ as substrate.

methylene)triphosphate $[pp(CH_2)pA]$, neither of which is a substrate
for AC (Ezra and Salomon, unpublished).

     To test whether desensitized AC can be resensitized, ovarian
plasma membranes preincubated for 10 or 40 min with LH + GTP were
washed and kept at 4°C in fresh assay mixture devoid of GTP.
Portions of the desensitized membrane preparation and of control
membranes were then incubated for 10 min at 30°C in the presence or
absence of p(NH)ppG and subsequently assayed for response to LH in
the presence of p(NH)ppG (Figure 10). Upon washing and further
incubation (10 min at 30°C) in GTP-free medium, activity of the
desensitized membranes increased slightly from 50 to 75 pmole/min/mg
protein. If, however, 10 μM p(NH)ppG was present during this period,
enzyme activity was stimulated, almost to the same extent as in
control membranes (142 pmole/min/mg protein). Thus, the desensitized
state is transient and the enzyme can be resensitized by further
incubation in GTP-free medium.

     To evaluate whether the reduced response of the desensitized
enzyme is associated with a reduction in receptor density, the
membrane preparation was desensitized with ^{125}I-hCG + GTP. The

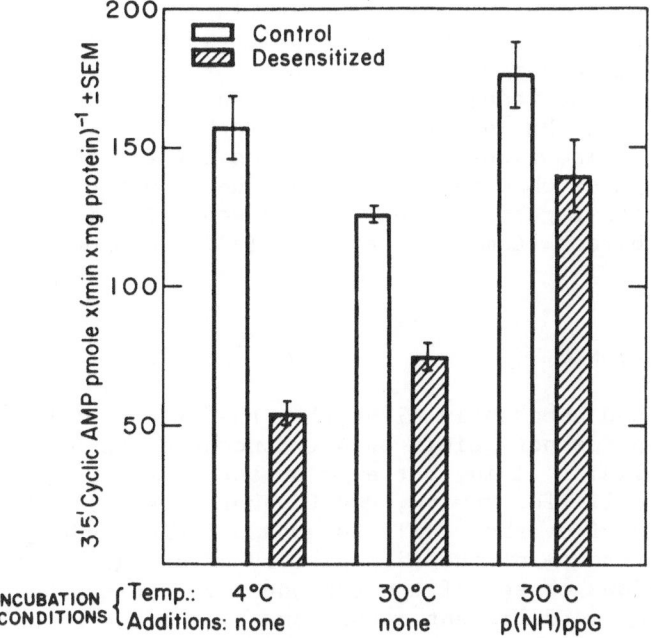

Figure 10. Resensitization of desensitized ovarian plasma membranes by incubation in GTP-free medium. Control and desensitized ovarian plasma membranes were prepared as described in Figure 6 using LH 0.1 μM and GTP 10 μM. The washed membrane preparations were suspended in AC assay mixture devoid of GTP and kept on ice. Portions of this suspension were futher incubated for 10 min at 30°C with ot without 10 μM p(NH)ppG. AC was subsequently assayed in the presence of LH 0.1 μM and p(NH)ppG 10 μM.

amount of ^{125}I-hCG bound in the absence of GTP (0.5±0.03 pmole/mg protein) was not significantly different from that bound in the presence of GTP (0.46±0.01 pmol/mg protein). The half lives of the receptor-hormone complex at 4°C, pH 4.6, in the two preparations were 14.5 and 15 min, respectively, indicating that no major change in the stability of the receptor-hormone complex is associated with the desensitized state of the enzyme. These results satisfy the third criterion for the definition of an uncoupled adenylate cyclase, as outlined at the beginning of this section.

In summary, a spontaneous process which requires the simultaneous presence of the hormone (LH or hCG) and GTP leads initially to stimulation of AC in ovarian plasma membranes and subsequently to a reduction in responsiveness of the enzyme to the hormone. In the case of the rat ovary, the reduction in AC activity during desensitization results from an uncoupling of AC from the receptor, rather than from down regulation of receptor density. In this respect, the process resembles the phenomenon of hormonally induced desensitization in the intact cell (Lamprecht et al., 1977). However, there are also important differences between the processes of desensitization, as observed in in vivo and in vitro systems, particularly with regard to kinetics and sensitivity to protein synthesis inhibitors (Lamprecht et al., 1977; Salomon and Ezra, unpublished).

GENERAL DISCUSSION

It is by now abundantly clear that the effect of hormones on any tissues depends not solely on the concentration of the hormone in the extracellular fluid, but also on the state of responsiveness of the target cell (for review, see Lindner et al., 1977). Thus, the sensitivity of ovarian cells to gonadotropins undergoes striking changes in the course of the life history of any given cell and during the various phases of the reproductive cycle. Here, we have considered two different mechanisms by which hormonal response of ovarian cells may be modulated, one depending on receptor density, the other on the efficiency of coupling of adenylate cyclase to the receptor. Similar mechanisms are likely to be operative in cells of different origin and with respect to other hormone-sensitive receptor systems. Obviously, the two examples given do not represent the only mechanisms by which cellular sensitivity to hormones can be altered.

The appearance of LH/hCG receptors in the pre-ovulatory follicle is a prerequisite for the subsequent response of granulosa cells to LH or hCG. The process is induced by FSH, probably in concert with estrogen (Richards and Midgley, 1976) and leads to a substantial (5- to 10-fold) increase in the number of LH receptors without substantially affecting the concentration of the catalytic subunits of AC. The resulting change in the numerical ratio of the two components is accompanied by a parallel increase in the responsiveness of the cyclase to LH/hCG. This result was not entirely expected, since it has been established that occupation of only a small fraction of LH-receptors is adequate to elicit a maximal response to the hormone.

In order to discuss these observations in molecular terms, we adopted the recent suggestions that membrane proteins, including those of the AC system (Rimon et al., 1978; Amsterdam et al., 1979a), are arranged in a fluid mosaic (Singer and Nicolson, 1972) and may interact with each other as a result of lateral mobility within the plane of the membrane (Orly and Schramm, 1976; Schlessinger et al., 1978; Amsterdam et al., 1979b). Thus, hormone occupied receptors

$(H \cdot R)$ (Figure 11) will collide with free GTP-binding protein (G) or cyclase (C)-associated CG.

Fruitful collision (Tolkovsky and Levitzki, 1978) will result in the activation of G by promoting the charging of this protein with GTP. The GTP-containing protein (G_{GTP}) will interact with C and cause its transition to an active form C*, resulting in catalysis of cyclic AMP formation from ATP. The turn-off reaction which cleaves GTP at the regulatory site (Cassel and Selinger, 1978) will eventually terminate the reaction chain and quench the response to the hormone.

Assuming constant concentrations for G and C in the membrane, the steady state level of active G_{GTP} and consequently of the active catalytic subunit C*, will be directly proportional to the concentration of HR. The concentration of HR in a given system (at fixed R) will be dependent on the concentration of H. However, in cells where the concentration of R increases with time, it is anticipated that the concentration of HR will increase proportionally as long as hormone concentration is not limiting. The concentration of HR required to elicit maximal AC activity (HR_{max}) is intrinsic to each system. In a given system, the concentration of either hormone or receptor may be too low to achieve the condition $HR = HR_{max}$ required for maximal cyclase activation. It is therefore easy to see that HR may approach HR_{max} even at low hormone concentrations, provided the total receptor concentration R_t is sufficiently high. In other words, at low receptor density, maximal AC activity may be achieved only at relatively high receptor occupancy (HR/R_t). On the other hand, if receptor density is high, an equal concentration of HR may be formed at a lower degree of occupancy, namely, at lower hormone concentrations.

The physiological implication of such a mechanism is that cells may gradually increase their response to tonic concentrations of hormones, simply by inserting new hormone receptors on the cell membrane. In the case of the maturing Graafian follicle, such a situation may allow response of granulosa cells to the low tonic LH levels present in the circulation well before the next LH-surge. In the case of down regulation, the same principle applies--namely, that reduction in receptor density is associated with desensitization. Even in desensitized cells, maximal stimulation may be attained, provided sufficiently high concentrations of hormone are applied (Catt et al., 1979).

The second example discussed in this review concerns a process that leads to attenuation of the hormonal response of AC in a cell-free system by a mechanism that does not require any change in receptor density. This desensitizing process was found to occur in purified ovarian plasma membranes and to require the presence of GTP together with the inducing hormone, LH or hCG. p(NH)ppG cannot

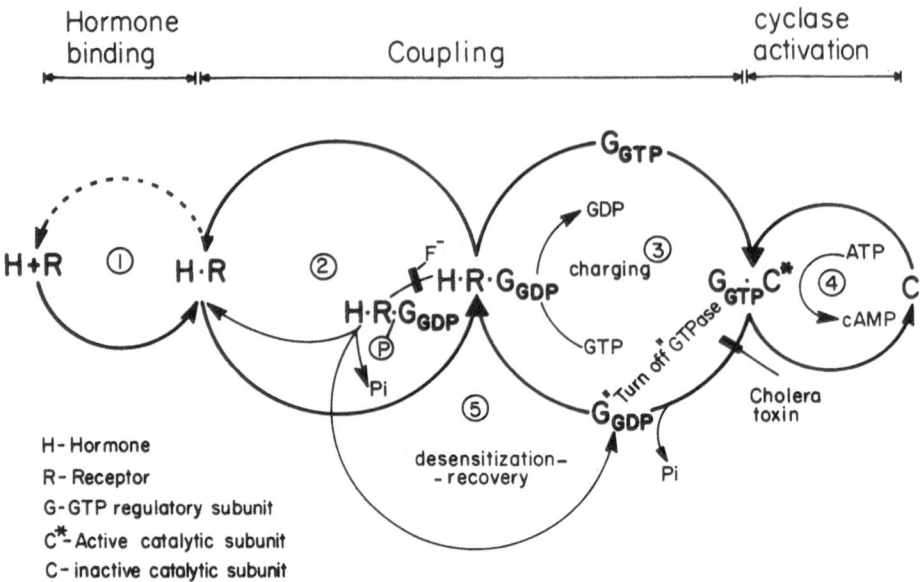

Figure 11.   Regulation of adenylate cyclase by the hormone receptor
complex. This scheme summarizes the current view of the reactions
that take place in the course of hormonal activation of AC (cycle
1-4, drawn in heavy lines) and GTP-dependent desensitization (cycle
5, thin line). AC activation: The hormone (H) binds to the membrane
receptor (R) in a reversible fashion (cycle 1). The HR complex is
able to interact reversibly with the GTP-binding protein (G) which
contains GDP and is in an inactive form (Cycle 2). The newly
formed complex $H \cdot R \cdot G_{GDP}$ in the presence of free GTP undergoes an
exchange reaction (Cassel and Selinger, 1978) in the course of which
the binding protein becomes charged with GTP to form active G_{GTP}.
This molecule further interacts with the catalytic subunit of
adenylate cyclase in its low-activity state (C) which now undergoes
transition to its activated state (C*) and catalyzes the formation
of cyclic AMP from ATP (cycle 4). Hydrolysis of GTP to GDP + Pi,
at the regulatory site (the turn-off GTPase reaction, cycle 3)
renders the complex inactive and cyclic AMP production terminates.
The GDP-containing G protein can now be reactivated (cycle 3) if
free GTP and $H \cdot R$ are present. Desensitization: At excess hormone
when $H \cdot R$ concentration is maximal for a long period the complex
$H \cdot R \cdot G_{GTP}$ may undergo a slow reaction, presumably autophosphorylation
by GTP. In the modified form this complex is inactive and the
cyclase response to fresh hormone is reduced. The reaction may be
blocked by NaF (Ezra and Salomon, 1980). No autophosphorylation
and hence no desensitization occurs when p(NH)ppG is substituted
for GTP.

substitute for GTP in the desensitizing process, though it is fully active in mediating hormonal stimulation. This discrepancy has led us to propose (Ezra and Salomon, 1980) that phosphorylation of a component of the enzyme system by GTP is likely to be associated with the desensitizing process. This suggestion is in line with an earlier proposal by Bockaert et al. (1976) who proposed that a phosphotransferase reaction that utilized ATP may be responsible for the desensitizing process. Further support for this idea came from recent studies by Hunzicker-Dunn et al. (1979), who reported that resensitization of a desensitized membrane preparation may be accelerated by exogenous phosphatase, presumably catalyzing dephosphorylation of the modified desensitized enzyme. This finding in turn suggests that the recovery from the desensitized state (Figure 10) that occurs spontaneously in GTP-free media may be due to a dephosphorylation reaction. That GTP is probably essential for the desensitization reaction in other cell types is also suggested by a recent report by Anderson and Jawarski (1979), who studied isoproterenol-sensitive AC in rat kidney cells.

Since desensitization of intact ovarian cells is specifically restricted to the homologous inducing hormone (Zor et al., 1976), it seems likely that the hormone receptor is associated in some form with the modification that leads to desensitization. The phosphorylated inactive form $H \cdot R_p G_{GDP}$ (Figure 11) may be incapable of further interaction with the catalytic subunit. The inactive complex includes the GTP-binding protein which is believed to mediate the phosphotransferase reaction, either to undergo self-phosphorylation or to catalyze phosphorylation of the receptor. The postulated involvement of the G protein in this reaction is compatible with the observation that desensitization and activation of AC have a similar concentration dependence on GTP. If inactivation by phosphorylation is confined to the receptor or to that fraction of the G protein associated with a particular hormone receptor, any excess of G will be free to interact with receptors for other hormones. This would explain why desensitization is usually restricted to the homologous hormone (Zor et al., 1976).

The desensitizing reaction (proposed to take place within the complex $H \cdot R \cdot G_{GTP}$) is slow relative to the formation of active G_{GTP}. If total receptor concentration R_t is much greater than HR_{max} and hormone concentrations are not exceedingly high, i.e., $HR \ll R_t$, no net desensitization may occur, since the small fraction of molecules that became phosphorylated may be effectively reactivated by dephosphorylation. However, if HR concentration approaches R_t and greatly exceeds HR_{max} ($HR \gg HR_{max}$), the fraction of the complex that is inactivated by phosphorylation (Figure 11; cycle 5) is large, leading to depletion of available free R. This relationship explains why high concentrations of hormone are frequently required for the desensitizing process to be observed.

Since in the developing ovary the responsiveness of AC to the hormone is directly proportional to the number of active receptors, it is conceivable that in other situations, too, a decline in responsiveness may result from a decrease in receptor density. In addition, the coupling reaction which mediates the hormonal stimulus may be subject to regulatory processes that lead to an autonomous attenuation of the primary hormonal signal.

Further work is needed to establish to what extent the mechanism of desensitization of ovarian membranes in vitro, which occurs within minutes, resembles that operating in ovarian cells in vivo or in organ culture, which requires hours. In the latter case, de novo protein synthesis and changes in cytoskeletal function have been implicated (Zor et al., 1979). It is also still unclear how the human corpus luteum of pregnancy is protected against the potentially desensitizing action of rising hCG levels before the luteoplacental shift of progestational maintenance is established (Lindner, 1979).

REFERENCES

Amir-Zaltsman, Y., and Salomon, Y., 1980, Studies on the receptor for luteinizing hormone in a purified plasma membrane preparation from rat ovary, Endocrinology (in press).

Amsterdam, A., Nimrod, A., Kohen, F., and Lindner, H. R., 1979a, Redistribution of receptors for human chorionic gonadotropin in cultured rat granulosa cells in relation to the cellular response to the hormone, in Molecular Mechanisms of Biological Recognition, M. Balaban, ed., pp. 419-428, Elsevier/North-Holland Biomedical Press, Amsterdam.

Amsterdam, A., Nimrod, A., Lamprecht, S. A., Burstein, Y., and Lindner, H. R., 1979b, Internationalization and degradation of receptor-bound hCG in granulosa cell cultures, Am. J. Physiol. 236(2):E129.

Anderson, W. B., and Jaworski, C. J., 1979, Isoproterenol-induced desensitization of adenylate cyclase responsiveness in a cell-free system, J. Biol. Chem. 254:4596.

Aurbach, G. D., Spiegel, A. M., and Gardner, J. D., 1975, β-Adrenergic receptors, cyclic AMP, and ion transport in the avian erythrocyte, Adv. Cyclic Nucl. Res. 5:117.

Azulai, R., and Salomon, Y., 1980, Photoinduced inactivation and uncoupling of gonadotropin receptors in rat ovarian plasma membrane, Biochim. Biophys. Acta, 628:76.

Baker, T. G., and Neal, P., 1970, Gonadotrophin-induced maturation of mouse Graafian follicles in organ culture, in Oogenesis, J. D. Biggers and A. W. Schuetz, eds., pp. 377-396, University Park Press, Baltimore, Butterworths, London.

Birnbaumer, L., 1973, Hormone-sensitive adenylyl cyclases. Useful models for studying hormone receptor functions in cell-free systems, Biochim. Biophys. Acta 300:129.

Birnbaumer, L., Yang, P. C., Hunzicker-Dunn, M., Bockaert, J., and Duran, J. M., 1976, Adenylyl cyclase activities in ovarian tissues. I. Homogenization and conditions of assay in Graafian follicles and corpora lutea of rabbits, rats, and pigs: Regulation by ATP, and some comparative properties, Endocrinology 99:163.

Bockaert, J., Hunzicker-Dunn, M., and Birnbaumer, L., 1976, Hormone-stimulated desensitization of hormone-dependent adenylyl cyclase, J. Biol. Chem. 251:2653.

Bramley, T. A., and Ryan, R. J., 1978a, Interactions of gonadotropins with corpus luteum membranes. I. Properties and distributions of some marker enzyme activities after subcellular fractionation of the superovulated rat ovary, Endocrinology 103:778.

Bramley, T. A., and Ryan, R. J., 1978b, Interactions of gonadotropins with corpus luteum membranes. VII. Association of hCG-binding and adenylate cyclase activities with a rabbit corpus luteum plasma-membranes, Mol. Cell. Endocr. 12:319.

Cassel, D., and Selinger, Z., 1977, Mechanism of adenylate cyclase activation by cholera toxin: Inhibition of GTP hydrolysis at the regulatory site, Proc. Natl. Acad. Sci. USA 74:3307.

Cassel, D., and Selinger, Z., 1978, Mechanism of adenylate cyclase activation through the β-adrenergic receptor: Catecholamine-induced displacement of bound GDP by GTP, Proc. Natl. Acad. Sci. USA 75:4155.

Cassel, D., Levkovitz, H., and Selinger, Z., 1977, The regulatory GTPase cycle of turkey erythrocyte adenylate cyclase, J. Cyclic. Nucl. Res. 3:393.

Catt, K. J., and Dufau, M. L., 1976, Basic concepts of the mechanism of action of peptide hormones, Biol. Reprod. 14:1.

Catt, K. J., Harwood, J. P., Aguilera, G., and Dufau, M. L., 1979, Hormonal regulation of peptide receptors and target cell responses, Nature 280:109.

Channing, C. P., and Kammerman, S., 1974, Binding of gonadotropins to ovarian cells, Biol. Reprod. 10:179.

Channing, C. P., and Tsafriri, A., 1977, Mechanism of action of luteinizing hormone and follicle-stimulating hormone on the ovary in vitro, Metabolism 26:413.

Dufau, M. L., Hayashi, K., Sala, G., Baukal, A., and Catt, K. J., 1978, Gonadal luteinizing hormone receptors and adenylate cyclase: transfer of functional ovarian luteinizing hormone receptors to adrenal fasciculata cells, Proc. Natl. Acad. Sci. USA 75:4769.

Ezra, E., and Salomon, Y., 1979, Interdependent action of lutropin and GTP in desensitizing lutropin-sensitive adenylate cyclase of the rat ovary, Isr. J. Med. Sci. 15:81.

Ezra, E., and Salomon, Y., 1980, Mechanism of desensitization of adenylate cyclase by lutropin: GTP dependent uncoupling of the receptor, J. Biol. Chem. 255:653.

Ezra, E., Lindner, H. R., and Salomon, Y., 1979, Lutropin induced desensitization of rat ovarian adenylate cyclase: A GTP-dependent process, in *Ovarian Follicular and Corpus Luteum Function*, C. P. Channing, J. M. Marsh, and W. A. Sadler, eds., pp. 711-715, Plenum Press, New York.

Harwood, J. P., Löw, H., and Rodbell, M., 1973, Stimulatory and inhibitory effects of guanyl nucleotides on fat cell adenylate cyclase, J. Biol. Chem. 248:6239.

Harwood, J. P., Conti, M., Conn, P. M., Dufau, M. L., and Catt, K. J., 1978, Receptor regulation and target cell responses: Studies in the ovarian luteal cell, Mol. Cell. Endocr. 11:121.

Hunzicker-Dunn, M., and Birnbaumer, L., 1976, Adenyl cyclase activities in ovarian tissue. II. Regulation of responsiveness to LH, FSH, and PGE_1 in the rabbit, Endocrinology 99:185.

Hunzicker-Dunn, M., Derda, D., Jungmann, R. A., and Birnbaumer, L., 1979, Resensitization of the desensitized follicular adenylyl cyclase system to luteinizing hormone, Endocrinology 104:1785.

Insel, P. A., Maguire, M. E., Gilman, A. G., Bourne, H. R., Coffino, P., and Melmon, K. L. 1976, Beta adrenergic receptors and adenylate cyclase: products of separate genes?, Mol. Pharmacol. 12:1062.

Koch, Y., Zor, U., Chobsieng, P., Lamprecht, S. A., Pomerantz, S., and Lindner, H. R., 1974, Binding of luteinizing hormone and human chorionic gonadotrophin to ovarian cells and activation of adenylate cyclase, J. Endocr. 61:179.

Lamprecht, S. A., Zor, U., Tsafriri, A., and Lindner, H. R., 1973, Action of prostaglandin E_2 and of luteinizing hormone on ovarian adenylate cyclase, protein kinase, and ornithine decarboxylase activity during postnatal development and maturity in the rat, J. Endocr. 57:217.

Lamprecht, S. A., Zor, U., Salomon, Y., Koch, Y., Ahrén, K., and Lindner, H. R., 1977, Mechanism of hormonally induced refractoriness of ovarian adenylate cyclase to luteinizing hormone and prostaglandin E_2, J. Cyclic Nucl. Res. 3:69.

Lee, C. Y., 1976, The porcine ovarian follicle: III. Development of chorionic gonadotropin receptors associated with increase in adenyl cyclase activity during follicle maturation, Endocrinology 99:42.

Lefkowitz, R. J., and Williams, L. T., 1978, Molecular mechanisms of activation and desensitization of adenylate cyclase coupled beta-adrenergic receptors, Adv. Cyclic Nucl. Res. 9:1.

Lindner, H. R., 1979, Mechanism and significance of luteal desensitization, in *Ovarian Follicular and Corpus Luteum Function*, C. P. Channing, J. M. Marsh, and W. A. Sadler, eds., pp. 703-710, Plenum Press, New York.

Lindner, H. R., Tsafriri, A., Lieberman, M. E., Zor, U., Koch, Y., Bauminger, S., and Barnea, A., 1974, Gonadotropin action on cultured Graafian follicles: Induction of maturation division of the mammalian oocyte and differentiation of the luteal cell, Rec. Prog. Hormone Res. 30:79.

Lindner, H. R., Amsterdam, A., Salomon, Y., Tsafriri, A., Nimrod, A., Lamprecht, S. A., Zor, U., and Koch, Y., 1977, Intraovarian factors in ovulation: determinants of follicular response to gonadotrophins, J. Reprod. Fert. 51:215.

Lineweaver, H., and Burk, D., 1934, The determination of enzyme dissociation constants, J. Am. Chem. Soc. 56:658.

Londos, C., Salomon, Y., Lin, M. C., Harwood, J. P., Schramm, M., Wolff, J. And Rodbell, M., 1974, 5'-Guanylylimidodiphophate, a potent activator of adenylate cyclase systems in eukaryotic cells, Proc. Nat. Acad. Sci. USA 71:3087.

Marsh, J. M., 1976, The role of cyclic AMP in gonadal steroidogenesis, Biol. Reprod. 14:30.

Mintz, Y., Amir, Y., Amsterdam, A., Lindner, H. R., and Salomon, Y., 1978, Properties of LH-sensitive adenylate cyclase in purified plasma membranes from rat ovary, Mol. Cell. Endocr. 11:265.

Nimrod, A., Tsafriri, A., and Lindner, H. R., 1977a, In vitro induction of binding sites for hCG in rat granulosa cells by FSH, Nature 267:632.

Nimrod, A., Bedrak, E., and Lamprecht, S. A., 1977b, Appearance of LH-receptors and LH-stimulable cyclic AMP accumulation in granulosa cells during follicular maturation in the rat ovary, Biochem. Biophys. Res. Commun. 78:977.

Orly, J., and Schramm, M., 1976, Coupling of catecholamine receptor from one cell with adenylate cyclase from another cell by cell fusion, Proc. Natl. Acad. Sci. USA 73:4410.

Perkins, J. P., 1973, Adenyl cyclase, Adv. Cyclic Nucl. Res. 3:1.

Pfeuffer, T., 1977, GTP-binding proteins in membranes and the control of adenylate cyclase activity, J. Biol. Chem. 252:7224.

Pohl, S. L., Birnbaumer, L., and Rodbell, M., 1971, The glucagon-sensitive adenyl cyclase system in plasma membranes of rat liver, I. Properites, J. Biol. Chem. 246:1849.

Richards, J. S., and Midgley, A. R., Jr., 1976, Protein hormone action: A key to understanding ovarian follicular and luteal cell development, Biol. Reprod. 14:82.

Rimon, G., Hanski, E., Braun, S., Levitzski, A., 1978, Mode of coupling between hormone receptors and adenylate cyclase elucidated by modulation of membrane fluidity, Nature 276:394.

Robison, G. A., Schmidt, M. J., and Sutherland, E. W., 1970, On the development and properties of the brain adenyl cyclase system, in Role of Cyclic AMP in Cell Function, P. Greengard and E. Costa, eds., pp. 11-30, Raven Press, New York.

Rodbell, M., 1975, On the mechanism of activation of fat cell adenylate cyclase by guanine nucleotides, J. Biol. Chem. 250: 5826.

Rodbell, M., Birnbaumer, L., Pohl, S. L., and Krans, H. M. J., 1970, Properties of the adenyl cyclase systems in liver and adipose cells: The mode of action of hormones, Acta Diabetologica Latina VII:9.

Rodbell, M., Birnbaumer, L., Pohl. S. L., and Krans, H. M. J., 1971, The glucagon-sensitive adenyl cyclase system in plasma membranes of rat liver. V. An obligatory role of guanyl nucleotides in glucagon action, J. Biol. Chem. 246:1877.

Rodbell, M., Lin, M. C., Salomon, Y., Londos, C., Harwood, J. P., Martin, B. R., Rendell, M., and Berman, M., 1975, Role of adenine and guanine nucleotides in the activity and response of adenylate cyclase systems to hormones: Evidence for multi-site transition states, Adv. Cyclic Nucl. Res. 5:3.

Rosen, O. M., and Rosen, S. M., 1968, The effect of catecholamines on adenyl cyclase of frog and tadpole hemolysates, Biochem. Biophys. Res. Commun. 31:82.

Ross, E. M., Haga, T., Holett, A. C., Schwarzmeier, J., Schleifer, L. S., and Gilman, A. G., 1977, Hormone-sensitive adenylate cyclase: Resolution and reconstitution of some components necessary for regulation of the enzyme, Adv. Cyclic Nucl. Res. 9:53.

Salomon, Y., 1978, Adenylate cyclase in the immature rat ovary: Induction of responsiveness to luteinizing hormone, in *FEBS Federation of European Biochemical Societies 11th Meeting Copenhagen*, P. Nicholls, ed., vol. 45, pp. 299-308, Pergamon Press, Oxford and New York.

Salomon, Y., 1979, Adenylate cyclase assay, Adv. Cyclic Nucl. Res. 10:35.

Salomon, Y., and Azulai, R., 1979, Inactivation and uncoupling of the gonadotropin receptor in rat ovarian plasma membranes by high intensity light and N,N' dicyclohexyl carbodiimide, in *Molecular Mechanisms of Biological Recognition*, M. Balaban, ed., pp. 429-441, Elsevier/North-Holland Biomedical Press, Amsterdam, New York, Oxford.

Salomon, Y., and Rodbell, M., 1975, Evidence for specific binding sites for guanine nucleotides in adipocyte and hepatocyte plasma membranes, J. Biol. Chem. 250:7245.

Salomon, Y., Lin, M. C., Londos, C., Rendell, M., and Rodbell, M., 1975, The hepatic adenylate cyclase system. I. Evidence for transition states and structural requirements for guanine nucleotide activation, J. Biol. Chem. 250:4239.

Salomon, Y., Yanovsky, A., Mintz, Y., Amir, Y., and Lindner, H. R., 1977, Synchronous generation of ovarian hCG binding sites and LH-sensitive adenylate cyclase in immature rats following treatment with pregnant mare serum gonadotropin, J. Cyclic Nucl. Res. 3:163.

Schimmer, B. P., 1972, Adenylate cyclase activity in adrenocorticotropic hormone-sensitive and mutant adrenocortical tumor cell lines, J. Biol. Chem. 247:3134.

Schlessinger, J., Schechter, Y., Cuatrecasas, P., Willingham, M. C., and Pastan, I., 1978, Quantitative determination of the lateral diffusion coefficients of the hormone-receptor complexes of insulin and epidermal growth factor on the plasma membrane of cultured fibroblasts, Proc. Natl. Acad. Sci. USA 75:5353.

Singer, S. J., and Nicolson, G. L., 1972, The fluid mosaic model of the structure of cell membranes, Science 175:720.

Sternweis, P. C., and Gilman, A. G., 1979, Reconstitution of cate-cholamine-sensitive adenylate cyclase, J. Biol. Chem. 254:3333.

Su, Y. F., Harden, T. K., and Perkins, J. P., 1979, Isoproterenol-induced desensitization of adenylate cyclase in human astro-cytoma cells, J. Biol. Chem. 254:38.

Tell, G. P., Haour, F., Saez, J. M., 1978, Hormonal regulation of membrane receptors and cell responsiveness: A review, Metabolism 27:1566.

Tolkovsky, A. M., and Levitzki, A., 1978, Mode of coupling between the β-adrenergic receptor and adenylate cyclase in turkey erythrocytes, Biochemistry 17:3795.

Zeleznik, A. J., Midgley, A. R., Jr., and Reichert, L. E., Jr., 1974, Granulosa cell maturation in the rat: increased binding of human chorionic gonadotropin following treatment with follicle-stimulating hormone, Endocrinology 95:818.

Zor, U., Lamprecht, S. A., Misulovin, A., Koch, Y., and Lindner, H. R., 1976, Refractoriness of ovarian adenulate cyclase to continued hormonal stimulation, Biochim. Biophys. Acta 428:761.

Zor, U., Strulovici, B., Lamprecht, S. A., Amsterdam, A. Oplatka, A., and Lindner, H. R., 1979, Effect of modulators of cyto-skeletal function on desensitization and recovery of PGE_2-responsive ovarian adenylate cyclase, Prostaglandins (in press).

ACKNOWLEDGEMENTS

We thank Drs. U. Zor and S. Handwerger for helpful discussions. This work was supported in part by a grant (to Y.S.) from the U.S.-Israel Binational Science Foundation (BSF), Jerusalem, and by grants (to H. R. L.) from the Rockefeller Foundation, the Ford Foundation, and the Population Council Inc., New York. Y. S. is the incumbent of the Charles and Tillie Lubin Career Development Chair and H. R. L. of the Adlai E. Stevenson II Chair of Endocrinology and Reproductive Biology. We wish to thank Mrs. Millicent Kopelowitz for excellent secretarial assistance.

TESTIS-DETERMINING H-Y ANTIGEN

AND THE INDUCTION OF THE HCG RECEPTOR

Ulrich Müller

Memorial Sloan-Kettering Cancer Center, New York
New York, U.S.A. and Institut für Humangenetik
und Anthropologie der Universität, Freiburg
Federal Republic of Germany

INTRODUCTION

The discovery of H-Y ("male specific") antigen is the result of a finding in the field of transplantation immunology (Eichwald and Silmser, 1955). In some highly inbred strains of the mouse, male skin grafts are rejected by female recipients, but not vice versa. Due to the genetic identity of animals within an isogenic strain, this rejection phenomenon must be attributed to an antigen coded or controlled by the Y chromosome (which is absent in the female). The term H-Y (histocompatibility-Y) refers to the dependence of this male-specific antigen on the Y chromosome.

Several methods exist for the detection of H-Y antigen (Wachtel and Koo, 1980). Many of them use anti-H-Y antibodies raised in isogenic rodents either by inoculating female animals with male spleen cells, or by grafting male skin on female hosts. The techniques most commonly applied are cytotoxicity assays. These tests are based on the finding that anti-H-Y antibodies are cytotoxic to male epithelial cells (Scheid et al., 1972), sperm (Goldberg et al., 1971) or certain lymphoma cells (Fellous et al., 1978) in the presence of complement. Absorption of H-Y antiserum with H-Y antigen positive cells reduces the cytotoxicity of the antiserum for the target cells, whereas absorption with H-Y antigen negative cells does not affect the lytic activity of the antiserum.

Application of these techniques showed that H-Y antigen is expressed on almost all cell types in males (= heterogametic sex) of all mammalian species tested so far, but not in females (Wachtel, 1977). Moreover, non-mammalian vertebrates such as birds (Wachtel et al., 1975a), reptiles (Zaborski et al., 1979), amphibians (Wachtel et al., 1975a), and even fish (Müller and Wolf, 1979; Pechan et al., 1979) express H-Y antigen in the heterogametic sex only. Evidently then, H-Y antigen is highly conserved in evolution; this indicates that the molecule has a persistent specific function (most likely in connection with sex differentiation). In addition, genetically female (XX) mammals that are sex-reversed to males such as Sxr, XX mice (Bennett et al., 1977) or human XX males (Wachtel et al., 1976; Müller and Bross, 1979) type H-Y positive. Based on these observations, a testis-differentiating function of H-Y antigen in mammals was postulated (Wachtel et al., 1975a; Ohno, 1976). Here, experiments supporting this hypothesis are described. Evidence is given that H-Y antigen induces the expression of the hCG receptor in male embryonic gonads. The function of the receptor for stimulation of fetal testosterone synthesis and thus for the differentiation of male genitalia is discussed. Finally, a model for the mechanism of H-Y action is suggested.

SECRETION AND BINDING OF H-Y ANTIGEN

In order for male-specific H-Y antigen to function as a testis-inducing substance, the following are required: 1) release of H-Y antigen by a certain organ(s) in order to be transferred to its gonadal target cells; 2) expression of a specific receptor of H-Y antigen on the gonads of both sexes by which H-Y antigen triggers testicular differentiation.

These requirements are indeed fulfilled by H-Y antigen (Table I). In vitro culture of different male organs shows that testicular tissues exclusively release H-Y antigen into the culture medium (Muller et al., 1978b). In the cytotoxicity test, the activity of anti-H-Y antiserum is highly reduced after absorption with testis supernatant but it is not influenced after absorption with culture media of non-gonadal male tissues such as spleen, liver, epididymis, and brain. Cycloheximid, an inhibitor of translation, blocks testicular secretion of H-Y antigen without influencing the expression of H-Y antigen on the cell surface during the culture period. Evidently the testis actively secretes H-Y antigen. [This function could be attributed to the Sertoli cells (Zenzes et al., 1978a).]

Testis cell secreted H-Y antigen and membrane-bound H-Y antigen seem to be identical, or very similar, rather than being molecules that merely share common antigenic sites. This is concluded from biochemical findings of Sertoli secreted H-Y antigen and H-Y antigen released by a male lymphoma cell line (Daudi cells*): both the

---

*Daudi cells synthesize H-Y antigen but have lost the ability to integrate it into the cell membrane. This is due to a defect in

TABLE I: Expression, binding and secretion of H-Y antigen by gonadal and non-gonadal cells or tissues of both sexes.

Tissue	Expression of (endogenous) H-Y antigen	Secretion of H-Y antigen	Binding of exogenous H-Y antigen
OVARY	−	−	+
TESTIS			
Leydig Cells	+	−	+
Sertoli cells	+	+	+
diploid germ cells	−	−	−
epididymal sperm	+	−	−
NON-GONADAL*			
male	+	−	−
female	−	−	−

* Liver, spleen, brain, epididymis, kidney

actively secreted antigen and the putative membrane-bound antigen have the same mol. wt. of about 18,000 daltons, and both seem to absorb anti-H-Y antiserum to the same extent in serological tests (Wachtel, S. S., personal communication).

The existence of a gonad-specific receptor of H-Y antigen as a prerequisite for testicular differentiation is suggested by binding studies (Muller et al., 1978a). The following procedure

the synthesis of β_2-microglobulin [a globular molecule (mol. wt. 12,000 daltons) of the outer cell membrane of almost all cell types (Vitetta and Capra, 1978)] which seems to be required for the expression of H-Y antigen on the cell surface (Beutler et al., 1978).

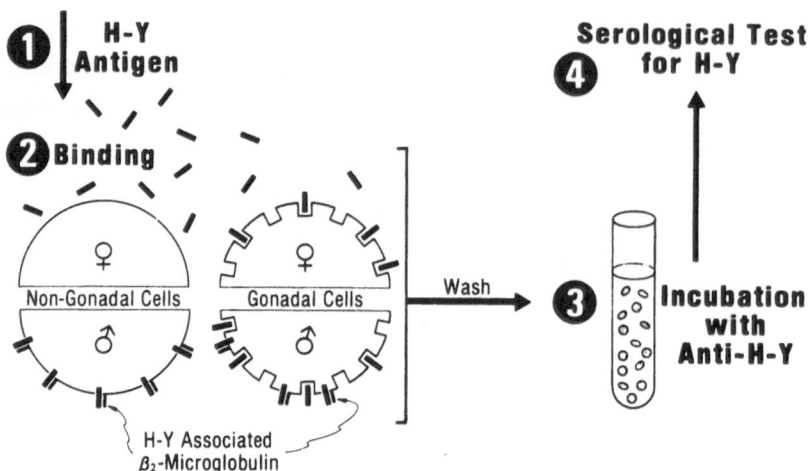

Figure 1.   Binding studies with H-Y antigen; experimental procedure.
(1) Source of H-Y antigen; epididymal fluid, supernatant of
cultured testes or Daudi cells. (2) Incubation of tissues with
H-Y antigen containing fluids for 30 min at 37°C. (3) After two
washes, absorption of H-Y antiserum with tissues. (4) Test of
residual cytotoxicity of absorbed antiserum for target cells.

is employed (Figure 1): Supernatants of either cultured testicular
cells or Daudi cells serve as source of H-Y antigen. The tissues
under study are homogenized and incubated with the H-Y antigen
containing fluid for 30 minutes at 37°C. After two washes, anti-
H-Y antiserum is absorbed with these tissues; it is subsequently
tested for residual cytotoxicity on target cells (e.g., male
epidermal cells or sperm). Ovarian cells loaded with H-Y antigen
become H-Y postive, whereas female non-gonadal tissues remain
negative, even after exposure to H-Y antigen. The amount of H-Y
antigen on testicular cells appears to increase after incubation
with H-Y antigen, but not the amount on male non-gonadal tissues.
Evidently, only the gonads of both sexes bind exogenous H-Y antigen.
In the testis, H-Y is bound by Sertoli and by Leydig cells (Zenzes
et al., 1978a).

    From these findings it is concluded that: 1) H-Y positive cells
which do not bind exogenous H-Y antigen, i.e., almost all male
mammalian cells, produce their own endogenous H-Y antigen;
2) gonadal cells are endowed with a specific receptor for H-Y

antigen. The existence of a gonad-specific receptor is substantiated by redistribution experiments with β_2-microglobulin (β_2-m, see note above). On the cell surface, H-Y antigen is associated with this molecule, and in fact β_2-m seems to be required for the expression of H-Y. Thus, removal of β_2-m from the cell membrane with anti-β_2-m antibody ("lysostripping") is associated with loss of H-Y antigen as well. Association of β_2-m and H-Y has been demonstrated for non-gonadal (Fellous et al., 1978; Beutler et al., 1978), as well as for gonadal cells (Müller et al., 1979b). However, the capacity of the gonads to bind exogenous H-Y antigen is not affected by removal of β_2-m, thus indicating independence of the gonad-specific receptor and the molecule necessary for the expression of endogenous H-Y antigen (β_2-m).

EXPERIMENTAL EVIDENCE FOR TESTIS-ORGANIZING FUNCTION OF H-Y ANTIGEN

Direct evidence of a testis-organizing function of H-Y antigen is provided in "Moscona-type" reaggregation experiments (Moscona, 1957). These experiments are based on the observation that in rotating cultures dispersed cells of the different organs and tissues reaggregate to form structures characteristic of the organ or tissue from which they originated. When ovarian cells from newborn rats are cultivated in this way, they organize ovarian structures; corresponding results are obtained with testicular cells. When anti-H-Y antiserum is added to a suspension of testicular cells of newborn rats or mice, however, testicular organization is blocked (presumably H-Y is lyso-stripped from the cells) and instead, ovarian structures are formed in the rotation culture (Zenzes et al., 1978c; Ohno et al., 1978). Conversely, testicular organization is obtained when ovarian cells are exposed to H-Y antigen during cultivation (Zenzes et al., 1978b). Supernatants of the cultured testis, or epididymal fluid, serve as sources of H-Y antigen (the latter contains large amounts of H-Y).

The testis-organizing function of H-Y antigen is borne out in another experiment (Ohno et al., in press). Indifferent gonads of genetic female (XX) bovines develop into testes in vitro when cultured in the presence of H-Y antigen from Daudi cells. Sertoli-like cells and tubular structures arise after three days of culture; a *tunica albuginea* is detectable five days after onset of the experiment. Sex-reversed gonads are clearly distinguishable from control gonads that have been cultured for the same period in the <u>absence</u> of H-Y antigen.

INDUCTION OF HCG RECEPTOR BY H-Y ANTIGEN

In the Moscona-type experiments ovarian cells not only reorganize histologically into testicular structures in the presence of

TABLE II: Expression of the hCG receptor in the gonads of rats.

Age	Testis	Ovary	'Ovarian'cells, sex-reversed in vitro by H-Y antigen
FETAL	+	—	?
NEWBORN	+	—	+
>7-10 DAYS	+	+	+

H-Y antigen, but they are converted functionally as well (Müller et al., 1978c). This is demonstrated by selecting as a testis-specific parameter the hCG receptor which is expressed in the testis of embryonic and newborn rats (Frowein and Engel, 1974), but not in the ovary before days 7-10 postnatally (Presl et al., 1972; Stebers et al., 1977; Bortolussi et al., 1979). After conversion of newborn ovarian cells into testicular structures by H-Y antigen, the hCG receptor becomes detectable (Table II). [Experimental procedures for the detection of the receptor are described elsewhere (Müller et al., 1978c). K_D and b_s were determined according to Scatchard, 1949).] HCG receptors first appear in reaggregates 4 hr after onset of the experiment and increase slightly in number up to 16 hr of culture. The number of binding sites (b_s = 0.67 moles/mg wet wt. x 10^{15}) and the dissociation constant (K_D = 3.8 moles/liter x 10^{10}) in the converted gonad are almost identical to those of newborn reaggregated control testes (b_s = 0.9 moles/mg wet wt. x 10^{15}; K_D = 5.2 moles/liter x 10^{10}). Appearance of the receptor is prevented by cycloheximid, indicating that protein synthesis is required for its expression, at least at the level of translation. Non-specific effects feigning H-Y antigen induction of the hCG receptor in these experiments are very unlikely. HCG receptors are not detectable even in the presence of H-Y antigen containing epididymal fluid when cycloheximid is added to the rotation culture, or when ovarian cells are kept in suspension for 16 hr so that reorganization is prevented. Specific binding of hCG also is not found in cells of non-gonadal organs after 16 hr exposure to epididymal fluid. Thus, the following possibilities can be excluded: external addition of soluble hCG receptors with the epididymal fluid, or addition of enzymes (e.g., neuraminidase) which could unmask precursors of the hCG receptor (Müller et al., 1979a).

The experiments described above provide evidence that H-Y antigen may also be involved in the induction of the hCG receptor in vivo during the processes of testicular Leydig cell differentiation. The relatively short period required for the induction of the receptors in vitro agrees well with findings in vivo. During testicular development, Leydig cells differentiate within a few hours from primordial precursors to a mature state expressing specific receptors of hCG (Catt et al., 1975).

ROLE OF THE HCG RECEPTOR IN MALE SEX DIFFERENTIATION

Normally a functional testis is required for the development of male genitalia (Jost, 1947; Jost, 1970). Testosterone, produced by Leydig cells of the fetal testis, induces the Wolffian ducts to form epididymis, ductus deferens, and seminal vesicles (Wilson, 1973); anti-Müllerian hormone secreted by Sertoli cells represses the constitutive (?) development of the Müllerian ducts into female genitalia (Josso et al., 1977). Differentiation of prostate and male external genitalia depends on dihydrotestosterone (DHT) metabolized from testosterone by the enzyme 5α-reductase (Imperato-McGinley et al., 1974; Wilson and MacDonald, 1978).

Considering a role of the hCG receptor in male sex differentiation, the question arises whether fetal, as well as postnatal testosterone secretion, is controlled by gonadotropins. Is the differentiation of male genitalia dependent on LH and/or hCG? Evidence for a role of gonadotropins in fetal testosterone secretion comes from the detection of specific hCG receptors in fetal testes of various animal species, including man (Catt et al., 1975; Frowein and Engel, 1974; Huhtaniemi et al., 1977), but not in fetal ovaries (Siebers et al., 1977). Fetal testes respond to gonadotropin stimuli by synthesizing cAMP and testosterone (Abramovich et al., 1974; Ahluwalia et al., 1974; Huhtaniemi, 1977), thereby demonstrating that the hCG receptors are functional. A close correlation is found between the appearance of specific hCG receptors and the onset of testosterone synthesis in embryonic testes of the rabbit (Catt et al., 1975). Recent findings suggest that at the very onset of testicular differentiation, the hCG receptors are not yet coupled with testosterone synthesis. Thus, testes of the embryonic rabbit do not respond to gonadotropin stimuli in vitro before the second or third day after Leydig cell differentiation, though specific binding of hCG is observed. These data, however, could indicate that the functional receptors at this early developmental stage are already saturated with endogenous hCG (George et al., 1978).

Most likely the hormone that physiologically stimulates testosterone synthesis is maternal hCG and not fetal LH, at least in earlier pregnancy. This may be concluded from several findings in human embryos: hCG is found in the circulation (Clements et al., 1976) as well as in the various organs of the embryo, including the testis (Huhtaniemi et al., 1978). Production of gonadotropins by the fetal pituitary is rather limited or even non-existent (Groom et al., 1971; Levina, 1972) when maximal testosterone levels are found (Abramovich and Rowe, 1973). In late embryonic life, fetal LH becomes more important for stimulation of the testis (Kaplan et al., 1976).

Thus hCG, by regulating testosterone synthesis in earlier fetal life, induces differentiation of male genitalia via the hCG receptor which itself may be under control of H-Y antigen.

HYPOTHETICAL MECHANISMS OF TESTICULAR DIFFERENTIATION

While a testis-inducing function of H-Y antigen is evident, nothing is known about the mechanism of H-Y antigen action. A proteo-hormone-like action is suggested by the finding that H-Y antigen is actively secreted and evidently transferred to its target cells where it is bound by a specific receptor of the cell membrane. The onset of testicular differentiation in male embryonic life might be restricted to the appearance of this gonad-specific receptor, which might occur constitutively at a certain stage of gonadal development in both sexes. In the male, H-Y antigen -- already detectable in the eight-cell embryo (Krco and Goldberg, 1976) -- is bound to this receptor either by cell contact during the processes of rearrangement of embryonic tissues or after having been shed from cell surfaces (almost all male cells express H-Y antigen). According to this notion, H-Y antigen should induce its own secretion in prospective Sertoli cells. However, a constitutive onset of secre- tion of H-Y antigen by the male gonad is also plausible. Binding of H-Y antigen and formation of the H-Y antigen-receptor complex might result in testis-cell specific functions. Cell-type specific antigens ("cognins") might be induced which are required for cell- cell recognition (Moscona and Hausman, 1977). These cognins would in turn mediate testicular morphogenesis. The induction of a testis- cell specific molecule, i.e., the hCG receptor, by H-Y antigen is consistent with that view.

SUMMARY

Experimental data strongly favor the view that H-Y antigen is the inducer of the mammalian testis. Thus H-Y antigen -- actively secreted by testicular Sertoli cells -- is bound by a gonad-specific receptor. The receptor is present in the gonads of both sexes; evidently, the receptor is a prerequisite of testicular induction. Reaggregation experiments in vitro using dissociated gonads of the newborn rat demonstrate that testicular cells reorganize into ovarian structures in the presence of H-Y antibody. Conversely, ovarian cells form testicular structures in the presence of H-Y antigen. The hCG receptor, a testis-specific parameter, is expressed in the sex-reversed "ovary." This indicates that morphological conversion is functional. Furthermore, indifferent XX gonads of the bovine develop into testes when cultured in medium containing H-Y antigen.

Physiologically the hCG receptor is required for testosterone production in the fetal testis. Most likely in early embryonic life maternal hCG (and not fetal LH) stimulates testosterone synthesis and therefore, differentiation of the male genitalia. Stimulation occurs after reaction of hCG and its receptor; which itself may be under the control of H-Y antigen.

REFERENCES

Abramovich, D. R., and Rowe, P., 1973, Foetal plasma testosterone levels at mid-pregnancy and at term, J. Endocrinol. 56:621.

Abramovich, D. R., Baker, T. G., and Neal, P., 1974, Effect of human chorionic gonadotrophin on testosterone secretion by the foetal human testis in organ culture, J. Endocrinol. 60:179.

Ahluwalia, B., Williams, J., and Verma, P., 1974, In vitro testosterone biosynthesis in the human fetal testis. II. Stimulation by cyclic AMP and human chorionic gonadotropin (hCG), Endocrinology 95:1411.

Bennett, D., Mathieson, B. J., Scheid, M., Yanagisawa, K., Boyse, E. A., Wachtel, S. S., and Cattanach, B. M., 1977, Serological evidence for H-Y antigen in Sxr, XX sex-reversed phenotypic males, Nature 265:255.

Beutler, B., Nagai, Y., Ohno, S., Klein, G., and Shapiro, I. M., 1978, The HLA-dependent expression of testis-organizing H-Y antigen by human male cells, Cell 13:509.

Bortolussi, M., Marini, G., Rolandi, M. T., Galli, S., and Munari, P. F., 1979, LH receptors in the rat ovary during sexual development, Acta Endocrinol. 91, Suppl. 225:287.

Catt, K. J., Dufau, M. L., Neaves, W. B., Walsh, P. C., and Wilson, J. D., 1975, LH-hCG receptors and testosterone content during differentiation of the testis in the rabbit embryo, Embryology 97:1157.

Clements, J. A., Reyes, F. I., Winter, J. S. D., and Faiman, C., 1976, Studies on human sexual development. III. Fetal pituitary and serum, and amniotic fluid concentrations of LH, CG, and FSH, J. Clin. Endocrinol. Metab. 42:9.

Eichwald, E. J., and Silmser, C. R., 1955, Communication, Transplant. Bull. 2:148.

Fellous, M., Günther, E., Kemler, R. Wiels, J., Berger, R. Guenet, J. L., Jakob, H., and Jacob, F., 1978, Association of the H-Y male antigen with β_2-microglobulin on human lymphoid and differentiated mouse teratocarcinoma cell lines, J. Exp. Med. 147-58.

Frowein, J., and Engel, W., 1974, Constitutivity of the hCG-receptor protein in the testis of rat and man, Nature 249:377.

George, F. W., Catt, K. J., Neaves, W. B., and Wilson, J. D., 1978, Studies on the regulation of testosterone synthesis in the fetal rabbit testis, Endocrinology 102:665.

Goldberg, E. H., Boyse, E. A., Bennett, D., Scheid, M., and Carswell, E. A., 1971, Serological demonstration of H-Y (male) antigen on mouse sperm, Nature 232:478.

Groom, G. V., Groom, M. A., Cooke, E. D., and Boyns, A. R., 1971, The secretion of immuno-reactive luteinizing hormone and follicle stimulating hormone by the human foetal pituitary in organ culture, J. Endocrinol. 49:335.

Huhtaniemi, I., 1977, Studies on steroidogenesis and its regulation in human fetal adrenal and testis, J. Steroid Biochem. 8:491.

Huhtaniemi, I. T., Korenbrot, C. C., and Jaffe, R. B., 1977, hCG binding and stimulation of testosterone biosynthesis in the human fetal testis, J. Clin. Endocrinol. Metab. 44:963.

Huhtaniemi, I. T., Korenbrot, C. C., and Jaffe, R. B., 1978, Content of chorionic gonadotropin in human fetal tissues, J. Clin. Endocrinol. Metab. 46:994.

Umperato-McGinley, J., Guerrero, L., Gautier, T., and Peterson, R. E., 1974, Steroid 5α-reductase deficiency in man: an inherited form of male pseudohermaphroditism, Science 186:1213.

Josso, N., Picard, J. Y., and Tran, D., 1977, The anti-mullerian hormone, Recent Prog. Horm. Res. 33:117.

Jost, A., 1947, Recherches sur la différenciation sexuelle de l'embryon de lapin. III. Rôle des gonades foetales dans la différenciation somatique, Arch. Anat. Microsc. Morphol. Exp. 36:271.

Jost, A., 1970, Hormonal factors in the sex differentiation of the mammalian foetus, Philos. Trans. R. Soc. Lond. [Biol.] 259:119.

Kaplan, S. L., Brumbach, M. M., and Aubert, M. L., 1976, The ontogenesis of pituitary hormones and hypothalamic factors in the human fetus: Maturation of central nervous system regulation of anterior pituitary function, Recent Prog. Horm. Res. 32:161.

Krco, C. J., and Goldberg, E. H., 1976, Detection of H-Y (male) antigen on 8-cell mouse embryos, Science 193:1134.

Levina, S. E., 1972, Times of appearance of LH and FSH activities in human foetal circulation, Gen. Comp. Endocrinol. 19:242.

Moscona, A. A., 1957, The development in vitro of chimeric aggregates of dissociated embryonic chick and mouse cells, Proc. Natl. Acad. Sci. USA 43:184.

Moscona, A. A., and Hausman, R. E., 1977, Biological and biochemical studies on embryonic cell-cell recognition, in *Cell and Tissue Interactions*, J. W. Lash and M. M. Burger, eds., pp. 173-185, Raven Press, New York.

Müller, U., and Bross, K., 1979, A highly sensitive peroxidase-antiperoxidase method for detection of H-Y antigen on cultivated human fibroblasts, Hum. Genet., in press.

Müller, U., and Wolf, U., 1979, Cross-reactivity to mammalian anti-H-Y antiserum in teleostean fish, Differentiation 14:185.

Müller, U., Aschmoneit, I., Zenzes, M. T., and Wolf, U., 1978a, Binding studies of H-Y antigen in rat tissue. Indications for a gonad-specific receptor, Hum. Genet. 43:151.

Müller, U., Siebers, J. W., Zenzes, M. T., and Wolf., U., 1978b, The testis as a secretory organ for H-Y antigen, Hum. Genet. 45:209.

Müller, U., Zenzes, M. T., Bauknecht, T. Wolf, U., Siebers, J. W., and Engel, W., 1978c, Appearance of the hCG-receptor after conversion of newborn ovarian cells into testicular structures by H-Y antigen in vitro, Hum. Genet. 45:203.

Müller, U., Engel, W., and Siebers, J. W., 1979a, LH/hCG receptor of the ovary during early postnatal development, Ann. Biol. Anim. Biochem. Biophys. 19(4B):1363.

Müller, U., Wolf, U., Siebers, J. W., and Günther, E., 1979b, Evidence for a gonad-specific receptor for H-Y antigen: Binding of exogenous H-Y antigen to gonadal cells is independent of β_2-microglobulin, Cell 17:331.

Ohno, S., 1976, Major regulatory genes for mammalian sexual development, Cell 7:315.

Ohno, S., Nagai, Y., and Ciccarese, S., 1978, Testicular cells lyso-stripped of H-Y antigen organize ovarian follicle-like aggregates, Cytogenet. Cell Genet. 20:351.

Ohno, S., Nagai, Y., Ciccarese, S., and Iwata, H., Testis-organizing H-Y antigen and the primary sex-determining mechanism of mammals, Recent. Prog. Horm. Res., in press.

Pechan, P., Wachtel, S. S., and Reinboth, R., 1979, H-Y antigen in the teleost, Differentiation 14:189.

Presl, J., Posisil, J., Figarová, V., and Wagner, V., 1972, Developmental changes in uptake of radioactivity by the ovaries, pituitary and uterus after ^{125}I-labelled human chorionic gonadotrophin administration in rats, J. Endocrinol. 52:585.

Scatchard, G., 1949, The attractions of proteins for small molecules and ions, Ann. N. Y. Acad. Sci. 51:660.

Scheid, M., Boyse, E. A., Carswell, E. A., and Old, L. J., 1972, Serologically demonstrable alloantigens of mouse epidermal cells, J. Exp. Med. 135:938.

Siebers, J. W., Peters, F., Zenzes, M. T., Schmidtke, J., and Engel, W., 1977, Binding of human chorionic gonadotropin to rat ovary during development, J. Endocrinol. 73:491.

Vitetta, E. S., and Capra, J. D., 1978, The protein products of the murine 17th chromosome: genetics and structure, Adv. Immunol. 26:148.

Wachtel, S. S., 1977, H-Y antigen: Genetics and serology, Immunol. Rev. 33:33.

Wachtel, S. S., and Koo, G. C., H-Y antigen in gonadal differentiation, in Mechanisms of Sex Differentiation in Animals and Man, C. R. Austin and R. G. Edwards, eds., Academic Press, London, (In press).

Wachtel, S. S., Koo, G. C., and Boyse, E. A., 1975a, Evolutionary conservation of H-Y ('male') antigen, Nature 254:270.

Wachtel, S. S., Ohono, S., Koo, G. C., and Boyse, E. A., 1975b, Possible role for H-Y antigen in the primary determination of sex, Nature 257:235.

Wachtel, S. S., Koo, G. C., Breg, W. R., Thaler, H. T., Dillard, G. M., Rosenthal, I. M., Dosik, H., Gerald, P. S., Saenger, P., New, M., Lieber, E., and Miller, O. J., 1976, Serologic detection of a Y linked gene in XX males and XX true hermaphrodites, New Engl. J. Med. 295:750.

Wilson, J. D., 1973, Testosterone uptake by the urogenital tract of the rabbit embryo, Endocrinology 92:1192.

Wilson, J. D., and MacDonald, P. C., 1978, Male pseudohermaphroditism due to androgen resistance: Testicular feminization and related syndromes, in The Metabolic Basis of Inherited Disease, J. B. Stanbury, J. B. Wyngaarden and D. S. Frederickson, eds., pp. 894–913, McGraw-Hill, New York.

Zaborski, P., Dorizzi, M., and Pieau, C., 1979, Sur l'utilisation de sérum anti-H-Y de Souris pour la détermination du sexe génétique chez Emys orbicularis L., C. R. Acad. Sci. [D] (Paris) 288:351.

Zenzes, M. T., Müller, U., Aschmoneit, I., and Wolf, U., 1978a, Studies on H-Y antigen in different cell fractions of the testis during pubescence. Immature germ cells are H-Y negative, Hum. Genet. 45:297.

Zenzes, M. T., Wolf, U., and Engel, W., 1978b, Organization in vitro of ovarian cells into testicular structures, Hum. Genet. 44:333.

Zenzes, M. T., Wolf, U., Gunther, E., and Engel. W., 1978c, Studies on the function of H-Y antigen: Dissociation and reorganization experiments on rat gonadal tissue, Cytogenet. Cell Genet. 20:365.

ACKNOWLEDGEMENTS

I am very grateful to Dr. S. S. Wachtel for critical reading and Ms. Karen Leahy for preparation of the manuscript.

This work was supported in part by NIH grants CA-09748, AI-11982, and by a grant from the Deutsche Forschungsgemeinschaft (Si 185/2).

PRESENCE OF AN HCG-LIKE SUBSTANCE IN NON-PREGNANT HUMANS

Glenn D. Braunstein, Joan Rasor,
and Maclyn E. Wade

Departments of Medicine and Obstetrics and
Gynecology, Cedars-Sinai Medical Center, and
UCLA School of Medicine, Los Angeles, Calif., U.S.A.

INTRODUCTION

In 1972, Vaitukaitis and co-workers developed a radioimmunoassay
that was relatively specific for hCG. This assay utilized an antiserum generated against the purified beta subunit of hCG, radioiodinated hCG or its beta subunit as a labeled ligand, and a highly
purified preparation of hCG as a standard. With this method, serum
concentrations of hCG as low as 1 ng (5 mIU)/ml could be measured in
the presence of physiologic quantities of luteinizing hormone (LH),
including those found during the mid-cycle LH surge in premenopausal
women and the large concentrations found in the serum of postmenopausal women (Vaitukaitis et al., 1972). Following the introduction
of this assay, a number of investigators examined the sera of patients
with a variety of nontrophoblastic neoplasms for the presence of
immunoreactive hCG (Braunstein, 1978; Braunstein, 1979). The combined
data from all of these studies indicated that immunoreactive hCG is
found in the sera of approximately 20% of patients with cancer
(Braunstein, 1979).

In several of these studies, control patients without disease or
with benign disorders were also examined for the presence of immunoreactive hCG in their circulation. As summarized in Table I, 2.6%
of the control subjects were found to have detectable levels of hCG
in their sera. Although the actual concentrations of hCG in the sera
of these control patients were generally at the lower limits of detection in the βhCG RIA and could have been due to nonspecific protein
effects or possibly extremely high levels of LH, this finding raised
the possibility that hCG production might not be confined to the
placental trophoblast or malignant tissue.

TABLE I: Incidence of hCG in sera of control patients without neoplasms.

Author	Year	Type of Control	Number of Patients	% Positive Patients
Braunstein et al.	1973a	Normal subjects; patients with benign disorders	433	0.7
Braunstein et al.	1973b	Ugandan Africans with benign disorders	97	2.1
Goldstein, Kosasa and Skarim	1974	Normal subjects; patients with benign disorders	115	0
Sheth et al.	1974	Benign breast disorders	22	0
Samaan et al.	1976	Normal subjects	15	0
Gailani et al.	1976	Normal subjects	70	1.4
Lange et al.	1976	Benign genito-urinary disorders	24	0
Vaitukaitis et al.	1976	Benign gastrointestinal tract disorders	106	9.4
Hagan et al.	1976	Normal subjects; patients with chronic renal failure	149	0
Franchimont et al.	1976, 1977	Normal blood bank donors and patients with non-neoplastic disease	1172	0.8
Williams et al.	1977	Framingham heart study controls	31	12.9
Coombes et al.	1977	Benign breast disease	9	0
Kahn et al.	1977	Normal subjects	87	0
Rutanen and Seppala	1978	Benign gynecologic disorders	104	14.4
Cowen et al.	1978	Normal; benign breast disorders	101	7.9
Dosogne-Guerin et al.	1978	Controls without cancer	56	1.8
			2690	2.6

In 1975, an hCG-like substance was identified in aqueous extracts of testicular tissue (Braunstein et al., 1975). Serial dilutions of the testicular extracts were parallel to the hCG standard in the βhCG RIA and the immunoreactive material co-chromatographed with hCG on a Sephadex G-100 column, and was adsorbed to concanavalin A covalently coupled to Sepharose. Subsequent studies by a number of other workers have demonstrated the presence of an immunoreactive hCG-like substance in human urine, pituitary, colon, liver, kidney, lung, stomach, heart, fibroblasts, and semen (Table II). Some of the investigators utilized radioimmunoassays that were specific for the unique carboxy-terminal portion of the hCG molecule (Chen et al., 1976; Robertson et al., 1978). HCG-like activity was also found in the rat Leydig cell radioreceptor assay (Yoshimoto et al., 1977, 1979a, 1979b) and by in vitro bioassay (Chen et al., 1976; Robertson et al., 1978; Asch et al., 1979). Acevedo and co-workers (1977) and Asch and associates (1977) demonstrated specific binding of rabbit anti-hCG or anti-beta hCG to human spermatozoa by double antibody immunofluorescence technique.

The immunoreactive material present in plasma and urine and extracts of the testis and pituitary have been found to co-chromatograph with purified hCG on columns of Sephadex or Ultragel (Braunstein et al., 1975; Chen et al., 1976; Robertson et al., 1978; Borkowski and Muquardt, 1979; Asch et al., 1979). Robertson and co-workers (1978) demonstrated that the hCG-like material present in pituitary and urinary extracts possessed pI values similar to those of hCG when subjected to isoelectrofocusing. The immunoreactive material present in urine extracts was found to be adsorbed to affinity chromatography columns containing antibodies to the carboxy-terminal portion of the beta subunit of hCG (Ayala et al., 1978), and the hCG-like substance in extracts of the colon, kidney, liver, lung, stomach, and heart was adsorbed to affinity columns containing anti-hCG (Yoshimoto et al., 1979a, 1979b). Together, these studies indicate that an hCG-like substance is widely distributed throughout normal human tissues and bodily fluids.

Few of these studies have critically examined the possibility of proteolytic enzyme interference in the radioligand methods utilized to detect and quantitate the hCG-like substance. In this regard, Richert and Ryan (1977a) demonstrated that a proteolytic enzyme from *Pseudomonas maltophilia* cross-reacted with antisera to intact hCG, as well as antisera to its beta subunit. They extended their studies (Richert and Ryan, 1977b) to show that a variety of serine proteases mimicked the hCG stimulation of adenylate cyclase activity in a membrane-enriched fraction of rat ovary. The studies that are most pertinent to the discussion of an hCG-like substance in normal human tissues are those of Maruo and co-workers (1979). These investigators demonstrated that serial dilutions of extracts of the stomach and hepatopancreas of the crab, *Ovalipes ocelatus*, were parallel to hCG in a homologus hCG radioimmunoassay, carboxy-

TABLE II: Summary of published studies of hCG-like substance in normal human tissues.

Author	Year	Tissue Studies	Assays Utilized*
Braunstein et al.	1975	Testis	RIA (βhCG, hCG)
Chen et al.	1976	Urine, pituitary	RIA (hCG, βhCG, COOH-βhCG); in vitro bioassay
Yoshimoto et al.	1977	Colon, liver	RIA (βhCG); RRA
Acevedo et al.	1977	Sperm	Immunofluorescence
Asch et al.	1977	Sperm, semen	Immunofluorescence; RIA (βhCG)
Dericks-Tan et al.	1977	Semen	RIA (βhCG)
Robertson et al.	1978	Plasma, pituitary, urine	RIA (COOH-βhCG); in vitro bioassay
Ayala et al.	1978	Urine	RIA (βhCG)
Krause	1978	Semen	RIA (βhCG)
Rosen et al.	1978	Fibroblasts in vitro	RIA (βhCG)
Chowdhury and Steinberger	1979	Testis, semen	RIA (βhCG)
Yoshimoto et al.	1979	Kidney, lung, liver, heart, stomach	RIA (βhCG); RRA
Borkowski and Muquardt	1979	Fractionated plasma	RIA (βhCG)
Asch et al.	1979	Sperm	RIA (βhCG); in vitro bioassay
Braunstein et al.	1979	Testis, ovary, lung, pituitary liver, kidney, spleen, stomach, small intestine	RIA (βhCG); RRA

* Abbreviations: RIA=radioimmunoassay; βhCG=hCG beta subunit radioimmunoassay; COOH-βhCG=carboxy terminal beta subunit radioimmunoassay; RRA=radioreceptor assay.

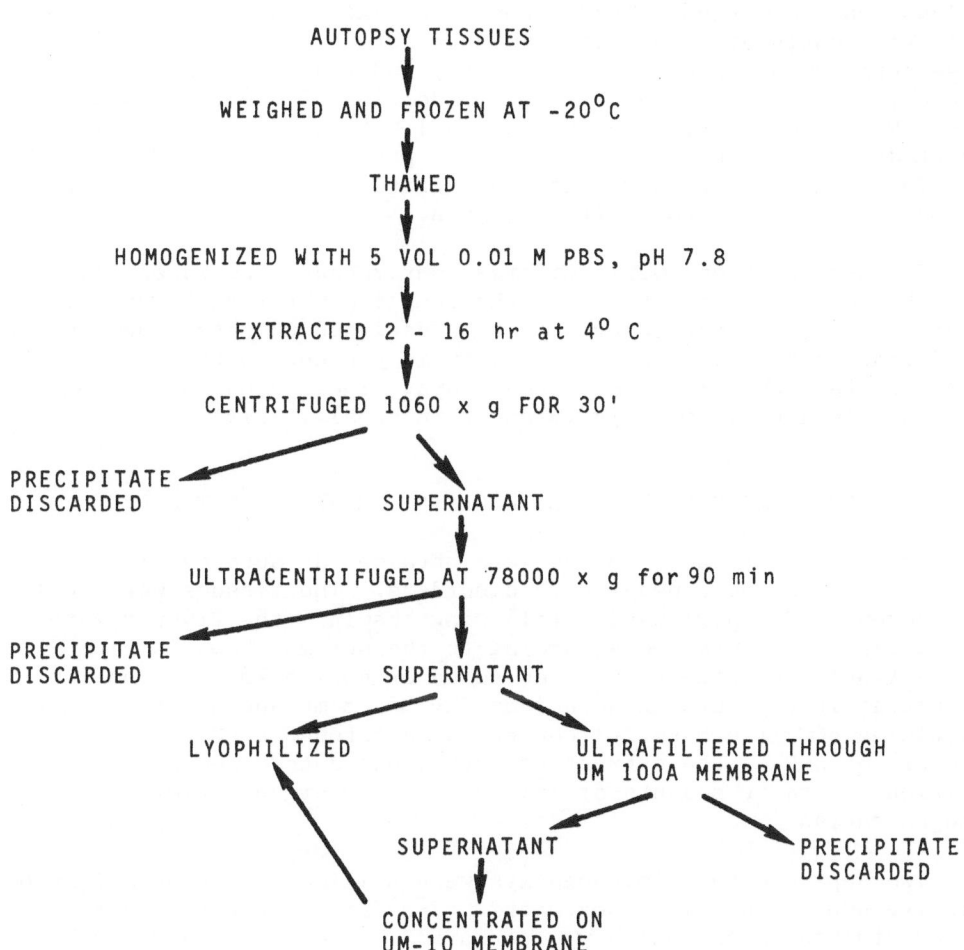

Figure 1. Procedure for extraction and concentration of hCG-like substance from normal human tissues.

terminal-βhCG radioimmunoassay and an hCG radioreceptor assay. Following incubation of the crab stomach extract with trypsin inhibitors, the hCG-like activity was markedly reduced in the RIA. Incubation of ^{125}I-hCG with the purified crab hCG-like factor resulted in degradation of the labeled ligand and led to false positive results for hCG in the hCG radioligand assays. Recently, Adejuwon and co-workers (1979) found that extracts of normal human colon and testis also contained immunoreactive hCG-like material whose activity by both radioimmunoassay and radioreceptor assay was markedly decreased by heat or by the addition of the trypsin inhibitor, N-α-p-tosyl-1-lysine chloromethyl ketone HCl (TLCK). Thus, any study purporting to demonstrate the presence of an hCG-like material in normal human tissues must critically examine the extracts for the presence of proteolytic enzymes.

The next sections will summarize our recent studies on the distribution and quantitation of the hCG-like material in normal human tissues, and our control studies designed to determine whether sufficient proteolytic enzyme activity is present in the extracts to interfere with our radioligand assays. These studies have been published in detail recently (Braunstein et al., 1979).

DISTRIBUTION OF AN HCG-LIKE SUBSTANCE IN NORMAL HUMAN TISSUES

Individual tissues samples were obtained at autopsy or surgery from patients without neoplastic disorders. The tissues were weighed and frozen -20°C until used. Following thawing, the tissues were homogenized and extracted according to the scheme shown in Figure 1. If the final supernatant appeared to be exceptionally viscous, it was ultrafiltered through an Amicon UM-100A membrane and the filtrate containing hCG-like material concentrated through a UM-10 membrane. Recovery of hCG by the extraction method was determined by the addition of tracer amounts of ^{125}I-hCG to the organs prior to homogenization.

Two separate radioimmunoassays were utilized to measure immunoreactive hCG in the tissue extracts. The first was the standard βhCG radioimmunoassay which was performed by reagents supplied by the Hormone Distribution Officer, NIAMDD NIH. The second assay also used an antiserum raised against a highly purified preparation of the beta subunit of hCG which had been prepared in our laboratory (Swaminathan et al., 1979). The antiserum used in this assay, SN-4-adsorbed, had been passed through an immunoadsorbant column containing partially purified human pituitary luteinizing hormone covalently coupled to Sepharose 4B. This antibody recognizes the secondary structure of hCG and requires that the disulfide bonds of the beta subunit be intact (Swaminathan and Braunstein, 1979). The cross-reactions of standard and purified hormone preparations in both of these assays are tabulated in Table III.

TABLE III: Cross-reaction of purified and standard hormone preparations in the βhCG and βLH radioimmunoassays.[a]

Hormone	ng required for 50% inhibition of ^{125}I-ligand binding		
	SB-6	SN-4-Adsorbed	Anti-LH-β
hCG (CR 117)	0.48	3.2	NP[b]
hCG-β (CR 115β)	0.20	2.1	NP
hCG-α (CR 117α)	105.7	>1000.0	>1000.0
LH (LER 960)	20.2	3000.0	3.57
LH (LER 907)	530.3	35000.0	118.2
LH-β (AFP-290-β)	5.0	>25.0	0.49
LH-β (LER 1793-β)	–	–	0.53
WHO-IRP-HPLH (68/40)	16.3	–	1.22
WHO-2nd IRP-HMG	2225.0	20655.0	110.0
WHO-1st IRP FSH/LH (69/104)	3133.3	–	350.0

[a]From Swaminathan and Braunstein, 1978 and Braunstein et al., 1979.

[b]NP: non-parallel.

The rat Leydig cell radioreceptor assay of Catt and co-workers (1971) was used to demonstrate binding of the hCG-like receptors. In this assay, purified alpha and beta subunits of hCG do not displace ^{125}I-hCG from the receptors (Catt et al., 1972).

The inhibition curves produced by serial dilutions of tissue extracts from the testis, ovary, pituitary, lung, liver, kidney, spleen, stomach, and placenta were parallel to that obtained with a purified hCG reference preparation in the hCG radioimmunoassay which utilizes the SB-6 antiserum (Figure 2, top). These extracts also demonstrated parallelism to the hCG standard in the βhCG radioimmunoassay containing the SN-4-adsorbed antiserum (Figure 2, bottom) and in the hCG radioreceptor assay (Figure 3). Most pancreatic extracts and some small intestinal extracts showed significant deviation from parallelism, as did extracts with protein concentrations greater than 70 mg/ml. A highly significant correlation (r = 0.99, p <0.001) was found between the immunoreactive hCG concentrations determined with the SB-6 antiserum and that found with the SN-4-adsorbed antiserum in the various tissues, with the exception of the pituitary extracts. The amount of immunoreactive reactive material measured with the SN-4-adsorbed antiserum in pituitary extracts was approximately 4% of

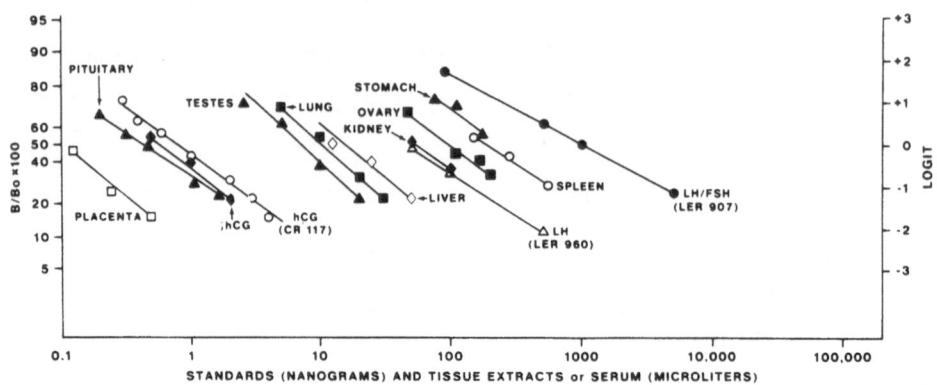

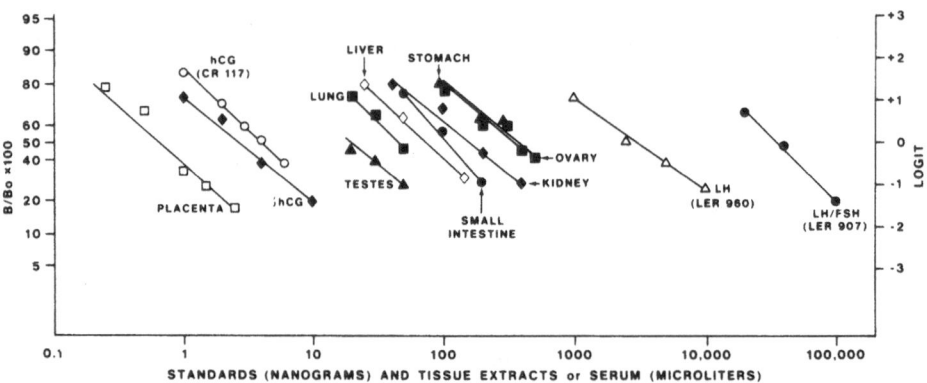

Figure 2. Dose-response curves for purified hormone preparations and extracts of normal human tissues in the hCG radioimmunoassays. (Top): hCG radioimmunoassay with SB-6 antiserum. (Bottom): hCG radioimmunoassay with SN-4-adsorbed antiserum. B represents counts bound in the presence of labeled and unlabeled ligand; Bo is counts bound in the presence of labeled ligand alone. From Braunstein et al., 1979.

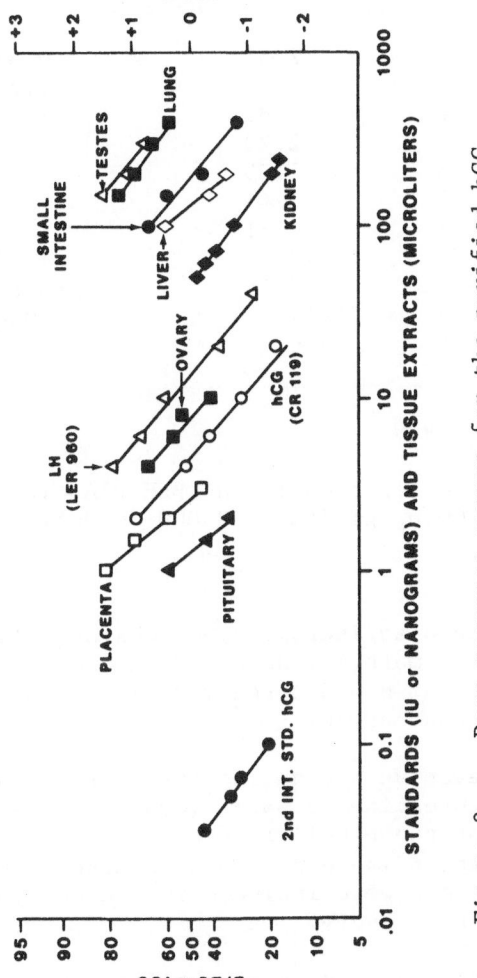

Figure 3. Dose-response curves for the purified hCG preparations (CR 119), the Second International Standard for hCG and serial dilutions of tissue extracts in the rat Leydig cell radioreceptor assay. CR 119 is expressed in terms of ng/tube, while the Second International Standard for hCG is depicted as IU/tube. From Braunstein et al., 1979.

TABLE IV: Concentration of hCG-like substance in normal human tissue.[a]

| Organ | N | hCG Content | |
| | | Median | Range |
			(ng/hCG/gm tissue)
Spleen	6	2.63	0.38-4.33
Kidney	8	4.51	1.72-7.19
Lung	6	2.69	1.68-8.38
Liver	7	2.23	<0.4-6.47
Small intestine	5	10.75	7.9-132.8
Stomach	1	3.45	--
Adrenal	1	1.31	--
Testes	77	19.93	1.44-51.74
Ovary	30	5.55	<0.64-122.9
Pituitary	3	20847.[b]	5954-28492
Placenta	5	5396.	1031-34940

[a]From Braunstein et al., 1979.

[b]Median LH concentration determined in the βLH RIA with LER 907 as the standard was 39,700 ng/gm (range 25000-54400).

that measured with the SB-6 antiserum. The substantially greater quantity of immunoreactive material detected in the pituitary extracts by the latter antiserum undoubtedly reflects the large amount of LH present in that organ.

Recovery of immunoreactive hCG during the extraction procedures varied from 23% (small intestine) to 96.7% (ovary). The median concentrations and ranges of the hCG-like material in the various tissues studied are given in Table IV. Only extracts that were parallel to the hCG standard were included in the analysis, and all values were corrected for recovery.

Immunoreactive LH was measured in a radioimmunoassay which utilizes a rabbit antiserum raised against the beta subunit of LH, ^{125}I-LH as a labeled ligand and a purified preparation of LH (LER 960) as the standard. The reagents for this assay were supplied by the Hormone Distribution Officer, NIAMDD NIH, Bethesda, Maryland, and the cross reactions of the various purified hormone preparations in this assay are shown in Table III.

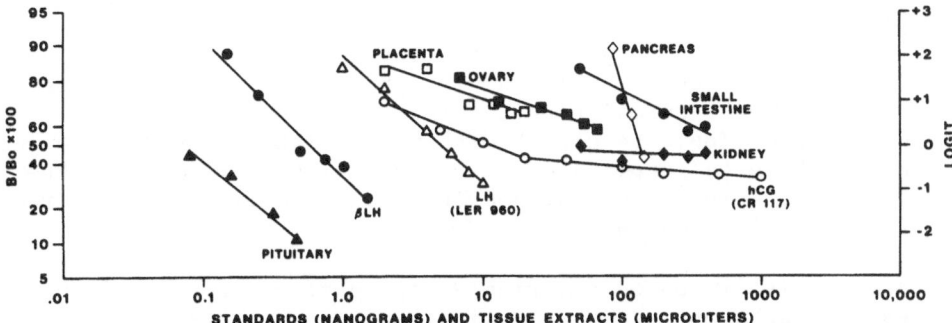

Figure 4.   Dose-response curves for purified hormone preparations and serial dilutions of extracts of normal human tissues in the βLH radioimmunoassay.   From Braunstein et al., 1979.

As would be anticipated, serial dilutions of the pituitary extracts gave parallel dose-response curves to the LH standard in this assay (Figure 4).   However, purified hCG demonstrated a two component curve.   Serial dilutions of placental, ovarian, renal, small intestinal, testicular, and pulmonary extracts were not parallel to the LH standard and more closely resembled the pattern seen with hCG.   Extracts of the pancreas had a steeper slope than either the hCG or LH standards (Figure 4).

These results indicate that an immunoreactive hCG-like material is present in a variety of normal human tissues.   The evidence that the substance is hCG-like includes the immunologic similarity noted in the different hCG immunoassay systems and in the rat Leydig cell radioreceptor assay.   The use of the LH-immunoadsorbed anti-beta hCG serum in the βhCG RIA eliminated the potential source of interference of immunoreactive LH.   The close correlation between the results obtained with the SB-6 and the SN-4-adsorbed antisera in all tissues except for the pituitary, indicates that both assays were measuring the same substance.   The lack of parallelism between serial dilutions of non-pituitary tissue extracts and the LH standards in the βLH radioimmunoassay, provides additional evidence that the immunoreactive material more closely resembles hCG than hLH.

CONCANAVALIN A BINDING STUDIES

Aliquots of the tissue extracts or purified hormone preparations were applied to 0.7 x 4 cm columns containing 0.25 ml Sephadex G-25 and 1.5 ml of concanavalin A covalently coupled to Sepharose 4B. The non-adsorbed substances were eluted with phosphate buffered saline, pH 7.8, containing 1% normal rabbit serum. The concanavalin A-adsorbed glycoproteins were eluted with 0.2 M alpha-D-methylglucoside (MeG) in phosphate buffered saline. One milliliter aliquots of the eluted fractions were collected, and the immunoreactive hCG measured in the βhCG radioimmunoassay.

These studies revealed a variable degree of adsorption of the immunoreactive substance to the lectin (Figure 5). A larger percentage of the immunoreactive material present in the testis, ovaries, placenta, and small intestine adsorbed to concanavalin A than that found in the lung, liver, or kidney. Several pancreatic extracts were chromatographed, and all of the immunoreactive material that could be recovered eluted prior to the application of the 0.2 M alpha-D-methylglucoside. As indicated in Figure 5, the amount of immunoreactive material recovered following concanavalin A-Sepharose chromatography varied with each tissue. Re-chromatography of the non-adsorbed fractions on fresh concanavalin A-Sepharose columns did not result in any additional binding to concanavalin A. Thus, the failure of complete binding of the immunoreactive substance to concanavalin A in each of the extracts could not be attributed to overloading of the column by tissue proteins. These results are similar to those of Yoshimoto and co-workers (1976, 1979a, 1979b).

These studies indicate that differences do exist between the predominate molecular species present in purified placental hCG and the immunoreactive material present in other tissues. Since concanavalin A adsorbs glycoproteins by interactions with the carbohydrate moiety of the protein (Dufau et al., 1972), the variable and incomplete adsorption of the immunoreactive substance in normal tissues suggests that there are differences in the degree of glycosylation of the hCG-like material from different tissues. Although all of the highly purified urinary hCG applied to the concanavalin A column was adsorbed and recovered, each of the tissue extracts, including the placenta, had material which was not adsorbed and which eluted prior to the addition of MeG.

Several investigators have indicated that the hCG that is present in the urine of pregnant women is actually composed of iso-hormones with variable amounts of sialic acid (Van Hell et al., 1968; Schuurs et al., 1968; Matthies and Diczfalusy, 1971). Since progressive removal of sialic acid from highly purified hCG results in more rapid clearance of hCG from serum (Van Hall, 1971; Tsuruhara et al., 1972; Moyle et al., 1975; Bahl, 1977), it would be anticipated

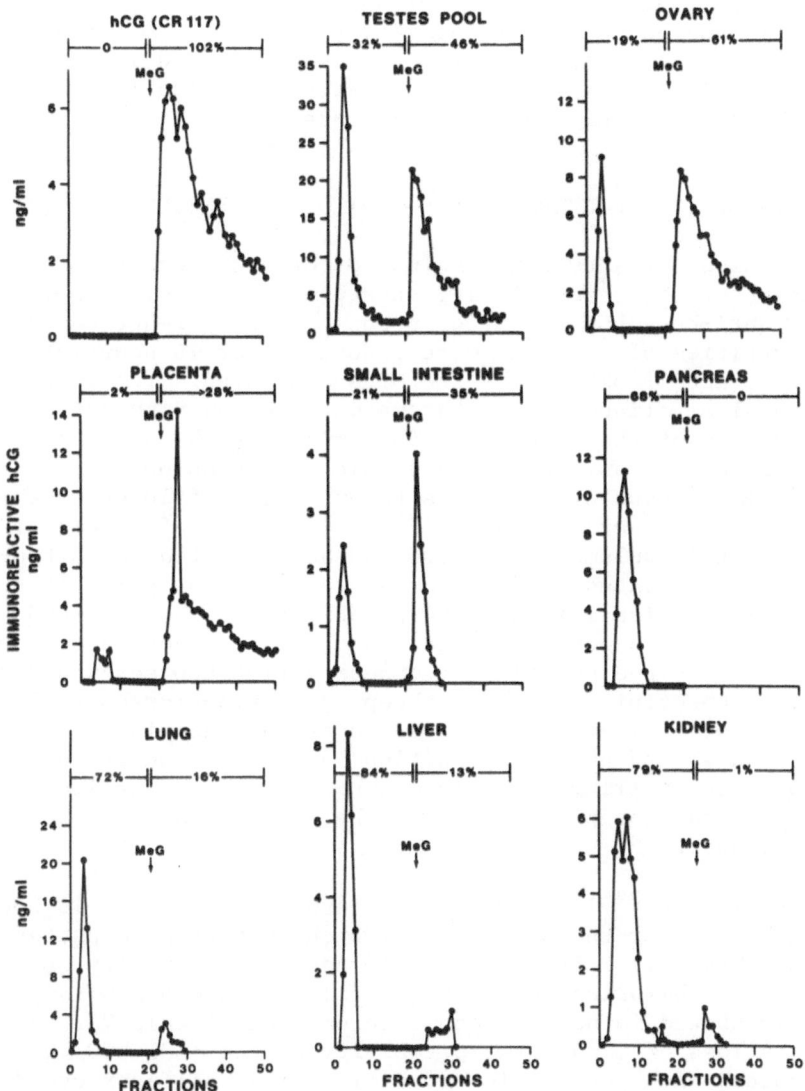

Figure 5. Concanavalin A-Sepharose column chromatography of purified hCG (CR 117) and extracts of normal human tissues. The immunoreactive hCG content was measured in the beta hCG radioimmunoassay with the SB-6 antiserum. The non-adsorbed material is depicted to the left of the arrow, while the concanavalin A-adsorbed immunoreactive substances are shown to the right of the arrow. The numbers above each chromatogram indicate the percentage recovery of immunoreactive hCG in the non-adsorbed and concanavalin A-adsorbed fractions respectively. MeG= 0.2 M α-D-methylglucoside. From Braunstein et al., 1979.

that the hCG-like material in normal tissues would be rapidly cleared from the circulation if it is incompletely glycosylated. This would explain the low frequency of detection of immunoreactive hCG in the sera of non-pregnant individuals without neoplasms. Indeed, in preliminary studies we have found that the hCG-like material present in pooled extracts of normal human testes is cleared more rapidly from the circulation of immature male rats following intravenous injection than is highly purified placental hCG.

EXAMINATION OF TISSUE EXTRACTS FOR PROTEOLYTIC ENZYME ACTIVITY

The tissue extracts were evaluated for the presence of proteo-lytic enzyme or other interfering substances which might alter the ^{125}I-hCG, anti-beta hCG serum, or second antibody reaction. First, tracer quantities of ^{125}I-hCG were incubated for 16 hours at 4°C with the extracts from each of the organs studied. Following the incubation, 1 ml aliquots were chromatographed on Sephadex G-100. The void volume of the column was determined by the peak elution volume of blue dextran, while the volume of exclusion for ^{125}I-hCG incubated with tissue extracts was taken as the effluent tube with the highest counts per minute of ^{125}I. The ratio of volume of exclusion to void volume was determined and compared to that obtained with ^{125}I-hCG incubated in 2.5% normal rabbit serum prior to chroma-tography. The residual immunoprecipitability of the ^{125}I-hCG following incubation with the organs and the Sephadex chromatography was determined by the addition of excess anti-β hCG serum and sub-sequent immunoprecipitation with sheep or goat anti-rabbit globulin. Non-specific precipitation was assessed by the addition of excess (10 IU) of unlabeled hCG. In addition, an evaluation of the degree of immunoprecipitability of ^{125}I-hCG which had been carried through the entire extraction procedure with the tissues was performed in a similar manner.

Incubation of ^{125}I-hCG with the tissue extracts for 16 hours at 4°C did not alter the Sephadex G-100 chromatographic pattern of the ligand (Table V). The residual immunoprecipitability of the labeled ligand following Sephadex gel filtration was similar to ^{125}I-hCG incubated in normal rabbit serum alone (Table V). However, there was a loss of immunoprecipitability of the ^{125}I-hCG that had been incubated with pancreatic and small intestinal extracts during the entire tissue extraction procedure (Table V), suggesting the presence of proteolytic enzymes in these tissues that could alter radioiodinated hCG.

A second control for proteolytic enzyme activity or other tissue factors that could alter the degree of adsorption of the hCG onto concanavalin A was carried out by incubating ^{125}I-hCG with tissue extracts for 16 hours at 4°C followed by concanavalin A chromato-graphy. Recovery of the ^{125}I-hCG in the non-adsorbed fractions and

TABLE V: Sephadex G-100 chromatography and immunoprecipitation studies of ^{125}I-hCG following incubation with tissues extracts.[a]

	Sephadex G-100		% IP[b] following
	Ve/Vo	% IP	extraction of organs with ^{125}I-hCG
^{125}I-hCG	1.23-1.40	100[c] (82.2-122.7)	100[c] (91.1-108.8)
ORGAN:			
Spleen	1.38	117	104.4
Kidney	1.37	104	93.2
Lung	1.35	114	111.4
Liver	1.34	110	111.7
Small Intestine	1.37	107	43.0
Pancreas	1.37	89	1.1
Pituitary	1.34	98	--
Ovary	1.32	114	91.5
Placenta	1.36	109	d

[a]From Braunstein et al., 1979.
[b]Ve=volume of exclusion; Vo=void volume; IP=immunoprecipitable.
[c]The immunoprecipitability of ^{125}I-hCG was assumed to be maximum when the tracer was chromatographed or extracted with 2.5% normal rabbit serum (NRS). The average value was designated 100% with the range from 4 experiments shown in parenthesis. The immuno-precipitability of the labeled ligand incubated or extracted with the same batch of ^{125}I-hCG incubated in NRS. This allows for the comparison of data obtained with ^{125}I-hCG that had been iodinated at different times.
[d]Excessive quantities of hCG prevented complete immunoprecipitation.

MeG (adsorbed) fractions was determined and compared to that found with ^{125}I-hCG incubated in 2.5% normal rabbit serum. The degree of residual immunoprecipitability of the ^{125}I-hCG which had been incubated with the tissues and which was adsorbed onto concanavalin A was established with the addition of excess anti-βhCG serum to the peak MeG effluent tubes, followed by precipitation with sheep or goat anti-rabbit globulin.

The results of the concanavalin A studies are shown in Table VI. The recovery of the ^{125}I-hCG in the non-adsorbed and adsorbed fractions and the residual immunoprecipitability of the ligand were similar for tracer that had been incubated in normal rabbit serum

TABLE VI: Concanavalin A chromatography and immunoprecipitation of ^{125}I-hCG following incubation with tissue extracts.

^{125}I-hCG in NRS	For 16 Hours^a % Recovered in Buffer Eluate (nonadsorbed)	% Recovered in MeG Eluate (adsorbed)	% Immuno-precipitable (after MeG)
	10.0 (7.0–12.5)	91.1 (81.0–104.8)	100^b (95.3–103.8)
ORGAN:			
Spleen	12.3	91.6	87.1
Kidney	12.8	89.7	97.6
Lung	12.5	97.7	96.9
Liver	11.1	95.3	100.3
Small Intestine	9.6	92.3	108.3
Pancreas	10.3	56.4	51.2
Pituitary	8.4	86.4	99.0
Ovary	11.4	90.4	92.5
Blood	12.1	91.5	98.1

^{a}From Braunstein et al., 1979.
^{b}The immunoprecipitability of ^{125}I-hCG was assumed to be maximum when the tracer chromatographed with 2.5% normal rabbit serum (NRS). The average value was designated 100% with the range from 5 experiments shown in parenthesis. The immunoprecipitability of the labeled ligand incubated with the organs was divided by that found with the same batch of ^{125}I-hCG incubated in NRS. This allows for comparison of data obtained with ^{125}I-hCG that had been iodinated at different times.
Abbreviations: MeG=0.2 M α-D-methylglucoside.

or extracts of the ovary, pituitary, lung, small intestine, liver, spleen, kidney, or pooled blood from male donors. Poor recovery and reduced immunoprecipitability of the ^{125}I-hCG was noted following incubation with pancreatic extracts, again suggesting that pancreatic extracts contained proteolytic enzymes that interfered with the radioligand assays.

A third control for the possibility of enzymatic degradation of ^{125}I-hCG by the tissue extracts consisted of high voltage electrophoresis and thin layer chromatography of ^{125}I-hCG which had been incubated with tissue extracts for 16 hours at 4°C. Both procedures were also carried out with ^{125}I-hCG which had been incubated with tissue extracts that had previously been boiled for 7 minutes in order to destroy any putative proteolytic enzyme activity. Under the conditions employed for both the high voltage electrophoresis and thin layer chromatography, unlabeled hCG did not move from the origin. High voltage electrophoresis of the ^{125}I-hCG following incubation with boiled and unboiled tissue extracts revealed that only the tracer incubated with the unboiled pancreatic extracts was sufficiently damaged to migrate away from the origin. Thin layer chromatography did not demonstrate fragments of hCG following incubation with the tissue extracts.

A fourth method of evaluating proteolytic enzyme activity was accomplished by comparing the content of immunoreactive hCG in the organ extracts before and after boiling for 20 minutes prior to the addition of the labeled ligand and first antibody in the βhCG radioimmunoassay. It was noted with some of the extracts that this procedure caused precipitation of proteins and the formation of a gel which undoubtedly lead to losses of hCG activity through nonspecific trapping. However, since the immunoreactive activity was lost to a similar degree in the nontrophoblastic tissue extracts, placental extracts and pregnancy serum (Table VII), we conclude that the reduction of immunoreactive hCG-like activity following the procedure is not primarily due to elimination of cross-reacting substances or destruction of proteolytic enzyme activity. It is of interest that Yoshimoto and co-workers (1979a, 1979b) found immunoreactive hCG in extracts of normal human tissues that had been extensively boiled.

Several proteolytic enzyme inhibitors were tested for their ability to inhibit the binding of serial dilutions of the tissue extracts in the βhCG radioimmunoassay. These inhibitors included: benzamidine, 156 µg/tube; n-α-p-tosyl-1-lysine chloromethyl ketone HCl (TLCK), 1 µg/tube and 2 mg/tube; apoprotinin, 44K IU/tube; ovalbumin, 100 µg/tube; soybean trypsin inhibitor 20 µg/tube; mercuric chloride, 272 µg/tube; and phenylmethylsulfonyl fluoride (PMSF), 174 g/tube. The dose-response curves for the immunoreactive hCG in the tissue extracts with the inhibitors, were compared with those found without the inhibitors.

None of the protease inhibitors significantly altered the dose-response curves of serial dilutions of the nontrophoblastic tissue extracts in comparison to their effect on placental extracts or pregnancy serum, with the exception of the pancreatic extracts, which gave inconsistent results with high non-specific counts. A summary of the studies with TLCK, 2 mg/tube, is given in Table VIII. It should be noted that this inhibitor was utilized by Maruo and co-workers (1979) and Adejuwon and colleagues (1979) to inhibit the activity of the crab stomach trypsin-like protease and hCG-like immunoreactivity in human testicular and colonic tissues.

TABLE VII: Effect of heating hCG or extracts at 90°C for 20 minutes.

Substance	N	% Change Mean	Range
hCG in NRS^a	2	-60.2	-48.7 to -71.7
hCG in NHP^b	1	-47.3	--
Pregnancy serum	4	-33.8	-95.4 to +28.3
Placenta	5	-41.5	-58.1 to +5.52
Testes	2	-20.6	-40.0 to -1.3
Ovary	1	-46.2	--
Small intestine	2	-26.3	-35.1 to -17.6
Stomach	2	-28.7	-62.7 to -45.1
Spleen	2	-62.1	-79.2 to -45.1
Kidney	2	-73.0	-85.3 to -60.7
Pituitary	2	- 7.2	-58.3 to +43.8
Lung	1	+ 1.9	--
Liver	1	-46.8	--
Urine	1	+13.2	--
Trypsin in NHP	1	All activity lost	--

^{a}Normal rabbit serum
^{b}Normal human plasma

TABLE VIII: Effect of N-α-p-tosyl-1-lysine chloromethyl ketone Hcl (TLCK), 2 mg/tube, on immunoreactive hCG concentration.

Substance	% Change with TLCK
hCG in NRS^a	+ 73.3
Pregnancy serum	+ 93.1
Placenta	+ 53.3
Testes	+ 22.6
Small intestine	+ 20.2
Stomach	+ 80.0
Spleen	+ 64.4
Kidney	+ 76.3
Pituitary	+293.1
Lung	+ 86.7
Liver	+116.2
Pancreas	- 18.3
Trypsin in NHP^b (20 mg/ml)	- 84.8

^{a}2.5% Normal rabbit serum
^{b}Normal human male plasma

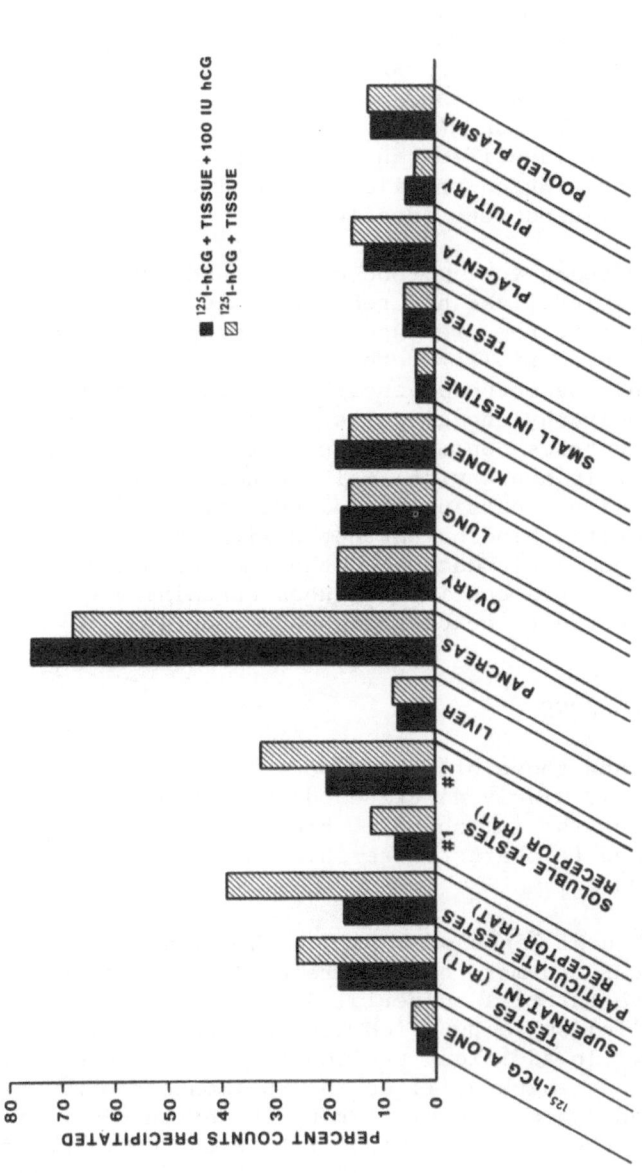

Figure 6. Percent counts precipitated of ^{125}I-hCG after incubation with tissue extracts for 16 hours in the presence (solid bars) or absence (hatched bars) of excess (100 IU) hCG. Precipitation of the labeled ligand was accomplished with 12.5% polyethylene glycol. Rat testicular hCG-receptor preparations were used for positive control purposes. The concentration of the rat soluble testes receptor #1 was equivalent to 0.1 gm testes, while #2 was equivalent to 0.46 gm. testes. From Braunstein et al., 1979.

EXAMINATION OF THE TISSUE EXTRACTS FOR SOLUBILIZED RECEPTORS

The extracts were also examined for the presence of solubilized receptors that could compete with the binding protein for ^{125}I-hCG in the radioligand assays. The Sephadex G-100 chromatography pattern of ^{125}I-hCG which had been incubated for 16 hours at 4°C with tissue extracts from each of the organs was compared to the elution pattern of ^{125}I-hCG chromatographed alone. No high molecular weight ^{125}I-hCG receptor complex was identified in the chromatograms following tissue incubation, and the elution profiles of the incubated and non-incubated labeled ligand were identical.

The polyethylene glycol method of Catt and Dufau (1975) for the precipitation of solubilized hCG receptors was also used in an attempt to demonstrate the presence of such receptors in the tissue extracts. Positive controls for the receptor assays were prepared from rat testis by the methods described by Catt and Dufau (1975). The addition of polyethylene glycol at a final concentration of 12.5% (ω/ν) to the tubes containing human tissue extracts that had been incubated for 16 hours with ^{125}I-hCG did not result in the background tubes with excess unlabeled hCG (Figure 6). A large amount of non-specific binding was noted with the pancreatic extracts, again suggesting enzymatic damage to the labeled hCG. Specific ^{125}I-hCG binding was present in the tubes containing the rat testicular extracts treated to concentrate hCG receptors.

SUMMARY AND CONCLUSIONS

Our studies and those of others (see Table II) indicate that an hCG-like material is widely distributed throughout the human body. Table IX summarizes the immunologic, biologic and physical studies that have been used to characterize the hCG-like substance in each of the organs studied.

There are several lines of evidence that indicate that the material being measured more closely resemble hCG, rather than LH. The immunoreactive material in serial dilutions of the extracts demonstrate parallelism to purified hCG, but not LH, in the βhCG radioimmunoassay. In addition, the quantities of hCG measured in the radioimmunoassay which utilizes the LH-immunoadsorbed anti-beta hCG serum, SN-4-adsorbed, are similar to those found with the SB-6 antiserum. Since the cross reaction of LH with the former antiserum is substantially less than that found with SB-6 (Table III), it is unlikely that the immunoreactive material present in non-pituitary tissue extracts is LH. Similarly, an hCG-like material has been detected in tissues with the use of carboxy-terminal-βhCG radio-immunoassays which do not recognize LH. The lack of parallelism between serial dilutions of nonpituitary tissue extracts and LH in

TABLE IX: Summary of immunologic and physical studies indicating that an hCG-like substance is present in non-trophoblastic tissues.

Fluid or Organ	βhCG-RIA	COOH-βhCG RIA[a]	RRA	Activity in in vitro bioassay	Adsorption to anti-hCG column	Co-elution with hCG on Sephadex	Similar pI by IEF[b]
Serum[c]	x	x				x	
Urine	x	x		x	x	x	x
Colon	x		x		x		
Heart	x		x		x		
Kidney	x		x		x		
Liver	x		x		x		
Lung	x		x		x		
Ovary	x		x				
Pituitary	x	x	x	x		x	x
Small intestine	x		x				
Spleen	x		x				
Stomach	x		x		x		
Testis[d]	x		x	x		x	

[a] carboxy-terminal βhCG radioimmunoassay
[b] isoelectrofocusing
[c] serum or plasma
[d] includes studies performed on sperm extracts or semen

the βLH radioimmunoassay provides further evidence that the immuno-reactive substance is not LH-like. Finally, there does not appear to be a correlation between the hCG immunoreactivity and LH immuno-reactivity when both are measured in the same sample (Robertson et al., 1978, Rutanen and Seppala, 1978; Borkowski and Muquardt, 1979).

The various immunoassays utilized suggest that the amino acid sequence and the secondary structure of the hCG-like material in nontrophoblastic tissues are similar, if not identical, to that produced by the placental trophoblast. However, the reduced binding of the hCG-like material in normal human tissues to concanavalin A suggests that there is incomplete glycosylation. This formulation would be compatible with current concepts of glycoprotein biosynthe-sis which indicate that the peptide sequence is synthesized under direct genetic control, while the carbohydrate attachment is a post-ribosomal event modulated by the glycosyl-transferase enzymes present in the Golgi apparatus of the cell (Schacter et al., 1970; Neutra and LeBlond, 1976; Eagon and Heath, 1977; Bielinska and Boime, 1978). However, only purification of the hCG-like material in nontrophoblastic tissues followed by amino acid sequence and carbo-hydrate studies will confirm whether the material is indeed hCG or merely hCG-like.

Despite the suggestions of Adejuwon and associates (1979), we were unable to demonstrate proteolytic enzyme interference in our radioligand assays in extracts of testis, ovary, pituitary, lung, liver, kidney, spleen, stomach, or placenta. Some small intestinal tissue samples also appeared to be free of significant proteolytic enzyme activity although others did degrade the labeled ligand during prolonged incubation. Out studies do show that the pancreatic extracts contained significant amount of proteolytic enzyme activity which altered the ^{125}I-hCG utilized in the various radioligand assays.

It is unknown if this material has any physiologic role in non-pregnant humans. It is also unclear whether the immunoreactive hCG-like material present in the various normal tissues is synthesized by each of these tissues, or represents binding or storage of the substance produced at a distant site. Direct evidence of production has been provided by Rosen and colleagues (1978) who noted the secretion of hCG or βhCG by normal human fibroblast cell lines grown in culture.

The production of this hCG-like material may represent incom-plete suppression in adult tissues of the fetal genome responsible for hCG production. Alternatively, the substance may be produced by relatively undifferentiated stem cells which are responsible for cell renewal in the various organs. Such cells may not have differ-entiated to the stage of repression of the hCG genome.

REFERENCE

Acevedo, H. F., Slifkin, M., Pouchet, G. R., and Rakhshan, M., 1977, Identification of the β subunit of choriogonadotropin in human spermatozoa, in *The Testis in Normal and Infertile Men*, P. Troen and H. R. Nankin, eds., pp. 185-192, Raven Press, New York.

Adejuwon, C. A., Segal, S. J., and Mitsudo, S., 1979, Protease inhibitor abolished the apparent hCG-like immunoactivity in human tissues, Abstracts of the 61st Annual Meeting of the Endocrine Society, Abstract #954, Endocrinology (Supplement).

Asch, R. H., Fernandez, E. O., and Pauerstein, C. J., 1977, Immunodetection of a human chorionic gonadotropin-like substance in human sperm, Fertil. Steril. 28:1258.

Asch, R. H., Fernandez, E. O., Siler-Khodr, T. M., and Pauerstein, C. J., 1979, Presence of a human chorionic gonadotropin-like substance in human sperm, Am. J. Obstet. Gynecol. (in press).

Ayala, A. R., Nisula, B. C., Chen, H., Hodgen, G. D., and Ross, G. T., 1978, Highly sensitive radioimmunoassay for chorionic gonadotropin in human urine, J. Clin. Endocrin. Metab. 47:767.

Bahl, O. P., 1977, Human chorionic gonadotropin, its receptor and mechanism of action, Fed. Proc. 36:2119.

Bielinska, M., and Boime, I., 1978, mRNA-dependent synthesis of a glycosylated subunit of human chorionic gonadotropin in cell-free extracts derived from ascites tumor cells, Proc. Natl. Acad. Sci. USA 75:1768.

Borkowski, A., and Muquardt, C., 1979, Human chorionic gonadotropin in the plasma of normal, nonpregnant subjects, N. Engl. J. Med. 301:298.

Braunstein, G. D., 1978, Use of human chorionic gonadotropin as a tumore marker in cancer, in *Immunodiagnosis of Cancer*, R. B. Herberman and K. R. McIntire, eds., pp. 383-409, Marcel Dekker, Inc., New York.

Braunstein, C. D., 1979, Human chorionic gonadotropin in non-trophoblastic tumors and tissues, in *Recent Advances in Reproduction and Regulation of Fertility*, G. P. Talwar, ed., pp. 389-397, Elsevier/North Holland Biomedical Press, Amsterdam.

Braunstein, G. D., Vaitukaitis, J. L., Carbone, P. P., and Ross, G. T., 1973a, Ectopic production of human chorionic gonadotropin by neoplasms, Ann. Intern. Med. 78:39.

Braunstein, G. D., Vogel, C. L., Vaitukaitis, J. L., and Ross, G. T., 1973b, Ectopic production of human chorionic gonadotropin in Ugandan patients with hepatocellular carcinoma, Cancer 32:223.

Braunstein, G. D., Rasor, J., and Wade, M. E., 1975, Presence in normal human testes of a chorionic-gonadotropin-like substance distinct from human luteinizing hormone, N. Engl. J. Med. 293:1339.

Braunstein, G. D., Kamdar, V., Rasor, J., Swaminathan, N., and Wade, M. E., 1979, Widespread distribution of a chorionic gonadotropin-like substance in normal human tissues, J. Clin. Endocrinol. Metab. (in press).

Catt, K. J., and Dufau, M. L., 1975, Gonadal receptors for luteinizing hormone and chorionic gonadotropin, in *Methods in Enzymology*, Vol. 37, B. W. O'Malley and J. G. Handman, eds., p. 167, Academic Press, New York.

Catt, K. J., Dufau, M. L., and Tsuruhara, T., 1971, Studies on a radioligand-receptor assay system for luteinizing hormone and chorionic gonadotropin, J. Clin. Endocrinol. Metab. 32:860.

Catt, K. J., Dufau, M. L., and Tsuruhara, T., 1972, Radioligand-receptor assay of luteinizing hormone and chorionic gonadotropin, J. Clin. Endocrinol. Metab. 34:123.

Chen, H. C., Hodgen, G. D., Matsuura, S., Canfield, R. E., and Ross, G. T., 1976, Evidence for a gonadotropin from nonpregnant subjects that has physical, immunological and biological similarities to human chorionic gonadotropin, Proc. Natl. Acad. Sci. U.S.A. 73:2885.

Chowdhury, M., and Steinberger, E., 1979, Effects of age and estrogen therapy on the immunoreactive human chorionic gonadotropin content of testes, Fertil. Steril. 31:328.

Coombes, R. C., Powles, T. J., Gazet, J. C., Ford, H. T., Nash, A. G., Sloane, J. P., Hillyard, C. J., Thomas, P., Keyser, J. W., Marcus, D., Zinberg, N., Stimson, W. H., and Neville, A. M., 1977, A biochemical approach to the staging of human breast cancer, Cancer 40:937.

Cowen, D. M., Searle, F., Ward, A. M., Benson, E. A., Smiddy, F. G., Eaves, G., and Cooper, E. H., 1978, Multivariate biochemical indicators of breast cancer: an evaluation of their potential in routine practice, Europ. J. Cancer 14:885.

Dericks-Tan, J. S. E., Bradler, H., and Taubert, H. D., 1977, Different concentrations of LH, FSH, PRL, and hCG-β in serum and seminal fluid, Acta Endocrinol. (KBH) 84:24.

Dosogne-Guerin, M., Stolarczuk, A., and Borkowski, A., 1978, Prospective study of α and β subunits of human chorionic gonadotropin in the blood of patients with various benign and malignant conditions, Europ. J. Cancer 14:525.

Dufau, M. L., Tsuruhara, T., and Catt, K. J., 1972, Interaction of glycoprotein hormones with agarose-concanavalin A, Biochem. Biophys. Acta 278:281.

Eagon, P. K., and Heath, E. C., 1977, Glycoprotein biosynthesis in myeloma cells, J. Biol. Chem. 252:2372.

Franchimont, P., Zangerle, P. F., Norgarede, J., Bury, J., Molter, F., Rutler, A., Hendrick, J.C., and Colletee, J., 1976, Simultaneous assays of cancer-associated antigens in various neoplastic disorders, Cancer 38:2278.

Franchimont, P., Zangerle, P. F., Hendrick, J. C., Reuter, A., and Colin, C., 1977, Simultaneous assays of cancer-associated antigens in benign and malignant breast diseases, Cancer 39:28-6.

Gailani, S., Chu, T. M., Nussbaum, A., Ostrander, M., and Christoff, N., 1976, Human chorionic gonadotropin (hCG) in nontrophoblastic neoplasms. Assessment of abnormalities of hCG and CEA in brochogenic and digestive neoplasms, Cancer 38:1684.

Goldstein, D. P., Kosasa, T. S., and Skarin, A. T., 1974, The clinical application of a specific radioimmunoassay for human chorionic gonadotropin in trophoblastic and nontrophoblastic tumors, Surg. Gynecol. Obstet. 138:747.

Hagen, C., Gilby, E. D., McNeilly, A. S., Olgaard, K., Bondy, P. K., and Rees, L. H., 1976, Comparison of circulating glycoprotein hormones and their subunits in patients with oat cell carcinoma of the lung and uremic patients on chronic dialysis, Acta Endocrinol. 83:26.

Hattori, M., Fukase, M., Yoshimi, H., Matsukura, S., and Imura, H., 1978, Ectopic production of human chorionic gonadotropin in malignant tumors, Cancer 42:2328.

Kahn, C. R., Rosen, S. W., Weintraub, B. D., Fajans, S. S., and Gorden, P., 1977, Ectopic production of chorionic gonadotropin and its subunits by islet-cell tumors. A specific marker for malignancy, N. Engl. J. Med. 297:565.

Krause, W., 1979, On the concentration of hCG-like material in human semen, Int. J. Androl. 2:43.

Lange, P. H., McIntire, K. R., Waldman, T. A., and Hakala, T. R., and Fraley, E., 1976, Serum alpha-fetoprotein and human chorionic gonadotropin in the diagnosis and management of nonseminomatous germ-cell testicular cancer, N. Engl. J. Med. 295:1237.

Maruo, T., Segal, S. J., and Koide, S. S., 1979, Studies on the apparent human chorionic gonadotropin-like factor in the crab Ovalipes ocellatus, Endocrinology 104:932.

Matthies, D.L., and Diczfalusy, E., 1971, Relationships between physico-chemical, immunological, and biological properties of human chorionic gonadotropin, Acta Endocrinol. (KBH) 67:434.

Moyle, W. R., Bahl, O. P., and Marz, L., 1975, Role of carbohydrate of human chorionic gonadotropin in the mechanism of hormone action, J. Biol. Chem. 250:9163.

Neutra, M., and LeBlond, C. P., 1966, Radioautographic comparison of the uptake of galactose-H^3glucose-H^3 in the Golgi region of various cells secreting glycoproteins or mucopolysaccharides, J. Cell Biol. 30:137.

Richert, N.D., and Ryan, R. J., 1977b, Proteolytic enzyme activation of rat ovarian adenylate cuclase, Proc. Nat. Acad. Sci. U.S.A. 74:4857.

Robertson, D. M., Suginami, H., Montez, H. H., Puri, C. P., Choi, S. K., and Diczfalusy, E., 1978, Studies on a human chorionic gonadotropin-like material present in non-pregnant subjects, Acta Endocrinol. 89:492.

Rosen, S. W., Weintraub, B. D., and Aaronsen, S., 1978, Nonrandom ectopic protein production by malignant cell lines: Direct evidence in vitro, Clin. Res. 26:537A.

Rutanen, E.M., and Seppala, M., 1978, The hCG-beta subunit radioimmunoassay in nontrophoblastic gynecologic tumors, Cancer 41:692.

Samaan, N. A., Smith, J. P., Rutledge, F. N., and Schultz, P. N., 1976, The significance of measurement of placental lactogen, human chorionic gonadotropin, and carcinoembryonic antigen in patients with ovarian carcinoma, Am. J. Obstet. Gynecol. 126:186.

Schacter, H., Jabbal, I., Hudgin, R. L., Pinteric, L., McGuire, E., and Roseman, S., 1970, Intracellular localization of liver sugar nucleotide glycoprotein glycosyl-transferases in a Golgi-rich fraction, J. Biol. Chem. 245:1090.

Schuurs, H., DeJager, W. M. E., and Homan, J. D. H., 1968, Studies on human chorionic gonadotropin. III immunochemical character-ization, Acta Endocrinol. (KBH) 59:120.

Seth, N. A., Saruiya, J. N., Ranadive, K. J., and Sheth, A. R., 1974, Ectopic production of human chorionic gonadotropin by human breast tumors, Br. J. Cancer 30:566.

Swaminathan, N., and Braunstein, G. D., 1978, Location of major antigenic sites of the beta subunit of human chorionic gonado-tropin, Biochemistry 12:5832.

Swaminathan, N., Rasor, J., and Braunstein, G. D., 1979, Preparation and properties of high titer antisera against the beta subunit of human chorionic gonadotropin, Mol. Immunol. 16:113.

Tsuruhara, T., Dufau, M. L., Hickman, J., and Catt, K., 1972, Biological properties of hCG after removal of terminal sialic acid and galactose residues, Endocrinology 91:296.

Vaitukaitis, J. L., Braunstein, G. D., and Ross, G. T., 1972, Radioimmunoassay which specifically measures human chorionic gonadotropin in the presence of human luteinizing hormone, Am. J. Obstet. Gynecol. 113:751.

Vaitukaitis, J. L., Ross, G. T., Braunstein, G. D., and Rayford, P. L., 1976, Gonadotropins and their subunits: Basic and clini-cal studies, Recent Prog. Horm. Res. 32:289.

Van Hall, E. V., Vaitukaitis, J. L., and Ross, G. T., 1971, Immuno-logical and biological activity of hCG following progressive desialyaction, Endocrinology 88:456.

Van Hell, H., Matthijsen, R., and Homan, J. D. H., 1968, Studies on human chorionic gonadotropin. I. Purification and some physico-chemical properties, Acta Endocrinol. (KBH) 59:89.

Williams, R. R., McIntire, K. R., Waldman, T. A., Feinleib, M., Go, V. L. W., Kannel, W. B., Dawber, T. R., Castelli, W. P., and McNamara, P. M., 1977, Tumor-associated antigen levels (carcinoembryonic antigen, human chorionic gonadotropin, and alpha-fetoprotein) antedating the diagnosis of cancer in the Framingham study, J. Natl. Cancer Inst. 58:1547.

Yoshimoto, Y., Wolfsen, A. R., and Odell, W. D., 1977, Human chorio-nic gonadotropin-like substance in nonendocrine tissues of normal subjects, Science 197:575.

Yoshimoto, Y., Wolfsen, A. R., Hirose, F., and Odell, W. D., 1979a, Human chorionic gonadotropin-like material: Presence in normal human tissues, Am. J. Obstet. Gynecol. 134:729.

Yoshimoto, Y., Wolfsen, A. R., and Odell, W. D., 1979b, Glycosyla-tion, a variable in the produciton of hCG by cancer, Am. J. Med. 67:414.

ACKNOWLEDGEMENTS

The secretarial assistance of Mrs. Helene Zauderer is greatly acknowledged. This work was supported in part from USPHS Research Grants CA-18362 and HD-13042.

APPARENT CHORIONIC GONADOTROPIN IMMUNOREACTIVITY IN

HUMAN NON-PLACENTAL TISSUES

Christopher A. Adejuwon, Samuel S. Koide, S. M. Mitsudo,
and Sheldon J. Segal

Center for Biomedical Research, The Population Council
The Rockefeller University, New York, New York, U.S.A.
and
Population Sciences, The Rockefeller Foundation
New York, New York, U.S.A.

INTRODUCTION

The human chorionic gonadotropin (hCG) is produced by cyto- and syncytiotrophoblast of human placenta (Yoshimoto et al., 1977) and by malignant tumors (Rosen et al., 1975; Vaitukaitis et al., 1976; Root et al., 1968; Becker et al., 1968). Recently, hCG-like material has been reported to be also in bacteria (Wuerthele-Caspe et al., 1974; Cohen and Strampp, 1976), normal human testis (Braunstein et al., 1975), pituitary gland (Chen et al., 1976; Robertson et al., 1978), liver and colon (Yoshimoto et al., 1977), and kidney, lung, ovary, pancreas, and spleen (Braunstein et al., 1978).

Since protease present in tissue samples may interfere with radioimmunoassay (RIA) and may even mimic the in vitro biological properties of hCG (Richert and Ryan, 1977), it is essential to eliminate the effects of this enzyme when analyzing tissue extracts for imputed hCG activity. Maruo et al. (1979) recently demonstrated that a trypsin-like protease is responsible for RIA dose-response curves parallel to hCG in extracts of the hepato-pancreas of the marine crab, *Ovalipes ocellatus*. These findings have prompted us to reinvestigate the presence of hCG-like material in normal and neoplastic human tissue samples, with experimental modification of the RIA system to differentiate between hCG and the effect of proteolytic enzymes on the radioligand assay.

PROCEDURES

Non-placental tissue specimens were obtained at surgery and stored at -20°C until use. HCG (CR119) and antiserum to hCGβ (SB-6) were gifts from the National Institute of Child Health and Human Development, Bethesda. Protease inhibitors [soybean trypsin inhibitor and N-α-p-tosyl-L-lysine chloromethyl ketone-HCl (TLCK)] and trypsin were purchased from Sigma Chemical Company.

Tissue Preparation

Tissues were weighed and homogenized into ten percent solutions with double distilled water, using the polytron tissue homogenizer model PCU-2-110. Homogenates were centrifuged at 12,000 g for 30 min at 4°C. The supernatant volume was measured, frozen in acetone-dry ice mixture and lyophilized. The lyophilized powder was weighed, gently crushed, and reconstituted into a small volume (1-4 ml) with 0.1 M phosphate buffered saline containing 0.1 percent azide. The reconstituted extract was centrifuged at 27,000 g for 30 min at 4°C. The clear supernatant was analyzed for hCG by RRI and subjected to heat treatment.

Radioimmunoassay

HCG (CR119) was iodinated by the method of Greenwood et al. (1963) to a specific activity of 40-60μCi/μg. HCG was determined by the double antibody technique (Vaitukaitis et al., 1972). The SB-6 antiserum (NICHD) used for the hCG assay was found to show 32% crossreactivity with hLH (LER 960, NICHD), and the sensitivity of the assay was 1.25 ng per ml assay fluid.

Heat Treatments

100 μl aliquots of tissue extracts or control samples were added to 500 μl of 0.1% bovine serum albumin (BSA) and heated at either 90° C for 20 min or at 55°C for varying periods of time (0, 15, 60, and 120 minutes). The remaining activity was determined in each case by RIA.

Treatment with Protease Inhibitors

Either 0.5 mg soybean trypsin inhibitor or 2.0 mg TLCK was added to each RIA tube (1 ml final volume) prior to incubation. The effect of each inhibitor on the slope of the hCG standard curve was determined separately.

RESULTS

Positive values for hCG by RIA were obtained in 33 of 41 non-placental human tissues (Table I), including several specimens of testis and colon, and individual tissues of normal kidney, kidney carcinoma, normal lung, lung adenocarcinoma, normal ovary, and ovarian metastatic adenocarcinoma. Treatment with TLCK reduced the hCG-like immunoreactivity in six samples of testis tissue by from 39% to over 90%, and in two samples of normal colon by 69% and 42%. TLCK reduced the hCG-like immunoreactivity of term placenta by only 16.8%, and a sample of colon cancer tissue by 25% (Table II). At the concentrations used, TLCK had no effect on the hCG standard curve (Figure 1). Another protease inhibitor, soybean trypsin inhibitor, was also tested at a dose that had no effect on the slope of the hCG standard curve. The reduction of hCG-like immunoreactivity of colon tissue was considerably less (18% inhibition) than achieved with TLCK.

Heat treatment at 90°C for 20 minutes profoundly lowered (greater than 75%) the hCG-like immunoreactivity in all normal non-placental tissues studied, but did not diminish greatly (16.5%) the activity present in a specimen of colon carcinoma. This pattern of heat treatment did not reduce the immunoreactivity of purified hCG (CR119) or the hCG present in term placenta, but virtually abolished the apparent activity of purified trypsin in the RIA system (Table III). Treatment with milder heat (55°C) for varying periods of time progressively reduced the hCG-like immunoreactivity in normal testis and in normal colon, but resulted in a progressive increase in the hCG immunoreactivity of purified hCG, term placenta, and tissue extracts of colon cancer (Figure 2).

DISCUSSION

The presence of hCG-like material in placenta, blood, and ovary can be expected on the basis of our present understanding of production, transport and target sites of this luteotropic hormone of pregnancy. Reports of its presence in other normal tissues, however, suggest either that the physiological significance of this hormone goes beyond its role in the maintenance of pregnancy, or that the sensitivity of present-day assay methods can detect minute quantities of the hormone which--while normally present in many tissues--have no physiological significance. The implications of either interpretation are considerable, so that careful weighing of the evidence for non-placental production of hCG is essential.

Earlier reports of a chorionic gonadotropin-like substance (distinct from hLH) in normal human tissue have been based on positive RIAs which may include the establishment of dose-response curves, showing a parallelism with purified hCG (Yoshimoto et al., 1977;

TABLE I: Immunoreactive hCG-like material in human tissues.

Tissue	Total Number of Samples	Samples Positive	hCG-like Immunoreactivity (ng/g wet tissue) Mean S. D.
Normal colon	18	15	2.27±4.48
Colon carcinoma	6	4	5.69±6.09
Normal testis	11	10	4.40±3.40
Normal kidney	1	1	1.09
Clear cell adeno-carcinoma of kidney	1	1	1.49
Normal lung	1	1	1.66
Well differentiated squamous cell carcinoma of lung	1	1	1.88
Metastatic adeno-carcinoma of ovary	1	0	-
Normal ovary	1	0	-
Term placenta	2	2	369.96±101.44

All assays were in duplicate; where individual samples are reported the value given is the average of the duplicate values.

TABLE II: Effect of TLCK on immunoreactive hCG-like material in human tissues.

Tissue	hCG-like Immunoreactive Material (ng/g wet weight tissue) Without TLCK*	With TLCK**	% Reduction
Normal testis	11.03	<1.10	>90.0%
" "	8.09	3.63	55.1%
" "	3.55	1.69	52.3%
" "	7.12	2.86	59.9%
" "	5.23	3.21	38.7%
" "	1.38	<0.48	>65.0%
Normal colon	12.75	3.95	69.0%
" "	13.77	7.99	42.0%
Colon carcinoma	11.35	8.47	25.4%
Term placenta	369.96	307.81	16.8%

*Standard RIA; uncorrected hCG-like activity

**2 mg TLCK per assay tube; corrected hCG-like activity

TABLE III: Effect of heat treatment on immunoreactive hCG-like material in human tissue, hCG, and trypsin.

| Sample | hCG-like Immunoreactive Material (ng/g weight wet tissue) | | % Change |
	Without Heat*	With Heat**	
Normal testis	11.03	<1.05	↓>90.5
" "	8.09	<0.87	↓>89.3
" "	3.54	<0.80	↓>77.4
" "	3.55	<0.52	↓>85.7
" "	7.12	<0.45	↓>93.7
" "	5.23	<0.63	↓>87.9
Normal Colon	12.75	<0.91	↓>92.9
" "	13.77	2.99	↓ 78.3
Colon carcinoma	11.35	9.48	↓ 16.5
Term placenta	369.96	510.55	↓138.1
10 mg Trypsin	0.08***	<0.01***	↓ 84.4
Controls	(Total Activity per Sample)		
2 ng hCG CR119	1.94	3.42	↑ 76.4
8 ng hCG CR119	7.89	39.33	↑398.5
32 ng hCG CR119	33.28	>64.00	↑>92.3

*Standard RIA; uncorrected hCG-like activity.

**Samples were heated at 90°C for 20 minutes; corrected hCG-like activity.

***pg per g enzyme.

Braunstein et al., 1975; Maruo et al., 1979). In some studies of non-placental hCG-like material, the degree of detail has been extended to include approximating the molecular weight by polyacrylamide gel electrophoresis and/or Sephadex column chromatography, as well as characterization of the carbohydrate moiety by Conconavalin A-affinity chromatography (Maruo et al., 1979). However, even with all these lines of evidence, the identification of the material as hCG can still be in doubt because of the dose-dependent effect of tissue proteases on the radioligand assay and the closeness of the molecular weight of some trypsin-like enzymes to the hCG subunits (Maruo et al., 1979). Indeed, as demonstrated by Richert and Ryan (1977), even the stimulatory effect of gonadotropins on rat ovarian adenylate cyclase activity can be simulated by the serine proteases, trypsin, chymotrypsin, and subtilisin (Richert and Ryan, 1977).

The results reported here demonstrate that a large part of the radioimmunoassayable hCG activity in samples of normal testis, colon, lung, and kidney can be eliminated by the addition of the protease inhibitor TLCK to the assay system or by pre-treatment of the tissue extract with heat under conditions that inactivate trypsin, but do not inactivate or reduce the immunoreactivity of purified hCG. Heat treatment of native hCG, to the contrary, increases significantly RIA activity. In the samples tested, activity increased by values within the range of approximately 75% to nearly 400%. This finding is unexplained, but may be due to the exposure of antigenic binding sites as a result of heat-induced unfolding of the hCG molecule. Alternatively, heat treatment may result in the dissociation of hCG into α- and β-subunits. Since the antiserum to the β-subunit was used in the RIA, the observed immunoreactivity of the dissociated β-subunit would be greater than that obtained with the intact hCG molecule (Wehmann and Nisula, 1979).

Preliminary observations using the RIA for another polypeptide hormone confirm that crude extracts of normal human tissues possess a non-specific, heat-labile substance that endows the test samples with apparent positive immunoreactivity. Five samples of normal human testis and one sample of normal colon were analyzed for human prolactin, using a standard RIA procedure (Serono human prolactin assay kit). All samples appeared to have immunoreactive human prolactin-like material (6.68 ± 5.29 ng/g wet weight). Unlike hCG, purified prolactin proved to be labile in the presence of TLCK (2 mg per assay tube) or at 90°C heat for 20 minutes. These procedures, therefore, could not be used to discriminate between apparent and true prolactin immunoreactivity. However, mild heat of 55°C for 15 min to 60 min does not reduce the immunoreactivity of purified human prolactin. Exposure to these conditions eliminated completely the apparent immunoreactivity of all samples of normal testis or colon tissue. A detailed report on tissue prolactin-like activity will be published elsewhere.

From the findings of this study, it may be concluded that most of the apparent radioimmunoassayable hCG activity in normal human tissue (other than placenta) is not indicative of active synthesis of hCG by these tissues. That active synthesis of hCG or "gene leakage" occurs in non-placental tissue is a postulate of considerable consequence which would need to be sustantiated by evidence beyond that obtained with radioimmunoassay or radioreceptor assay.

REFERENCES

Becker, K. L. Cottrell, J. C., Moore, C. F., Winnacker, J. L., Matthews, M. J., and Katz, S., 1968, Endocrine studies in a patient with a gonadotropin-secreting bronchogenic carcinoma, J. Clin. Endocrinol. Metab. 28:809.

Braunstein, G. D., Kamdar, V., Rasor, J., Swaminathan, N., and Wade, M. E., 1978, Widespread distribution of a chorionic gonadotropin-like substance in normal human tissues, Abstr. 44, Endocrinology (Suppl) 102:96.

Braunstein, G. D., Rasor, J., Wade, M. E., 1975, Presence in normal human testis of a chorionic gonadotropin-like substance distinct from human luteinizing hormone, N. Eng. J. Med. 293:1339.

Canfield, R. E., Birken, S., Morse, J. H., and Morgan, F. J., Human chorionic gonadotropin, in Peptide Hormone, J. A. Parsons, ed., pp. 299-315, University Park Press, Baltimore, Marvland.

Chen, H. G., Hodgen, G. D., Matsuura, S., Canfield, R. E., and Ross, G. T., 1976, Evidence for a gonadotropin from nonpregnant subjects that has physical, immunological, and biological similarities to human chorionic gonadotropin, Proc. Natl. Acad. Sci. U.S.A. 73:2885.

Cohen, H., and Strampp, A., 1976, Bacterial synthesis of substance similar to human chorionic gonadotropin, Proc. Soc. Exp. Biol. Med. 152:408.

Greenwood, F. C., Hunter, W. M., Glover, J. S., 1963, The preparation of ^{125}I-labeled human growth hormone of high specific radioactivity, Biochem. J. 89:114.

Maruo, T., Segal, S. J., and Koide, S. S., 1979, Studies on the apparent human gonadotropin-like factor in the crab Ovalipes ocellatus, Endocrinology 104($):932.

Reichert, L. E., Jr., and Lawson, G. M., Jr., 1973, Molecular weight relationships among the subunits of human glycoprotein hormones, Endocrinology 92(4):1034.

Richert, N. D., and Ryan, R. J., 1977, Specific gonadotropin binding to pseudomonas maltophilia, Proc. Natl. Acad. Sci. U.S.A. 74:878.

Robertson, D. M., Suginami, H., Montez, H. H., Puri, C. P. Choi, S. K., and Diczfalusy, E., Studies on human chorionic gonadotropin-like material present in nonpregnant subjects, Acta Endocrinologica 89:492.

Root, A. W., Bongiovanni, A. M., and Eberlein, W. R., 1968, A testicular-interstitial-cell-stimulating gonadotropin in a child with hepatoblastoma and sexual precocity, J. Clin. Endocrinol. Metab. 28:1317.

Rosen, S. W., Weintraub, B. D., Vaitukaitis, J. L., Sussman, H. H., Hershman, J. M., Muggia, F. M., 1975, Placental proteins and their subunits as tumor markers, Ann. Int. Med. 82:71.

Vaitukaitis, J. L., Braunstein, G. D., and Ross, G. T., 1972, A radioimmunoassay which specifically measures human chorionic gonadotropin in the presence of human luteinizing hormone, Am. J. Obstet. Gynecol. 113:751.

Vaitukaitis, J. L., Ross, G. T., Braunstein, G. D., and Rayford, P. L., 1976, Gonadotropins and their subunits: basic and clinical studies, Rec. Prog. Hor. Res. 32:289.

Wehman, R. E., and Nisula, B. C., 1979, Metabolic clearance rates of the subunits of human chorionic gonadotropin in man, J. Clin. Endocrinol. Metab. 48:753.

Wuerthele-Caspe Livingston, V., and Livingston, A. M., 1974, Some cultural, immunological and biochemical properties of progenitor cryptocides, Trans. N.Y. Acad. Sci. 36:569.

Yoshimoto, Y., Wolfson, A. R., and Odell, W. D., 1977, Human chorionic gonadotropin-like substance in non-endocrine tissues of normal subjects, Science 197:575.

ACKNOWLEDGEMENTS

We thank the Tumor Procurement Center, Memorial Sloan-Kettering Cancer Center, New York for the specimens of surgical tissues. This work was performed as part of the Contraceptive Development Program of the International Committee for Contraceptive Research of the Population Council. C.A.A. is supported by a Rockefeller Foundation Fellowship Award in Reproductive Biology.

GONADOTROPIN PRODUCED BY A MICROORGANISM

S. S. Koide, T. Maruo, H. Cohen, and S. J. Segal

Center for Biomedical Research, The Population Council
The Rockefeller University, New York, New York, U.S.A.
Wampole Laboratories, Cranbury, New Jersey, U.S.A., and
Population Sciences, The Rockefeller Foundation
New York, New York, U.S.A.

INTRODUCTION

Production of a factor resembling chorionic gonadotropin (CG) by a microorganism named *Progenitor cryptocides* was reported by Livingston and Livingston (1974) and Cohen and Strampp (1976). The factor was tentatively identified as a CG-like substance based on hemagglutination inhibition assay, radioimmunoassay (RIA), and radio-receptor assay (RRA) methods. Recently, with use of immuno-cytochemical techniques, Acevedo and associates (1978, 1979) and Slifkin et al. (1979) demonstrated that CG-like immunoreactive substance is present in the cell wall of several microorganisms which were isolated from patients bearing malignant neoplasms. Furthermore, Richert and Ryan (1977a) reported that the media in which *Pseudomonas maltophilia* were cultured may contain a protein which cross-reacts with antisera to hCG and hCGβ. Other microorganisms which were reported to produce or contain CG-like factor are *Escherichia Coli* (Cohen and Strampp, 1976), *Staphylococcus epidermidis* (Affronti et al., 1977a, b; Affronti and Charoenvit, 1979) and *Staphylococcus faecalis* (Koide et al., 1979).

These reports were based on assay methods subject to errors by interfering substances such as proteases and non-gonadotropin immunoreactive substances (Richert and Ryan, 1977a, b; Maruo et al., 1979). In the present report, data will be presented to show that a microorganism produces a biologically active gonadotropin which possesses physicochemical properties resembling hCG.

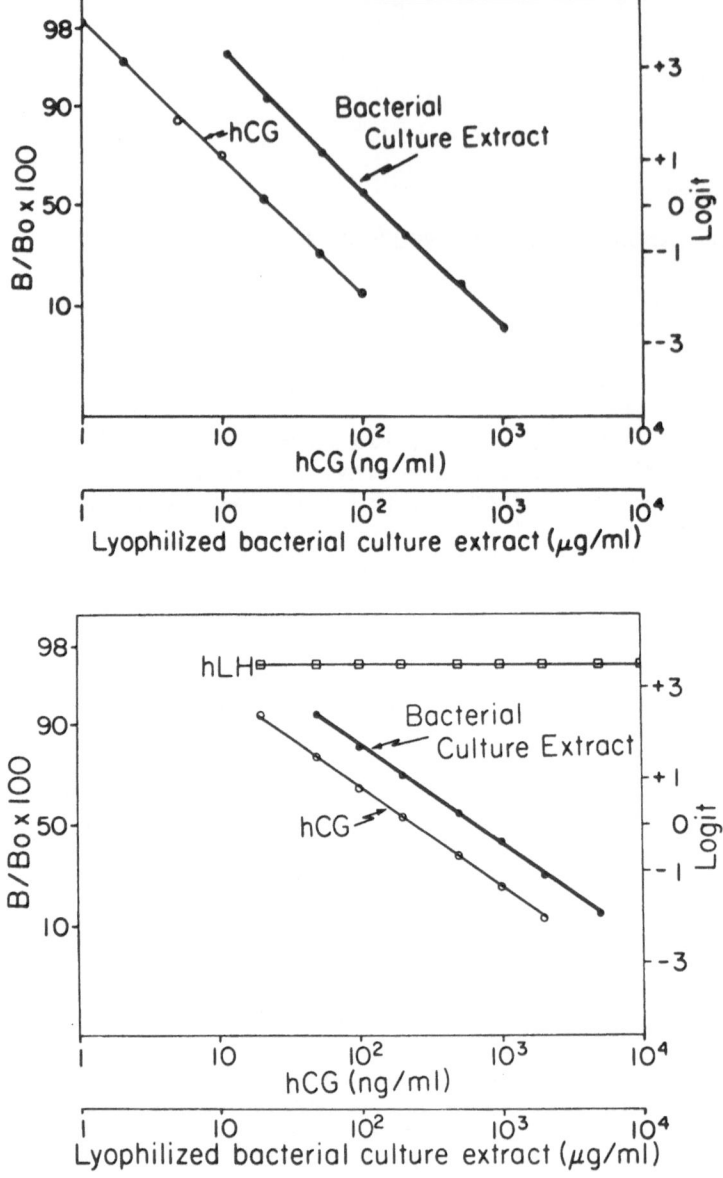

Figures 1 and 2.   Dose response curves for: (Top) hCG (CR-119) and
the lyophilized bacterial culture extract in the RRA; (Bottom) hCG
(CR-119), hLH (LER 960), and the lyophilized bacterial culture
extract in the RIA using antiserum to hCGβ-COOH-Terminal peptide
(H93). Results are shown as the log dose of the hCG reference
preparation (ng per ml) or of the lyophilized extract (µg per ml)
plotted against the logit transformation of the response. B = cpm
bound in the presence of ^{125}I-hCG and unlabeled ligand; B_O = cpm
bound in the presence of ^{125}I-hCG alone.

DETERMINATION OF GONADOTROPIN-LIKE FACTOR

Preparations of an acetone powder of the microorganism named *Progenitor cryptocides* were obtained from Biomedical Laboratories, Seattle, and from Dr. V. W. C. Livingston, Livingston Clinic, San Diego, prepared by a method described in the report of Livingston and Livingston (1974). An extract of the acetone powder was prepared and assayed for CG-like activity by RRA and RIA utilizing the homologous assay systems (Figures 1 and 2). RIA was also performed with antiserum raised against hCGβ-carboxyl-terminal peptide (Chen et al., 1976) (Figure 2). To exclude interference by proteases in the assay systems, the following inhibitors were added separately to the reaction mixtures: N-α-p-tosyl-L-lysine chloromethyl ketone (TPCK) (1 mM); leupeptin (1 mM); antipain (1 mM), and soybean trypsin inhibitor (0.1%). The addition of these protease inhibitors to the RRA and RIA systems did not influence the results. Acetone powder preparation of *Streptococcus faecalis* [American Type Culture Collection (ATCC) 12818] did not show any displacement of ^{125}I-hCG in the RRA and RIA systems.

TIME COURSE OF PRODUCTION OF CG-LIKE FACTOR

The production of gonadotropin-like factor by *Progenitor cryptocides* was determined at various periods of incubation (Figure 3). The highest amount was found in the 24 hr culture incubated at 22°C or 37°C, which subsequently decreased as the incubation continued. This finding is at variance with the reports of Livingston and Livingston (1974) and Affronti et al. (1977a, b). They indicated that the production of CG-like factor by *Progenitor cryptocides* and *Staphylococcus epidermidis*, respectively, reached the highest level after several days of culture (stationary phase). The present observation that the amount of CG-like factor found in the culture decreased with prolonged incubation suggests that it was destroyed, probably by the action of proteases. However, it should be pointed out that the assay for CG-like factor in the acetone-precipitated preparation was not affected by the addition of protease inhibitors, as described above.

PURIFICATION OF THE CG-LIKE FACTOR

The factor was purified to validate whether it is similar to or different from human chorionic gonadotropin (hCG). The steps of purification included gel filtration on Sephadex G-100 (Figure 4), affinity chromatography on Concanavalin A-Sepharose (Con A-S) (Figure 5), and ion-exchange chromatography on DEAE-Sephadex A-50 (Figure 6). A salient observation was that during gel filtration on Sephadex G-100, a protein peak was eluted at the position corresponding to that of ^{125}I-hCG used as a marker, suggesting that

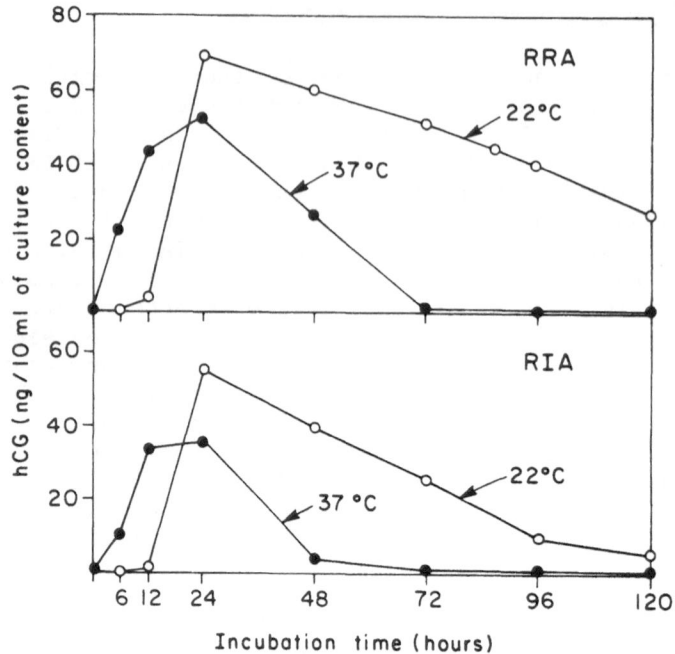

Incubation time (hours)

Figure 3.   Time course of production of CG-like factor in *Progenitor cryptocides* cultured in trypticase soy medium.   Incubation temperatures of 22°C and 37°C.   Aliquots were removed periodically and acetone powder prepared.   Extracts of the acetone powder preparations were assayed for CG-like factor by RIA and RRA.

the molecular weights of the two substances are similar (Figure 4). In addition, a second substance was eluted which showed immunoreactivity with anti-hCGβ and antiserum (H93) raised against the carboxyl-terminal peptide of hCGβ (Chen et al., 1976) (Figure 4). The position of the second material was retarded compared to ^{125}I-hCGβ used as a marker.   The present finding suggests that this second substance is hCGβ-like by immunoreactivity, but smaller in size.   It is of interest to note that no substance showing immunoreactivity with anti-hCGα was detected.   That the CG-like factor did absorb to Con A-S (Figure 5) suggests that it probably contains mannose and/or glucose moieties.   The CG-like factor was eluted as a single immunoreactive peak at a conductivity of 4.0-6.0 mS on a DEAE-Sephadex A-50 column (Figure 6).

At this stage of purification, one can conclude tentatively that two immunoreactive factors are produced by the microorganism. One is a CG-like factor with properties resembling hCG and possesses the following characteristics: immunoreactivity to antisera raised

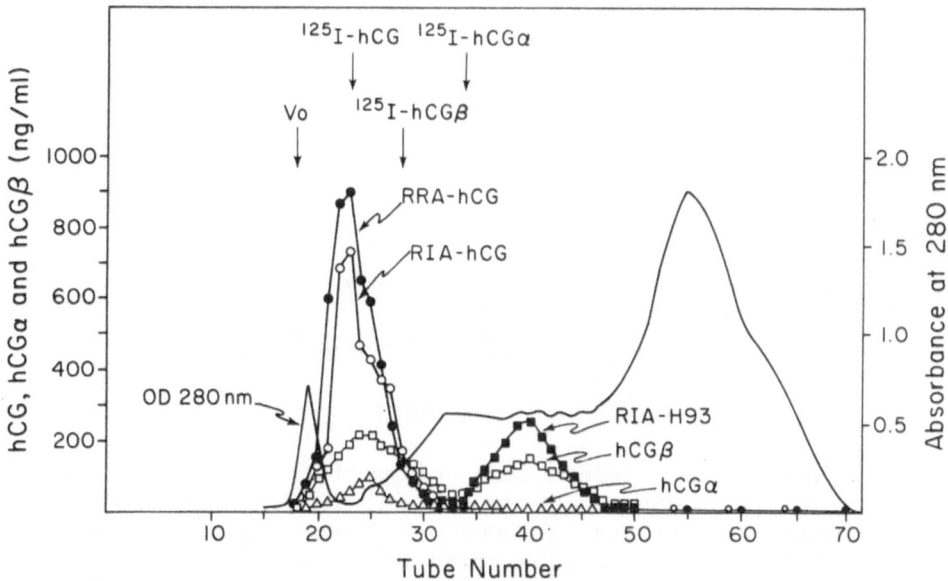

Gel Filtration on Sephadex G-100

Figure 4. Sephadex G-100 elution profile of the bacterial culture extract. Each 2.0 ml fraction was assayed by the RRA and by the RIA systems for hCG, hCGα, hCGβ, and hCGβ-COOH-terminal peptide. Protein content of the eluted fractions was measured by absorbancy at 280 nm. V_o represents void volume determined by elution of blue dextran. The vertical arrows indicate the elution positions of ^{125}I-hCG, ^{125}I-hCGβ, and ^{125}I-hCGα.

against hCG, hCGβ, hCGα, and hCGβ-carboxyl-terminal peptide (H93); receptor activity; a glycoprotein containing mannose and/or glucose; and mol. wt. similar to hCG by gel filtration. The second factor is possibly a CGβ-like fragment, since it shows immunoreactivity to antisera raised against hCGβ and to hCGβ-carboxyl-terminal peptide (H93), and apparently has a lower mol. wt. than standard ^{125}I-hCGβ.

YIELD AND RELATIVE POTENCY OF PURIFIED PRODUCT

The yield and relative potency of the CG-like factor determined by RIA and RRA are shown in Table I. The amount of purified product obtained was less than 0.06% of the starting material. The potency measured by RIA and RRA increased about 380-fold.

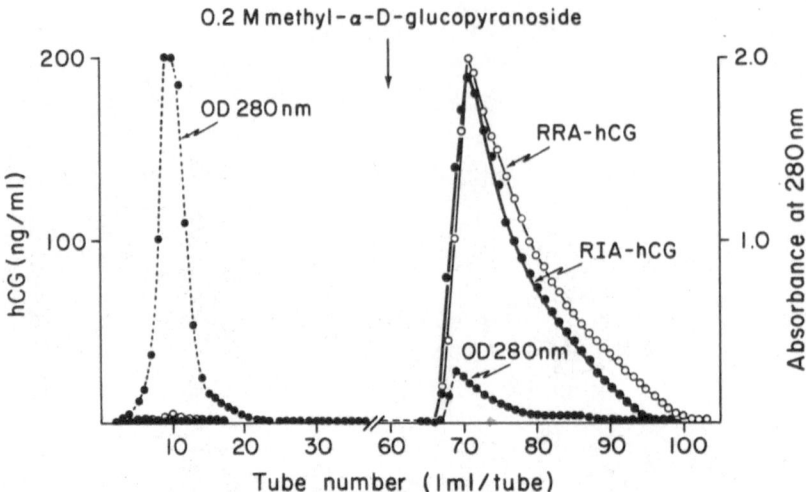

Figure 5. Elution on Con A-Sepharose column chromatography of the
CG-containing fraction obtained from Sephadex G-100 column. Fractions
1-59 were eluted with PBS and followed by a second elution with PBS
containing 0.2 M methyl-α-D-gluco-pyranoside. Each 1 ml fraction
was assayed for hCG by the RRA and RIA systems. Protein content was
estimated by measurement of absorbancy at 280 nm.

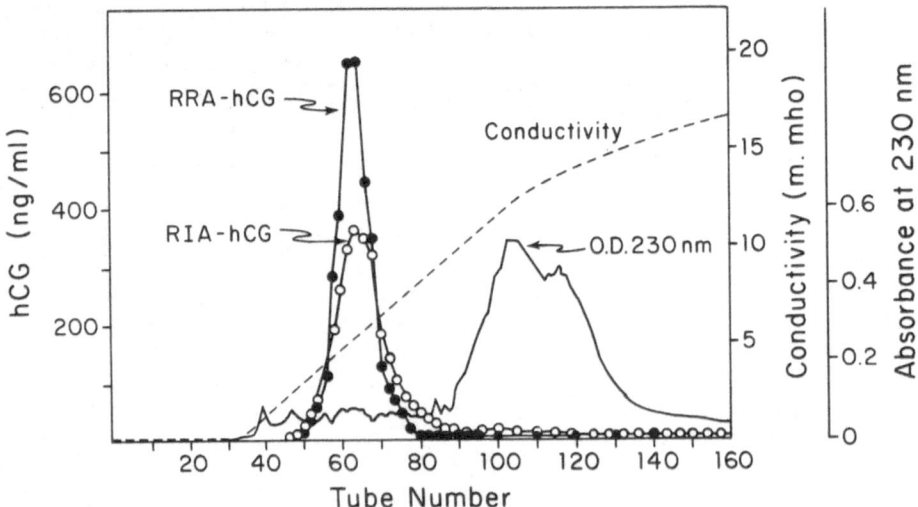

Figure 6. Elution profile of the Con A-adsorbed CG fraction on DEAE-
Sephadex A-50 column chromatography. Adsorbed protein on the column
was eluted with a linear 300 ml gradient from 0-0.5 M NaCl in 0.0. M
Tris-HCl buffer (pH 7.4); each 2.0 ml fraction was assayed for hCG
by RRA and RIA. Protein content was measured by absorbancy at 230 nm.

TABLE I: Yield and relative hCG potency of CG-like factor at each purification step.

Fraction	Yield		hCG Potency (IU/mg)	
	(mg protein)	(%)	RRA	RIA
Lyophilized Extract	1000.0	100.0	8.5 ± 0.5	5.3 ± 0.3
Sephadex G-100	31.2	3.1	231 ± 11	150 ± 7
Con A-Sepharose	6.4	0.6	880 ± 45	542 ± 27
DEAE-Sephadex	0.6	0.06	3580 ± 160	2260 ± 102

Relative hCG potency (mean ± SD) was determined by the RRA and homologous hCG RIA using the Second International Standard hCG as a reference preparation.

To establish that the partially purified product did not contain any protease activity, the CG-like material (1 mg) obtained from gel filtration on Sephadex G-100 was incubated with ^{125}I-hCG (5 x 10^5 cpm) used as a tracer in the RIA and RRA for 60 min at 37°C. The radioactive hCG was recovered intact on analysis by gel filtration of the reaction mixture on Sephadex G-100. The present result indicates that at this step of purification the factor did not contain any proteases or proteolytic activity.

ELECTROPHORESIS OF THE PURIFIED CG-LIKE FACTOR ON POLYACRYLAMIDE GEL

The purified factor was analyzed by electrophoresis on poly-acrylamide gel (PAGE) by the method of Ornstein (1964a) and Davis (1964b). The factor separated into two bands at positions distant from authentic hCG (data not shown).

Isoelectric focusing analysis (Nguyen and Chrambach, 1977) of the purified CG-like factor showed two major bands. One of the bands focused at pH 6.9 and the other at pH 7.1. A faint band was noted at pH 7.9. Authentic hCG has been reported to have an isoelectric point corresponding to pH 2.95 (Got, 1960), pH 2.6 ± 0.6, and 4.8 ± 0.8 (Hammond et al., 1970); six bands range from 3.8 to 5.4 (Graesslin et al., 1973). Hence, the higher pI of the bacterial CG-like factor (pH 6.9 and 7.1) might reflect lower sialic acid content compared to authentic hCG.

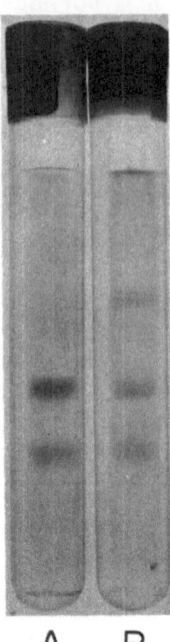

A   B

Figure 7. SDS–polyacrylamide gel electrophoresis. Gel A shows the electrophoretic pattern of hCG (CR-119) (20 µg) which dissociated in SDS-gel into α- and β-subunits. Gel B represents electrophoretic pattern of the purified bacterial CG-factor (20 µg) obtained from DEAE-Sephadex A-50 chromatography. The migration is toward the anode at the bottom of the figure.

To determine whether or not the bacterial CG-like factor is composed of subunits, the purified product was analyzed by electrophoresis on sodium dodecyl sulfate (SDS) polyacrylamide gel (Weber and Osborn, 1969) (Figure 7). The factor separated into two bands which correspond to the subunits of hCG. An additional minor band was found which was retarded compared to standard hCG (Figure 7). To validate that the observed bands correspond to the subunits of hCG, the gel was sliced into 2.2 mm segments. Each segment was homogenized in 500 µl of phosphate buffer solution (PBS) (pH 7.4). The homogenate was centrifuged at 3000 x g for 20 min and the supernatant assayed by the respective homologous hCG RIA systems. Segments 11, 22, and 28 showed immunoreactivities with hCG, hCGβ, and hCGα, respectively (Figure 8). Thus, segments 22 and 28 corresponded to the position of β- and α-subunits run in parallel (Figure 8). Segment 11, however, is probably a species of CG-like

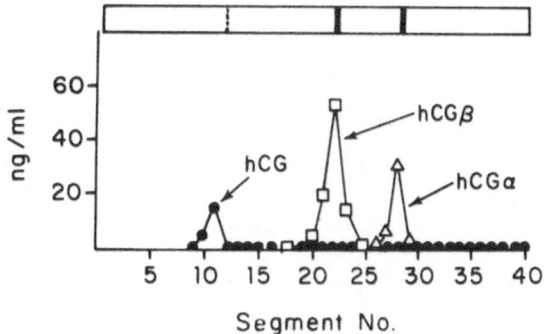

Segment No.

Figure 8. Localization of the immunoreactivity of hCGα and hCGβ in the gel prepared in the same manner as Gel B (Figure 7). Each 2.2 mm segment of the gel was homogenized in PBS and the supernatant was assayed for hCG, hCGα, and hCGβ by the respective homologous RIAs.

factor which did not undergo dissociation under the experimental conditions used. The mobility of this band was retarded compared with standard hCG, and resembles the large species of hCG isolated from human placenta (Maruo et al., 1979). The present results demonstrate that the bacterial CG-like factor is composed of two subunits corresponding to the respective subunits of standard hCG, and possibly a large, undissociated CG-like factor.

BIOLOGICAL ACTIVITY

The biological potency of the bacterial factor was determined by the rat uterine and ovarian weight assays referred to by Diczfalusy and Loraine (1955) (Figure 9). The potency, as determined by RRA and RIA, is shown in Table I. The biological potencies of the CG-like factor determined by the uterine and ovarian weight assay methods were 380 (320-490) IU/mg protein and 880 (780-1020) IU/mg, respectively.

The biological potency of the purified bacterial factor (380 IU/mg and 880 IU/mg) is low compared to that of standard hCG (>10,000 IU/mg) (Morgan et al., 1974). The low activity might be due to the sialic acid content, since desialyated hCG has low in vivo biological activity due to its rapid metabolic clearance (Van Hall et al., 1971; Tsuruhara et al., 1972). On the other hand,

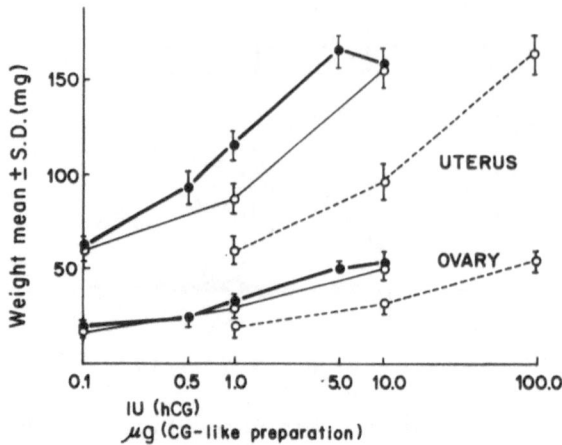

Figure 9. Dose-response curves of standard hCG and bacterial CG-like preparations determined by measuring the uterine and ovarian weights in immature female rats. ——●—— : Second International Standard hCG; --o-- : CG-like preparation obtained from Sephadex G-100; ——o—— : CG-like preparation from DEAE-Sephadex A-50.

the potency measured by RRA (3580 ± 160 IU/mg) and RIA (2260 ± 102 IU/mg) approaches that of standard hCG (about 22% and 35%). It is known that desialyated hCG retains its full activity in the RRA and RIA systems.

CONCLUSION

A noteworthy observation is that considerable amounts of CGβ-like material were detected in fractions eluted by gel filtration on Sephadex G-100 (Figure 4), whereas no free α-subunit-like factor was detected in the bacterial preparation. In most situations where free subunits of hCG were measured, substantial amounts of free α-subunit were found, as in sera of pregnant women (Ashitaka et al., 1974), and human placental extracts (Vaitukaitis, 1974; Maruo, 1976) without detectable free hCGβ. Hence, in placental tissues, the biosynthesis of hCGβ is rate-limiting while the situation in the microorganism may reflect a different mechanism regulating the biosynthesis of CG-like material.

Acevedo et al. (1978, 1979) reported that hCG-like immunoreactive protein can be demonstrated in several microorganisms isolated from urine and tissues of patients bearing neoplastic tumors. Richert and Ryan (1977a) reported that the microorganism *Pseudomonas maltophilia* has receptors for ^{125}I-hCG and that the culture media may contain a factor which immunoreacts with anti-hCGα and anti-hCGβ. However, the apparent immunoreactivity might be due to a protease and a soluble hCG-binding substance (Richert et al., 1978).

The production of a mammalian hormone (CG-like factor) by a microorganism is an unusual phenomen. The questions raised by the present study relative to factors influencing evolution are not unlike those arising from the commonality of various enzymes involved in intermediate metabolism across the range of living organisms. Does a single gene or gene-set pass through the broad sweep of evolution, or does the same gene arise de novo at different points in the phylogenetic sequence? It is possible that the CG-gene has an early origin in evolution, long before the need for its role in eutherians to support the function of the corpus luteum, and that the CG-like factor in earlier living forms may have a completely different function, e.g., proteolytic activity or cell wall structure. The fact that there is homology in the peptide sequence between the β-subunit of gonadotropin and some proteases (Kurosky et al., 1977) suggests the possibility that these or related proteases might be an ancestral form of CG. In this regard, it is interesting to note that proteases can mimic the action of CG by stimulating cAMP production by the pseudo-pregnant ovary in vitro (Richert and Ryan, 1977a, b).

An alternate view is that the production of CG by a microorganism is an expression of a mammalian gene as a consequence of a natural process of recombination of DNA, i.e., the insertion of a mammalian gene into the bacteria in the form of plasmid DNA. This contention is supported by the finding that microorganisms claimed to have the capacity to produce CG-like factor have thus far been isolated from the urine, blood, and tissues of patients with advanced cancer (Livingston and Livingston, 1974; Acevedo et al., 1978) (Table I). These observations suggest that the microorganisms must be associated with human tissues making hCG in order to acquire the capability of producing CG-like factor. It is conceivable that evolutionary trends might be influenced or modified by the insertion of genes into the DNA of prokaryotic and/or eukaryotic cells by a process of recombination of plasmid DNA or by infection with phage or viruses. Thus, mutants, variants, or strains may arise endowed with the capacity to produce or recreate toxins, enzymes, and other metabolites to enable the organism to cope with the ever-changing environment.

REFERENCES

Acevedo, H. F., Slifkin, M., Pouchet-Melvin, G. R., Campbell-Acevedo, E. G., 1979, Choriogonadotropin-like antigen in the anaerobic bacterium, *Eubacterium lentum*, isolated from rectal tumor,

Infection and Immunity 24:920.

Acevedo, H. F., Slifkin, M., Pouchet, K. R., and Pardo, M., 1978, Immunohistochemical localization of a choriogonadotropin-like protein in bacteria isolated from cancer patients, Cancer 41:1217.

Affronti, L. F., Chu, L., and Brumbaugh, R., 1977a, Production of a human gonadotropin-like substance by bacterial tumor isolates, Abst. Ann. Meeting Am. Sci. Microbiol., New Orleans, p. 84.

Affronti, L. F., Grow, L., Brumbaugh, R., and Chu, Y. M., 1977b, Further characterization of a bacterial tumor isolate: Production of a human chorionic gonadotropin-like substance, Abst. 5227, Fed. Proc. 36:1256.

Affronti, L/ F., and Charoenvit, Y., 1979, Bacterial tumor isolates, Proc. Am. Soc. Microbiol.

Ashitaka, Y., Nishimura, R., Endo, Y., and Tojo, S., 1974, Subunits of human chorionic gonadotropin and their radioimmunoassays, Endocrinol. Jap. 21:429.

Birken, S., and Canfield, R. E., 1978, Structural and immunochemical properties of human choriogonadotropin, in Structure & Function of Gonadotropins, K. W.. McKerns, Ed., pp. 47-80, Plenum Press, New York.

Chen, H. C., Hodgen, G. D., Matsuura, S., Lin, L. J., Gross, E., Reichert, L. E., Jr., Birken, S., Canfield, R. E., and Ross, G. T., 1976, Evidence for a gonadotropin from nonpregnant subjects that has physical, immunological and biological similarities to human chorionic gonadotropin, Proc. Natl. Acad. Sci. 73:2885.

Cohen, H., and Strampp, A., 1976, Bacterial synthesis of substance similar to human chorionic gonadotropin, Proc. Soc. Exp. Biol. Med. 152:408.

Davis, B. J., 1964, Disc electrophoresis-II. Method and application to human serum proteins. Ann. N. Y. Acad. Sci. 121:404.

Diczfalusy, E., and Loraine, J. A., 1955, J. Clin. Endocrinol. Metab. 15:424.

Got, R., 1960, Récentes acquisitions sur la gonadotropine choriale humaine, Pathol. Biol. 8:1583.

Graesslin, D., Weise, H. C., and Braendle, W., 1973, The microhetero-geneity of human chorionic gonadotropin (hCG) reflected in the β-subunit, FEBS Letters 31:214.

Hammond, J. M., Bridson, W. E., and Kohler, P. O., 1970, Physical properties of human chorionic gonadotrophin (CG) produced in tissue culture (TG)), Abst. of the Endocr. Soc., 52nd Meeting.

Koide, S. S., Maruo. T., Cohen, H., and Segal, S. J., 1980, Chorio-gonadotropin in evolution, in Hormones Adaptation and Evolution, S. Ishii, ed., pp. 295-301, Japan Science Society Press,Tokyo/ Springer Verlag, Berlin.

Kurosky, A., Markel, D. E., Peterson, J. W., and Fitch, W. M., 1977, Primary structure of cholera toxin β-chain: glycoprotein hormone analog? Science 195:299.

Livingston, V. W. C., and Livingston, A. M., 1974, Some cultural, immunological, and biochemical properties of *Progenitor cryptocides*, Trans. N. Y. Acad. Sci., Series II 36:569.

Maruo, T., 1976, Studies on in vitro synthesis and secretion of human chorionic gonadotropin and its subunits, Endocrinol. Jap. 23:119.

Maruo, T., Ashitaka, Y., Mochizuki, M., and Tojo, S., 1974, Chorionic gonadotropin synthesized in cultivated trophoblast, Endocrinol. Jap. 21:499.

Maruo, T., Segal, S. J., and Koide, S. S., 1977, Evidence for synthesis of a polypeptide similar to human chorionic gonadotropin in aquatic organisms, Biol. Bull. 153:438.

Maruo, T., Segal, S. J., and Koide, S. S., 1979, Studies on the apparent human chorionic gonadotropin-like factor in the crab *Ovalipes ocellatus*, Endocrinology 104:932.

Maruo, T., Segal, S. J., and Koide, S. S., 1980, Evidence for in vitro biosynthesis of a large molecular species of chorionic gonadotropin, Acta Endocrinologica (In press).

Nguyen, N. Y., and Chrambach, A., 1977, Stabilization of pH gradient formed ampholyte, Anal. Biochem. 82:226.

Ornstein, L., 1964, Disc electrophoresis-I. Background and theory, Ann. N. Y. Acad. Sci. 121:321.

Richert, N. D., and Ryan, R. J., 1977a, Specific gonadotropin binding to *Pseudomonas maltophilia*, Proc. Nat. Acad. Sci. 74:878.

Richert, N. D., and Ryan, R. J., 1977b, Proteolytic enzyme activation of rat ovarian adenylate cyclase, Proc. Nat. Acad. Sci. 74:4857.

Richert, N. D., and Ryan, R. J., 1977c, Protease inhibitors block hormonal activation of adenylate cyclase, Biochem. Biophys. Res. Commun. 78:799.

Richert, N. D., Bramley, G. A., and Ryan, R. J., 1978, in *Novel Aspects of Reproductive Physiology*, C. H. Spilman and J. W. Wilks, eds., pp. 81-106, SP Medical and Scientific Books, Spectrum Publications, Inc., New York/London.

Slifkin, M., Pardo, M., Pouchet-Melvin, G. R., and Acevedo, H. F., 1979, Immuno-electron microscopic localization of a chorionic gonadotropin-like antigen in cancer-associated bacteria, Oncology 36:208.

Tsuruhara, T., Dufau, M. L., and Hickman, J., 1972, Biological properties of hCG after removal of terminal sialic acid and galactose residues, Endocrinology 91:296.

Van Hall, E. V., Vaitukaitis, J. L., and Ross, G. T., 1971, Immunological and biological activity of hCG following progressive desialyzation, Endocrinology 88:456.

Vaitukaitis, J. L., 1974, Changing placental concentrations of human chorionic gonadotropin and its subunits during gestation, J. Clin. Endocrinol. Metab. 38:755.

Weber, K., and Osborn, M., 1969, The reliability of molecular weight determination by dodecyl sulfate-polyacrylamide gel electrophoresis, J. Biol. Chem. 244:4406.

ACKNOWLEDGEMENTS

We are grateful to Dr. V. Livingston and Mr. J. Majnarich for the acetone powder preparation of *Progenitor cryptocides*. We thank Drs. Y. Y. Tsong and C. C. Chang for providing the purified hCG and antisera raised against hCG, hCGα, and hCGβ. We appreciate the cooperative assistance of Ms. J. Bell, Dr. A. Strampp, and Dr. K. Horiuchi in culturing the microorganism. T. Maruo is the recipient of a Rockefeller Foundation Fellowship in Reproductive Biology.

IMMUNODETECTION OF CHORIOGONADOTROPIN-LIKE

ANTIGEN IN BACTERIA ISOLATED FROM CANCER PATIENTS

Hernan F. Acevedo, Elizabeth A. Campbell-Acevedo
and Malcolm Slifkin

Division of Experimental Pathology, Department of
Laboratory Medicine, Allegheny General Hospital,
Pittsburgh, Pennsylvania 15212, U. S. A.

INTRODUCTION

As early as 1948, Virginia (Wuerthele-Caspe) Livingston and her associates have published a series of papers describing a pleomorphic, acid-fast bacterium which they isolated from cancer tissues and body fluids of patients with malignant neoplasms. Livingston and Alexander-Jackson (1970) published a full description of the organism(s) and proposed the name *Progenitor cryptocides* as a new taxon within the *Actinomycetales*. They reported that this bacterium crossreacts antigenically with *Mycobacterium tuberculosis*, with which it shares the property of acid fastness.

Based on the reported presence of a human choriogonadotropin (CG)-like protein in the serum of numerous patients with different types of cancer (Dailey and Marcuse, 1969; Beck et al., 1970; Braunstein et al., 1973), and on her particular views concerning the nature of cancer, primarily in respect to her consideration of *P. cryptocides* as an etiologic agent of the disease, Livingston and her associates tested their bacterial isolates for the presence of the hormone. Their investigations demonstrated that these bacteria, when cultured in vitro, produced a substance immunologically similar to the human trophoblastic hormone (Livingston and Livingston, 1974).

It was not until two years later that Cohen and Strampp (1976) reported that they obtained two cultures of the so-called *P. cryptocides* from Dr. Livingston, and confirmed the production of a CG-like material by radioimmunoassay (RIA) using specific antibody to the β-subunit of CG according to Vaitukaitis et al. (1972). These investigators also demonstrated the glycoprotein nature of the material

435

by its chromatographic behavior on Concanavalin A-Sepharose columns (Dufau et al., 1972a) and the presence of in vitro biological activity by the radioreceptor analysis (Saxena et al., 1974) and by the testosterone stimulating assay (Dufau et al., 1972b).

Working independently, Affronti and his associates (1975, 1976) have also described the isolation of two CG-like protein producing microorganisms. One was identified as a *Staphylococcus epidermidis* strain obtained from patients with advanced carcinoma of the breast, and the other was an *Escherichia coli* strain isolated from patients with adenocarcinoma of the colon.

Because of the findings by us and others of the de novo biosynthesis and expression of a membrane-associated CG-like "antigen" by all experimental animal malignant cells tested in vivo and in vitro (Acevedo et al., 1978a; Acevedo et al., 1978b; Malkin et al., 1978; Slifkin et al., 1978) as well as in the great majority of cultured cells, frozen sections, and/or touch imprints of human malignant neoplasms that have been studied (Naughton et al., 1975; McManus et al., 1976; Ghosh and Cox, 1976; Schlegel-Haueter et al., 1978; Rabson et al., 1973; Chou, 1978), we initiated an investigation of the presence of the CG-like antigen in bacteria by immunohistochemical techniques, including immunoelectronmicroscopy, in order to study the presence and localization of the immunoreactive material. Transmission electronmicroscopy was also utilized in order to study the ultrastructural characteristics of the microorganisms expressing the material as compared to the characteristics of their counterparts that do not express the compound(s).

While this work was being carried out, Richert and Ryan (1977a) at the Mayo Medical School isolated from the ovarian fluid of a sow two Gram-negative, motile bacteria identified as *Pseudomonas maltophilia* and *Enterobacter cloacae*. Subsequent outgrowth of the isolated strains in liquid media demonstrated that this porcine *P. maltophilia* was capable of binding ^{125}I-labeled CG, whereas *E. cloacae* showed no gonadotropin binding. Among several strains of different bacteria utilized as controls, the investigators used a *P. maltophilia*, strain 13637, obtained from the American Type Culture Collection (ATCC). This bacterial strain also demonstrated similar CG-binding properties. The authors concluded that CG-binding was not widespread among all Gram-negative organisms, nor was it a common feature of all Pseudomonads. They also suggested that the CG-binding was not an artifact of the culturing conditions, because all bacteria tested were grown under identical conditions. Their preliminary data also indicated that the bacterial culture medium contained a large molecule that crossreacted with antiserum to complete CG and to its β-subunit, and a smaller heat-labile molecule that appeared to stimulate rat ovarian adenylate cyclase. Further work done by these investigators demonstrated that the material that was responsible for the CG-binding and stimulates adenylate cyclase has the structure of serine proteases (Richert and Ryan, 1977b;

Richert and Ryan, 1977c; Richert and Ryan, 1977d). But one of the most important aspects concerning *P. maltophilia* ATCC 13637 was the fact that this culture was the only *P. maltophilia* that Richert and Ryan used as "control" (1977a), and that they did not disclose in their publication that this bacterial strain was originally isolated from the nasopharyngeal region of a patient with mouth cancer (The American Type Culture Collection, Catalog of Strains I, 1978, Hugh and Ryschenkow, 1961).

Our investigations were initiated by obtaining nine samples of what we will designate as "cancer associated bacteria." All these bacteria were obtained from cancer patients at the Livingston Clinic in San Diego, California. All the patients were advanced cases, and included carcinoma, sarcomas and lymphomas. One of the cultures was obtained from neoplastic tissue, and the remaining were isolated from the urine samples. Two of these cultures were sent to us by Dr. A. Strampp, and were the ones on which she and Dr. Cohen made their original studies (Cohen and Strampp, 1976).

We also obtained six additional cultures from Dr. Lewis F. Affronti, George Washington University Medical Center, Washington, D.C. These six bacterial strains were isolated from cancer tissue, three of them from patients with untreated Stage II carcinoma of the breast, and the other three from patients with carcinoma of the colon. The procedures for the primary isolation of all these bacteria were those previously described by Livingston and Alexander-Jackson (1970) and by Diller and Donnelly (1970).

To avoid any bias in these preliminary studies, we also obtained from ATCC the already mentioned strain 13637 of *P. maltophilia* described in 1961 as having been isolated from a patient with mouth cancer (Hugh and Ryschenkow, 1961), strain 25559 of *Eubacterium lentum*, an obligate anaerobe originally isolated in 1938 from a rectal tumor, and strain 12818 of *Streptococcus faecalis*, originally isolated from a patient with a squamous cell carcinoma of the gingival ridge (Hugh, 1959). Through the courtesy of Dr. Christine Poojies, Department of Microbiology, Pennsylvania State University, University Park, Pa., and Dr. Ellis L. Kline, Department of Biology, Edinboro State College, Edinboro, Pa., we also obtained virulent and non-virulent cultures of *Agrobacterium tumefaciens*, strains H-38-9 and H-38-7 respectively. Pathogenic strains of the Gram-negative *A. tumefaciens* induce crown-gall tumors in many (mostly dicotyledonous) plants because of the Ti plasmids present in these microorganisms (Van Larabeke et al., 1975; Watson et al., 1975).

All the nine cultures originating with Dr. Livingston's patients, as well as two of the three microorganisms isolated from breast carcinoma patients by Dr. Affronti were identified as *Staphylococcus epidermidis*, biotype III. The remaining culture corresponded to a *S. epidermidis*, biotype I.

Two of the three microorganisms isolated by Dr. Affronti and his associates from patients with carcinoma of the colon were identified as *Escherichia coli*. The third bacterium was identified as *Pseudomonas aeruginosa*.

Using two immunohistochemical methods, the indirect fluorescein-labeled and the indirect peroxidase-labeled techniques (sandwich technique or double antibody technique) and utilizing a specific antiserum to the β-subunit of CG, as well as to the total CG as first antibody, we were able to demonstrate the presence of CG-like immunoreactive material in the walls (membranes) of 16 of 19 "cancer associated bacteria," that is, the 12 strains of *S. epidermidis*, the two strains of *E. coli*, ATCC 13637 strain of *P. maltophilia* and ATCC 25559 strain of the anaerobic *E. lentum*. The CG-like "antigen" was undetectable in the other samples of "cancer associated bacteria," Dr. Affronti's *P. aeruginosa* isolated from carcinoma of the colon, ATCC 12818 strain of *S. Faecalis* and the pathogenic strain of *A. tumefaciens*, thus demonstrating that not all cancer associated bacteria were able to synthesize the CG-like immunoreactive compound, at least in detectable amounts (Acevedo et al., 1978c; Acevedo et al., 1979).

Furthermore, the nonpathogenic strain of *A. tumefaciens* as well as 20 strains from ATCC (Table I) and 29 strains of laboratory isolate "controls" (Table II) were consistently negative for the presence of the antigen, thus demonstrating the lack of, and/or extremely low expression of the information for the synthesis of the CG-like antigen.

The importance of the negative results observed in the three strains of "cancer associated bacteria" as well as in the 50 strains of "noncancer" controls was greatly enhanced by the fact that the "screening" for the presence of the CG-like immunoreactive material in all bacteria was done utilizing antiserum to total CG, which is not a monospecific antiserum.

Possible morphologic differences between the CG-like material producing "cancer associated bacteria" (the "producers") and their "nonproducing" counterparts were also investigated by a study of the ultrastructural characteristics by transmission electronmicroscopy of the "producer" and "nonproducer" *S. epidermidis*. Only an increasing thickness of the cell wall of the "producer" *S. epidermidis* was apparent (Acevedo et al., 1978c). Gas chromatographic analysis (Holdeman and Moore, 1972) of short and long chain fatty acids used as "fingerprinting" did not reveal any difference between the "producers" and the "nonproducers." Acid fastness was not demonstrated.

Immunoelectronmicroscopy has also demonstrated the association of the CG-like immunoreactive material with the membranes of the

TABLE I: "Control bacteria" from American Type Culture Collection

Aeromonas hydrophilia subsp. *formicans*	ATCC 13137
Clostridium haemoliticum	ATCC 9650
Clostridium novyi Type A	ATCC 19402
Propionibacterium acnes (C. parvum)	ATCC 11829
Escherichia coli	ATCC 25922
Fusobacterium nucleatum	ATCC 25586
Haemophilus aegyptus	ATCC 1116
Lactobacillus casei	ATCC 7469
Mycoplasma hominis Type I	ATCC 23114
Moraxella lacunata	ATCC 17967
Pseudomonas aeruginosa	ATCC 27853
Pseudomonas maltophilia	ATCC 13270
	ATCC 13636
	ATCC 17448
	ATCC 17666
Pseudomonas testosteroni	ATCC 11996
Serratia marcescens	ATCC 13880
Staphylococcus epidermidis	ATCC 14970
Streptobacillus moniliformis	ATCC 14647
Streptococcus mutans	ATCC 25175

TABLE II: "Control bacteria" laboratory isolates

Acinetobacter anitrates
Aeromonas hydrophilia
Bordetella bronchiseptica
Neisseria gonorrhoeae   (10 strains)

Pseudomonads:

a) *P. aeruginosa*
b) *P. cepacia*
c) *P. fluorescens*
d) *P. maltophilia*
e) *P. putrefaciens*
f) *P. stutzeri*

Staphylococci:

a) *S. aureus*   (2 strains)
b) *S. epidermidis*   (8 strains)

bacterial walls in the two strains of "cancer associated bacteria" that have been studied, the $E.$ $coli$ and the ATCC 25559 strain of the anaerobe $E.$ $lentum$ (Slifkin et al., 1979).

Because of the important biological and physiological implications of all these findings, we have undertaken a systematic investigation for the presence and localization of the CG-like antigen in bacteria in order to determine (1) to what extent bacteria not associated with cancer to the best of our knowledge, express the CG-like antigen, (2) if the presence of the antigen is limited to bacteria isolated from humans and animals with cancer, and (3) the clinical frequency of the phenomenon.

As part of this investigation, we have examined for the presence of the CG-like material, eight strains of $E.$ $coli$, two strains of Eubacteria, 13 strains of Pseudomonads, three strains of $S.$ $epidermidis$, nine strains of Propionibacteria (Coryneforms), six strains of $Streptococcus$ $pyogenes$ $(S.$ $hemolyticus$), eight strains of Mycobacteria, and single strains of $Clostridium$ $tetani,$ $Staphylococcus$ $aureus,$ $Streptococcus$ $faecalis$ and $Vibrio$ $cholerae.$ The possible presence of free α-subunit of CG was also investigated in all bacteria that have revealed definitive CG-like immunoreactive material. The results of this work are presented here.

MATERIALS AND METHODS

Bacteria

Seven of eight $E.$ $coli$ cultures were obtained from ATCC. They were strains 11775 (a neotype strain), 8739, 10536, 13207, 11698 (an α-type), 11696 (a β-type), and 4350 (a member of subspecies $communior$). The other $E.$ $coli$ culture, designated as strain TZ, was a laboratory isolate, obtained from the urine of a 22 year old woman in her 32nd week of pregnancy. The two strains of Eubacteria were $E.$ $multiforme,$ ATCC strain 25552, and $E.$ $ruminantium,$ ATCC strain 17233. The $S.$ $epidermidis$ cultures, also from ATCC, were strains 27626 and 21787. The importance of the examination of these bacteria is obvious, since some of the "cancer associated bacteria" that were previously found to express the CG-like antigen were identified as $E.$ $coli,$ $E.$ $lentum$ and $S.$ $epidermidis$ (Affronti et al., 1975; Affronti et al., 1976; Acevedo et al., 1978c; Acevedo et al., 1979). Of the 13 strains of Pseudomonads, eight were ATCC strains 9027, 14502, 14886, 15523, 23997, 25314, 27312 and 19582 of $P.$ $aeruginosa,$ two were ATCC strains 11250 and 12842 of $P.$ $Fluorescens,$ and the remaining were $P.$ $aureofaciens$ ATCC strain 13986, $P.$ $allo$-$precipitans$ strain 19860 and $P.$ $syringae$ (aptata) ATCC strain 10205.

TABLE III: List of strains: Coryneforms

	VPI Strain No.	Other Designations*	Origin
P. acnes, type I	6630	*C. parvum*, Prevot 3594	Blood culture
	6630	*C. parvum*, Prevot 1317	Blood culture
			Malignant histiocytosis (histiocytic leukemia)
P. acnes, type II	1966	NASA strain X3	–
	6265	Gundersen Clinic, LaCrosse, WI	Surgical head wound
	6632	*C. parvum*, Prevot 2355-A	Abcess of neck
	6637	*C. parvum*, Prevot 2508	Blood culture
	6649	*C. parvum*, Prevot 2501	Sinusitis
P. avidum, type I	0665	CDC 2598 A	Exudate
P. avidum, type II	4982	London Hospital London, England	"Normal" skin

* NASA: National Aeronautics and Space Administration
  CDC: Center for Disease Control

The characteristics of the nine strains of Propionibacteria (Coryneforms) are detailed in Table III. These anaerobic bacteria were obtained through the courtesy of Dr. C. S. Cummins, from the Anaerobe Laboratories of the Virginia Polytechnic Institute (VPI) and State University, Blacksburg, Virginia, and most of them are collectively referred to as *Corynebacteria*. It is important to note that one of these bacterial strains, VPI 6660, was "cancer associated," since it was originally isolated from the blood of a patient with histiocytic leukemia. The study of the Coryneforms was done because *C. parvum* vaccines are being widely used in cancer therapy. The strains listed in Table III were selected on the basis of the findings of Cummins and Linn (1977) which described a high reticulo-stimulating activity of vaccines prepared from these microorganisms as judged by the degree of spleen hypertrophy produced after their injection into mice. The different strains of *S. pyogenes* were investigated because they are also being utilized in the preparation of vaccines for cancer treatment (Aoki et al., 1976; Kimura et al., 1976). Table IV lists the strains studied, all obtained from ATCC.

The characteristics of the different strains of *M. tuberculosis* and BCG are listed in Table V. The Japanese strain of BCG was obtained through the courtesy of Dr. L. F. Affronti. All the others were provided by Dr. Ray G. Crispen, Director, Institute for Tuberculosis Research (ITR), University of Illinois, Chicago. The decision to investigate *M. tuberculosis* and BCG is obvious, since the antagonism between cancer and infectious disease, particularly tuberculosis, has been recognized since the 19th century. This basic clinical observation, and the subsequent experimental work that ultimately demonstrated the immunological crossreactivity between BCG and some experimental and human malignant neoplasms, constituted the basis for the wide use of BCG vaccines as an adjuvant in the therapy of cancer (Crispen, 1974; Baldwin and Primm, 1978).

S. aureus, Cowan's serotype I, ATCC strain 12598, was selected for testing because of the great amount of Protein A that these bacteria contain in their cell walls. About 90% of all *S. aureus* strains produce such protein A which combines with the Fc portion of IgG. By means of the Fc/protein A reaction, most IgG in human and rabbit serum can be absorbed by preparations of *S. aureus* (Forsgreen and Sjoquist, 1966; Lind and Mansa, 1968; Kronwall and Williams, 1969; Ankerst et al., 1974).

V. Cholerae, ATCC strain 14035, a neotype strain of *V. cholerae asiaticae*, was selected for investigation because of the reported possibility that the cholera toxin β-chain may be a glycoprotein hormone analog. Recent work by Kurowsky et al. (1977) on the determination of the primary structure of cholera toxin β-chain and its comparison with the β-chains of CG, LH, FSH and TSH, has shown that the overall chemical similarity of the toxin β-chain to the polypeptide hormones was not statistically different from random. However,

TABLE IV: List of strains: *Streptococcus pyogenes*

ATCC. No.	Other designations	Origin, if known
Lancefield's Group A		
21059	*S. hemolyticus*	Human source. Production of anti-tumor agent (U.S. Pat. 3,477,914)
21060	*S. hemolyticus*	Derived from *S. pyogenes* ATCC 21059. Production of anti-tumor agent (U.S. Pat. 3, 477,914)
21547	*S. hemolyticus*	Human source. Production of anti-tumor agent (U.S. Pat. 3,786,141)
27762	A. Bernheimer C203U	Derived from *S. pyogenes* ATCC 14289
Type 3		
21546	*S. hemolyticus* A. Bernheimer C203S	Production of anti-tumor agent(U.S. Pat.3,810,819)
Type II		
21548	*S. hemolyticus*, strain Blackmore	Production of anti-tumor agent(U.S. Pat.3,810,819)

these investigators found that a comparison of the first 40 amino-acid residues of the cholera toxin β-chain to those of the glycoprotein hormones revealed a segment (CAGY) which was chemically similar. For this reason, it has been suggested that the CG-like immunoreactivity demonstrated by some of the strains of "cancer associated bacteria" could be due to such homologous sequence. *Chlostridium tetani*, ATCC strain 19406, was also examined because of the possibility of a small degree of crossreactivity between antiserum to the β-subunit of CG and tetanus toxin. Finally, the culture of *Streptococcus faecalis*, designated as AK strain was obtained through the courtesy of Dr. S. S. Koide, Center for Biomedical Research of the Population Council, The Rockefeller University, New York. This

TABLE V: List of strains: *Mycobacteria*

Name	ATCC No.	Other	Origin
M. tuberculosis:	27294	–	Human lung isolate. Neotype strain.
	–	"Wild"	Laboratory isolate.
M. bovis:	–	Japanese strain	Research Institute of Tuberculosis, Tokyo*
	–	10553 BCG strain	ITR, Univ. of Ill.
	–	7495 BCG strain	ITR, Univ. of Ill.
	–	1029(S)1 BCG strain	ITR, Univ. of Ill.
	–	9-8(S)104 BCG strain	ITR, Univ. of Ill.
	–	1122S BCG strain	ITR. Univ. of Ill.

* Obtained from milk of infected cattle and originally isolated by Calmette at the Pasteur Institute.

microorganism was isolated from the urine of an advanced case of adenoid cystic carcinoma of the nasopharynx.

Bacteriological Methods

All bacteria were identified by standard morphological, physiological, nutritional and biochemical tests (Washington et al., 1974) including gas chromatographic procedures as described by Holdeman and Moore (1972). Biotyping of *S. epidermidis* was performed according to the method of Baird-Parker (1974). *Enterobacteriaceae* were also identified by a computerized system (Auto Microbic System, Vintek Systems, Inc., Hazelwood, Missouri).

The anaerobic bacteria were grown on 5% sheep blood agar with Columbia base (BBL) for 48 to 72 hours at 35°C in anaerobic jars (Gas Pak, BBL). They were also grown in pre-reduced peptone yeast glucose broth under similar conditions. The aerobic bacteria were grown on 5% sheep blood agar with Columbia base for 18 hours at 35°C.

Immunological Reagents

Purified and specific antibodies were obtained from different sources, thus providing a way for monitoring quality control and reproducibility. Rabbit antiserums to total CG was supplied by Dr. Vernon C. Stevens, The Ohio State University College of Medicine, and was also obtained commercially from Cappel Laboratories, Downington, Pa. These antisera are not monospecific and crossreact significantly with LH irrespective of species.

Rabbit antisera to β-CG were also supplied by Dr. Stevens (H-9); by Dr. Morris L. Givner (475-7-T), Department of Endocrinology and Immunochemistry, Ayerst Research Laboratories, Montreal; by Serono Laboratories, Inc. Braintree, Mass., and by Dr. Steven Birken (R-126), Department of Medicine, College of Physicians and Surgeons of Columbia University, New York. Crossreactivity of these antisera with pure LH, as determined by RIA, varies from 0.16% to 5%, depending on the source (McBride and Truang, 1978). Antiserum R-141, an anti-CGβ COOH-terminal peptide, was supplied by Dr. Birken. This is a sialic acid sensitive antiserum that at a given concentration does not bind the native hormone, only asialo CG. Antisera to the α-subunit of CG (R-111 and R-112) were also supplied by Dr. Birken. These are high titer antisera without crossreactivity with the β-subunit of CG. All these antisera were used as first antibodies.

The second antibodies, fluorescein-labeled goat antirabbit IgG, peroxidase-labeled goat antirabbit IgG, and the peroxidase-antiperoxidase complex (PAP) were obtained commercially from Cappel Laboratories and from Gibco Laboratories, Grand Island, New York. Nonimmunized rabbit serum (NRS), total as well as IgG fraction, light and heavy chains, and rabbit antihorse antiserum, utilized as controls, were also obtained from Cappel Laboratories.

The indirect immunoperoxidase reaction requires 3-3'-diaminobenzidine-tetrahydrochloride (DAB) as peroxidase stain, 3.5 mg in 10 ml of phosphate buffered saline (PBS) with 0.015 ml of 30% hydrogen peroxide, and Permount is used as mounting media. 95% glycerine in PBS (Bacto Fluid, Difco Laboratories, Detroit, Mich.) is used as mounting media for the indirect immunofluorescein reaction.

Neuraminidase (Mucopolysaccharide N-acetylneuraminylhydrolase, 3.2.1.18) was obtained from Behring Diagnostics, Somerville, N.J. This brand of *V. cholerae* neuraminidase (VCN) does not contain proteases, aldolase or lecithinase C. The solution contains no preservatives, and has an activity of 500 U/ml.

Incubations were done by suspending the microorganisms (moderate turbidity) in 0.2 ml sterile water and adding 50 μl of VCN. Tests and controls were incubated for 30 minutes at 37°C and then centrifuged in clinical centrifuge for 10 minutes at 2000 rpm.

After discarding the supernatant, the samples were washed three times with sterile water. After the last wash, the microbes were suspended in 0.2 ml of sterile water and vortexed briefly for mixing. 25 µl aliquots from these suspensions were used for immuno-chemical analysis.

Controls

The standard controls for immunohistochemistry were always used with all antisera. Therefore, utilization of CG-absorbed first antibody, for example, was done as an indication of the specificity of the first antibodies, anti-total CG or anti-βCG. The absorption was done by incubating the first antibody at 37°C for a period of 30 to 45 minutes with an excess of CG. Commercial (APL^R, Ayerst Laboratories brand of human CG) as well as a pure preparation (CR-119, a gift from NICHD and Dr. Robert Canfield, Columbia University, New York) were utilized.

Replacement of the first antibody 1) by non-immunized rabbit serum (NRS), 2) by rabbit antihorse antiserum (immunized rabbit serum), and 3) by PBS, were routinely used as tests for specificity, mainly of the second antibody.

A negative reaction obtained in the control test in which the first antibody has been replaced by PBS, is not only an indication of specificity of the second antibody, but it also indicates: 1) the absence of endogenous peroxidase or endogenous fluorescence, depending on the reactive used, 2) the absence of protein A type material that will bind with the Fc fragment of the second antibody, and 3) the absence of Fc receptors on the surface of the cell.

If interference by endogenous peroxidase is proven by incubat-ing the cell preparation with DAB, the enzyme can be eliminated by a 15-30 minute incubation prior to immunostaining, either with 0.3% hydrogen peroxide in absolute methanol (Streefkerk, 1972) or with 0.074% HCl in ethanol (Weir et al., 1974). Fc receptors may be blocked by incubating with fragment Fc IgG, available from Cappel Laboratories. Possible interference of membrane-bound serine proteases (Kurowsky et al., 1977) with anti-β-CG is eliminated by heating the preparation at 55° to 90°C (Adejuwon et al., 1979) for 20 minutes prior to immunostaining.

These standard controls for immunohistochemistry are of great importance because, due to the nature of the test that required the use of concentrated antisera (1:5 to 1:160) it is inappropriate to rely on data obtained by RIA at dilutions utilized for such a test as proof of characterization. Therefore, as we (Acevedo et al., 1978a) and Taylor (1978) have proposed, and as has been stressed at the Workshop in Immunoperoxidase Techniques in Diagnostic Pathology

(DeLellis et al., 1979), known positive and negative cell controls are also used.

The positive cell control used is the cultured human malignant trophoblast (BeWo cell). The great amount of CG produced by this cell (about 1000 IU/24 hr/10^8 cells) plus the fact that it also synthesizes practically every polypeptide hormone, fragments, enzymes, etc., makes this cell ideal for testing the specificity of first and second antibodies, as well as the complete reaction. We also use another established cultured malignant cell, sarcoma-180 (ATCC CCL 8) and *E. coli* strain M3, which have been demonstrated to express the immunoreactive material. As negative cell controls we are using proven "nonproducing" bacteria.

Immunohistochemical Methods

For examination, a drop of sterile water is placed in each one of the circles of a Fluoro Slide (Curtin Matheson). Then, the surface of a colony of the respective microorganisms is gently touched with a bacteriological loop and mixed into the drop of water in each circle. After air drying, the preparations are labeled following previously described techniques (Bain and Ezrin, 1970; LeLeux and Robin, 1971; Mazurkiewicz and Nakane, 1972; Petruz, 1972; Moriarty et al., 1973; McManus et al., 1976; Acevedo et al., 1978a; DeLellis et al., 1979; McLean and Nakane, 1974).

For the indirect immunofluorescein reaction, a drop of the first antibody is applied to cover the preparation of one of the circles of the slide. The preparation on the other circle is used as control and PBS or any other replacement of the first antibody is added to cover it. The samples are then incubated at room temperature in a moist atmosphere chamber for 30 minutes. The slides are then gently rinsed with PBS, placed in staining dishes containing PBS and gently agitated on a clinical rotator (Eberbach Corporation, Ann Arbor, Michigan) for three 5-minute washes. After completion of this time, the slides are removed and drained briefly. Without allowing the preparation to dry, each sample is then treated with one or more drops of the fluorescein-labeled second antibody. The 30 minutes incubation is repeated, followed by rinses and washes, as above. The slides are then well drained, and a drop of BACTO fluid and coverslip are applied. Samples are then ready for examination with the ultraviolet microscope. When present, the CG-like antigen is recognized by an apple green fluorescence at the foci of the protein. From the moment of reconstitution of the fluorescein-labeled second antibody, all the work must be done in a darkened laboratory.

The procedure followed for the indirect immunoperoxidase reaction is identical to the method used for the indirect immunofluorescein reaction up to the rinses and washes done following incubation with the second antibody, this time peroxidase-labeled. The preparations are subsequently fixed in denatured alcohol for 15 minutes, washed twice in PBS for 5 minutes and stained with freshly prepared DAB for 10 minutes. Two 5 minute and two 10 minute PBS washings are followed by a 1 minute distilled water rinse. Dehydration is then performed by washing twice for 1 minute in 95% alcohol, followed by 3 slow dips in absolute methanol, and two 1 minute washings in xylene. With the xylene still on the slide, Permount and coverslip are then applied. The presence of the trophoblastic-like protein is indicated by a brown-to-almost-black granular or continuous staining, depending on the concentration of the antigen.

The trophoblastic-like protein(s) is considered to be present only when the indirect fluorescein-labeled and the indirect peroxidase-labeled immunohistochemical reactions are positive by light microscope.

The use of the two immunohistochemical reactions is an important time saver in the screening process, since it eliminates the possibility of equivocal reactions due to either intrinsic peroxidase content or natural fluorescence. Nonspecific fluorescence does not constitute a problem, since it is easily recognized by an experienced observer, and it can be eliminated by the use of appropriate filters and/or counterstaining.

Instruments

The optical system for examining the preparations subjected to the indirect immunofluorescein reaction consists of a Leitz-Ortholux microscope fitted with a darkfield condenser, 10X ocular and achromatic oil immersion objectives (100X and 95X:NA 1.0), and a lamphousing with an Osram HBO mercury vapor bulb. A BG-12 excitor filter is used in combination with a barrier filter No. 47. Photographs are made with a 35 mm Leitz camera using Eastman Kodak Ektachrome 400 fast color film with exposure times from 20 to 40 seconds.

RESULTS

With the exception of three bacterial strains, $S.$ $faecalis$ AK, $S.$ $epidermidis$ ATCC 21787, and $S.$ $aureus$, Cowan's serotype I, ATCC 12598, the other 49 strains of biologically and physiologically important microorganisms that were screened for the presence of the CG-like antigen were consistently negative when tested by either one of the immunohistochemical reactions using commercial antiserum (Cappel Laboratories) to total CG as first antibody, indicating a lack of or an extremely low expression of the information for the synthesis of the CG-like immunoreactive material. Fig. 1 shows an example of the reaction of a "positive cell control," $E.$ $coli$ M3, and Fig. 2 its corresponding reagent control. The negative reaction given by $E.\ coli$ TZ utilized as a "negative cell control" is shown in Fig. 3.

The three bacterial strains presenting a postive reaction when screened with one of the immunohistochemical reactions were subsequently tested with the second reaction and subjected to all the controls described above. The results obtained with the "cancer associated" $S.\ faecalis$ AK and ATCC strain 21787 of $S.\ epidermidis$ strongly suggested the presence of a CG-like immunoreactive material. An example of the results is given by Figs. 4, 5 and 6, illustrating the positive indirect immunofluorescein reaction displayed by the $S.\ epidermidis$, its corresponding NRS control, and its postive indirect immunoperoxidase reaction respectively. Further testing of both bacterial strains with specific antiserum to the β-subunit of CG from different sources, demonstrated unequivocally the presence of a CG-like immunoreactive material in the microorganisms (Figs. 7 and 8).

In contrast to the clearcut results obtained with $S.\ faecalis$ AK and $S.\ epidermidis$ ATCC strain 21787, the ATCC strain 12598 of $S.\ aureus$, Cowan's serotype I, demonstrated postive reactions not only in the test samples, but also in all the control reactions that were performed (Figs. 9, 10 and 11). These results indicated that the positivity of all the immunohistochemical reactions at the concentrations of antisera utilized, were due primarily to the great amount of protein A produced by this particular strain of $S.\ aureus$, and demonstrated that protein A also binds goat IgG (Fig. 11). Protein A is abundant in the growth media, and these bacteria absorb antisera to total CG, as well as to its β-subunit as demonstrated by direct agglutination tests, when the antisera are applied to bacteria killed and treated according to the method of Ankerst et al. (1974). The fact that protein A appears to be loosely bound to the cell wall (Baird Parker, 1972) explains some negative results obtained when using antisera at higher dilutions.

Treatment with neuraminidase did not produce noticeable effects in the reactions performed with the antiserum to total CG in the CG-producing bacteria tested. In contrast, VCN treated CG-producing bacteria showed a positive immunohistochemical reaction using antiserum R-141, an anti-CGβ COOH-terminal peptide, while the untreated bacteria, at equal concentration of antiserum did not exhibit immunoreactivity.

When antiserum to the α-subunit of CG was used, all the CG-producers tested, $E.\ coli$ M3, $P.\ maltophilia$ ATCC strain 13637, $S.\ faecalis$ AK, and $S.\ epidermidis$ 21787 gave positive results with both immunohistochemical reactions. An example of one of the reactions is illustrated in Fig. 12, while Fig. 13 shows the corresponding control, and Fig. 14, the negative cell control. Parallel

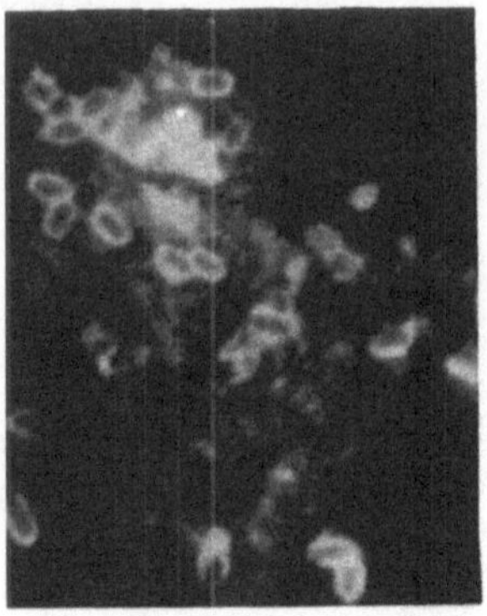

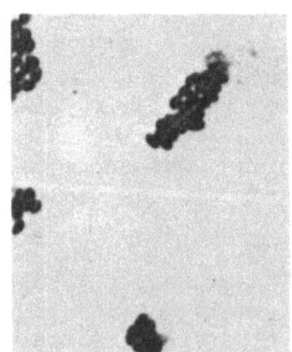

Fig. 1 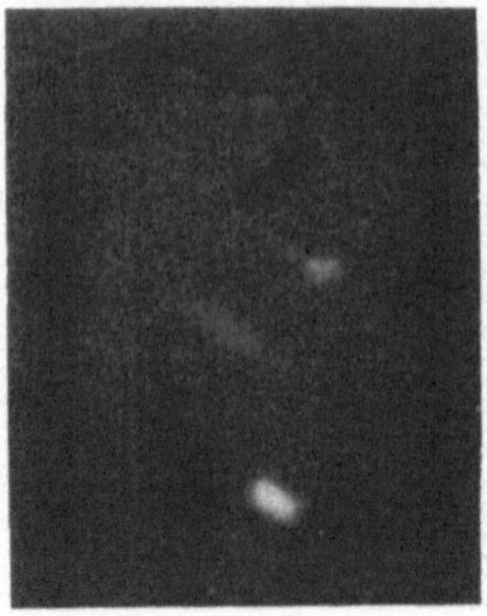   Fig. 2 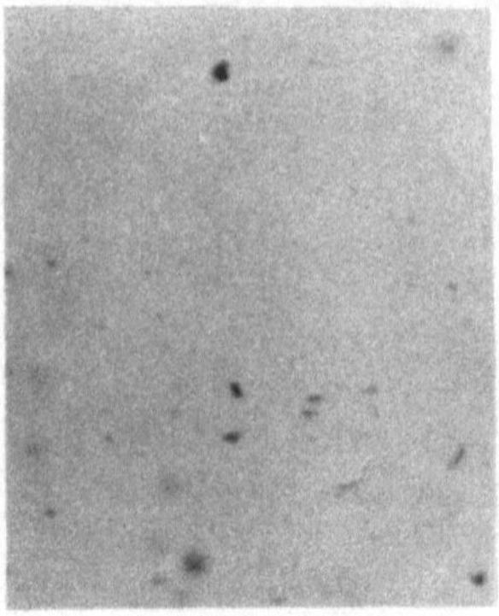   Fig. 3

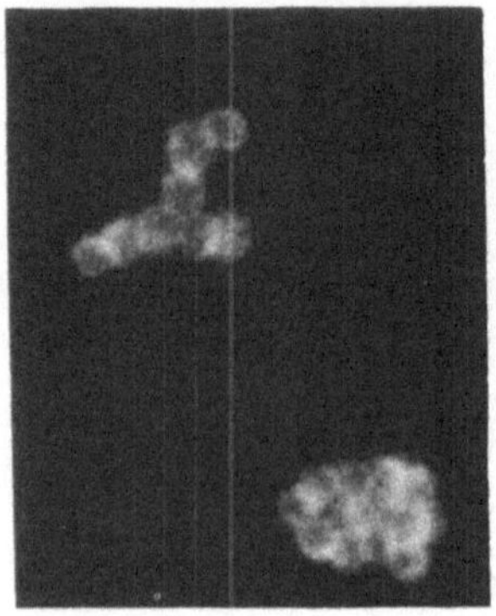

Fig. 4 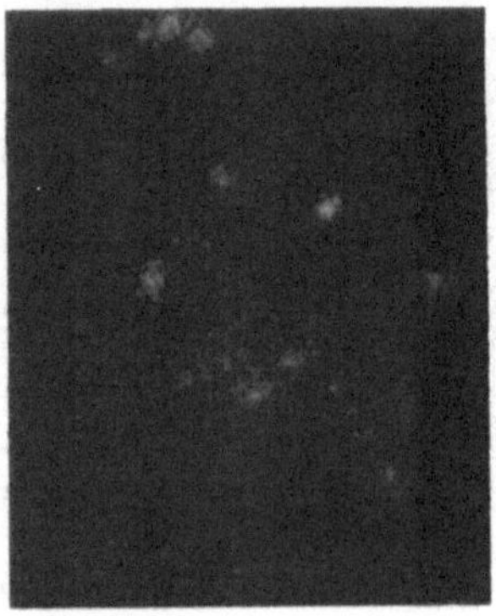   Fig. 5 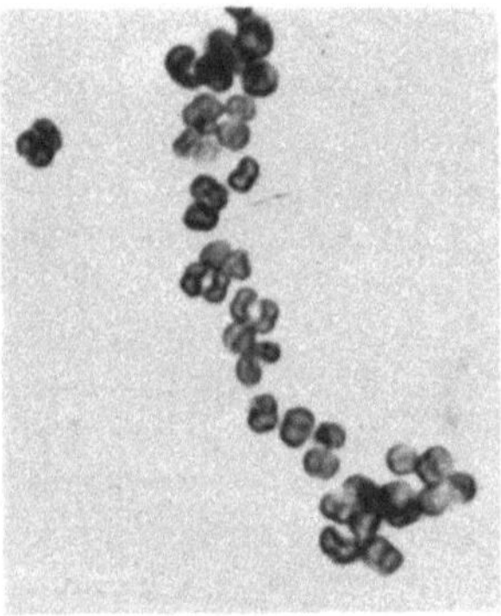   Fig. 6

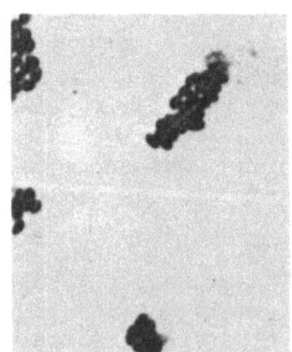

Fig. 7 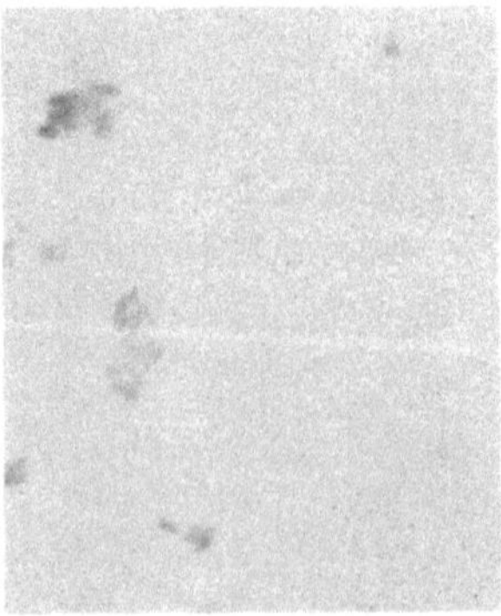   Fig. 8

Figure 1: "Positive cell control," indirect immunofluorescein reaction, *E. coli* strain M3. Antiserum to CG 1:20; fluorescein-labeled goat antirabbit IgG 1:20.

Figure 2: PBS control (reagent control) of *E. coli* M3.

Figure 3: "Negative cell control," indirect immunoperoxidase reaction, *E. coli* strain TZ. Antiserum to CG 1:20; peroxidase-labeled goat antirabbit IgG 1:40.

Figure 4: *S. epidermidis* ATCC 21787, indirect immunofluorescein reaction. Antiserum to CG 1:20; fluorescein-labeled goat antirabbit IgG 1:20.

Figure 5: *S. epidermidis* ATCC 21787, normal rabbit serum control of indirect immunofluorescein reaction.

Figure 6: *S. epidermidis* ATCC 21787, indirect immunoperoxidase reaction. Antiserum to CG 1:20, peroxidase-labeled goat antirabbit IgG 1:20.

Figure 7: *S. faecalis* AK, indirect immunoperoxidase reaction utilizing antiserum to CGβ (1:10).

Figure 8: PBS control (reagent control) of reaction of Figure 7.

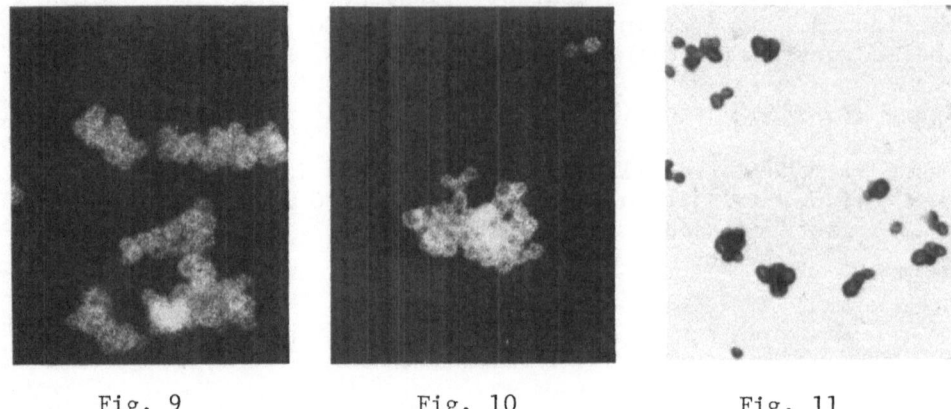

Fig. 9   Fig. 10   Fig. 11

Figure 9: *S. aureus* ATCC 12598, Cowan's serotype I. Indirect immunofluorescein reaction, test conditions identical to Figure 1.

Figure 10: Reagent control of the reaction of Figure 9. First antibody replaced by NRS.

Figure 11: *S. aureus* ATCC 12598. Reagent control of the indirect immunoperoxidase reaction. First antibody replaced by PBS.

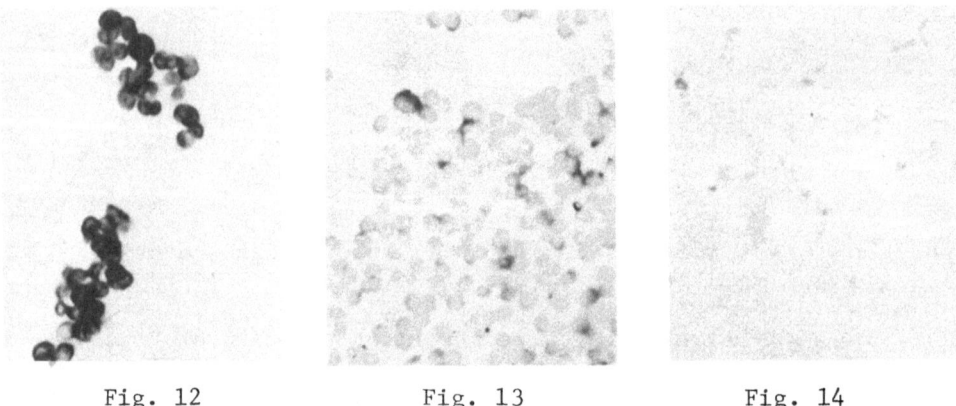

Fig. 12   Fig. 13   Fig. 14

Figure 12: *S. epidermidis* ATCC 21787. Indirect immunoperoxidase reaction with antiserum to CGα as first antibody (1:5).

Figure 13: PBS control (reagent control) of reaction of Figure 12.

Figure 14: "Negative cell control," indirect immunoperoxidase reaction, *E. coli* TZ. Antiserum to CGα as first antibody (1:5).

titrations of the bacterial strains also revealed immunoreactivity at different concentrations of anti-αCG. The results obtained suggested that these bacterial strains synthesize an α-CG-like material, and that their rate of production appears to be different to that of the CG and/or β-CG-like antigen.

DISCUSSION

Antibody to the complete hormone has been used in the screening procedure because it is highly sensitive, relatively inexpensive, and commercially available. However, it is not a monospecific antibody, because it crossreacts with LH. If there is no reaction when this antiserum is used as first antibody, the results are conclusive, and there is no need to use the more specific (and more expensive), somewhat less sensitive antiserum to the β-subunit of CG.

The negative immunohistochemical reactions of 49 of the 52 strains of microorganisms examined, are of important physiologic and biochemical significance, and have provided definitive answers to some of the criticisms that have been expressed in relation to our previous findings. The fact that the screening testing of bacteria in all our work has been done with the non-monospecific commercially available antiserum greatly enhances the significance of all the negative findings, especially since one of the 49 bacterial strains giving a negative reaction, VPI strain 6660 of *P. acnes*, originated from a patient with cancer (Table III). The results obtained in this phase of our investigation, added to our previous findings, provided further support for our theory that the expression of the CG-like antigen is not a ubiquitous finding (Acevedo et al., 1978c; Acevedo et al., 1979).

We have also postulated that the natural presence of the CG-like immunoreactive material in those particular bacterial strains can only be explained by its de novo biosynthesis. While it is recognized that, in general, the simple demonstration of a product within a cell or on its surface is not necessarily evidence of its in situ biosynthesis, it provides a tenable working hypothesis in the absence of other explanations for its presence, such as phagocytosis or absorption by specific receptors and/or nonspecific binding.

In the case of all the bacterial strains expressing the CG-like antigen, phagocytosis and/or absorption of the material by specific or nonspecific binding from the site of origin are entirely ruled out. First, because all the bacteria examined to date are subcultures of the original isolates. Second, the reaction is not an artifact of the culturing conditions because all bacteria tested, the "producers" as well as their nonproducing counterparts were grown in the same media under identical conditions, and third, because different growth media are used depending on the microorganisms (i.e., aerobes, obligate anaerobes), and RIA of the medium or of ultrafiltrates of the medium have given negative results for the presence of the antigen.

It has also been suggested that the positive reactions exhibited by the strains of "cancer associated bacteria" could be due to a bacterial contamination of the immunizing agent, CGβ or its fragments and the adjuvant, which could give reactive antibodies to bacteria. If contamination with production of bacterial antibodies iccurred, such antiserum would have reacted, for example, with most, if not all of the *E. coli*, Mycobacteria, or *S. epidermidis* tested, and not only with certain ones, as our results have shown.

The negative results obtained with the Coryneforms, the BCG strains of Mycobacteria and the *S. pyogenes* strains, all bacteria that are or have been utilized in the production of anti-tumor vaccines, demonstrated that the antibodies elicited by such vaccines are without activity toward CG or a CG-like material.

The results shown by the protein A producing *S. aureus*, have provided definitive evidence that the positive reactions given by strains of "cancer associated bacteria," under experimental conditions used, are not due to a protein A type of reaction. Our results have also demonstrated that the amount of protein A produced by a given strain of *S. aureus* is the limiting factor for its testing for the presence of CG-like antigen.

The negative results demonstrated by *V. cholerae* have also eliminated the possibility that, under the experimental conditions used, the expression of the CG-like antigen by those special bacterial strains could be due to crossreactivity with a glyco-protein analog or homolog of the cholera toxin β-chain.

S. faecalis, strain AK, and *S. epidermidis*, ATCC strain 21787 were the only two bacterial strains from the 52 that were tested, that demonstrated the expression of the CG-like antigen. While the origin of the AK strain of *S. faecalis* was well established, the origin of the *S. epidermidis* strain, so far, has been impossible to trace. It is only known that this bacterium came from the Kikkoman Shoyu Co., Ltd. (U.S. Patent 3,932,671, listed herein as *Tetracoccus soyae*) and is used for the production of protein hydrolysates, mainly of soya sauce.

The positive results observed with the antibodies to the α-subunit of the trophoblastic hormone, as well as to the CGβ-COOH terminal, gave further evidence for the production of a CG-like material. The detection of α-CG-like immunoreactive material is of great significance because there is not possible interference with serine proteases, since the CAGY sequence is only present in the β-subunit of CG.

The immunohistochemical findings have been corroborated by the recent findings of Maruo, Cohen and Koide (1979) demonstrating that the material obtained from cultures of microorganisms isolated from cancer patients and showing immunoreactivity to CG possessed biophysical, biochemical and biological characteristics of the hormone, including in vivo biological activity in the rat uterine weight assay. These investigators concluded that except for a difference in biological potency, all the properties of the bacterial material and native human CG were entirely similar.

The findings of a de novo bacterial synthesis of a material so similar to the human trophoblastic hormone has great implications, because it constitutes the first demonstration of the "natural synthesis" of a "hormone-like" material by prokaryotes. The biological importance of this finding is greatly enhanced because of the considerable evidence that now exists of the in vitro and in vivo production of biochemically similar and biologically active CG-like material by cancer cells in human and other species (Rabson et al., 1973; Tormey et al., 1975; Goldstein, 1976; Perlin et al., 1976; Kurman et al., 1977; Acevedo et al., 1978a; Schlegel-Haueter et al., 1978; Hatori et al., 1978), as well as in spermatozoa (Acevedo et al., 1977; Asch et al., 1979), rabbit morulae (Asch et al., 1978) and blastocyst (Channing et al., 1978), and by the fact that to date, every bacterium that has been shown to express the CG-like material, has always been isolated from a patient with cancer.

The biological and physiological implications of such an occurrence in the fields of bacteriology, genetics, molecular biology, oncology and reproductive physiology are obvious, since none of the current knowledge in these fields can explain the phenomenon observed with the bacterial systems, nor its apparent relation to cancer.

REFERENCES

Acevedo, H. F.., Slifkin, M., Pouchet, G. R., and Rakhshan, M., 1977, Identification of the β-subunit of choriogonadotropin (CG) in human spermatozoa, in *The Testis in Normal and Infertile Men*, P. Troen and H. R. Nankin, ed., pp. 185-192, Raven Press, N.Y.
Acevedo, H. F., Slifkin, M., Pouchet, G. R., and Rakhshan, M., 1978a, Human chorionic gonadotropin in cancer cells. I. Identification in *in vitro* and *in vivo* cancer cell systems, in *Detection and Prevention of Cancer*, Part 2, Vol. I, H. E. Nieburgs, ed., pp. 937-963, Marcel Dekker, Inc., New York.

Acevedo, H. F., Slifkin, M., Pardo, M., and Pouchet, G. R., 1978b, Choriogonadotropin (CG)-like antigen in rat prostatic carcinoma: Immunohistochemical detection and fine structure studies, Prog. 3rd Internatl. Conf. on Differentiation and Neoplasia, Minneapolic, MN, Aug. 28-Sept. 1, Abst. 124.

Acevedo, H. F., Slifkin, M., Pouchet, G. R., and Pardo, M., 1978c, Immunohistochemical localization of a choriogonadotropin-like protein in bacteria isolated from cancer patients, Cancer 41: 1217.

Acevedo, H. F., Slifkin, M., Pouchet-Melvin, G. R., and Campbell-Acevedo, E. A., 1979, Choriogonadotropin-like antigen in the anaerobic bacterium, Eubacterium lentum, isolated from rectal tumor, Infection and Immunity 24:920.

Adejuwon, C. A., Segal, S. J., and Mitsudo, S., 1979, Protease inhibitor abolishes the apparent hCG-like immunoactivity in human tissues, Prog. of the 61st Annual Mtg., The Endocrine Society, Anaheim, CA, June 13-15, Abst. 954.

Affronti, L. F., Grow, L., and Begell, F., 1975, Characterization of bacterial tumor isolates, Fed. Proc. 34(3); 1043, Abst. 4676.

Affronti, L. F., Grow, L., Brumbaugh, R. and Orton, K., 1976, Bacterial tumor isolates, Abst. Anl. Mtg. Am. Soc. Microbiol., Atlantic City, NJ, May 3-8, Abst. E-56.

Ankerst, J., Christensen, P., Kjellen, L., and Kronvall, G., 1974, A routine diagnostic test for IgA and IgM antibodies to Rubella virus: Absorption of IgG with Staphylococcus aureus, J. Infect. Dis. 130:268.

Aoki, T., Kvedar, J. P., Hollis, V. W., Jr., and Bushar, G. S., 1976, Streptococcus pyogenes preparation OK-432: Immunoprophylactic and immunotherapeutic effects on the incidence of spontaneous leukemia in AKR mice, J. Natl. Cancer Inst. 56:687.

Asch, R. H., Fernandez, E. O., and Pauerstein, C. J., 1977, Immuno-dectection of hCG-like substance in human sperm, Fertility and Sterility 28:1258.

Asch, R. H., Fernandez, E. O., Magnasco, L. A., and Pauerstein, C. J., 1978, Demonstration of a chorionic gonadotropin-like substance in rabbit morulae, Fertility and Sterility 29:444.

Asch, R. H., Fernandez, E. O., Siler-Khodr, T. M., and Pauerstein, C. J., 1979: Presence of an hCG-like substance in human sperm. Am. J. Obstet. Gynec. In press.

Bain, J., and Ezrin, C., 1970, Imunofluorescent localization of the LH of the human adenophypophysis, J. Clin. Endocr. 30:181.

Baird-Parker, A. C., 1972, Classification and identification of Staphlococci and their resistance to physical agents, in The Staphlococci, J. O. Cohen, ed., pp. 1-20, John Wiley and Sons, Inc., New York.

Baird-Parker, A. C., 1974, The basis for the present classification of staphylococci and micrococci, Ann. N.Y. Acad. Sci. 236:7.

Baldwin, R. W., and Pimm, M. V., 1978, BCG in tumor immunotherapy, Adv. Cancer Res. 28:91.

Beck, J. S., Porteous, I. B., and Ullyot, J. L., 1970, Gonadotropin-secreting bronchial carcinoma: Aberrant endocrine activity or trophoblastic differentiation? J. Path. 101:59.

Braunstein, G. D., Vaitukaitis, J. L., Carbone, P. P., and Ross, G. T., 1973, Ectopic production of human chorionic gonadotropin by neoplasms. Ann. Int. Med. 78:39.

Channing, C. P., Stone, S. L., Sakai, C. N., Haour, F., and Saxena, B. B., 1978, A Stimulating effect of the fluid from preimplantation rabbit blastocysts upon luteinization of monkey granulosa cell cultures, J. Reprod. Fert. 54:215

Chou, J. Y., 1978, Regulation of the synthesis of human chorionic gonadotropin by strains of HeLa Cells in culture, In Vitro 14:775.

Cohen, H. and Strampp, A., 1976, Bacterial synthesis of substance similar to human chorionic gonadotropin, Proc. Soc. Exp. Biol. Med. 152:408.

Crispen, R. G., 1974, BCG vaccine in perspective, Seminars in Oncology, 1:311.

Cu-mins, C. S., and Linn, D. M., 1977, Reticulostimulating properties of killed vaccines of anaerobic Coryneforms and other organisms. J. Natl. Cancer Inst. 59:1679.

Dailey, J. E., and Marcuse, P. M., 1969, Gonadotropin secreting giant cell carcinoma of the lung, Cancer 24:388.

DeLellis, R. A., Sternberger, L. A., Mann, R. B., Banks, P. M., and Nakane, P. K., 1979, Immunoperoxidase techniques in diagnostic pathology, Report of a Workshop sponsored by the National Cancer Institute, Am. J. Clin. Path. 71:483.

Diller, I. C., and Donnelly, A. J., 1970, Experiments with mammalian tumor isolates, Ann. N.Y. Acad. Sci. 174:655.

Dufau, M. L., Tsuruhara, T., and Catt, K. J., 1972a, Interaction of glycoprotein hormones with Agarose-Concanavalin-A, Biochem. Biophys. Acta 278:281

Dufau, M. L., Catt, K. J., and Tsuruhara, T., 1972b, Sensitive gonadotropin responsive system and radioimmunoassay of testosterone production by the rat testis in vitro, Endocrinology, 90:1032.

Forsgren, A., and Sjoquist, J., 1966, "Protein A" from S. Aureus. I. Pseudo-immune reation with human famma globulin, J. Immunol. 97:822.

Ghosh, N. K., and Cos, R. P., 1976, Production of human chorionic gonadotropin in HeLa cell cultures, Nature 259:416.

Goldstein, D. P., 1976, Chorionic Gonadotropin, Cancer 38:453.

Hattori, M., Fukase, M., Yoshimi, H., Matsukura, S. and Imura, H., 1978, Ectopic production of human chorionic gonadotropin in malignant tumors, Cancer 42:2328.

Holdeman, L. V., and Moore, W. E. C. (ed.), 1972, Anaerobic Laboratory Manual, The Virginia Polytechnic Institute and State University Anaerobic Laboratory, Blacksburg, Va.

Hugh, R., 1959, Motile streptococci isolated from the oro-pharyngeal region, Can. J. Microbiol. 5:351.

Hugh, R., and Ryschenkow, E., 1961, *Pseudomonas maltophilia*, an alcaligenes-like species, J. Gen. Microbiol. 26:123.

Kimura, I., Ohnoshi, T., Yashara, S., Sugiyama, M., Urabe, Y., Jujii, M., and Machida, Kr., 1976, Immunochemotherapy in human lung cancer using the streptococcal agent OK-432, Cancer 27:2201.

Kronvall, G., and Williams, R. C., Jr., 1969, Differences in anti-protein A activity among IgG subgroups, J. Immunol. 103:828.

Kurman, R. J., Scardino, P. T., McIntire, K. R., Waldemann, T. A., and Javadpour, N., 1977, Cellular localization of α-fetoprotein and human chorionic gonadotropin in germ cell tumors of the testis using an indirect immunoperoxidase technique. A new approach to classification utilizing tumor markers, Cancer 40: 2136.

Kurowsky, A., Markel, D. E., Peterson, J. W., and Fitch, W. M., 1977, Primary structure of cholera toxin β-chain. A glycoprotein hormone analog? Science 195:299.

LeLeux, P., and Robin, C., 1971, Immunohistochemistry of individual adenohypophyseal cells, Acta endocr. (Kbh) Supp. 153:168.

Lind, I., and Mansa, B., 1968, Further investigation of specific and non-specific adsorption of serum globulins to *Staphylococcus aureus*. Acta Pathol. Microbiol. Scand. (B). 73:637.

Livingston, (W-C) V., and Alexander-Jackson, E., 1970, A specific type of organism cultivated from malignancy: bacteriology and proposed classification, Ann. N.Y. Acad. Sci. 174:636.

Livingston, (W-C) V., and Livingston, A. M., 1974, Some cultural immunological and biochemical properties of *Progenitor cryptocides*, Trans. N.Y. Acad. Sci. 36:569.

Malkin, A., Kellen, J. A., Kolin, A., Cameron, R., and Farber, E., 1978, The immunohistochemical detection of chorionic gonadotropin in experimental rat hepatomas, Scand. J. Immunol. 8:Suppl. 8, 603.

Maruo, T., Cohen, H., and Koide, S. S., 1979, Studies on choriogonadotropin from a microorganism, Prog. of the 61st Annual Mtg., The Endocrine Society, Anaheim, Calif., June 13-15, Abst. 951.

Mazurkiewicz, J. E., and Nakane, P. K., 1972, Light and electron microscopic localization of antigens in tissue embedded in polyethyleneglycol with a perioxidase-labeled antibody method, J. Histochem. Cytochem. 20:969.

McBride, J. H., and Truong, K., 1978, Further comments on estimating choriogonadotropin in serum, Clin. Chem. 24:2207.

McLean, I. W., and Nakane, P. K., 1974, Periodate-Lysine-Paraformaldehyde fixative: A new fixative for immunoelectronmicroscopy, J. Histochem. Cytochem. 22:1077.

McManus, L. M., Naughton, M. A., and Martinex-Hernandez, A., 1976, Human chorionic gonadotropin in human neoplastic cells, Cancer Res. 36:3476.

Moriarty, G. C., Moriarty, D. M., and Sternberger, A., 1973, Ultrastructural immunocytochemistry with unlaveled antibodies and the peroxidase-antiperoxidase couples. A technique more sensitive than radioimmunoassay, J. Histochem. Cytochem. 21:825.

Naughton, M. A., Merrill, D. A., McManus, L. M., Fink, L. M., Berman, E., White, M.J., and Martinez-Hernandez, A., 1975, Localization of the β-chain of human chorionic gonadotropin in human tumor cells and placental cells, Cancer Res. 35:1887.

Perlin, E., Engeler, J. E., Edson, J., Karp, D., McIntire, R., and Waldman, T. A., 1976, The value of serial measurement of both human chorionic gonadotropin and alpha-fetoprotein for monitoring germinal cell tumors, Cancer 37:215.

Petrusz, P., 1972, Light microscopic localization of binding sites for human chorionic gonadotropin in luteinized rat ovaries by a peroxidase-labeled antibody method, J. Histochem. Cytochem. 21:279.

Tabson, A. S., Rosen, S. W., Tashjian, A. H., Jr., and Weintraub, B. D., 1973, Production of human chorionic gonadotropin in vitro by a cell line derived from a carcinoma of the lung, J. Natl. Cancer Inst. 50:669.

Richert, N. D., and Ryan, R. J., 1977a, Specific gonadotropin binding to Pseudomonas maltophilia, Proc. Natl. Acad. Sci. U. S. A. 74:878.

Richert, N. D., and Ryan, R. J., 1977b, A new bacterial stimulant of rat ovarian adenylate cyclase activity. Prog. 58th Annual Meet. The Endocrine Society, Chicago, Ill., June 8-10, Abst. 85.

Richert, N. D., and Ryan, R. J., 1977c, Protease inhibitors block hormonal activation of adenylate cyclase, Biochem. Biophys. Res. Comm. 78:799.

Richert, N. D., and Ryan, R. J., 1977d, Proteolytic enzyme activation of rat ovarian adenylate cyclase. Proc. Natl. Acad. Sci. U. S. A. 74:4857.

Samaan, N. A., Smith, J. P., Rutledge, F. N., and Schulta, P. N., 1976, The significance of measurement of human placental lactogen, human chorionic gonadotropin and carcinoembryonic antigen in patients with ovarian carcinoma, Am. J. Obstet. Gynec. 126:186.

Saxena, B. B., Hasan, S. H., Haour, F., and Schmidt-Gollwitzer, M., 1974, Radioreceptor assay of human chorionic gonadotropin: Detection of early pregnancy, Science 184:793.

Schlegel-Haueter, S., Robinson, J. D., and Cho, J. Y., 1978, Characterization of human chorionic gonadotropin synthesized by human cell lines, Prog. 60th Annual Meet., The Endocrine Society, Miami, FA, June 14-16, Abst. 43.

Slifkin, M., Acevedo, H. F., Pardo, M., Pouchet, G. R., and Rakshan, M., 1978, Human chorionic gonadotropin in cancer cells. II. Ultrastructural localization, in Detection and Prevention of Cancer, Part 2, Vol. I, H. E. Nieburgs, ed., pp. 965-979, Marcel Dekker, Inc., New York.

Slifkin, M., Pardo, M., Pouchet-Melvin, G. R., and Acevedo, H. F., 1979: Immunoelectronmicroscopic localization of a choriogonadotropin-like antigen in cancer associated bacteria, Oncology 36:208.

Streefkerk, J. C., 1972, Inhibition of erythrocyte pseudoperoxidase activity by treatment with hydrogen peroxide following methanol, J. Histochem. Cytochem. 20:829.

Taylor, C. R., 1978, Immunohistological approach to tumor diagnosis, Oncology 35:189.

The American Type Culture Collection, Catalog of Strains, 13th Edition, 1978, H. D. Hatt and M. J. Gantt, ed., Rockville, Md.

Tormey, D. C., Waalkes, T. P., Ahman, D., Gehrke, C. W., Zumwatt, R. W., Snyder, J., and Hansen, H., 1975, Biological markers in breast carcinoma. I. Incidence of abnormalities of CEA, hCG, three polyamines and three minor nucleosides, Cancer 35: 1095.

Vaitukaitis, J. L., Braunstein, G. D., and Ross, G. T., 1972, A radioimmunoassay which specifically measures human chorionic gonadotropin in the presence of human luteinizing hormone, Am. J. Obstet. Gynec. 113:751.

Van Larabeke, N., Genetello, Ch., Schell, J., Schilperoort, R. A., Hermans, A. K., Hernalsteens, J. P., and Van Montagu, M., 1975, Acquisition of tumor-inducing ability by non-oncogenic Agrobacteria as a result of plasmid transfer, Nature 255:742.

Washington, J. A., II, Martin, W. J., and Karlson, A. G., 1974, Identification of bacteria, in Laboratory Procedures in Clinical Microbiology, J. A. Washington, II, ed., pp. 53-124, Little, Brown and Co., Boston.

Watson, B., Currier, T. C., Gordon, M. P., Chilton, M-D., and Nester, E. W., 1975, Plasmid required for virulence of Agrobacterium tumefaciens, J. Bact. 123:255.

Weir, E. E., Pretlow, II, T. G., Pitts, A., and Williams, E. E., 1974, Determination of endogenous peroxidase activity in order to locate cellular antigens by peroxidase-labeled antibodies, J. Histochem. Cytochem. 22:55.

ACKNOWLEDGEMENTS

Supported by contributions in memory of Brooke D. Cadwallader, the Carolyn Reich Memorial Fund and the Cancer Research Foundation (Pittsburgh, Pa.), and by the Research Development Program Grant RD-52 of the American Cancer Society.

A BACTERIAL FACTOR CROSS-REACTING WITH ANTI-CG

S. S. Koide, T. Maruo, H. F. Acevedo,
E. A. Campbell-Acevedo, and M. Slifkin

Center for Biomedical Research, The Population Council
The Rockefeller University, New York, New York, U.S.A.
and Division of Experimental Pathology, Department of
Laboratory Medicine, Wm. H. Singer Memorial Research
Institute of the Allegheny General Hospital, Pittsburgh,
Pennsylvania, U.S.A.

INTRODUCTION

In the present communication, data will be presented to show
that a strain of *Streptococcus faecalis* produces a factor having
immunoreactivity to antiserum raised against the β-subunit of human
chorionic gonadotropin (hCG). The partially purified factor dis-
places the β-subunit in the homologous $CG\beta$ radioimmunoassay (RIA)
system. In addition, the expression of $CG/CG\beta$, as well as of $CG\alpha$
immunoreactive substances in the microorganism, was demonstrated by
immunohistochemical techniques.

ORIGIN AND IDENTIFICATION OF THE MICROORGANISM

The bacteria was isolated from the urine (No. 5491) of a patient
(A.K. No. 082788) with advanced adenoid cystic carcinoma of the
nasopharynx and ethmoid sinus, who was confined at Queens Hospital,
Hawaii. Staining reaction, culture properties, and fermentation
tests of the microorganism were characteristic of *S. faecalis*,
designated as AK strain. The identity of the bacteria was also
confirmed by the Department of Infectious Diseases of Memorial
Hospital, New York and the Department of Laboratory Medicine of the
Allegheny General Hospital, Pittsburgh, Pa.

DETERMINATION OF CG-LIKE FACTOR

The microorganism was grown in trypticase soy broth (TSB) at 37°C for 25 hr. Acetone powder of the culture was prepared. The powder was re-suspended in distilled water, dialyzed, centrifuged, and assayed in a homologous RIA for CGβ. The supernatant contained about 3.4 ng/ml of extract obtained from 10 ml of TSB culture. To verify that the bacterial culture contains immunoreactive CGβ-like factor, acetone powder was prepared from 1 liter of culture and processed as described above. The extract was analyzed by gel filtration on Sephadex G-100 (Figure 1). A substance showing CGβ-immunoreactivity was detected. The elution of this substance was

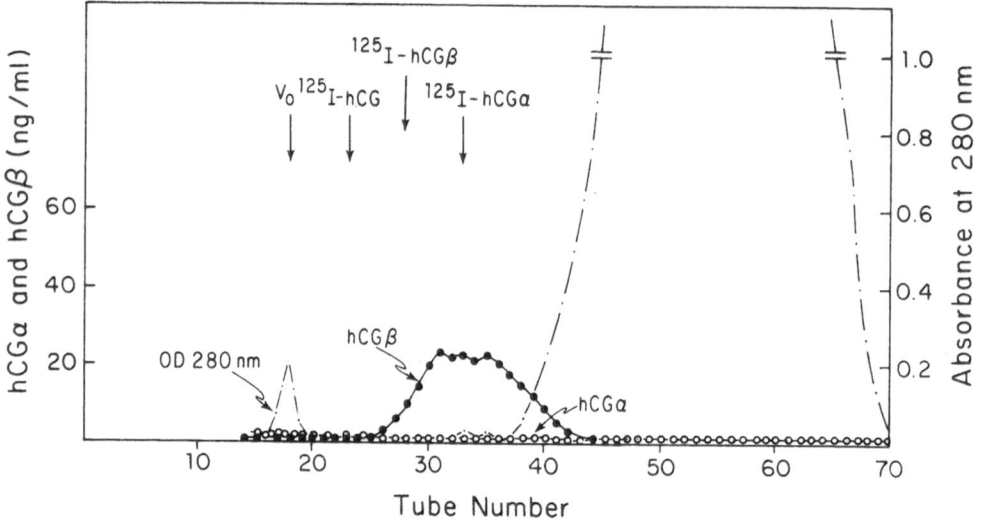

Figure 1. Elution profile of an acetone powder extract of a culture of *Streptococcus faecalis* AK strain purified on Sephadex G-100. Lyophilized powder obtained from the bacterial culture (100 mg) was dissolved in 2.0 ml of 0.01 M tris-HCl buffer (pH 7.4), 0.15 M NaCl, and the mixture applied to a column (1.5 x 85 cm) of Sephadex G-100, equilibrated at 4°C with 0.01 M tris-HCl, 0.15 m NaCl. Each 2.0 ml fraction was assayed by RIA for hCG, hCGα, and hCGβ. Protein content of the eluted fractions was estimated by measuring absorbance at 280 nm. V_0 represents void volume determined by elution of blue dextran. The vertical arrows indicate the elution positions of ^{125}I-hCG, ^{125}I-hCGβ, and ^{125}I-hCGα.

retarded compared to ^{125}I-hCGβ used as a marker, indicating that its mol. wt. is less than that of standard hCGβ. This observation suggested that the substance might be a fragment of CGβ or that it has a low carbohydrate content. It should be noted that no free CGα-like material was detected in the extract. Furthermore, a culture of a strain of S. faecalis, Lancefield's Group D, isolated from a patient with advanced epidermoid cancer of the gingival ridge (ATCC No. 12818) did not contain any immunoreactive CG-like material.

IMMUNOHISTOCHEMICAL ANALYSIS

Immunodetection of CG/CGβ and CGα membrane-associated material was performed using the indirect fluorescein-labeled and the indirect peroxidase-labeled techniques (sandwich technique or double antibody technique), and utilizing antiserum to the complete hormone, as well as antisera to its β- and α-subunits. Procedures, optical system used, and origin and characteristics of the reagents have been published in detail in the chapter of Acevedo et al. Air dried preparations of the AK strain of S. faecalis demonstrated the presence of CG/CGβ and of CGα-like immunoreactive material by the indirect peroxidase-labeled techniques. Moreover, ATCC 12818 strain of S. faecalis has been previously demonstrated by us to be negative for the presence of the membrane-associated CG-like immunoreactive material (Acevedo et al., 1978).

CONCLUSION

The present results suggest that the culture media of the AK strain of S. Faecalis isolated from the urine of a patient with adenoid cystic carcinoma of the nasopharynx contains a factor which cross-reacts with antiserum raised against CGβ. The substance appears to be smaller than ^{125}I-hCGβ. A similar type of CGβ-like substance was detected in a culture of the so-called Progenitor cryptocides analyzed by gel filtration on Sephadex G-100. It is conceivable that these two substances might be related.

The above findings, added to detection of membrane-associated CG/CGβ and CGα immunoreactive material, support the thesis that biosynthesis of CG is an expression of separate genes for each subunit (Daniels-McQueen et al., 1978). Shedding of a preponderance of β-subunit by this microorganism is unusual since in most conditions studied, significant amounts of free α-subunit are found [sera of pregnant women and placenta (Vaitukaitis, 1974; Ashitaka et al., 1974, 1977; Maruo, 1976; Good et al., 1977; Benveniste et al., 1979)]. Present results also raise the possibility that the rate-limiting step in regulation of production of CG-like factor by microorganisms differs from that of human placenta, i.e., synthesis of α-subunit may be the rate-limiting step, rather than production of β-subunit.

REFERENCES

Acevedo, H. F., Slifkin, M., Pouchet, G. R., and Pardo, M., 1978, Immunohistochemical localization of a choriogonadotropin-like protein in bacteria isolated from cancer patients, Cancer 41:1217.

Acevedo, H. F., Campbell-Acevedo, E. A., and Slifkin, M., 1980, Immunodetection of choriogonadotropin-like antigen in bacteria isolated from cancer patients, in The Chorionic Gonadotropin Molecule, S. J. Segal, ed., Plenum Press, New York.

Ashitaka, Y., Nishimura, Y., Endo, Y., and Tojo, S., 1974, Subunits of human chorionic gonadotropin and their radioimmunoassays, Endocrinol. Japon. 21:429.

Ashitaka, Y., Nishimura, R., Futamura, K., and Tojo, S., 1977, Alpha-subunits of human chorionic gonadotropin in fluid of molar vesicles, Endocrinol. Japon. 24:115.

Benveniste, R., Lindner, J., Puett, D., and Rabin, D., 1979, Human chorionic gonadotropin α-subunit from cultured choriocarcinoma (JEG) cell: Comparison of the subunit secreted free with that prepared from secreted human chorionic gonadotropin, Endocrinology 103:581.

Daniels-McQueen, S., McWilliams, D., Birken, S., Canfield, R., Landfield, T., and Boime, I., 1978, Identification of mRNAs encoding the α and β subunits of human choriogonadotropin, J. Biol. Chem. 253:7109.

Good, A., Ramos-Uribe, M., Ryan, R. J., and Kempers, R. D., 1977, Molecular forms of human chorionic gonadotropin in serum, urine, and placental extracts, Fertil. Steril. 28:846.

Maruo, T., 1976, Studies on in vitro synthesis and secretion of human chorionic gonadotropin and its subunits, Endocrinol. Japon. 23:119.

Vaitukaitis, J. L., 1974, Changing placental concentrations of human chorionic gonadotropin and its subunits during gestation, J. Clin. Endocrinol. Metab. 38:755.

ACKNOWLEDGEMENTS

We are grateful to Drs. N. Oishi and S. Oyama and Ms. E. Ayling, Queens Hospital, and to Dr. D. Armstrong and Ms. J. Bell, Memorial Hospital, for assistance in culturing and identification of the microorganisms.

This work was performed as part of the Contraceptive Development Program of the International Committee for Contraceptive Research of the Population Council. T. Maruo is the recipient of a Rockefeller Foundation Fellowship in Reproductive Biology.

HCG PRODUCTION BY NON-PLACENTAL TISSUE AND ITS SIGNIFICANCE

Brij B. Saxena

Department of Medicine and Department of Obstetrics
and Gynecology, Cornell University Medical College,
New York, New York, U.S.A.

INTRODUCTION

Human chorionic gonadotropin (hCG), a glycoprotein hormone,
is synthesized and secreted by the syncytiotrophoblast cells of
the placenta. HCG is found in the blood, urine, amniotic fluid
(Clements et al., 1976), and fetal tissue (Bruner, 1951). The main
function of hCG in early pregnancy is to stimulate the corpus luteum
to secrete progesterone to support the endometrium. The role of hCG
in stimulating fetal testicular androgen has also been implicated
(Jaffe et al., 1977).

The development of highly specific and sensitive radioimmunoassays (RIA) of hCG by the use of antisera raised against the
hormone-specific β-subunit (Vaitukaitis et al., 1972), and the
radio-receptor assays (RRA) of hCG by the use of specific gonadal
"receptor" (Saxena et al., 1974), as well as the in vitro bioassays
by the measurement of testosterone and progesterone in Leydig cells
(Catt et al., 1972) and granulosa cell cultures (Channing et al.,
1978), respectively, has provided a reliable detection of as little
as one mIU of hCG. The application of these assays has permitted
the detection of hCG as early as the peri-implantation phase of
pregnancy (Landesman and Saxena, 1976), and in patients with early
stages of trophoblastic disease and ectopic tumors, thus significantly improving the diagnosis and management of the disease (Dawood
et al., 1977). The hCG molecules produced by the placenta, choriocarcinoma, and hydatidiform mole appear to be chemically similar,
as shown by amino acid and carbohydrate analyses (Tables I and II).
HCG and large molecular weight immunoreactive species of hCG, as
well as immunoreactive α- and β-subunits of hCG, have also been
identified in human chorionic tissues and in cancer cell lines

TABLE I: Composition of choriogonadotropin.

Amino Acid	hCG-hydatidiform mole[a]	hCG[b]	hCG-choriocarcinoma[c]
	Based on 4 His residues/molecule		
Lys	10.4	9.3	10.1
His	4.0	4.0	4.0
Arg	10.6	14.2	14.3
Asp	16.9	16.1	15.6
Thr	16.8	15.6	15.8
Ser	16.8	17.9	17.9
Glu	19.3	16.8	17.1
Pro	25.6	26.3	27.4
Gly	13.3	11.6	9.7
Ala	12.2	11.6	10.9
$\frac{1}{2}$Cys	11.1	18.5	17.7
Val	17.1	15.9	16.2
Met	3.5	3.6	3.6
Ileu	6.3	5.1	5.5
Leu	15.6	13.7	13.7
Tyr	6.3	5.9	5.7
Phe	7.6	5.2	5.3

[a]Choy et al., 1979, JBC 254:1159.
[b]Bahl, 1969, JBC 244:567.
[c]Canfield et al., 1971, Rec. Prog. Horm. Res. 27:121.

TABLE II: Composition of choriogonadotropin.

Carbohydrate	hCG-hydatidiform mole[a]	hCG[b]
	Based on 4 His residues/molecule	
Fucose	0.4	0.6
Galactose	6.7	5.3
Mannose	2.1	5.3
GalNAc	0.5	2.2
GlcNAc	5.4	8.9
Sialic acid	6.1	9.0
Total Carbohydrate	21.2	31.3

[a]Choy et al., 1979, JBC 254:1159.
[b]Bahl, 1969, JBC 244:567.

cultivated in vitro (Benveniste et al., 1979). The large molecular weight species of hCG supposedly represents precursors which are converted to smaller molecular weight-biologically active hCG molecules. In a recent study, Yoshimoto et al. (1979) have reported the presence of non-glycosylated material in the normal tissues. It is suggested that the hCG molecule with its protein moiety alone is present in all cells. The protein moiety of hCG in the placenta is glycosylated. It may be of interest to mention that hCG-like material has also been encountered in bacteria isolated from the urine of patients with cancer (Cohen and Strampp, 1976). The detection of hCG in the blood and tissue of normal subjects has been implicated in the genesis of cancer cells (Acevedo et al., 1977). The presence of hCG-like material in the blastocyst (Haour and Saxena, 1974) and sperm (Asch et al., 1979), however, acquires a significant role in reproduction and fertility regulation.

HCG IN NEOPLASTIC TISSUES

In general, excluding pregnancy, the sperm hCG levels over 1 ng/ml, serum hCG-β levels over 1.5 ng/ml, and serum hCG-α levels over 3.5 ng/ml are considered pathological (Franchimont et al., 1978). HCG secretion by normal or neoplastic trophoblastic cells, by terato-carcinomas (Odell et al., 1967) and by 10% to 20% of variety of neoplasms, e.g., carcinoma of the lung, pancreas, and colon, has been reported (Braunstein et al., 1973a; Vaitukaitis et al., 1976). The presence of hCG together with alfa-fetoprotein has been detected in testicular, ovarian, and extra-gonadal malignant germ cell tumors (Pederson, 1978). In patients with gonadal tumors, the ectopic secretion of hCG is found in 42% of the patients with adenocarcinoma of the ovary and in 51% of the patients with testicular tumors (Rochman, 1978). Eleven out of 130 patients with testicular seminoma have increased serum hCG levels (Javadpour et al., 1978a). Schultz et al. (1978) have studied 67 patients with malignant germ cell neoplasia of the testis and found hCG elevation in 38% of the 34 patients without seminoma. In 60 patients of seminoma, four exhibited elevated serum hCG levels (Javadpour et al., 1978c). After retroperitoneal lymph node dissection and chemotherapy, the hCG levels returned to normal.

Gonadotropin production is also extended to a number of non-endocrine tumors (Vaitukaitis, 1978), such as hepatoblastoma (Hung et al., 1963; Root et al., 1968), and bronchogenic carcinoma (Fusco and Rosen, 1966; Faiman et al., 1967; Rosen et al., 1968) (Table III). Vaitukaitis (1978) reports an adenocarcinoma of the stomach in a post-menopausal woman producing quantities of hCG comparable to those observed in the first trimester of pregnancy. In patients with non-gonadal tumors, the highest incidence of hCG is found in association with the pancreatic carcinoma (33%), gastric adeno-carcinoma (22%), and lung carcinoma (9%). Hattori et al. (1978)

TABLE III: HCG and hCG-β in plasma, urine, and tissue extracts
of patients with malignancy.

Site of Malignancy	Blood	Tissue	Reference*
	% sample positive for hCG or hCGβ		
Lung	6	34	1
Esophagus	0	67	1
Stomach	19	67	1
Liver	17	100	2
Pancreas	33	33	1, 2
Rectum, Colon	11	0	1
Duodenum	–	100	1
Retroperitoneum	–	100	1
Lymph Node	–	0	1
Mediastinum	–	0	1
Uterus	–	67	1
Adrenal	–	0	1
Testis	51	0	1
Normal Controls	1		2

*1: Hattori et al., 1978 Cancer 42:2328.
 2: Javadpour, 1978, Urology 12:177.

TABLE IV: HCG, hCG-α and hCG-β in patients with carcinoma of
the bladder.[1]

	hCG	hCG-α	hCG-β
Blood ng/ml	280	41	72
Tissue ng/g wet tissue	5414	5188	10,910
Urine ng/ml	489	569	501

[1]The control values of normal males are as follows: hCG, n.d.-1.25;
 hCG-α, n.d.-1.2; hCG-β, n.d. Kawamura et al., 1978, Cancer 42:2773.

report that 10 percent plasma samples from patients with malignant tumors contain hCG (Table III). The gonadotropin produced by these tumors is similar to hCG or LH (Braunstein et al., 1973a; Braunstein et al., 1973b). Gynecomastia has been associated with ectopic gonadotropin secretion in patients with carcinoma of the lung (Fusco and Rosen, 1966), adrenal gland (Rose et al., 1968), and liver (Hung et al., 1963). As shown in Table IV, hCG, hCG-β, and hCG-α are detected in the blood, urine, and tissue from the malignant neoplasm of a patient with bladder carcinoma with a terminal stage of gynecomastia (Kawamura et al., 1978). Tumors of the gastrointestinal tract have been among those associated with the highest circulating levels of ectopically secreted hCG. In studies of pineal tumors, the concentration of the subunits of hCG may be increased, but it is not sufficiently abnormal to provide a useful index of tumor activity (Barber et al., 1978).

HCG IN NORMAL TISSUE

Extracts of human testes obtained at autopsy (Braunstein et al., 1975), urinary concentrates, pituitary extracts, and blood from non-pregnant subjects (Chen and Hodgen, 1976; Robertson et al., 1978) contain a substance which is immunologically similar to hCG, elutes from columns of Sephadex G-100 and Ultrogel ACA-54 with K_d similar to hCG, has an isoelectric point similar to that of hCG, and exhibits in vitro biological activity similar to hLH and hCG. A post-menopausal urinary gonadotropin preparation contains in vitro hCG-like biological activity in the RRA: the source of hCG is assumed to be of the pituitary origin. A large concentration of immuno-reactive α-subunit, co-chromatographing with TSH-, LH-, or FSH-α has also been detected in extracts of normal pituitary tissue (Prentice and Ryan, 1975; Kourides et al., 1975).

An immunoreactive hCG-like substance has been identified in extracts of liver and colon (Yoshimoto et al., 1977) and recently in kidney, liver, lung, colon, and stomach of normal subjects (Yoshimoto et al., 1979). The colon and liver CG do not bind to Con-A Sepharose columns, indicating little carbohydrate content, which may explain the lack of in vivo bioactivity of the material.

Recently, hCG-like material was found in almost 20% of 200 serum samples obtained randomly during the luteal phase from women of known fertility and who were using IUDs (Landesman et al., 1976). However, these women did not develop clinical signs of pregnancy. Beling et al. (1976) applied a hemagglutination inhibition test with a sensitivity of 30 IU per liter to urine sample collected during the second half of the cycle, and found that 32 out of 73 samples contained hCG. Both urine and blood samples were also examined for hCG by a specific RIA and RRA. There were 14 hCG positives in 92

cases, of whom two demonstrated clinical signs of pregnancy, and
hCG could be demonstrated in serum when urinary levels exceeded
100 IU/ml. These results were not confirmed by another group of
workers (Sharpe et al., 1977) in either the blood or urine of
women with IUDs using RIA of hCG having cross-reaction with LH in
the range of 15 to 50 mIU. In a recent study by other investigators
(Hodgen et al., 1978), a more specific RIA, as well as bioassay and
RRA of hCG, detected transitory hCG-like activity in the urine of
women wearing IUDs. The current disagreement on the presence of
hCG in women with IUDs appears to be partly due to the low levels
of perhaps partially glycosylated hCG and the use of assays at the
limit of their sensitivity. The ubiquitous presence of hCG-like
material in normal cells may indicate a vestigial evolutionary
genome which may be expressed in all adult cells.

TUMOR MARKERS

HCG has served as a cancer marker in the diagnosis of trophoblastic neoplasms (Weintraub and Rosen, 1973a; Bagshawe, 1975;
Vaitukaitis, 1978; Franchimont et al., 1978). Use of highly sensitive RIA and RRA of hCG in serum or urinary concentrates has further
increased the rate of early detection of trophoblastic disease and
other hCG-secreting tumors. There is evidence for the production
of free subunits of hCG by the neoplasms, hence to rule out active
disease, specific RIAs for hCG and its free α- and β-subunits are
suggested to be performed during therapy when the hCG levels fall
below 10 mIU/ml (Saxena and Landesman, 1978). HCG and α-feto-protein
(AFP) have been used as biological markers for detecting, staging,
and monitoring the managment of non-seminomatous testicular tumors
(Javadpour, 1978c; Javadpour, 1978b; Wajsman and Murphy, 1978).
The RRA and RIA have increased the sensitivity of hCG measurement
so signigicantly that up to 60% of patients with non-seminomatous
tumors were found to have elevated levels of hCG (Wajsman and Murphy,
1978) and the RIA of hCG in the urine of patients with non-
seminomatous testis tumor has been found to be of significant
prognostic value. In addition to trophoblastic and testicular tumors,
elevated levels of hCG have also been used as a guide in non-endocrine
tumors such as gastric, pancreatic, and breast carcinoma. Serum hCG
levels have been found to be elevated in 48.5% of patients with
breast carcinoma (Tormey et al., 1977). In the same study, 35.7%
patient serum pre-operatively, and 27.2% post-operatively showed hCG.
The use of hCG as a pre- and post-operative marker in breast cancer
is being explored. The concept of specific tumor markers has now
been extended to the subunits. A few tumors have been found to
ectopically secrete only one of the subunits of hCG. An elevated
level of hCG or its subunits may indicate the presence of active
disease; however, a normal level does not exclude active disease
being present. Current evidence on the presence of hCG-like material
in normal tissues in the range of 10-120 mIU/g (Yoshimoto et al.,

1979) necessitates serial measurement of hCG not only to detect levels significantly above the basal levels, but also to observe fluctuations compatible with the clinical status of the disease during the course of treatment. The serum concentration of immunoreactive hCG-α in a patient with an adenocarcinoma of the stomach, exceeded 20,000 ng/ml (Rosen and Weintraub, 1974). The secretion of only hCG-β has been found in patients with a pancreatic tumor (Weintraub et al., 1972; Weintraub and Rosen, 1973b). HCG-β is also the predominant form present in a patient with a lung tumor (Vaitukaitis, 1978). The α-subunit of hCG was used to localize a recurrent metastatic tumor for the first time by Javadpour et al., in 1978(c).

HCG-LIKE MATERIAL IN THE RABBIT BLASTOCYST

There is evidence that the blastocyst and the uterus exchange information prior to implantation (Psychoyos, 1967). The maintenance of the corpus luteum of pregnancy in the presence of blastocysts in the oviduct and after transplantation of the blastocyst under the kidney capsule in the rabbit (Zielmaker and Verhamme, 1978) suggests that the blastocyst is the source of luteotropic stimuli prior to implantation. A greater increase in the secretion of progesterone in pregnant rabbits than in pseudo-pregnant rabbits (Figure 1) on days 4-6 (Fuchs and Beling, 1974; Singh and Adams, 1978; Varma et al., 1979) and the secondary rise of CG-LH-like material in the serum of pregnant rabbits on days 3 and 4 postcoitum, further suggest the maternal recognition of the fetus prior to implantation. Huff and Eik-Nes (1966), Dickman and Dey (1974), and Perry et al. (1973) have provided the evidence of steroidogenesis in rabbit, rat, mice, hamster, and pig embryos prior to implantation. Dickman and Dey (1976) suggested that the steroidogenesis in the rabbit blastocyst may be activated locally by a gonadotropin material of the blastocyst origin. The detection of gonadotropic material on the surface of the mouse (Wiley, 1974) and rabbit morulae (Asch et al., 1978), as well as of the rabbit blastocyst (Varma et al., 1979) has been documented (Figure 2). The presence of a luteotropic substance in the pre-implantation rabbit blastocyst fluid has also been demonstrated by RIA (Fujimoto et al., 1975), by RRA (Haour and Saxena, 1974), and by the ability of the blastocyst fluid to stimulate morphological luteinization and progesterone synthesis in porcine and simian granulosa cell cultures (Channing et al., 1978).

However, Harrington and Rothermel (1977) found little difference in the plasma progesterone levels in pregnant and pseudo-pregnant animals. Holt et al. (1976) and Sundaram et al. (1975) failed to stimulate testosterone production by the decapsulated rat testes and progesterone from rabbit ovarian tissue when incubated with day 6 rabbit blastocyst in vitro. The reason for these discrepancies

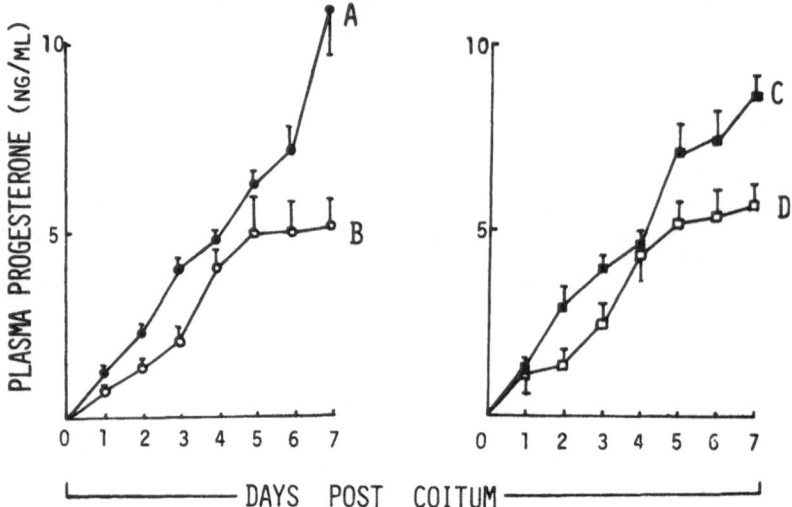

Figure 1.   Plasma progesterone levels in the rabbit: A = pregnant;
B = pseudopregnant; C = 4-day blastocysts transferred day 4;
D = sham transfer. (Singh and Adam, 1978, J. Reprod. Fert. 53:331.)

may partly be due to the mode of collection of blastocysts and
differences in the methodology used. The incubation of very small
quantities of luteotropic material in the blastocyst or its fluid
for extended periods at 37°C in crude tissue homogenate can cause
proteolytic destruction of the luteotropic material. Holt et al.
(1976) might not have attained a 20% concentration of the blastocyst
fluid in vitro granulosa cell cultures which is necessary to obtain
a response, a shown by Channing et al. (1978). Adams (1970) has
also shown that in vivo the presence of at least four blastocysts
in the uterus is neceesary to maintain the corpus luteum of pregnancy
in the rabbit. Further investigations have therefore been undertaken
independently in our laboratory, as well as those of Dr. Ricardo
Asch at San Antonio and Dr. Cornelia Channing of the University of
Maryland, on the existence of luteotropic substances in the rabbit
blastocyst fluid prior to implantation.

Adult female as well as normal male New Zealand rabbits (3-4
kg) were maintained at room temperature in 12 hr of light (0600 to
1800 h). The animals were provided with compressed food and water
ad libitum. After mating, the female rabbits were examined for the
presence of sperm in the vagina and the ovulation was confirmed by

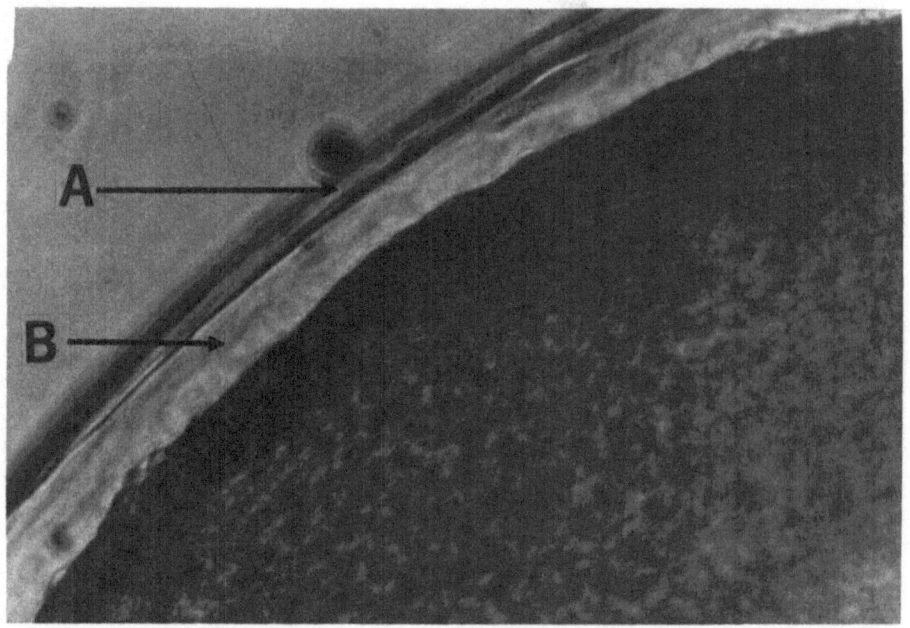

Figure 2. Photograph of a portion of a rabbit blastocyst stained with FITC conjugated γ-globulin isolated from antibodies to hCG-β. A: zona pellucida; B: layer of trophoblastic cells.

the presence of corpora lutea in the ovary at the time of laparotomy in all rabbits. The day of mating was designated as day 0. Blastocysts were also recovered by laparotomy (Figure 3) performed under sterile conditions on day 6 after mating, as described earlier (Saxena, 1979). The animals were remated after 4 weeks to collect more blastocysts. Excess saline adhering to the blastocysts was aspirated. The blastocysts were ruptured by a needle to release the fluid and centrifuged at 5000 rpm at 4°C for 30 min. The supernatants from all the blastocysts were pooled and made 10^{-6}M in PMSF and 20 KIU in Trasylol per ml. The blastocyst fluid was stored at -20°C. Four batches of 2.5, 3.2, 4.5, and 14.4 ml fluid representing 155, 193, 271, and 843 blastocysts, respectively, were purified by chromatography on Con-Canavalin-A-Sepharose (Con A-S) and gel filtration on Sephadex G-100.

In a typical experiment, 4.5 ml of the lyophilized blastocyst fluid was dissolved in one ml of 0.01 M Tris-HCl buffer of pH 7.5 containing 0.1 M NaCl, and centrifuged. The supernatant was applied to a 0.7 x 20 cm column of Con A-S 4B (Figure 4) which was previously

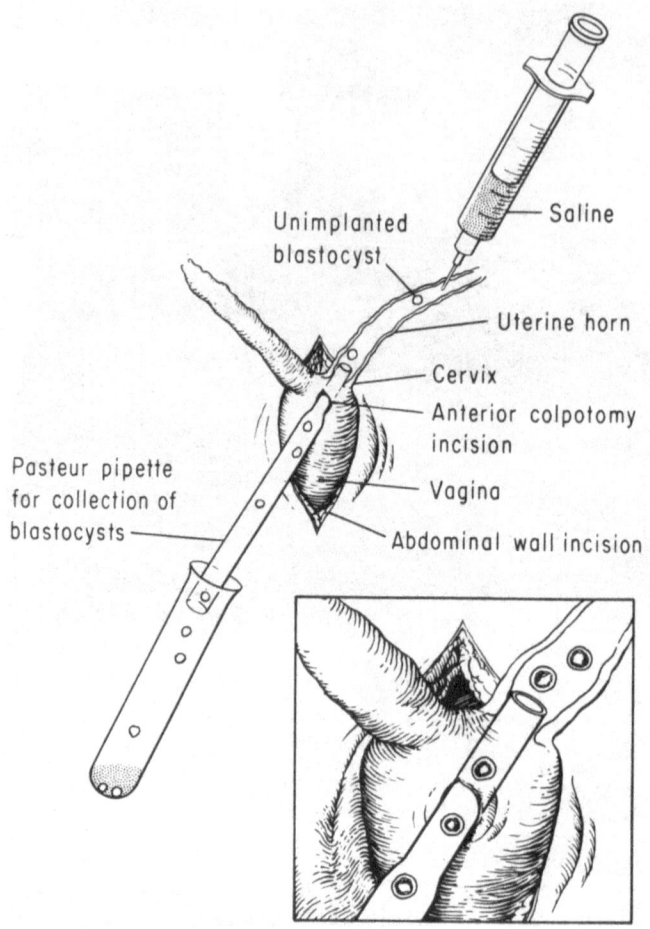

Figure 3. Diagramatic representation of laparotomy performed on day 6 in rabbits. The animals were anesthesized with sodium pentobarbitol (25 mg/kg body weight) given via the ear vein. A 100 x 7 mm Pasteur pipet was cut, narrowed and fire polished at one end to give a 4.5 mm diameter and was used to collect the blastocysts from each uterine horn. An anterior colpotomy was performed and the narrow end of the pipet was inserted through the cervix into the uterine horn. The uterine lumen was flushed from the opposite end with 5 ml saline. The blastocysts were collected into a polystyrene tube. The colpotomy incision was closed with interrupted silk (00) sutures and the abdominal incision was closed in layers. These rabbits were remated 3-4 times, at 4 week intervals, after recovery from each laparotomy.

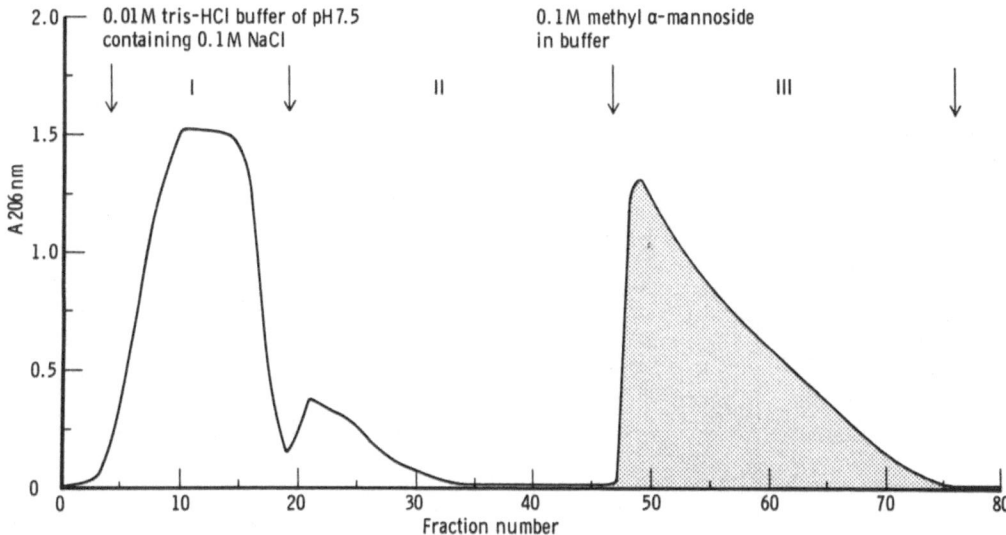

The shaded area indicates fraction containing the luteotropic activity

Figure 4. Chromatography of blastocyst fluid on Concanavalin-A Sepharose 4B. 1 ml fractions were collected and the eluate was monitored at 206 nm.

equilibrated with 0.01 M Tris-HCl buffer of pH 7.5 in 0.1 M NaCl. After the elution of the unabsorbed fraction with the above buffer, the column was eluted with 0.1 M α-methyl mannoside in the same buffer (Agarwal and Goldstein, 1972). The fractions obtained during the purification procedures were assayed for hCG-like activity in the RRA. The adsorbed fraction III from the Con A-S column containing the hCG-like activity was lyophilized, dissolved in 0.5 ml of 0.1 M ammonium bicarbonate buffer and fractionated on a 1 x 115 cm column of Sephadex G-100, equilibrated in the same buffer. The gel filtration of fraction III yielded three fractions (Figure 5). Fraction II, containing hCG-like activity, was further fractionated on Sephadex G-10 column (Figure 6).

Aliquots of 10, 20, 50, and 80 µl blastocyst fluid from rabbits were assayed for hCG-LH-like material by the RRAs of LH-hCG as described earlier (Saxena et al., 1974). The purified fractions containing hCG-like activity were assayed by RRA and RIA (Saxena, 1979; Asch et al., 1979), as well as in vitro bioassays measuring progesterone synthesis in monkey granulosa cells (Channing et al., 1978) and testosterone production by the rat Leydig cell homogenate

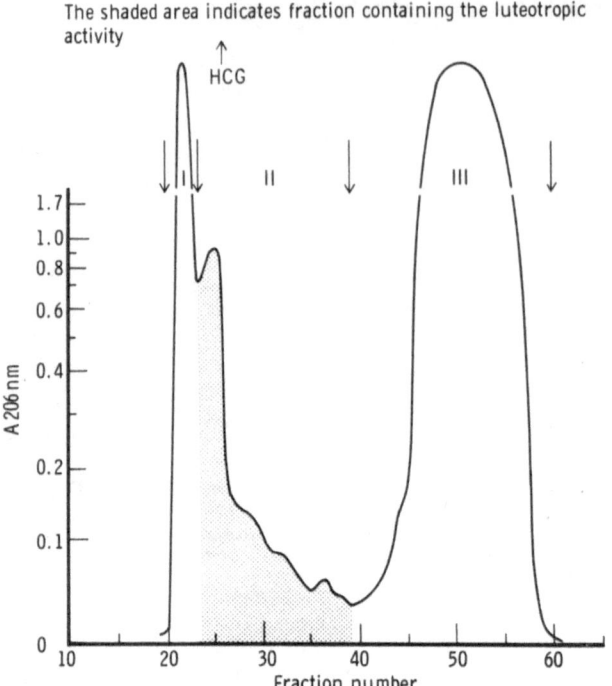

Figure 5.   Gel filtration on Sephadex G-100 of fraction III from Con-A-Sepharose.

(Catt et al., 1972). The blastocyst fluid and fraction III from Con A-S column were assayed for protease activity by the method of Denker and Fritz (1979) using Bz-L-phe-L-Val-L-arg-NHNp and Tos-Gly-L-Pro-L-arg-NHNp as substrates, and were found to contain very weak (1-3 mIU/mg) protein and undetectable protease activity respectively.

It has been demonstrated that the hCG-like material in the pre-implanted rabbit blastocyst fluid is undialyzable and susceptible to proteolytic degradation, suggesting that the luteotropic activity is associated with a large molecular weight protein moiety (Haour and Saxena, 1974; Channing et al., 1978). An average of 16.6 ± 3 µl fluid was present in each blastocyst. Serial dilutions of the rabbit blastocyst fluid yield dose-response curves similar to the hCG standard in RIAs and RRAs (Varma et al., 1979; Asch et al., 1979) In Figure 7, the logit-log relationship of the standard curve with hCG is presented. The presence of 10, 20, 50, and 100 µl of blasto-cyst fluid yielded a slope of -0.72 which was similar to that of

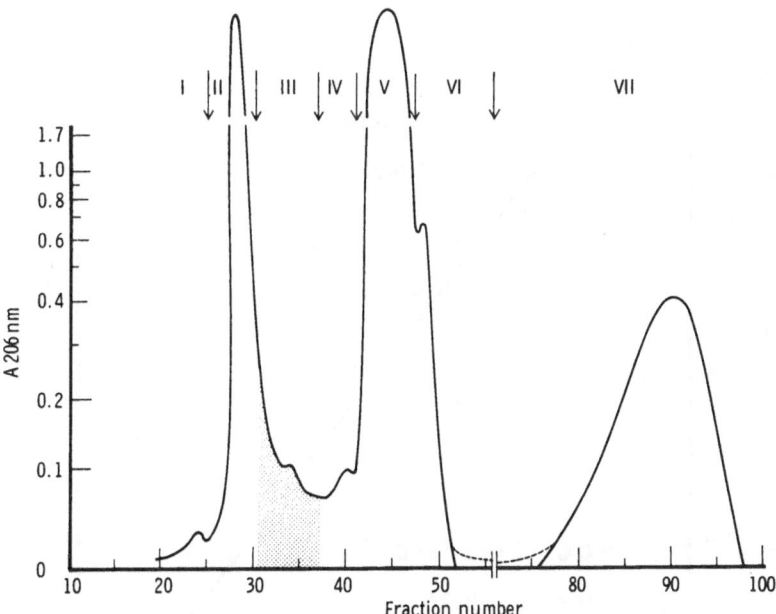

The shaded area indicates fraction containing the luteotropic activity

Figure 6. Gel filtration on Sephadex G-10 of fraction II from Sephadex G-100 column.

hCG-LH (Varma et al., 1979). Estimates from 16 independent RRAs using bovine corpus luteum yielded 0.83-1.0 ng hCG-LH-like luteotropin per blastocyst. Each ml of blastocyst fluid contained 1234 µg protein and 87 ng of hCG-like material as determined by RRA. In the absence of the estimates of the secretory and clearance rates, the estimates of the hCG-LH-like material produced prior to or at the time of implantation are at present only tentative. The hCG-like material of the blastocyst fluid are adsorbed on to Concanavalin-A and eluted with 0.1 M methyl-α-mannoside, indicating the glycoprotein nature of the hCG-like material (Saxena, 1979; Asch et al., 1979).

Chromatography of Con A-S column (Figure 3) yielded hCG-like activity in the adsorbed Fraction III. Gel filtration of the fraction III on a columm of Sephadex G-100 yielded hCG-like activity in fraction II (Figure 4). In the gel filtration studies, the K_{av} of the hCG-like material eluted from Sephadex G-100 column was similar to that of hCG. An immunoreactive material was eluted from the rabbit blastocyst fluid in the region corresponding to native hCG;

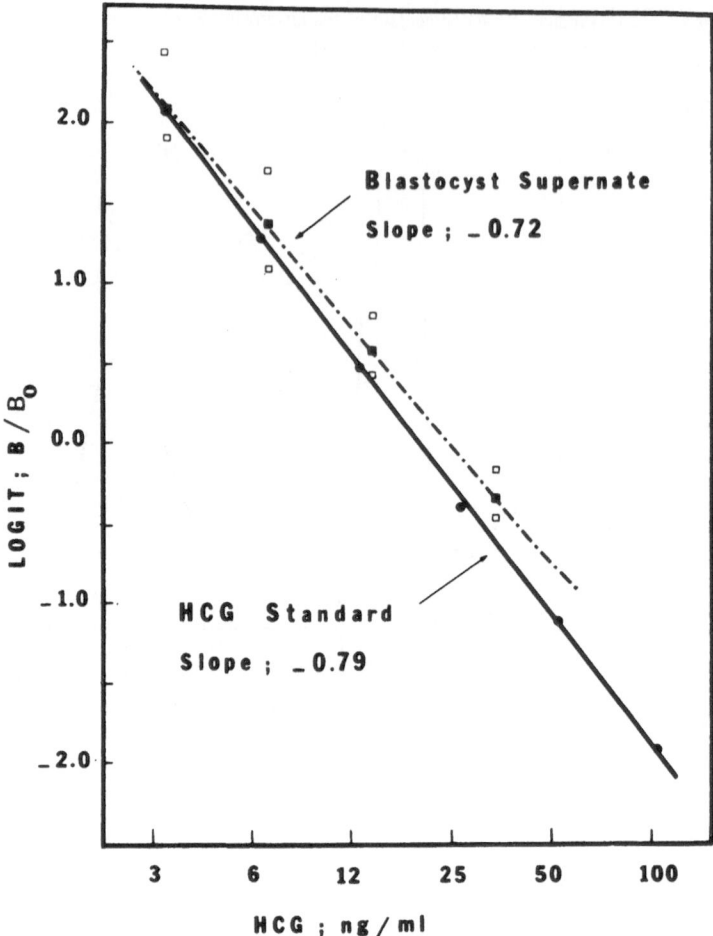

Figure 7.   Dose-response curve for human chorionic gonadotropin (hCG) and the supernatant of the ruptured and centrifuged blastocysts expressed as logit-log transformation. The ratio B/B_0 is the ratio of ^{125}I-labeled hCG bound in the membrane receptor to the total ^{125}I-labeled hCG. Open squares represent duplicate experiments.

no activity was detected in the extracts from unfertilized ova and non-pregnant uterus (Asch et al., 1979). It should be emphasized that during purification, fractions rich in salt yield false inhibition in both RIA and RRA. After dialysis these fractions showed no hCG-like activity. The yield and activity of hCG-like material during the purification of the fluid is shown in Table V.

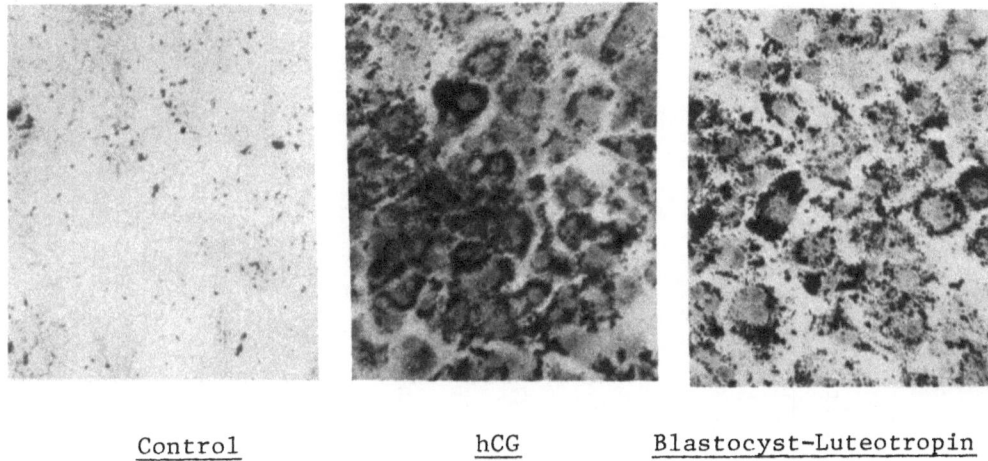

| Control | hCG | Blastocyst-Luteotropin |

Figure 8. Luteinization of monkey granulosa cells by partially purified blastocyst luteotropin. (Oil red O stain + hematoxylin.)

Fractionation by chromatography on Con A-S and gel filtration on Sephadex G-100 increased the specific activity from 0.07 ng to 2 ng hCG-like material per μg protein in the blastocyst fluid, representing a 28-fold purification and a 60% recovery of the hCG-like material of the blastocyst fluid. The luteinization of monkey granulosa cells by the partically purified blastocyst luteotropin similar to hCG is shown in Figure 8. The hCG-like activity of the purified blastocyst luteotropin in the RIA and RRA, as well as in rat Leydig cell testosterone production (Figure 9) and monkey granulosa cell progesterone assay, respectively, was 2.0, 0.78, 1.4, and 2.5 ng hCG-like material/μg protein (Table VI). Hence, the purified material needs at least 500-fold purification to achieve homogeneity. A preliminary amino acid analysis of the purified material indicates preponderance of Asp and Gln similar to those in hCG; however, approximately 50% lower quantities of Pro, ½Cys, Lys, and Arg then in hCG. The carbohydrate composition of the purified blastocyst luteotropin reveals the presence of mono-saccharide units similar to that of hCG, except significantly lower quantities of sialic acid (Saxena, 1979) which may accelerate the clearance rate of the blastocyst luteotropic material and thus create difficulties in detection in peripheral circulation.

Eutherian mammals may be divided into two groups, one where the ovary is the main source of progesterone, for example, in the rabbit; the other, where the placenta is the prime source of progesterone, e.g., in man. The ovary, however, provides the

TABLE V: Yield and activity of fractions obtained during purification of blastocyst fluid.

Fraction	Yield[a]	hCG-like activity[a] (RRA of hCG-LH)	Total Activity	Recovery
	μg protein/ml B.F.	ng/μg protein	ng/ml B. F.	%
Blastocyst Fluid	1234	0.07	87	100
Con-A-Sepharose III	247	0.31	76	87
Sephadex G-100-II	70	0.84	59	68
Sephadex G-10-III	26	2.0	53	61

[a]Average of three determinations.

TABLE VI: HCG-like activity measured by different assays.*

Fraction	RRA	RIA**	(T) Production	(P) Production***
			ng hCG/μg protein	
Sephadex G-10-III (purified blastocyst luteotropin)	2.0	0.78	1.4	2.5

*PMSF 10 and 0.01% sodium azide were used in the assay buffer to inhibit enzymatic or other degradation.
**Antisera to hCG-β subunit.
***Day 5/culture/day.

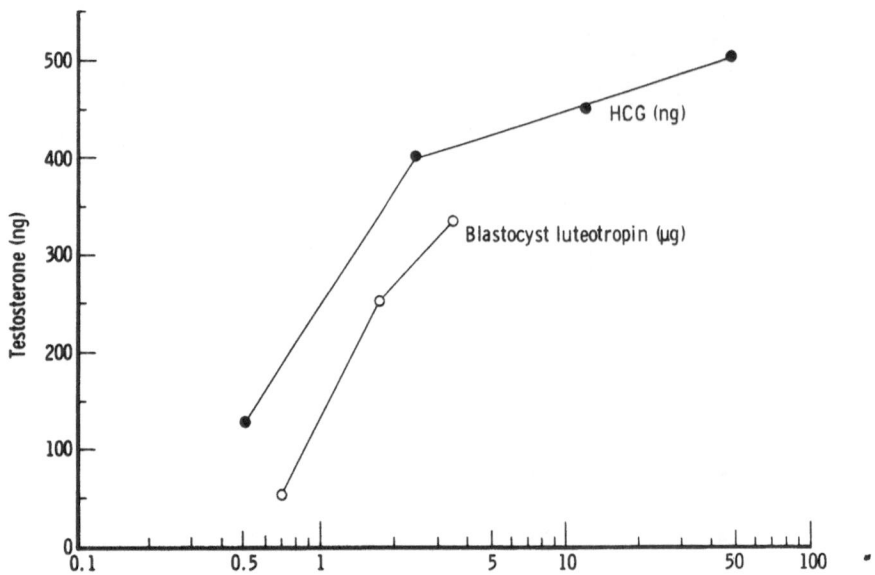

Figure 9. Production of testosterone by rat Leydig cells stimulated with hCG and partially purified blastocysts luteotropin.

initial sustenance to the pregnancy, the corpus luteum being maintained by luteotropic stimuli originating from the fertilized blastocyst in the reproductive tract. The fact that the blastocyst can implant at sites different from the endometrium -- for example, in ectopic pregnancies -- and produce hCG, strongly suggests that it is the blastocyst which carries the message and is equipped to synthesize hCG. If the hCG-like substance is produced in the rabbit blastocyst, its presence in the blood suggests an active transport of material through the uterine wall before implantation and prior to the establishment of vascular connections. It is interesting to note that exogenous hCG introduced in rabbit uteri and the human reproductive tract appears in the peripheral circulation within 30 minutes and six hours, respectively (Saxena et al., 1977).

The estrogen alone as an alternate luteotropic agent in the rabbit cannot be invoked since 17β-estradiol level remains constant throughout the pre- and post-ovulatory phases in the rabbit, and the presence of a secondary support during pre-implantation may account for the maintenance of the corpus luteum of gestation. In the presence of endogenous LH, the rate of progesterone secretion is dependent on the number of corpora lutea and the quantity of luteotropin. The number of corpora lutea being 13 ± 1 in pregnant, and 12 ± 2 in pseudo-pregnant, rabbits (Saxena, 1979). The higher secretion of progesterone on days 3 and 5 in pregnant rabbits may be due to the locally stimulated steroidogenesis by the embryonic luteo-tropin, as has previously been suggested by Dickman et al. (1976). In rats, Chatterton et al. (1975) have provided in vivo experimental evidence for the secretion by the unimplanted blastocyst of a sub-stance with activity different from and more effective in promoting progesterone synthesis than the pituitary prolactin.

The existence of luteotropic or anti-luteolytic substances prior to or at the time of implantation has also been indicated in sheep (Moor and Rowson, 1966), monkey (Hodgen et al., 1974), and human (Saxena et al., 1974). For example, hCG has been detected by RIA in the monkey uterine venous effluent at the time of implantation (Hodgen et al., 1974). Moudgal et al. (1978) compared the serum progesterone levels of pregnant monkeys with those of cycling monkeys (*Macaca radiata*) and revealed that the levels in the former tend to be higher just prior to establishment of implantation, thus suggesting the presence of a stimulus to corpus luteum from the unimplanted blastocyst. This is consistent with the findings of the secretion of a gonadotropin-like material by the pre-implanted blastocyst in the rhesus monkey by Batta and Channing (1979). HCG-like material has also been detected in the serum of women on days 6-8 after conception by a specific RIA of hCG using antibody against hormone-specific β-subunit (Kosasa et al., 1974) and by RRA (Saxena et al., 1974). Such an early detection of hCG strongly suggests the synthe-sis of hCG during the peri-implantation phase. Obviously, due to the absence of vascularization, the levels in the peripheral circu-lation are low and are sometimes difficult to detect unless very sensitive in vitro and in vivo assays are utilized.

A role of pre-implantation luteotropic material in the regula-tion and maintenance of the corpus luteum of gestation may be postulated in the following. After the establishment of the corpora lutea, a luteotropic substance from the blastocyst may bind to the receptor in the corpus luteum to sustain the secretion of proges-terone. The binding of the hCG-like material is facilitated by prolactin, which has also been shown to be present in the rabbit (Saxena, 1979) and mouse blastocyst (McCommack and Glasser, 1979). Low levels of hCG-like material in the presence of an augmenting effect of prolactin are sufficient since the saturation of only 5% of the total receptor may be necessary to fully sustain the secretion of the corpus luteum. Excessive quantities of hCG may result in the down-regulation of the receptor and luteolysis of the corpus luteum. The presence of hCG-like material in the sperm as the precursor of the blastocyst luteotropin has also been suggested (Acevedo et al., 1977; Asch et al., 1979). A possible role of hCG-like material as a barrier to immunological rejection of the blasto-cyst has also been considered (Beer and Billingham, 1978). It may be of interest to mention that hCG-β immunized marmoset monkeys (Hearn, 1978) who ovulate show that implantation occurs only when the antibody titers are low. The exact chemical nature, source, and mode of action of hCG-like material of the pre-implanted blastocyst origin, however, need to be further investigated. Obviously, further knowledge in this area is of great significance from the standpoint of current studies on the development of a contraceptive vaccine (Talwar, 1978) in particular, and in the search of new avenues of fertility regulation in general.

REFERENCES

Acevedo, H. F., Slifkin, M., Pouchet, G. R., and Rakshan, M., 1977, Identification of the β subunit of choriogonadotropin in human spermatozoa, in *The Testis in Normal and Infertile Men*, P. Troen and H. R. Nankin, eds., p. 185, Raven Press, New York.

Adams, C. E., 1970, Maintenance of pregnancy relative to the presence of few embryos in the rabbit, J. Endocrinol. 48:243.

Agarwal, B. B. L., and Goldstein, I. J., 1972, Concanavalin-A, the Jack Bean (Canavalia ensidormis) Phytohemagglutinin, in *Methods in Enzymology*, Volume XXVIII, pp. 313-318, Academic Press, New York.

Asch, R. H., Fernandez, E. O., Magnasco, L. A., and Pauerstein, C. J., 1978, Demonstration of a chorionic gonadotropin-like substance in rabbit morulae, Fertility Sterility 29:123.

Asch, R. H., Fernandez, E. O., Siler-Khodr, T. M., and Pauerstein, C. J., 1979, Presence of an hCG-like substance in human sperm, Am. J. Obstet. Gynecol., in press.

Bagshawe, K., ed., 1975, *Medical Oncology, Medical Aspects of Malignant Disease*, Blackwell Scientific Publications, Oxford, England.

Barber, S. G., Smith, J. A., Cove, D. H., Smith, S. C. H., and London, D. R., 1978, Marker for pineal tumors, Lancet 2 372:8085.

Batta, S. K., and Channing, C. P., 1979, Preliminary evidence for the secretion of a preimplantation gonadotropin by the preimplantation rhesus monkey blastocyst, Life Sciences, in press.

Beer, A. E., and Billingham, R. E., 1978, Immunoregulatory aspects of pregnancy, Federation Proc. 37:2374.

Beling, C. G., Dederqvist, L. L., and Fuchs, F., 1976, Demonstration of gonadotropin during the second half of the cycle in women using intrauterine contraception, Am. J. Obstet. Gynecol. 125:855.

Beneviste, R., Conway, M. C., Puett, D., and Rabinowitz, D., 1979, Heterogeneity ofhCG-α secreted by cultured choriocarcinoma (JEG) cells, J. Clin. Endocrin. Metab. 48:85.

Braunstein, G. D., Vaitukaitis, J. L., Carbone, P. P., and Ross, G. T., 1973a, Ectopic production of human chorionic gonadotropin by neoplasms, Ann. Inter. Med. 78:39.

Braunstein, G. D., Grodin, J. M., Vaitukaitis, J. L., and Ross, G.T., 1973b, Secretory rates of human chorionic gonadotropin by normal trophoblast, Am. J. Obstet. Gynecol. 115:447.

Braunstein, G. D., Raser, J., and Wade, M. E., 1975, Presence in normal human testes of a chorionic gonadotropin-like substance distinct from human luteinizing hormone, N. Eng. J. Med. 293:1339.

Bruner, J. A., 1951, Distribution of chorionic gonadotropin in mother and fetus at various stages of pregnancy, J. Clin. Endocrin. Metab. 11:360.

Catt, K. J., Dufau, M. L., and Vaitukaitis, J. L., 1972, Radioligand receptorassay of LH and chorionic gonadotropin, J. Clin. Endocrin. Metab. 34:123.

Channing, C. P., Stone, S. L., Sakai, C. N., Haour, F., and Saxena, B. B., 1978, A stimulatory effect of the fluid from preimplantation rabbit blastocysts upon luteinization of monkey granulosa cell cultures, J. Reprod. Fertil. 54:477.

Chatterton, R/ J/. McDonald, G. J., and Ward, D. A., 1975, Effects of blastocysts on rat ovarian steroidogenesis in early pregnancy, Biol. Reprod. 13:77.

Chen, H. C., and Hodgen, G. D., 1976, Primate chorionic gonadotropins: Antigenic similarities to the unique carboxyl-terminal peptide of hVH-β subunit, J. Clin. Endocin. Metab. 43:1414.

Clements, J. A., Reyes, F. I., Winter, J. S. D., and Faiman, C., 1976, Studies on human sexual development. III. pituitary and serum and amniotic fluid concentrations of LH, CG, and FSH, J. Clin. Endocrin. Metab. 42:9.

Cohen, H., and Strampp, A., 1976, Bacterial synthesis similar to human chorionic gonadotropin, Proc. Soc. Exp. Biol. Med. 152:408.

Dawood, M. Y., Saxena, B. B., and Landesman, R., 1977, Human chorionic gonadotropin and its subunits in hydatidiform mole and choriocarcinoma, Obstet. & Gynecol. 50:172.

Denker, H. W., and Fritz, H., 1979, Enzymic characterization of rabbit blastocyst protinase with synthetic substrates of trypsin-like enzymes, Hoppe-Seyler's Z. Physiol. Chem. Bd. 360, S 107-113. February.

Dickman, A., and Dey, S. K., 1974, Steroidogenesis in the preimplantation rat embryo and its possible influence on the morula-blastocyst transformation and implantation, J. Reprod. Fertil. 37:91.

Dickman, A., Dey, S. K., and Sen-Gupta, J., 1976, A new concept: Control of early pregnancy by steroid hormones originating in the preimplantation embryo, J. Vitam. Horm. 34:215.

Faiman, C., Colwell, J. A., Ryan, R. J., Hershman, J. M., and Shields, T. W., 1967, Gonadotropin secretion from a bronchogenic carcinoma: demonstration by radioimmunoassay, N. Eng. J. Med. 277:1395.

Franchimont, P., Reuter, A., and Gaspard, U., 1978, Ectopic production of hCG and its α and β subunits in Current Topics in Experimental Endocrinology, L. Martini and V. H. T. James, eds., Vol. 3, pp. 202-216, Academic Press, New York.

Fuchs, A. R., and Beling, C. G., 1974, Evidence of early ovarian recognition of blastocysts in rabbits, Endocrinology 95:1054.

Fujimoto, S., Euker, J. S., Riegle, G. D., and Dukelov, W. R., 1975, On a substance cross-reacting with luteinizing hormone in the preimplantation blastocyst fluid of the rabbit, Proc. Japan Acad. Sci. 51:123.

Fusco, F. D., and Roasen, S. W., 1966, Gonadotropin producing anaplastic large cell carcinomas of the lung, N. Eng. J. Med. 275:507.

Haour, F., and Saxena, B. B., 1974, Detection of a gonadotropin in rabbit blastocyst before implantation, Science 185:444.

Harrington, F. E., and Rothermel, J. D., 1977, Daily changes in peripheral plasma testosterone concentrations in pregnant and pseudopregnant rabbits, Life Sciences 20:1333.

Hattori, M., Fukase, M., Yoshimi, H., Matsukara, S., and Imura, H., 1978, Ectopic production of human chorionic gonadotropin in malignant tumors, Cancer 42:2328.

Hearn, J. P., 1978, Long term suppression of fertility by immunization with hCG-β subunit and its reversabilty in female marmoset monkeys, in Recent Advances in Reproduction and Regulation of Fertility, G. P. Talwar, ed., p 427, Elsevier/North Holland Bio-Medical Press, Amsterdam.

Hodgen, G. D., Tullner, W. W., Vaitukaitis, J. L., Ward, D. N., and Ross, G. T., 1974, Specific radioimmunoassay of chorionic gonadotropin during implantion in rhesus monkeys, J. Clin. Endocrin. Metab. 39:457.

Hodgen, G. D., Chen, H. C., Dufau, M. L., Klien, T. A., and Mishell, D. R., 1978, Transitory hCG-like activity in the urine of some IUD users, J. Clin. Endocrin. Metab. 46:698.

Holt, J. A., Heise, W. F., Wilson, S. M., and Keyes, P. L., 1976, Lack of gonadotropin activity in the rabbit blastocyst prior to implantation, Endocrinology 98:904.

Huff, R., and Eik-Ness, K., 1966, Metabolism in vitro of acetate and certain steroids by six-day-old rabbit blastocysts, J. Reprod. Fertil. 11:57.

Hung, W., Blizzard, R. M., Migeon, C. J., Camacho, A. M., and Nyhan, W. L., 1963, Precocious puberty in a boy with hepatoma and circulating gonadotropin, J. Pediatrics 63:895.

Jaffe, R. B., Seron-Ferre, M., Huhtaniemi, I., and Korenbrot, C., 1977, Regulation of the primal fetal adrenal gland and testis, in vitro and in vivo, J. Steroid Biochem. 8:479.

Javadpour, N., 1978a, Biological tumor markers in management of testicular and bladder cancer, Urology 12:177.

Javadpour, N., 1978b, Current concepts in management of testicular tumor, Urol. Survey 28:89.

Javadpour, M., McIntire, K. R., and Waldman, T. A., 1978z, HCG and AFP in sera and tumor cells of patients with testicular seminoma: A prospective study, Cancer 42:2768.

Javadpour, N., McIntire, K. R., Waldman, T. A., and Bergman, S. M., 1978b, The role of α-fetoprotein and human chorionic gonadotropin in seminoma, J. Urol. 120:687.

Javadpour, N., McIntire, K. R., Waldman, T. A., Scardino, P. T., Bergman, S. and Anderson, T., 1978c, The role of RIA of serum AFP and hCG in intensive chemotherapy and surgery of metastatic testicular tumors, J. Urol. 119:759.

Kawamura, J., Machida, S., Yoshida, O., Oseko, F., Imura, H., and Hattori, M., 1978, Bladder carcinoma associated with ectopic production of gonadotropin, Cancer 42:2773.

Kosasa, T. S., Levesque, L. A., Goldstein, D. P., and Taymor, M. L., 1974, Clinical use of a solid phase radioimmunoassay specific for hCG, J. Obstet. Gynecol. 119:784.

Kourides, I. A., Weintraub, B. D., Ridgway, E. C., and Maloff, F., 1975, Pituitary secretion of free alpha and beta subunits of human thyrotropin in patients with thyroid disorders, J. Clin. Endocrin. Metab. 40:872.

Landesman, R., and Saxena, B. B., 1976, Results of the first 1000 radioreceptorassays for the determination of human chorionic gonadotropin: A new, rapid, reliable, and sensitivie pregnancy test, Fertil. Steril. 27:357.

Landesman, R., Coutinho, E., and Saxena, B. B., 1976, Detection of hCG in blood of regularly bleeding women using copper IUDs, Fertil. Steril. 28:1258.

McCormack, S. A., and Glasser, S. R., 1979, Hormone production by preimplantation and midpregnancy rat trophectoderm in vitro, Abstr. presented at the Seminar on Cellular and Molecular Aspects of Implantation, Houston, Texas.

Moudgal, R. N., Mukku, V. R., Prahlad, S., Murty, G. S. R. C., and Li, C. H., 1978, Passive immunization with an antibody to the β-subunit of ovine luteinizing hormone as a method of early abortion - A feasibility study in monkeys (Macaca Radiata), Fertil. Steril. 30:223.

Moor, A. M., and Rowson, L. E. A., 1966, The corpus luteum of the sheep: Functional relationship between the embryo and the corpus luteum, J. Endocrinol. 34:233.

Odell, W. D., Hertz, R., Lipsett, M. B., Ross, G. T., and Hammond, C. B., 1967, Endocrine aspects of trophoblastic neoplasms, Clin. Obstet. Gynecol. 10:290.

Pederson, B. N., 1978, Clinical use of AFP and hCG in testicular tumors of germ-cell origin, Lancet 2 8098:10.

Perry, J. S., Heap, R. B., and Amoroso, E. C., 1973, Implantation: Pig blastocyst produces steroid hormones, Nature 245:45 (London).

Prentice, L. G., and Ryan, R. J., 1975, LH and its subunits in human pituitary, serum and urine, J. Clin. Endocrin. Metab. 40:303.

Psychoyos, A., 1967, The hormonal interplay controlling egg-implantation in the rat, in Advances in Reproduction Physiology, A. McLanen, ed., pp. 257-277, Academic Press, New York.

Robertson, D. M., Suginami, H., Montes, H. H., Puri, C. P., Choi, S. K., and Diczfalusy, E., 1978, Studies on a CG-like material present in nonpregnant subjects, Acta Endocrinol. 89:492.

Rochman, H., 1978, Tumor associated markers in clinical diagnosis, Ann. Clin. Lab. Sci. 8:167.

Root, A. W., Borgiovanni, A. M., Eberlain, W. R., 1968, A testicular-interstitial-cell-stimulating gonadotropin in a child with hepatoblastoma and sexual precocity, J. Clin. Endocrin. Metab. 28:1317.

Rose, L. I., Williams, G. H., Jagger, P. I., and Lauler, D. P., 1968, Feminizing tumor of the adrenal gland with positive 'chorionic like" gonadotropin test, J. Clin. Endocrin. Metab. 28:903.

Rosen, S. W., and Weintraub, B. D., 1974, Ectopic production of the isolated alpha subunit of the glycoprotein hormones. A quantitative marker in certain cases of cancer, N. Eng. J. Med. 290:1441.

Rosen, S. W., Becker, C. E., Schlaff, S., Easton, J., and Gluck, M. C., 1968, Ectopic production before clinical recognition of bronchogenic carcinoma, N. Eng. J. Med. 279:640.

Saxena, B. B., 1979, Current studies of a gonadotropin-like substance in preimplanted rabbit blastocyst, in Recent Advances in Reproduction and Regulation of Fertility, G. P. Talwar, ed., pp. 319-332, Elsevier/North Holland Biomedical Press, Amsterdam.

Saxena, B. B., and Landesman, R., 1978, Diagnosis and management of pregnancy by the radioreceptorassay of human chorionic gonadotropin, Am. J. Obstet. Gynecol. 131:97.

Saxena, B. B., Hasan, S. H., Haour, F., and Schmidt-Gollwitzer, M., 1974, Radioreceptorassay of human chorionic gonadotropin: Early detection of pregnancy, Science 184:793.

Saxena, B. B., Kaali, S., and Landesman, R., 1977, The transport of chorionic gonadotropin throught the reporductive tract, Eur. J. Obstet. Gynecol. 7:1.

Schultz, H., Sell, A., Norgaard-Pederson, B., and Arends, J., 1978, Serum AFP and hCG as markers for the effect of postoperative radiation therapy and/or chemotherpay in testicular cancer, Cancer 42:2182.

Sharpe, R. M., Wrixon, W., Hobson, B. M., Corker, C. S., McLean, H. A., and Short, R. V., 1977, Absence of hCG-like activity in the blood of women fitted with intrauterine contraceptive devices, J. Clin. Endocrin. Metab. 45:496.

Singh, M. M., and Adams, C. E., 1978, Luteotropic effect of the rabbit blastocyst, J. Reprod. Fertil. 53:331.

Sunduram, K., Connell, K. G., and Passatino, T., 1975, Implication of absence of hCG-like gonadotropin in the blastocyst for control of corpus luteum. Function in pregnant rabbit, Nature 256:739.

Talwar, G. P., 1979, ed., Recent Advances in Reproduction and Regulation of Fertility, Elsevier/North Holland Biomedical Press, Amsterdam.

Tormey, D. C., Waalkes, P. T., and Simon, R. M., 1977, Biological markers in breast carcinoma, Cancer 39:2391.

Vaitukaitis, J. L., 1978, Glycoprotein hormones and their subunits immunological and biological chaterizations, in Structure and

Function of the Gonadotropins, K. W. McKerns, ed., pp. 339-360, Plenum Press, New York.

Vaitukaitis, J. L., Braunstein, G. D., and Ross, G. T., 1972, A radioimmunoassay which specifically measures human chorionic gonadotropin in the presence of human luteinizing hormone, Am. J. Obstet. Gynecol. 113:751.

Vaitukaitis, J. L., Boss, G. T., Braunstein, G. D., and Rayford, P. L., 1976, Gonadotropins and their subunits: Basic and clinical studies, Recent Prog. Horm. Res. 32:289.

Varma, S. K., Dawood, M. Y., Haour, F., Channing, C. P., and Saxena, B. B., 1979, Gonadotropin-like substance in the preimplanted rabbit blastocyst, Fertil. Steril. 31:68.

Wajsman, A., and Murphy, G. P., 1978, The current management of advanced testicular cancers, Urological Survey 28:4:127.

Weintraub, B. D., and Rosen, S. W., 1973a, Competitive radioassays and "specific" tumor markers, Metabolism 22:1119.

Weintraub, B. D., and Rosen, S. W., 1973b, Ectopic production of the isolated β=subunit of human chorionic gonadotropin, J. Clin. Inves. 52:3135.

Weintraub, B. D., Kadasky, Y. M., and Rosen, S. W., 1972, Ectopic production of human chorionic gonadotropin (hCG) and its free beta subunit (hCG-β), Clin. Res. 20:444.

Wiley, L. D., 1974, Presence of gonadotropin on the surface of preimplanted mouse embryo, Nature 252:715.

Yoshimoto, Y., Wolfsen, A. R., and Odell, W. D., 1977, Human chorionic gonadotropin-like substance in non-endocrine tissues of normal subjects, Science 197:575.

Yoshimoto, Y., Wolfsen, A. R., Hirose, F., and Odell, W. D., 1979, Human chorionic gonadotropin-like material. Presence in normal tissues, Am. J. Obstet. Gynecol. 134:729.

Zielmaker, G. H., and Verhamme, C. M. P. M., 1978, Luteotropic activity of ectopically developing rat blastocysts, Acta Endocrinol. 88:589.

INDEX